Brain Damage in the Preterm Infants

Brain Damage in the Preterm Infants

Editor: Jerome Holyfield

AMERICAN
MEDICAL PUBLISHERS
www.americanmedicalpublishers.com

AMERICAN
MEDICAL PUBLISHERS
www.americanmedicalpublishers.com

Cataloging-in-Publication Data

Brain damage in the preterm infants / edited by Jerome Holyfield.
p. cm.
Includes bibliographical references and index.
ISBN 978-1-63927-943-2
1. Premature infants--Diseases. 2. Brain damage. 3. Brain-damaged children. I. Holyfield, Jerome.
RJ496.B7 B73 2023
618.928--dc23

American Medical Publishers,
41 Flatbush Avenue,
1st Floor, New York,
NY 11217, USA

ISBN 978-1-63927-943-2 (Hardback)

Contents

Preface

Premature birth or preterm birth refers to the birth of a baby before completing 37 weeks of gestation, as opposed to full term delivery of approximately 40 weeks. Preterm birth may lead to various problems such as increased threat of morbidity and mortality, brain damage, and cerebral palsy. There are various factors that lead to the development of brain injury in preterm infants. Factors such as perinatal asphyxia, infection/inflammation, chronic hypoxia, and exposure to treatments such as mechanical ventilation, and corticosteroids causes severe damage to parts of the brain. One of the conditions which are caused due to brain damage in preterm infants is cerebral palsy. The Children suffering from cerebral palsy (CP) face problem with hearing, speaking, sensation and vision. A child with cerebral palsy has impaired muscle tone, reflexes, motor development, and coordination. Brain damage can be prevented partly through maternal immunization and minimization of head traumas in children. This book aims to shed light on some of the unexplored aspects of preterm birth and related brain damage, and the recent researches related to it. Researchers and students engaged in this area of study will be greatly assisted by it.

This book is a result of research of several months to collate the most relevant data in the field.

When I was approached with the idea of this book and the proposal to edit it, I was overwhelmed. It gave me an opportunity to reach out to all those who share a common interest with me in this field. I had 3 main parameters for editing this text:

1. Accuracy - The data and information provided in this book should be up-to-date and valuable to the readers.

2. Structure - The data must be presented in a structured format for easy understanding and better grasping of the readers.

3. Universal Approach - This book not only targets students but also experts and innovators in the field, thus my aim was to present topics which are of use to all.

Thus, it took me a couple of months to finish the editing of this book.

I would like to make a special mention of my publisher who considered me worthy of this opportunity and also supported me throughout the editing process. I would also like to thank the editing team at the back-end who extended their help whenever required.

Editor

1

The Cerebrospinal Fluid Inflammatory Response to Preterm Birth

*James P. Boardman[1,2], Graeme Ireland[1], Gemma Sullivan[1], Rozalia Pataky[1], Bobbi Fleiss[3,4,5], Pierre Gressens[3,4,5] and Veronique Miron[1]**

[1] MRC Centre for Reproductive Health, The Queen's Medical Research Institute, The University of Edinburgh, Edinburgh, United Kingdom, [2] Centre for Clinical Brain Sciences, Chancellor's Building, The University of Edinburgh, Edinburgh, United Kingdom, [3] Centre for the Developing Brain, Division of Imaging Sciences and Biomedical Engineering, King's College London, London, United Kingdom, [4] PROTECT, INSERM, Université Paris Diderot, Sorbonne Paris Cité, Paris, France, [5] PremUP, Paris, France

***Correspondence:**
Veronique Miron
V.Miron@ed.ac.uk;
veronique.miron@ed.ac.uk

Background: Preterm birth is the leading risk factor for perinatal white matter injury, which can lead to motor and neuropsychiatric impairment across the life course. There is an unmet clinical need for therapeutics. White matter injury is associated with an altered inflammatory response in the brain, primarily led by microglia, and subsequent hypomyelination. However, microglia can release both damaging and trophic factors in response to injury, and a comprehensive assessment of these factors in the preterm central nervous system (CNS) has not been carried out.

Method: A custom antibody array was used to assess relative levels of 50 inflammation- and myelination-associated proteins in the cerebrospinal fluid (CSF) of preterm infants in comparison to term controls.

Results: Fifteen proteins differed between the groups: BDNF, BTC, C5a, FasL, Follistatin, IL-1β, IL-2, IL-4, IL-9, IL-17A, MIP-1α, MMP8, SPP1, TGFβ, and TNFβ ($p < 0.05$). To investigate the temporal regulation of these proteins after injury, we mined a gene expression dataset of microglia isolated from a mouse model of developmental white matter injury. Microglia in the experimental model showed dynamic temporal expression of genes encoding these proteins, with an initial and sustained pro-inflammatory response followed by a delayed anti-inflammatory response, and a continuous expression of genes predicted to inhibit healthy myelination.

Conclusion: Preterm CSF shows a distinct neuroinflammatory profile compared to term controls, suggestive of a complex neural environment with concurrent damaging and reparative signals. We propose that limitation of pro-inflammatory responses, which occur early after perinatal insult, may prevent expression of myelination-suppressive genes and support healthy white matter development.

Keywords: preterm birth, brain injury, inflammation, cerebrospinal fluid, microglia, myelination

INTRODUCTION

Preterm birth is closely associated with white matter injury and life course impairments including cerebral palsy, learning difficulty, autism spectrum disorder, and psychiatric disease (Volpe, 2009; Johnson and Marlow, 2017). A characteristic feature of white matter injury is oligodendrocyte dysmaturation, which is driven in part by immune dysregulation, and results in hypomyelination (Back and Miller, 2014; Hagberg et al., 2015). Magnetic resonance imaging studies show that generalized atypical white matter tract development is often apparent in preterm infants at term-equivalent age (Batalle et al., 2017; Telford et al., 2017), which suggests that interventions to prevent injury and support normal myelination may need to be applied during the perinatal period. Therefore a priority is to better understand the immune mediators and receptors that drive preterm white matter injury in order to identify therapeutic targets that promote healthy white matter development.

Neuropathological analyses of post-mortem tissue have shown robust activation of central nervous system (CNS)-endogenous immune cells, microglia, which express pro-inflammatory markers (iNOS, TNFα, IL-1β, and IL-6) (Yoon et al., 1997; Haynes et al., 2009); and systemic inflammation due to co-morbidities of preterm birth such as chorioamnionitis and necrotizing enterocolitis, is associated with abnormal white matter on magnetic resonance imaging *in vivo* (Shah et al., 2008; Anblagan et al., 2016; Barnett et al., 2018).

Elevated levels of inflammatory proteins in blood or cerebrospinal fluid (CSF) are associated with perinatal brain injury and increased risk of adverse neurodevelopmental outcome (Yoon et al., 1996; Nelson et al., 1998; Savman et al., 1998; Bartha et al., 2004; Viscardi et al., 2004; Carlo et al., 2011; Armstrong-Wells et al., 2015; Basu et al., 2015). However, protein levels in plasma do not always correlate with those in the CSF in preterm infants with white matter injury, demonstrating that blood analyses may not reflect events in the CNS (Ellison et al., 2005; Rajkumar et al., 2018). Furthermore, a comprehensive assessment of inflammation-associated factors in preterm CSF has not been carried out. Here, we asked whether a large-scale measurement of inflammatory markers in preterm CSF, including measures of factors known to be detrimental or supportive of white matter development, could provide a broader understanding of the neuropathology of preterm brain injury.

MATERIALS AND METHODS

Participants

We recruited two groups of neonates from the Royal Infirmary of Edinburgh between June 2014 and September 2015 who required CSF sampling, usually for the evaluation of suspected meningitis: 17 preterm neonates with mean (SD) postmenstrual age (PMA) at birth 27.14 (2.14) weeks; and 20 term infants with mean (SD) PMA at birth 39.86 (1.86) weeks. The mean (SD) PMA at CSF sampling was 29.29 (2.86) weeks for preterm infants and 40.29 (2.0) weeks for term infants. There were no significant differences in the proportion of infants with CSF contaminated by blood defined as red blood cell count >1000 cells/mm^3 (50% versus 42%, $p = 0.73$). Methods for sampling and storage of CSF, and the clinical phenotype of participants including plasma C-Reactive Protein, full blood count, CSF total protein and glucose concentrations and CSF microscopy have been reported previously (Pataky et al., 2017). No infant in either group had meningitis; 10 out of 17 of the preterm infants and 8 out of 20 of the term infants were classified as having blood stream infection (BSI) at the time of CSF sampling, defined as either (1) blood culture grew a pathogenic bacterial species; or (2) the blood culture was negative or grew coagulase negative Staphylococcus (CoNS) *and* the infant had one or more signs of generalized infection (apnoea, temperature instability, feeding intolerance, worsening respiratory distress, or hemodynamic instability) *and* the attending neonatologist treated with IV antibiotics for ≥ 5 days. The difference in proportion of infants with BSI in each group was not statistically significant ($p = 0.33$).

This study was carried out in accordance with the recommendations of UK National Research Ethics Service with written informed consent from all subjects. All subjects gave written informed consent in accordance with the Declaration of Helsinki. The protocol was approved by the South East Scotland Research Ethics Committee (14/SS/044). Written parental informed consent was obtained for CSF sampling, and the study was approved by the UK National Research Ethics Service (14/SS/044).

Custom Antibody Microarray

A custom antibody array ("G-series" from Tebu-bio/RayBiotech) against 50 human analytes was generated to detect relative levels of: activin-A (INHBA), Brain-derived neurotrophic factor (BDNF), bone morphogenetic protein (BMP)2, BMP4, BMP7, betacellulin (BTC), cluster of differentiation (CD)200, Complement 5a (C5a), C-reactive protein (CRP), Fas ligand (FasL), follistatin, furin, Galectin-3 (Gal3), granulocyte macrophage colony-stimulating factor (GM-CSF), insulin-like growth factor-1 (IGF-1), interferon-gamma (IFNγ), insulin, interleukin (IL)-1α, IL-1β, IL-2, IL-4, IL-5, IL-6, IL-8, IL-9, IL-10, IL-12p40, IL-12p70, IL-13, IL-17A, IL-17B, IL-17C, IL-17F, IL-18, monocyte chemoattractant protein-1 (MCP1), macrophage inflammatory protein 1-alpha (MIP1α), MIP1β, matrix metalloproteinase (MMP) 8, MMP-9, nerve growth factor (NGF)-β, neurotrophic factor 3 (NT3), Osteopontin (SPP1), placental growth factor (PLGF), regulated on activation, normal t cell expressed and secreted (RANTES), stem cell factor (SCF), tumor necrosis factor (TNF)-α, TNFβ, transforming growth factor-beta (TGFβ), urokinase-type plasminogen-activator (uPA), vascular endothelial growth factor-C (VEGF-C). Arrays were carried out according to the manufacturer's instructions. Briefly, antibodies printed onto sub-arrays were dried at room temperature (RT) for 2 h, then blocked for 30 min. Fifty microliters of CSF from each case was incubated with one sub-array for 2 h at RT, then washed with gentle rocking. Sub-arrays were then incubated with biotin-conjugated sandwich antibodies for 2 h at RT, washed thoroughly, then incubated with streptavidin-Cy3. Following washes in water, slides were read at 532 nm excitation frequency.

Antibody Array Data Analysis

Detected values of Cy3 intensity were normalized to an internal median background level on each slide. Analytes of interest were defined as those where the median value of the preterm group was outside the interquartile range of the controls. For analyses designed to generate hypotheses about group differences for gene expression studies, the distribution of values according to gestation category (preterm versus term) was investigated using independent samples Mann–Whitney U test, individual test p-values are reported, and a threshold of <0.05 was used to select proteins for microglia gene expression analysis. Analyses were performed using SPSS 21.0 (SPSS Inc., Chicago, IL, United States).

Animal Protocol

Experimental protocols were approved by the Bichat-Robert Debre (France) ethical committee under the reference 2011-14/676-0053, and met the guidelines for the United States Public Health Service's Policy on Humane Care and Use of Laboratory Animals (NIH, Bethesda, MD, United States). We housed the OF1 strain mice (Charles River; L'Arbresle, France) under a 12 h light-dark cycle with *ad libitum* food and water. On P1 pups were sexed, all males were kept but litters were maintained at 9–11 pups. Assessments of injury and outcomes were made only in male animals as females do not display white matter injury in response to this paradigm. The preponderance to injury in males is similar to what is observed in preterm born infants (O'Driscoll et al., 2018). Neonatal received twice a day (bid) from P1 to P4 and once on P5 a 5 μl intra-peritoneal (ip) injection of 10 μg/kg/injection recombinant mouse IL-1β in phosphate buffered saline (PBS; R&D Systems, Minneapolis, MN, United States) or PBS alone (control). IL-1β exposure, as reported previously, sets up a complex systemic inflammatory response (Favrais et al., 2011) and then a complex central neuroinflammatory response (Krishnan et al., 2017; Van Steenwinckel et al., 2018). This leads to microgliosis, oligodendrocyte maturation arrest, hypomyelination and cognitive deficits (Favrais et al., 2011; Schang et al., 2014; Krishnan et al., 2017; Van Steenwinckel et al., 2018) reminiscent of what is observed in preterm born infants (Billiards et al., 2008; Verney et al., 2012; Caldinelli et al., 2017; Spittle et al., 2017).

Neural Tissue Dissociation and Magnetic-Activated Cell Sorting

At P1, P5, and P10, we collected brains for cell dissociation and CD11b-positive cell enrichment using a magnetic coupled antibody extraction technique (MACS), as previously described (Schang et al., 2014; Krishnan et al., 2017) and according to the manufacturer's protocol (Miltenyi Biotec, Bergisch Gladbach, Germany). In brief, we pooled brains (n = 4 at P1, n = 3 at P5, and n = 2 at P10) and after removing the cerebellum and olfactory bulbs they were dissociated using the Neural Tissue Dissociation Kit. A total of six samples per group and per time point were generated with at least four independent litters per group. Using anti-CD11b MicroBeads we captured the CD11b+ cells and after elution, we centrifuged the isolated cells for 5 min at 600 g and then conserved them at −80°C. The purity of MACSed CD11B+ fraction has been validated using FACS analysis of CD11B fluorescence, and with RT-qPCR of the positive and negative cell fractions as previously described (Schang et al., 2014; Krishnan et al., 2017) and revealed the negative fraction has gene expression levels 98% lower than found in the respective primary cultures of astrocytes, neurons, and oligodendrocytes.

Microarray Analysis

As previously published, Miltenyi Biotec (France) performed microarrays (Mouse Agilent Whole Mouse Genome Oligo Microarrays, 8 × 60K) on 6 samples per time point per group for CD11b enriched cell samples from P1, P5, and P10 mice exposed to IL-1β or PBS; a total of 24 samples (Krishnan et al., 2017). Preparation of samples for array analysis has been previously described (Husson et al., 2005; Chhor et al., 2013; Krishnan et al., 2017). The Agilent feature extraction software was used to process microarray image files. We only included signal intensities above background. Signal intensity values were background subtracted and uploaded following instructions by Miltenyi Biotec GmbH (Stefan Tomiuk) and PerkinElmer (Matt Hudson) into GeneSifter Analysis Edition v4.0[1] for further analysis as previously described (Gustavsson et al., 2007). The pre-processed signal intensity values were median normalized, and the gene expression in neuroinflammatory and PBS controls were compared at P1, P5, and P10 using t-test (p < 0.05) with Benjamini-Hochberg multiple testing correction.

RESULTS

Differential Levels of Inflammation-Associated Proteins in Pre-term vs. Term Infant Cerebrospinal Fluid

To conduct a comprehensive assessment of CNS inflammatory state in preterm infants and associate this with factors affecting myelination, we designed an antibody array assessing expression of 50 proteins with functions in regulating inflammation and myelination (**Table 1**). This approach was optimal to assess relative protein levels in neonatal CSF because it allowed high-content simultaneous screening of low volumes of fluid with high sensitivity and a broad range of detection.

We found that 28 protein levels had a median value in CSF from preterm infants that was outside the interquartile range of the controls (**Table 1**, bold type); these represented proteins with known functions in enhancing or resolving inflammation, as well impairing or supporting myelination (**Table 1**). The distribution of 15 proteins differed in preterm CSF from that of the controls (p-value <0.05), and 5 analytes were increased in preterm CSF at a threshold of p < 0.01: C5a, interleukin (IL)-9, osteopontin (SPP1), Fas ligand (FasL), and follistatin. These data demonstrate that preterm CSF has a distinct inflammatory profile compared to term controls that includes both pro-inflammatory and anti-inflammatory proteins, as well as those which can support or impair myelination.

[1]http://jhu.genesifter.net/login

TABLE 1 | Median (IQR) normalized fluorescence intensity of 50 cerebrospinal fluid analytes from term control infants and preterm infants.

Analyte	Function	Control			Preterm		*p*-Value
		Median	IQR	Q1–Q3	Median	IQR	
C5a (*Hc*)	⊙	**1378.5**	**1382.5**	**680.8–2063.3**	**3592.6**	**2540.3**	**0.001****
CRP	⊙	28446.4	20206.4	15120.2–35326.6	35217.1	18532.5	0.133
GM-CSF (*Csf2*)	⊙	**255.6**	**91.2**	**212.2–303.5**	**330.2**	**284.2**	**0.125**
IFNγ	⊙O	403.2	127.0	328.4–455.4	402.4	159.3	0.916
IL-1α	⊙	**490.5**	**81.4**	**450.6–532.0**	**581.9**	**546.13**	**0.220**
IL-1β	⊙O	**52.1**	**73.3**	**10.0–83.3**	**108.8**	**338.8**	**0.014***
IL-2	⊙	**413.1**	**77.8**	**367.7–445.5**	**520.5**	**298.0**	**0.030***
IL-6	⊙■	580.0	3259.5	413.8–3673.3	706.2	8133.4	0.869
IL-8	⊙	19466.8	55521.7	16192.7–71714.4	18370.4	79637.3	0.707
IL-9	⊙O	**188.8**	**76.1**	**136.9–213.1**	**242.6**	**233.23**	**0.005****
IL-12p40	⊙	62.5	87.3	22.8–110.1	83.3	206.6	0.167
IL-12p70	⊙	**164.3**	**80.0**	**110.1–190.0**	**220.1**	**219.8**	**0.177**
IL-17A	⊙■	**202.1**	**45.4**	**182.5–227.9**	**296.4**	**225.6**	**0.028***
IL-17B	⊙	104.6	20.0	96.3–116.3	107.0	125.4	0.798
IL-17C	⊙	508.8	99.8	456.7–556.5	546.2	246.9	0.052
IL-17F	⊙	72.5	73.2	22.8–96.0	62.6	214.0	0.619
IL-18	⊙	**80.9**	**49.6**	**50.0–81.0**	**101.8**	**129.0**	**0.326**
MCP-1 (Ccl2)	⊙	116104.0	10004.9	112697.7–122702.6	109752.5	40956.0	0.283
MIP1α (Ccl3)	⊙	**211.5**	**282.6**	**118.0–400.6**	**1054.5**	**4168.5**	**0.015***
MIP1β (Ccl4)	⊙	**6715.4**	**17113.7**	**5549.0–22562.7**	**26868.7**	**31793.7**	**0.133**
PIGF	⊙	**593.2**	**375.6**	**438.0–813.6**	**948.0**	**1180.7**	**0.056**
RANTES	⊙	182.8	1590.6	115.7–1706.3	736.4	14673.8	0.244
TNFα	⊙■O	**1095.9**	**167.4**	**1036.8–1204.2**	**1242.3**	**935.8**	**0.074**
TNFβ	⊙	**452.6**	**68.8**	**404.4–473.3**	**504.0**	**380.4**	**0.011***
uPA	⊙	8733.4	8969.4	4470.1–13439.5	12527.5	18004.0	0.149
CD200	♦	98.9	61.3	58.4–119.7	113.6	163.9	0.326
IL-4	♦	**402.7**	**80.7**	**340.7–421.4**	**430.6**	**176.6**	**0.042***
IL-5	♦	299.9	58.6	271.5–330.1	301.9	258.2	0.798
IL-10	♦■	481.6	787.9	429.1–1216.9	917.7	6406.5	0.341
IL-13	♦	382.8	93.4	336.2–429.5	416.3	330.8	0.104
Activin-A (INHBA)	■♦	**238.2**	**62.7**	**204.9–267.6**	**271.1**	**314.6**	**0.257**
BDNF	■	**101.6**	**18.6**	**95.3–113.9**	**145.8**	**191.5**	**0.024***
BTC	■	**304.7**	**49.3**	**273.3–322.6**	**354.0**	**256.7**	**0.045***
β-NGF	■	**206.4**	**169.2**	**119.1–288.2**	**339.6**	**550.56**	**0.117**
NT-3	■	**85.7**	**55.20**	**49.9–105.1**	**106.7**	**147.0**	**0.283**
Furin	■O	360.4	580.5	189.6–770.1	464.7	995.9	0.537
Galectin-3	■	1598.1	1419.0	859.2–2278.2	1069.9	4638.26	0.892
IGF-1	■	2005.4	574.4	1685.3–2259.6	2048.0	662.5	0.812
Insulin (*Ins1*)	■	**180.6**	**70.3**	**149.0–219.3**	**253.8**	**271.8**	**0.074**
SCF (*Kitl*)	■	346.7	287.7	230.9–518.6	419.4	631.8	0.326
SPP1	■⊙	**1209.4**	**1828.0**	**766.5–2594.4**	**3064.4**	**4333.1**	**0.007****
TGFβ	■♦	**706.2**	**122.0**	**640.7–762.7**	**919.0**	**600.0**	**0.013***
VEGF-C	■	250.6	100.1	209.6–309.7	233.7	312.5	0.641
BMP2	O	191.5	168.6	100.5–269.1	140.3	301.7	0.752
BMP4	O	116.1	90.1	72.4–162.5	106.0	173.1	0.845
BMP7	O	**196.5**	**211.8**	**156.2–232.0**	**246.0**	**221.5**	**0.104**
FasL	O	**290.1**	**159.6**	**203.1–362.7**	**967.0**	**1484.7**	**0.001****
Follistatin (*Fst*)	O	**920.6**	**286.0**	**754.3–1040.3**	**1683.0**	**1192.8**	**0.007****
MMP8	O⊙	**319.7**	**187.2**	**219.5–406.7**	**416.7**	**1319.90**	**0.026***
MMP-9	⊙	**156.4**	**126.2**	**110.8–237.0**	**244.8**	**1378.6**	**0.125**

*Bold type highlights analytes with median concentration in CSF from preterm infants that was outside the IQR of analyte concentration from controls; *$p < 0.05$, **$p < 0.01$. ⊙Pro-inflammatory function; ♦ anti-inflammatory function; ■supporting oligodendrocyte lineage responses and myelination; O impairing oligodendrocyte lineage responses and myelination.*

Mapping of Dynamic Regulation of Inflammatory and Myelination-Associated Proteins During Experimental Developmental Brain Injury

To better understand how the proteins elevated in preterm infant CSF are regulated after injury, we mined an existing dataset in which dynamic changes in microglia gene expression were measured in an experimental model of developmental white matter injury. In this model, damage was induced by intraperitoneal injections of recombinant IL-1β (10 μg/ml) prior to the onset of myelination (twice daily from postnatal day [P]1 to P4 and one injection at P5) (**Figure 1A**). This paradigm mimics the pathophysiology of human perinatal brain injury by chronically impairing oligodendrocyte differentiation and myelination, as evidenced by immunostaining of myelin proteins, the oligodendrocyte lineage and electron microscopy (Favrais et al., 2011; Krishnan et al., 2017).

We analyzed microglia gene expression at the time of inflammation initiation (P1), during the subsequent phase when oligodendrocyte differentiation is impaired (P5), and when hypomyelination is observed (P10). Eleven of 15 proteins we found to be altered in human preterm CSF were significantly regulated at the mRNA level by microglia during the course of white matter injury (**Figure 1B**). At P1, microglia from IL-1β-treated mice showed an upregulation of pro-inflammatory genes *Il1b* and *Tnf* and concomitant downregulation of anti-inflammatory gene *Il4* (**Figure 1C**). *Tgfb1*, which supports oligodendrocyte lineage survival, proliferation, and differentiation (Dutta et al., 2014; Palazuelos et al., 2014), was upregulated simultaneously with *Mmp8*, which is associated with myelin damage (Folgueras et al., 2008; **Figure 1C**). At P5, microglia upregulated pro-inflammatory genes C5a (*Hc*), *Il1b*, *Il2*, *Il17a*, and showed a sustained downregulation of *Il4* (**Figure 1D**). Also upregulated were genes predicted to inhibit oligodendrocyte health and differentiation: *Mmp8* (Folgueras et al., 2008), *Fasl* (associated with oligodendrocyte death) (Wosik et al., 2003), and *Fst* (which would inhibit activin-A-driven oligodendrocyte differentiation) (Dillenburg et al., 2018; **Figure 1D**). At P10, *Il1b*, *Tnf*, and *Fasl* were still upregulated, however, concomitant upregulation of *Il4* and pro-myelination gene *Spp1* (Osteopontin) may indicate late attempts to resolve inflammation and counter white matter damage (**Figure 1E**). *Il1b* and *Il4*, prototypical pro- and anti-inflammatory cytokines respectively, were found to be regulated in expression throughout injury, with a sustained upregulation of *Il1b* and a delayed *Il4* response (**Figure 1F**). With regards to genes regulating myelination, although pro-survival/myelination genes *Tgfb1* and *Spp1* were slightly upregulated early and late in injury, respectively, genes whose products are predicted to impair white matter health were upregulated at all time points (**Figure 1G**). This data suggest that the proteins enriched in human preterm CSF are dynamically expressed by microglia following developing white matter insult, with an initial and sustained pro-inflammatory response followed by a delayed anti-inflammatory response, and a continuous expression of genes predicted to inhibit healthy myelination.

DISCUSSION

In this study, we identified a distinct inflammatory signature in preterm CSF relative to term controls. A comprehensive and sensitive measure of CSF protein levels by antibody array identified 15 factors which were relatively increased in preterm samples, and which have been previously associated with regulating inflammation and myelination. This revealed a complex preterm neural environment, with concurrent pro- and anti-inflammatory responses, and pro- and anti-myelination factors. Data-mining of microglia transcriptomes in the context of experimental perinatal brain injury revealed that microglia can express the majority of these factors following insult, and they are dynamically regulated over time, mirroring the complexity of inflammatory and myelination-regulating factors measured in the human samples. Although some of these genes are expressed by microglia in healthy developing brain (*Il1b, Ccl3, Tnf, Spp1,* and *Tgfb1*) (Zhang et al., 2014), the rapid increase of pro-inflammatory gene expression in microglia in this experimental model shortly after the first injection of IL-1β, concomitant with sustained expression of genes predicted to impair myelination, highlight the importance of early intervention to limit damage to the developing white matter.

Five proteins were increased in preterm CSF vs. controls at the threshold $p < 0.01$: C5a, IL-9, SPP1, FasL, and Follistatin. C5a is a component of the complement cascade which we previously showed to be increased in human preterm CSF by enzyme-linked immunoabsorbant assay (Pataky et al., 2017), validating our novel approach of using antibody array to identify differentially expressed proteins in CSF samples. Although C5a has been associated with normal brain development (Benard et al., 2008) and neuroprotection (Biggins et al., 2017), it may have damaging functions as inhibition of its receptor C5aR attenuates excitotoxic perinatal brain injury (Pedroni et al., 2013) and C5a is increased in the CSF of children with demyelinating disease (Horellou et al., 2015). In addition, we identified IL-9 as a novel preterm birth-associated CNS cytokine in humans. Although we found it is not regulated by microglia in the IL-1β injury model, it may be expressed by other cell types such as Th9 lymphocytes. In experimental models it has roles in mast cell activation and excitotoxicity (Patkai et al., 2001), neonatal cortical neuronal apoptosis (Fontaine et al., 2008), autoimmune demyelination (Li et al., 2011), and regulation of astrocyte chemokine production (Ding et al., 2015); our data support a role for IL9 in the human inflammatory response to preterm birth. In addition, its expression can be driven by TGFβ (Beriou et al., 2010), which when overexpressed by microglia is associated with hypomyelination (Nobuta et al., 2012). IL-9 may also have direct actions on oligodendrocyte lineage cells, as these express the IL-9 receptor and IL-9 treatment inhibits their differentiation *in vitro*, although, notably, it can encourage differentiation if co-supplied with IFN-γ (Ding et al., 2015).

The remaining three highly enriched proteins have been implicated in regulating the oligodendrocyte lineage and myelination. Osteopontin (SPP1) in particular has been suggested as a blood biomarker for neonatal encephalopathy (Graham et al., 2018) and it is highly induced by hypoxic

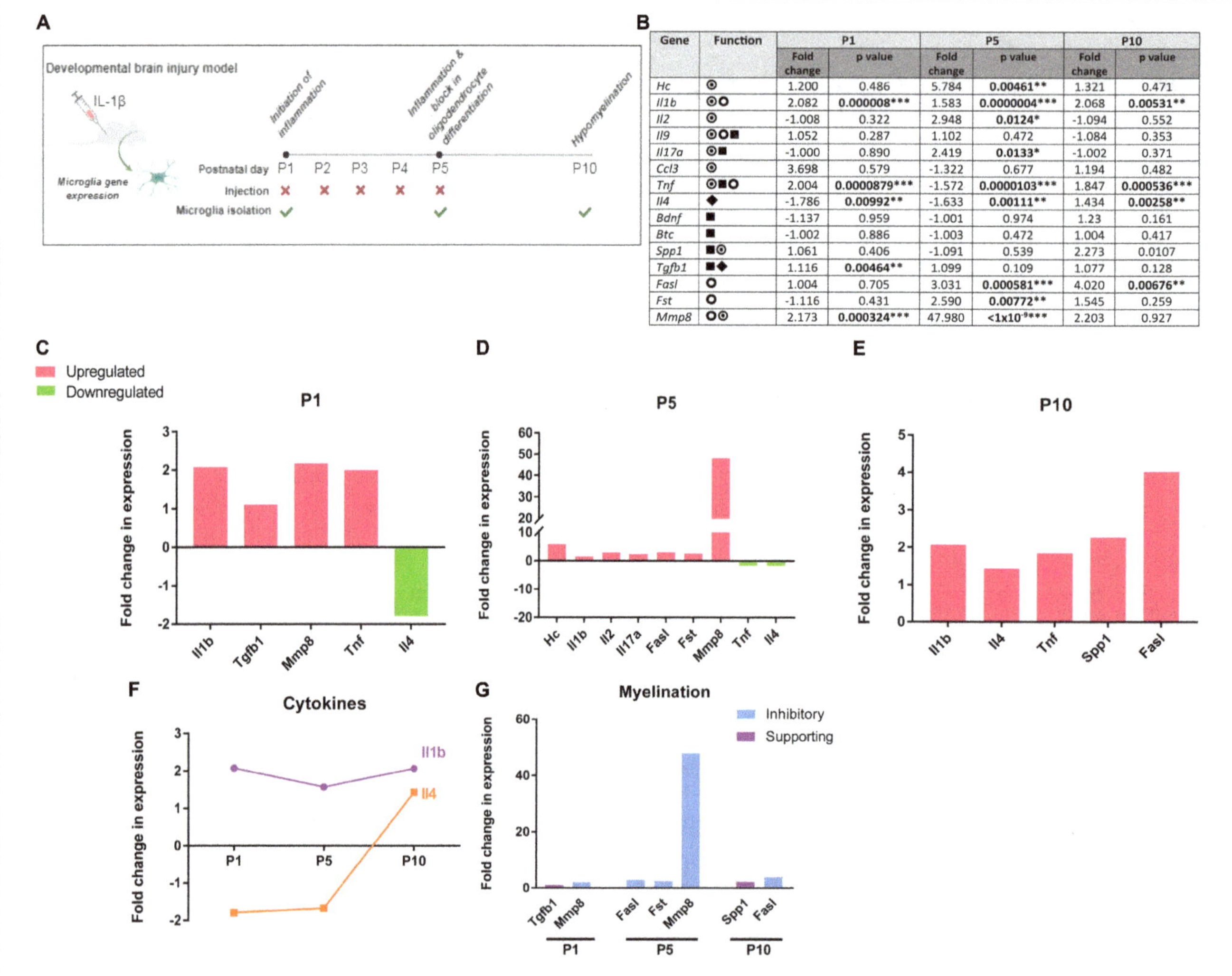

Gene	Function	P1		P5		P10	
		Fold change	p value	Fold change	p value	Fold change	p value
Hc	⊙	1.200	0.486	5.784	**0.00461****	1.321	0.471
Il1b	⊙○	2.082	**0.000008*****	1.583	**0.0000004*****	2.068	**0.00531****
Il2	⊙	-1.008	0.322	2.948	**0.0124***	-1.094	0.552
Il9	⊙○■	1.052	0.287	1.102	0.472	-1.084	0.353
Il17a	⊙■	-1.000	0.890	2.419	**0.0133***	-1.002	0.371
Ccl3	⊙	3.698	0.579	-1.322	0.677	1.194	0.482
Tnf	⊙■○	2.004	**0.0000879*****	-1.572	**0.0000103*****	1.847	**0.000536*****
Il4	◆	-1.786	**0.00992****	-1.633	**0.00111****	1.434	**0.00258****
Bdnf	■	-1.137	0.959	-1.001	0.974	1.23	0.161
Btc	■	-1.002	0.886	-1.003	0.472	1.004	0.417
Spp1	■⊙	1.061	0.406	-1.091	0.539	2.273	0.0107
Tgfb1	■◆	1.116	**0.00464****	1.099	0.109	1.077	0.128
Fasl	○	1.004	0.705	3.031	**0.000581*****	4.020	**0.00676****
Fst	○	-1.116	0.431	2.590	**0.00772****	1.545	0.259
Mmp8	○⊙	2.173	**0.000324*****	47.980	**$<1 \times 10^{-9}$*****	2.203	0.927

FIGURE 1 | Dynamic expression of human preterm CSF signature proteins at the gene expression level in microglia following experimental brain injury. **(A)** Mouse model of developmental white matter injury. **(B)** Fold change in gene expression in microglia isolated from IL-1β mouse model of developmental white matter injury, values at postnatal (P) day 1, 5, and 10 indicated, with *p*-values **p*<0.05, ***p* < 0.01, and ****p* < 0.001; ⊙ pro-inflammatory function, ◆ anti-inflammatory function, ■ supporting oligodendrocyte lineage responses and myelination, ○ impairing oligodendrocyte lineage responses and myelination. **(C–E)** Fold change in expression of genes in microglia isolated from IL-1β injury model compared to vehicle control, at postnatal days (P) 1, 5, and 10. Significantly upregulated genes shown in magenta, significantly downregulated genes shown in green. **(F)** Dynamic regulation of *Il1b* and *Il4* over the course of injury. **(G)** Fold change in expression over vehicle control for genes associated with impairing myelination (blue) and those supporting myelination (purple).

injury, where a protective role is suggested by decreased oligodendrogenesis in a knockout mouse subjected to hypoxic-ischemic injury (van Velthoven et al., 2011). This beneficial role may be dependent on mode of neural injury or age, as in adult mice SPP1 exacerbates autoimmune-mediated demyelination and is not required for regeneration of myelin on previously myelinated axons (Zhao et al., 2008). Nonetheless, it can directly increase myelin protein expression and myelination *in vitro* (Selvaraju et al., 2004). Another protein we detected in preterm CSF which may directly modulate myelination is follistatin, which sequesters activin-A to prevent its binding to activin receptors. This would be predicted to impair myelination, as we have recently shown these receptors to be required for oligodendrocyte differentiation and myelin maturation in healthy white matter development and following injury (Dillenburg et al., 2018). Lastly, the increase in Fas ligand in preterm CSF may indicate direct targeting of oligodendrocytes, as it has been associated with induction of oligodendrocyte death in a variety of neurological disorders (Austin and Fehlings, 2008).

Our study has some limitations. Although no infant in the study group had meningitis, a proportion of preterm and term infants had BSI at the time of CSF sampling. Therefore, it is possible that systemic inflammation contributed to observed alterations in the CSF inflammatory profile, although this potential confounding effect is likely to be balanced across the groups.

Our study was not designed to investigate the effect of astrocyte-mediated cytokine production, which could contribute to neuroinflammation as has been suggested by some experimental perinatal white matter injury models

(Nobuta et al., 2012; Shiow et al., 2017). In future work, investigating gene expression in other cell types including astrocytes and neurones may be informative.

Altogether, these findings identify a CSF signature in response to preterm birth, which reflects a complex environment that can both drive injury and support myelination. The pathological outcome of preterm birth may thus reflect a balance between damaging and reparative factors, which implies that effective therapies may need to operate on multiple targets. We propose that early therapeutic intervention could pre-empt the robust pro-inflammatory response and boost pro-repair mechanisms to support healthy myelination.

AUTHOR CONTRIBUTIONS

JB co-designed the study, analyzed the patient data, and contributed to writing the manuscript. GI and GS analyzed the patient samples. BF and PG co-designed the study, carried out the animal experiments, and generated the microglial gene expression dataset. RP collected the human CSF samples. VM co-designed the study, analyzed the microglia gene expression dataset, and co-wrote the manuscript. All authors read and approved the final manuscript.

FUNDING

This work was supported by Theirworld (www.theirworld.org), the MRC Centre for Reproductive Health (MRC G1002033), and a Career Development Award from the Medical Research Council (V.E.M.; MR/M020827/1). The funding body had no role in the design of the study or sample collection, analysis, and interpretation of data, or in writing the manuscript.

ACKNOWLEDGMENTS

The authors are grateful to the parents and carers who consented to take part in the study, and to clinical colleagues at the Neonatal Intensive Care Unit of the Royal Infirmary of Edinburgh for referring patients. The diagram in **Figure 1A** was created with BioRender.

REFERENCES

Anblagan, D., Pataky, R., Evans, M. J., Telford, E. J., Serag, A., Sparrow, S., et al. (2016). Association between preterm brain injury and exposure to chorioamnionitis during fetal life. *Sci. Rep.* 6:37932. doi: 10.1038/srep37932

Armstrong-Wells, J., Donnelly, M., Post, M. D., Manco-Johnson, M. J., Winn, V. D., and Sébire, G. (2015). Inflammatory predictors of neurologic disability after preterm premature rupture of membranes. *Am. J. Obstet. Gynecol.* 212, 212.e1–212.e9. doi: 10.1016/j.ajog.2014.09.016

Austin, J. W., and Fehlings, M. G. (2008). Molecular mechanisms of fas-mediated cell death in oligodendrocytes. *J. Neurotrauma* 25, 411–426. doi: 10.1089/neu.2007.0436

Back, S. A., and Miller, S. P. (2014). Brain injury in premature neonates: a primary cerebral dysmaturation disorder? *Ann. Neurol.* 75, 469–486. doi: 10.1002/ana.24132

Barnett, M. L., Tusor, N., Ball, G., Chew, A., Falconer, S., Aljabar, P., et al. (2018). Exploring the multiple-hit hypothesis of preterm white matter damage using diffusion MRI. *Neuroimage Clin.* 17, 596–606. doi: 10.1016/j.nicl.2017.11.017

Bartha, A. I., Foster-Barber, A., Miller, S. P., Vigneron, D. B., Glidden, D. V., Barkovich, A. J., et al. (2004). Neonatal encephalopathy: association of cytokines with MR spectroscopy and outcome. *Pediatr. Res.* 56, 960–966. doi: 10.1203/01.Pdr.0000144819.45689.Bb

Basu, S., Agarwal, P., Anupurba, S., Shukla, R., and Kumar, A. (2015). Elevated plasma and cerebrospinal fluid interleukin-1 beta and tumor necrosis factor-alpha concentration and combined outcome of death or abnormal neuroimaging in preterm neonates with early-onset clinical sepsis. *J. Perinatol.* 35, 855–861. doi: 10.1038/jp.2015.86

Batalle, D., Hughes, E. J., Zhang, H., Tournier, J. D., Tusor, N., Aljabar, P., et al. (2017). Early development of structural networks and the impact of prematurity on brain connectivity. *Neuroimage* 149, 379–392. doi: 10.1016/j.neuroimage.2017.01.065

Benard, M., Raoult, E., Vaudry, D., Leprince, J., Falluel-Morel, A., Gonzalez, B. J., et al. (2008). Role of complement anaphylatoxin receptors (C3aR, C5aR) in the development of the rat cerebellum. *Mol. Immunol.* 45, 3767–3774. doi: 10.1016/j.molimm.2008.05.027

Beriou, G., Bradshaw, E. M., Lozano, E., Costantino, C. M., Hastings, W. D., Orban, T., et al. (2010). TGF-beta induces IL-9 production from human Th17 cells. *J. Immunol.* 185, 46–54. doi: 10.4049/jimmunol.1000356

Biggins, P. J. C., Brennan, F. H., Taylor, S. M., Woodruff, T. M., and Ruitenberg, M. J. (2017). The alternative receptor for complement component 5a, C5aR2, conveys neuroprotection in traumatic spinal cord injury. *J. Neurotrauma* 34, 2075–2085. doi: 10.1089/neu.2016.4701

Billiards, S. S., Haynes, R. L., Folkerth, R. D., Borenstein, N. S., Trachtenberg, F. L., Rowitch, D. H., et al. (2008). Myelin abnormalities without oligodendrocyte loss in periventricular leukomalacia. *Brain Pathol.* 18, 153–163. doi: 10.1111/j.1750-3639.2007.00107.x

Caldinelli, C., Froudist-Walsh, S., Karolis, V., Tseng, C. E., Allin, M. P., Walshe, M., et al. (2017). White matter alterations to cingulum and fornix following very preterm birth and their relationship with cognitive functions. *Neuroimage* 150, 373–382. doi: 10.1016/j.neuroimage.2017.02.026

Carlo, W. A., McDonald, S. A., Tyson, J. E., Stoll, B. J., Ehrenkranz, R. A., Shankaran, S., et al. (2011). Cytokines and neurodevelopmental outcomes in extremely low birth weight infants. *J. Pediatr.* 159, 919.e3–925.e3. doi: 10.1016/j.jpeds.2011.05.042

Chhor, V., Le Charpentier, T., Lebon, S., Oré, M. V., Celador, I. L., Josserand, J., et al. (2013). Characterization of phenotype markers and neuronotoxic potential of polarised primary microglia in vitro. *Brain Behav. Immun.* 32, 70–85. doi: 10.1016/j.bbi.2013.02.005

Dillenburg, A., Ireland, G., Holloway, R. K., Davies, C. L., Evans, F. L., Swire, M., et al. (2018). Activin receptors regulate the oligodendrocyte lineage in health and disease. *Acta Neuropathol.* 135, 887–906. doi: 10.1007/s00401-018-1813-3

Ding, X., Cao, F., Cui, L., Ciric, B., Zhang, G. X., and Rostami, A. (2015). IL-9 signaling affects central nervous system resident cells during inflammatory stimuli. *Exp. Mol. Pathol.* 99, 570–574. doi: 10.1016/j.yexmp.2015.07.010

Dutta, D. J., Zameer, A., Mariani, J. N., Zhang, J., Asp, L., Huynh, J., et al. (2014). Combinatorial actions of Tgfbeta and activin ligands promote oligodendrocyte development and CNS myelination. *Development* 141, 2414–2428. doi: 10.1242/dev.106492

Ellison, V. J., Mocatta, T. J., Winterbourn, C. C., Darlow, B. A., Volpe, J. J., and Inder, T. E. (2005). The relationship of CSF and plasma cytokine levels to cerebral white matter injury in the premature newborn. *Pediatr. Res.* 57, 282–286. doi: 10.1203/01.pdr.0000148286.53572.95

Favrais, G., van de Looij, Y., Fleiss, B., Ramanantsoa, N., Bonnin, P., Stoltenburg-Didinger, G., et al. (2011). Systemic inflammation disrupts the developmental program of white matter. *Ann. Neurol.* 70, 550–565. doi: 10.1002/ana.22489

Folgueras, A. R., Fueyo, A., García-Suárez, O., Cox, J., Astudillo, A., Tortorella, P., et al. (2008). Collagenase-2 deficiency or inhibition impairs experimental autoimmune encephalomyelitis in mice. *J. Biol. Chem.* 283, 9465–9474. doi: 10.1074/jbc.M709522200

Fontaine, R. H., Cases, O., Lelièvre, V., Mesplès, B., Renauld, J. C., Loron, G., et al. (2008). IL-9/IL-9 receptor signaling selectively protects cortical neurons against developmental apoptosis. *Cell Death Differ.* 15, 1542–1552. doi: 10.1038/cdd.2008.79

Graham, E. M., Everett, A. D., Delpech, J. C., and Northington, F. J. (2018). Blood biomarkers for evaluation of perinatal encephalopathy: state of the art. *Curr. Opin. Pediatr.* 30, 199–203. doi: 10.1097/mop.0000000000000591

Gustavsson, M., Mallard, C., Vannucci, S. J., Wilson, M. A., Johnston, M. V., and Hagberg, H. (2007). Vascular response to hypoxic preconditioning in the immature brain. *J. Cereb. Blood Flow Metab.* 27, 928–938. doi: 10.1038/sj.jcbfm.9600408

Hagberg, H., Mallard, C., Ferriero, D. M., Vannucci, S. J., Levison, S. W., Vexler, Z. S., et al. (2015). The role of inflammation in perinatal brain injury. *Nat. Rev. Neurol.* 11, 192–208. doi: 10.1038/nrneurol.2015.13

Haynes, R. L., Folkerth, R. D., Trachtenberg, F. L., Volpe, J. J., and Kinney, H. C. (2009). Nitrosative stress and inducible nitric oxide synthase expression in periventricular leukomalacia. *Acta Neuropathol.* 118, 391–399. doi: 10.1007/s00401-009-0540-1

Horellou, P., Wang, M., Keo, V., Chrétien, P., Serguera, C., Waters, P., et al. (2015). Increased interleukin-6 correlates with myelin oligodendrocyte glycoprotein antibodies in pediatric monophasic demyelinating diseases and multiple sclerosis. *J. Neuroimmunol.* 289, 1–7. doi: 10.1016/j.jneuroim.2015.10.002

Husson, I., Rangon, C. M., Lelièvre, V., Bemelmans, A. P., Sachs, P., Mallet, J., et al. (2005). BDNF-induced white matter neuroprotection and stage-dependent neuronal survival following a neonatal excitotoxic challenge. *Cereb. Cortex* 15, 250–261. doi: 10.1093/cercor/bhh127

Johnson, S., and Marlow, N. (2017). Early and long-term outcome of infants born extremely preterm. *Arch. Dis. Child.* 102, 97–102. doi: 10.1136/archdischild-2015-309581

Krishnan, M. L., Van Steenwinckel, J., Schang, A. L., Yan, J., Arnadottir, J., Le Charpentier, T., et al. (2017). Integrative genomics of microglia implicates DLG4 (PSD95) in the white matter development of preterm infants. *Nat. Commun.* 8:428. doi: 10.1038/s41467-017-00422-w

Li, H., Nourbakhsh, B., Cullimore, M., Zhang, G. X., and Rostami, A. (2011). IL-9 is important for T-cell activation and differentiation in autoimmune inflammation of the central nervous system. *Eur. J. Immunol.* 41, 2197–2206. doi: 10.1002/eji.201041125

Nelson, K. B., Dambrosia, J. M., Grether, J. K., and Phillips, T. M. (1998). Neonatal cytokines and coagulation factors in children with cerebral palsy. *Ann. Neurol.* 44, 665–675. doi: 10.1002/ana.410440413

Nobuta, H., Ghiani, C. A., Paez, P. M., Spreuer, V., Dong, H., Korsak, R. A., et al. (2012). STAT3-mediated astrogliosis protects myelin development in neonatal brain injury. *Ann. Neurol.* 72, 750–765. doi: 10.1002/ana.23670

O'Driscoll, D. N., McGovern, M., Greene, C. M., and Molloy, E. J. (2018). Gender disparities in preterm neonatal outcomes. *Acta Paediatr.* doi: 10.1111/apa.14390 [Epub ahead of print].

Palazuelos, J., Klingener, M., and Aguirre, A. (2014). TGFbeta signaling regulates the timing of CNS myelination by modulating oligodendrocyte progenitor cell cycle exit through SMAD3/4/FoxO1/Sp1. *J. Neurosci.* 34, 7917–7930. doi: 10.1523/jneurosci.0363-14.2014

Pataky, R., Howie, F. A., Girardi, G., and Boardman, J. P. (2017). Complement C5a is present in CSF of human newborns and is elevated in association with preterm birth. *J. Matern. Fetal Neonatal Med.* 30, 2413–2416. doi: 10.1080/14767058.2016.1251896

Patkai, J., Mesples, B., Dommergues, M. A., Fromont, G., Thornton, E. M., Renauld, J. C., et al. (2001). Deleterious effects of IL-9-activated mast cells and neuroprotection by antihistamine drugs in the developing mouse brain. *Pediatr. Res.* 50, 222–230. doi: 10.1203/00006450-200108000-200108010

Pedroni, S. M., Gonzalez, J. M., Wade, J., Jansen, M. A., Serio, A., Marshall, I., et al. (2013). Complement inhibition and statins prevent fetal brain cortical abnormalities in a mouse model of preterm birth. *Biochim. Biophys. Acta* 1842, 107–115. doi: 10.1016/j.bbadis.2013.10.011

Rajkumar, R., Bhaya, B., Mamilla, D., Czech, T., Kisseih, E., Saini, A., et al. (2018). A preliminary evaluation of glial cell line-derived neurotrophic factor (GDNF) levels in cerebrospinal fluid across various gestational ages and clinical conditions of the neonate. *Int. J. Dev. Neurosci.* 65, 61–65. doi: 10.1016/j.ijdevneu.2017.10.001

Savman, K., Blennow, M., Gustafson, K., Tarkowski, E., and Hagberg, H. (1998). Cytokine response in cerebrospinal fluid after birth asphyxia. *Pediatr. Res.* 43, 746–751. doi: 10.1203/00006450-199806000-00006

Schang, A. L., Van Steenwinckel, J., Chevenne, D., Alkmark, M., Hagberg, H., Gressens, P., et al. (2014). Failure of thyroid hormone treatment to prevent inflammation-induced white matter injury in the immature brain. *Brain. Behav. Immun.* 37, 95–102. doi: 10.1016/j.bbi.2013.11.005

Selvaraju, R., Bernasconi, L., Losberger, C., Graber, P., Kadi, L., Avellana-Adalid, V., et al. (2004). Osteopontin is upregulated during in vivo demyelination and remyelination and enhances myelin formation in vitro. *Mol. Cell. Neurosci.* 25, 707–721. doi: 10.1016/j.mcn.2003.12.014

Shah, D. K., Doyle, L. W., Anderson, P. J., Bear, M., Daley, A. J., Hunt, R. W., et al. (2008). Adverse neurodevelopment in preterm infants with postnatal sepsis or necrotizing enterocolitis is mediated by white matter abnormalities on magnetic resonance imaging at term. *J. Pediatr.* 153, 170.e1–175.e1. doi: 10.1016/j.jpeds.2008.02.033

Shiow, L. R., Favrais, G., Schirmer, L., Schang, A. L., Cipriani, S., Andres, C., et al. (2017). Reactive astrocyte COX2-PGE2 production inhibits oligodendrocyte maturation in neonatal white matter injury. *Glia* 65, 2024–2037. doi: 10.1002/glia.23212

Spittle, A. J., Walsh, J. M., Potter, C., Mcinnes, E., Olsen, J. E., Lee, K. J., et al. (2017). Neurobehaviour at term-equivalent age and neurodevelopmental outcomes at 2 years in infants born moderate-to-late preterm. *Dev. Med. Child Neurol.* 59, 207–215. doi: 10.1111/dmcn.13297

Telford, E. J., Cox, S. R., Fletcher-Watson, S., Anblagan, D., Sparrow, S., Pataky, R., et al. (2017). A latent measure explains substantial variance in white matter microstructure across the newborn human brain. *Brain Struct. Funct.* 222, 4023–4033. doi: 10.1007/s00429-017-1455-6

Van Steenwinckel, J., Schang, A. L., Krishnan, M. L., Degos, V., Delahaye-Duriez, A., Bokobza, C., et al. (2018). Loss of the Wnt/β-catenin pathway in microglia of the developing brain drives pro-inflammatory activation leading to white matter injury. *bioRxiv* [Preprint]. doi: 10.1101/334359

van Velthoven, C. T., Heijnen, C. J., van Bel, F., and Kavelaars, A. (2011). Osteopontin enhances endogenous repair after neonatal hypoxic-ischemic brain injury. *Stroke* 42, 2294–2301. doi: 10.1161/strokeaha.110.608315

Verney, C., Pogledic, I., Biran, V., Adle-Biassette, H., Fallet-Bianco, C., and Gressens, P. (2012). Microglial reaction in axonal crossroads is a hallmark of noncystic periventricular white matter injury in very preterm infants. *J. Neuropathol. Exp. Neurol.* 71, 251–264. doi: 10.1097/NEN.0b013e3182496429

Viscardi, R. M., Muhumuza, C. K., Rodriguez, A., Fairchild, K. D., Sun, C. C., Gross, G. W., et al. (2004). Inflammatory markers in intrauterine and fetal blood and cerebrospinal fluid compartments are associated with adverse pulmonary and neurologic outcomes in preterm infants. *Pediatr. Res.* 55, 1009–1017. doi: 10.1203/01.pdr.0000127015.60185.8a

Volpe, J. J. (2009). Brain injury in premature infants: a complex amalgam of destructive and developmental disturbances. *Lancet Neurol.* 8, 110–124. doi: 10.1016/S1474-4422(08)70294-1

Wosik, K., Antel, J., Kuhlmann, T., Brück, W., Massie, B., and Nalbantoglu, J. (2003). Oligodendrocyte injury in multiple sclerosis: a role for p53. *J. Neurochem.* 85, 635–644. doi: 10.1046/j.1471-4159.2003.01674.x

Yoon, B. H., Romero, R., Kim, C. J., Koo, J. N., Choe, G., Syn, H. C., et al. (1997). High expression of tumor necrosis factor-alpha and interleukin-6 in periventricular leukomalacia. *Am. J. Obstet. Gynecol.* 177, 406–411. doi: 10.1016/S0002-9378(97)70206-0

Yoon, B. H., Romero, R., Yang, S. H., Jun, J. K., Kim, I. O., Choi, J. H., et al. (1996). Interleukin-6 concentrations in umbilical cord plasma are elevated in neonates with white matter lesions associated with periventricular leukomalacia. *Am. J. Obstet. Gynecol.* 174, 1433–1440. doi: 10.1016/S0002-9378(96)70585-9

Zhang, Y., Chen, K., Sloan, S. A., Bennett, M. L., Scholze, A. R., O'Keeffe, S., et al. (2014). An RNA-sequencing transcriptome and splicing database of glia, neurons, and vascular cells of the cerebral cortex. *J. Neurosci.* 34, 11929–11947. doi: 10.1523/jneurosci.1860-14.2014

Zhao, C., Fancy, S. P., ffrench-Constant, C., and Franklin, R. J. (2008). Osteopontin is extensively expressed by macrophages following CNS demyelination but has a redundant role in remyelination. *Neurobiol. Dis.* 31, 209–217. doi: 10.1016/j.nbd.2008.04.007

2

Supine vs. Prone Position with Turn of the Head does not Affect Cerebral Perfusion and Oxygenation in Stable Preterm Infants ≤32 Weeks Gestational Age

Dietmar Spengler, Elisa Loewe and Martin F. Krause*

Department of Pediatrics, University Hospital Schleswig-Holstein, Kiel, Germany

***Correspondence:**
Martin F. Krause
martin.krause@uksh.de

Intraventricular hemorrhage (IVH) is a frequent major damage to the brain of premature babies ≤32 weeks gestational age, and its incidence (20–25%) has not significantly changed lately. Because of the intrinsic fragility of germinal matrix blood vessels, IVH occurs following disruption of subependymal mono-layer arteries and is generally attributed to ischemia-reperfusion alterations or venous congestion, which may be caused by turn of the head. Therefore, supine position with the head in a midline position is considered a standard position for preterm infants during their first days of life. We asked whether a change in body position (supine vs. prone) linked with a turn of the head by 90° in the prone position would change blood flow velocities and resistance indices in major cerebral arteries and veins of stable premature babies at two different time points (t0, day of life 2, vs. t1, day 9). Moreover, we assessed cerebral tissue oxygenation (cStO2) by near-infrared spectroscopy and determined correlations for changes in velocities and oxygenation. Twenty one premature infants [gestational age 30 (26–32) weeks] with sufficiently stable gas exchange and circulation were screened by ultrasonography and near-infrared spectroscopy. Peak systolic and end-diastolic blood flow velocities in the anterior cerebral arteries (29 ± 6 m/s vs. 28 ± 7 peak flow at t0, 36 ± 8 vs. 35 ± 7 at t1), the basilar artery, the right and the left internal carotid artery, and the great cerebral vein Galen (4.0 ± 0.8 m/s vs. 4.1 ± 1.0 maximum flow at t0, 4.4 ± 0.8 vs. 4.4 ± 1.0 at t1) did not show significant differences following change of body and head position. Also, there were no differences in $cStO_2$ (83 ± 7% vs. 84 ± 7 at t0, 76 ± 10 vs. 77 ± 11 at t1) and in vital signs such as heart rate and blood pressure. We conclude that change in body position with turn of the head in the prone position does not elicit significant alterations in cerebral blood flow velocities or in oxygenation of cerebral tissues. Maturational changes in arterial flow velocities and $cStO_2$ are not correlated. For this subgroup of premature infants at low risk of IVH our data do not support the concept of exclusive preterm infant care in supine position.

Keywords: cerebral blood flow velocity, regional cerebral oxygenation, body position, turn of head, near-infrared spectroscopy, intraventricular hemorrhage

INTRODUCTION

Intraventricular hemorrhage (IVH) is a frequent major damage to the brain of premature infants ≤32 weeks of gestational age (WGA)/<1500 g birthweight, and despite great advances in neonatal care its incidence (20–25%) has not significantly changed within the last two decades (Humberg et al., 2017).

Long-term neurodevelopmental outcome depends on the immaturity of the infant and the degree of parenchymal damage by IVH ranging from mild germinal matrix bleeding to widespread periventricular hemorrhagic infarction. Neurologic sequelae of IVH include all degrees of motor deficits, cognitive deficits, learning disabilities, and seizure disorders: in high-risk premature infants <1000 g birthweight Sherlock et al. (2005) found a cerebral palsy incidence of 6% in infants with grade I IVH, 24% with grade II IVH, and 100% with grade IV IVH at 8 years of age.

The risk of bleeding is inversely correlated to gestational age and may be attributed to the following three factors: vascular immaturity of the germinal matrix, deficient extravascular matrix, and cerebral blood flow disturbances (Inder et al., 2018). First, vascular immaturity bases on the observation that the germinal matrix blood vessels are composed of endothelial cells only and lack muscle tissue and collagen. This immature microvascular network contains large diameter blood vessels without arterial or venous specification, is deficient in tight junction proteins (e.g., claudin and zonula occludens protein-1), and continues to be subject to involution and remodeling until the 37th WGA (Ballabh et al., 2005; Anstrom et al., 2007). Then, the extravascular matrix is rich in fibrinolytic activity (in contrast to developmental shortfalls in platelet and coagulation factor function), but lacks direct contact with perivascular structures due to slow astrocytic development (Rao et al., 2016) making the germinal matrix a gelatinous friable tissue deficient of mesenchymal and glial elements. Finally and most important, perfusion disturbances such as fluctuating cerebral blood flow (e.g., ischemia-hyperperfusion), a pressure-passive state of the cerebral perfusion, and sudden increases in cerebral venous pressure make the premature infant subject to germinal matrix bleeding (Baburamani et al., 2012).

As the internal jugular veins are the major blood outflow tract of the brain, turn of the head associated compromise of the venous blood drainage might lead to venous congestion, increased intracranial pressure, reduced cerebral oxygenation, and ultimately germinal matrix IVH (de Bijl-Marcus et al., 2017). Therefore, the head midline position has been advocated for many years for preventing the occurrence or extension of IVH in routine neonatal care, but an updated Cochrane systematic review was unable to support this approach due to a lack of adequate studies (Romantsik et al., 2017). In routine care of the respiratory and hemodynamically stable mature infant, however, prone position is preferred for reasons of improved oxygenation (secondary to augmented functional residual capacity) (Bhat et al., 2003), saturation stability (Heimann et al., 2010), airway patency (Francois et al., 1992), drainage of oropharyngeal secretions (Pickens et al., 1989; Waisman, 2006), reduction in obstructive apnea (Heimann et al., 2010), and improved quality of sleep (Bhat et al., 2006).

Our aim was to study the impact of supine position with the head in a midline position vs. prone position with turn of the head by 90° on arterial peak and end-diastolic flow, on resistance indices in cerebral arteries, and maximum flow in cerebral veins because this practical approach to stable preterm infant nursing has not been investigated before. In addition, we assessed cerebral oxygen saturation by near-infrared spectroscopy to capture any compromise in blood supply by a supportive technique, and compared the results of two different times of examination [t0 on day 2 (median) vs. t1 on day 9].

MATERIALS AND METHODS

The detailed study protocol was approved by the institutional ethics commission of the medical faculty of the Christian-Albrechts-University, Kiel (reference number A 102/13), in accordance with the World Medical Association's Declaration of Helsinki. The parents or the legal guardians of the infants admitted to the neonatal intensive care unit of the university hospital gave their written informed consent that could be withdrawn any time. A total of 32 premature infants ≤32 weeks of gestational age with sufficiently stable oxygenation/circulation (two infants on invasive mechanical ventilation with low pressures and FiO_2 <0.3) in a calm resting state [grade 1–3 according to Prechtl (Cioni and Prechtl, 1990)] were recruited to avoid motion-related inaccuracies in data acquisition and sampling. Exclusion criteria following the initial screening were all conditions of low blood pressure [i.e., below the 95% confidence limit for systolic and diastolic blood pressure for age 2 and 9 days (Zubrow et al., 1995)] with or without the administration of catecholamines, large patent ductus arteriosus [defined by the following three criteria: LA:Ao-ratio of >1.6:1, ductal diameter > 2.0 mm, retrograde diastolic flow in descending Ao > 30% of forward flow (Skinner, 2000)], congenital heart disease, IVH ≥ grade 2 on an initial ultrasound examination immediately after birth, and all kinds of congenital malformations. Two infants of 27 WGA were diagnosed with unilateral IVH grade 1 on day 2 that was almost completely reabsorbed on day 9.

In each infant two sets of investigations were carried out on day 2 (median, range 1–3; t0) and on day 9 (8–11; t1) of life to capture any maturational changes in all measured parameters. 6/21 infants received their t0 evaluations on day 1. The cerebral tissue oxygen saturation ($cStO_2$) was assessed by the application of an infant frontal adhesive sensor to the Invos 5100C near-infrared spectroscopy device (Somanetics Corp., Troy, MI, United States). The $cStO_2$ sensor was always taped to the middle of the forehead with the connecting flexible hose running to the right side. To assess cerebral perfusion an Acuson X300 (Siemens Healthcare, Erlangen, Germany) connected to a 9 MHz sector transducer was used to examine the side up anterior cerebral artery (ACA), the basilar artery (BA), the right and the left carotid artery (RICA and LICA), and the great cerebral vein Galen (GCV, the largest vessel in the midline inferior to the splenium of the corpus callosum) by sagittal and coronal sections performed via the great fontanelle as the acoustic window. For the Doppler measurements, the angle of insonation was kept $<30°$ to reduce the error of velocity measurements and was manually corrected to a minimum (**Figure 1**). Color Doppler ultrasound was used to clearly identify the different blood vessels, and all recordings were cross-checked by two experienced ultrasound investigators (DS, EL). From the arterial flow profiles the peak systolic velocity (PSV) and the end-diastolic velocity (EDV) were identified, and a resistance index (RI) was calculated by PSV-EDV/PSV. Venous flow profiles of the GCV were measured in pairs using a sagittal and a coronal approach to correct for any bias in low flow venous patterns. For comparisons the maximum systolic velocities (MSV) were used to compensate for possible waveform fluctuations (Ikeda et al., 2015). The ultrasound examinations started from either the supine or the prone position without any head-up angulation, and within the examination time of 25–35 min the body position was changed (from supine with the head in a midline position to prone with a turn of the head to the right or left by 90°, or *vice versa*). The same side of head turning was used for the t0 and the t1 examinations.

We also assessed pCO_2 (mmHg) and hemoglobin concentrations (g/dl) in capillary blood prior to each ultrasound investigation.

For statistics we applied a paired t-test to compare the data obtained from different body positions and from different time windows by the use of Prism 5 software (GraphPad, La Jolla, CA, United States). Pearson correlation of PSV and NIRS as independently measured variables were calculated. A *p*-value <0.05 was considered statistically significant.

RESULTS

Of the 32 preterm infants, 2 were excluded after withdrawal of informed consent; the registration of the Doppler profiles were greatly disturbed by motion-associated artifacts in 1 infant; complete sets of Doppler ultrasound recording (i.e., missing t1 recordings) were not available in two infants; in six infants the acquisition of t1 parameters could not be accomplished because of back transport to the referring hospitals. The data presented here base on the examination of 21 infants with each infant serving as its own control.

Among these 21 infants 10 (48%) were girls and 11 (52%) were boys. The gestational age was 29 ± 2 weeks, and the average weight was 1211 ± 342 g. 19/21 (90%) infants had received antenatal steroids. None of the infants was diagnosed with perinatal asphyxia (defined by an umbilical artery pH <7.1, and a 5-min Apgar score <5), even though 4/21 (19%) were prenatally screened with an absent end-diastolic umbilical artery flow. The co-morbidities are listed on **Table 1**. As mentioned above only infants with sufficiently stable oxygenation ($SpO_2 \geq 92\%$, $FiO_2 \leq 0.25$) and circulation (blood pressure above lower 95% CL, capillary refill ≤ 2 s) were screened for inclusion to this study depending on the vote of the attending neonatologist. When starting $cStO_2$ recordings and Doppler ultrasound examinations, the saturation by pulsed oximetry was 96% ± 2 at t0 and 97% ± 1 at t1; the heart rate was 148 bpm ± 14 at t0 and 161 ± 14 at t1; the blood pressure was 53 ± 8 mmHg (systolic)/30 ± 6 (diastolic) at t0 and 59 ± 9/35 ± 7 at t1. The results of the blood gases were: pCO_2 39 ± 6 mm Hg at t0 and 40 ± 4 at t1; hemoglobin 17.2 ± 2.8 g/dl at t0 and 14.6 ± 2.5 at t1.

PSV, EDV, and RI from the four arteries investigated (ACA, BA, RICA, LICA) are shown in **Figure 2**. There were no statistically significant differences between supine and prone position at t0 and at t1 except of RI of ACA at t1 ($p < 0.05$, **Figure 2B**). In contrast PSV and EDV (and RI) differences of all 4 arteries between t0 and t1 suggest maturational changes and come along with an increase in blood pressure level.

Maximum systolic velocities of the GCV was obtained by the use of two different approaches (sagittal vs. coronal) to the anterior fontanel as the acoustic window yielding no differences between supine vs. prone position, t0 vs. t1, and sagittal vs. coronal (**Figure 3**).

Figure 4 displays the results of the $cStO_2$ recordings without differences between supine vs. prone position, however, between t0 and t1 recordings. The calculation of correlation of PSV/EDV and $cStO_2$ yielded values of $r = 0.38$ to -0.14 (not significant). Despite differences in physiologic stability in the infants with early t0 scans (i.e., day 1) the flow velocity and $cStO_2$ analyses of

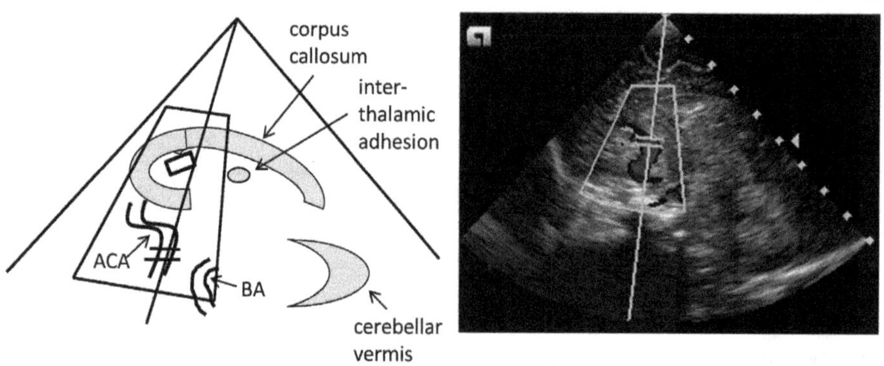

FIGURE 1 | Standard sagittal plane of the cerebral color Doppler ultrasound investigation performed through the anterior fontanel. This midline sagittal image shows the corpus callosum, the interthalamic adhesion, and the cerebellar vermis as reference structures. ACA, anterior cerebral artery; BA, basilar artery.

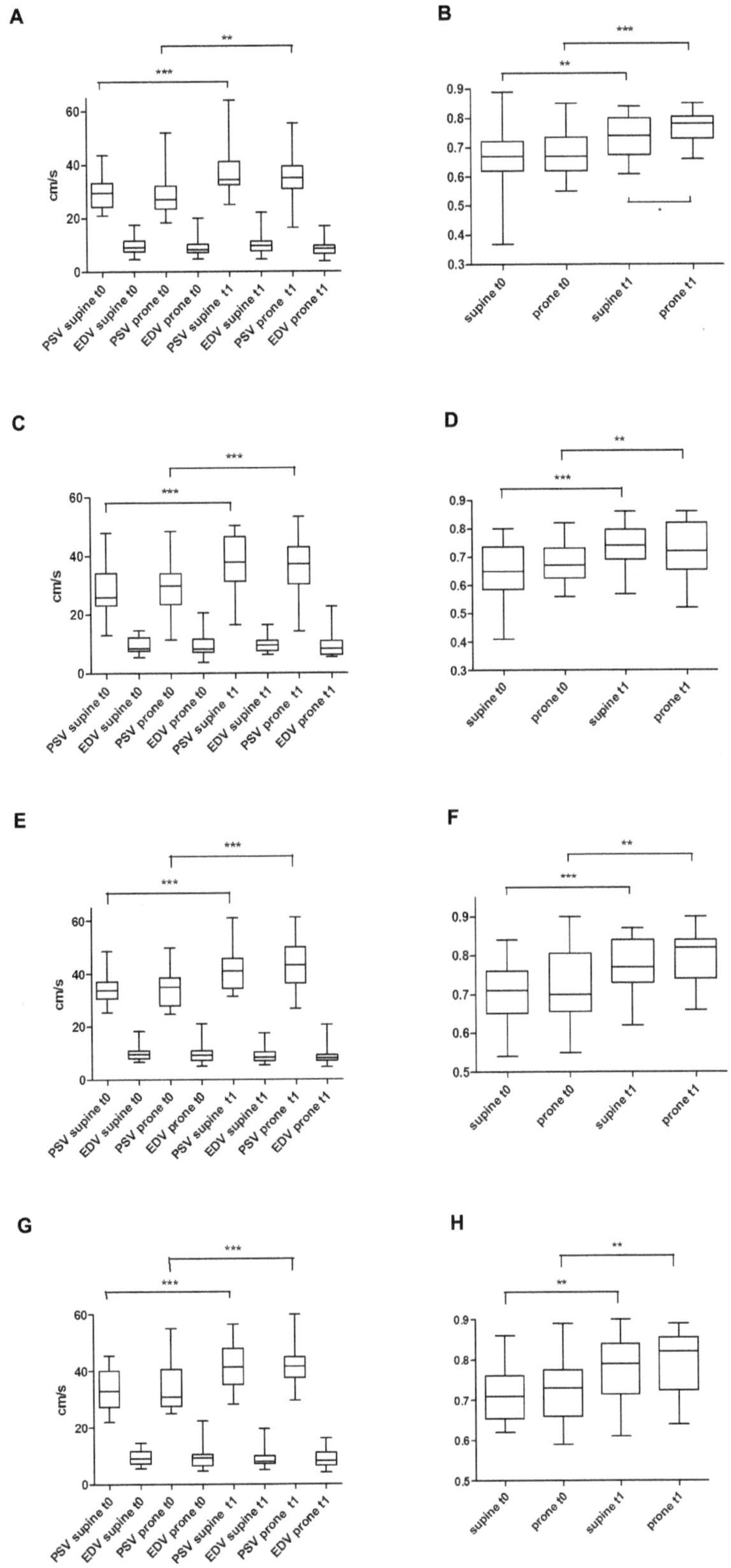

FIGURE 2 | Peak systolic velocity (PSV) and end-diastolic velocity (EDV) at two different times (t0, t1) and two different body positions (supine vs. prone) of the side up anterior cerebral artery (ACA) **(A)**; resistance indices of ACA **(B)**; PSV and EDV of the basilar artery (BA) **(C)**; resistance indices of BA **(D)**; PSV and EDV of the right internal carotid artery (RICA) **(E)**; resistance indices of RICA **(F)**; PSV and EDV of the left internal artery (LICA) **(G)**; resistance indices of LICA **(H)**. $^{*}p < 0.05$; $^{**}p < 0.01$; $^{***}p < 0.001$.

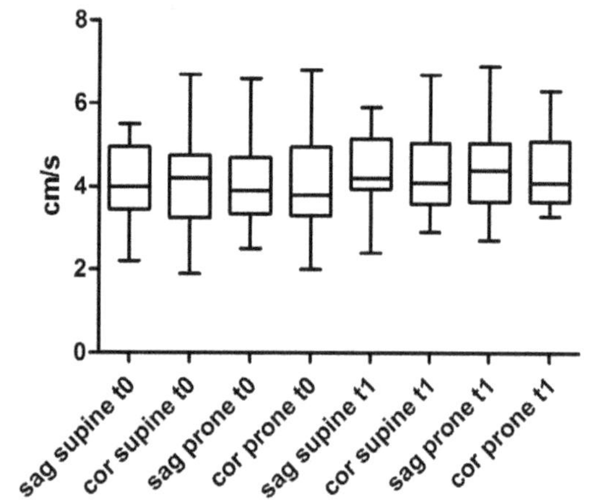

FIGURE 3 | Maximum systolic flow (MSV) of the great cerebral vein (GCV) using a sagittal (sag) and a coronal (cor) approach to the anterior fontanel as an acoustic window at two different times (t0, t1) and two different body positions (supine vs. prone).

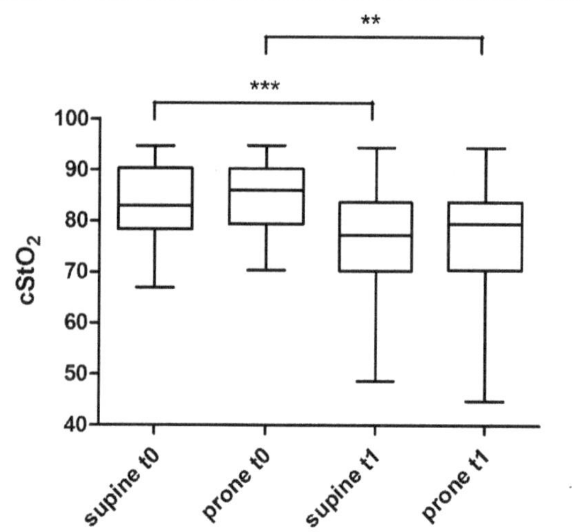

FIGURE 4 | $cStO_2$ (cerebral tissue oxygen saturation) recordings by NIRS technique from a frontal probe at two different times (t0, t1) and two different body positions (supine vs. prone). $^{**}p < 0.01$; $^{***}p < 0.001$.

this subgroup do not show significant differences when compared to the group examined on day 2 and 3 (data not shown).

DISCUSSION

Our data demonstrate that arterial and venous blood flow velocities do not depend on body position comparing supine with the head in a midline position vs. prone with a turn of the head by 90° position. In contrast we show that PSV and EDV are subject to maturational changes with increases in PSV (and RI) comparing t0 vs. t1. These changes were not observed in venous flow patterns which remained stable over time and were independent of the approach to the anterior fontanel as an acoustic window (sagittal vs. coronal). PSV and $cStO_2$ were not correlated and need to be interpreted individually.

TABLE 1 | Comorbidities of the study group.

	t0* (*n* = 21)	**t1 (*n* = 21)**
IVH grade I**	2 (9%)	2 (9%)
RDS***	18 (85%)	11 (52%)
Large PDA****	0	0
Apnea/bradycardia	12 (57%)	16 (76%)
Infection (antibiotic use)	15 (71%)	3 (14%)

**t0 examinations on day 2 (median, range 1–3); t1 examinations on day 9 (8–11). **IVH, intraventricular hemorrhage; infants with IVH ≥ grade II were excluded from the study. ***RDS, respiratory distress syndrome, mild to moderate; two infants received invasive mechanical ventilation at t0. ****Large PDA (defined by LA:Ao-ratio of >1.6:1, ductal diameter >2.0 mm, retrograde diastolic flow in descending Ao > 30% of forward flow).*

It needs to be stressed that these findings concern a subgroup of premature infants with sufficient respiratory and hemodynamic stability and may not be generalized. Infants at greatest risk of IVH typically are <28 weeks gestational age, <1000 g body weight, in their first 3–5 days of life, on invasive mechanical ventilation, equipped with umbilical lines, diagnosed with PDA or other hemodynamic instabilities, treated with specific medication for PDA closure, and often times without antenatal corticosteroids administration. Explicitly, this kind of infants was not included into this study to avoid possible undesired side effects by changes in body and head position.

However, newer technologies such as assisted non-invasive ventilation and surfactant application by different LISA (less invasive surfactant application) maneuvers allow us to provide sufficient respiratory support in a growing high-risk subgroup of premature infants as described above not receiving invasive ventilation and not being equipped with umbilical lines. Nursing in prone position with turn of the head to stabilize respiratory function is therefore mandatory and carried out in our institution beyond 96 h of age also in this subgroup of premature infants given the fact that a Cochrane Systematic Review (Romantsik et al., 2017) could not show differences in germinal matrix IVH, severe IVH, and neonatal mortality comparing supine vs. prone position.

Our findings are in line with 6 studies (Lawson et al., 1987; Buckley et al., 2009; Ancora et al., 2010; Al-Abdi et al., 2011; Elser et al., 2012; Liao et al., 2015) investigating the effect of body position (including body/head elevation) or turn of the head on oxidative phosphorylation, cerebral blood flow velocities and $cStO_2$; however, the current study is the only study using both interventions simultaneously (i.e., change from supine to prone and from midline to turn of the head by 90° positions, or *vice versa*). The alteration of cerebral blood flow following turn of the head was studied by Lawson et al. (1987) in preterm and term infants using ^{31}phosphorus nuclear magnetic resonance spectroscopy. The phosphocreatine/inorganic phosphate ratio did not change regardless of head-turning or supine vs. prone body position in both cohorts. Buckley et al. (2009) studied body/head elevation by 12° in 4 premature infants of 26 WGA and found no significant change in PSV, EDV, and diffuse correlation spectroscopy. They calculated a weak correlation (Pearson's r^2 = 0.13–0.58) of PSV/EDV and spectroscopy when performing body/head elevation. NIRS was used by Ancora et al. (2010) when studying 24 premature infants ≤32 WGA in six consecutive positions: supine/neutral head/bed 0°, supine/head-turning 90°/bed 0°, supine/head-turning 90°/bed + 30°, supine/neutral head/bed + 30°, prone/head minimally turned/bed + 30°, prone/head minimally turned/bed 0°. Changes in tissue hemoglobin/tissue oxygenation indices were not observed. Al-Abdi et al. (2011) assessed the incidence of IVH comparing preterm infants positioned supine with the head either in a neutral or turn of the head by 90° position and described a similar incidence (26% vs. 20%). Cerebral oxygen saturation was studied by Elser et al (Elser et al., 2012) in six different body positions involving supine/lateral/prone positions, body elevation by 15°, and turn of the head by 15–45° without any change in oxygenation (range 69–76%). Finally, Liao et al. (2015) assessed cerebral oxygen saturations in elevated supine position by 30° changing the head position several times from midline to the left/right 90° head-turning position. The range in average saturation (71–75%) was even closer as in the previous publication.

Fluctuations in the venous perfusion waveform of the GCV appear as a strong predictor of IVH in preterm infants. Ikeda et al. (2015) categorized four different GCV flow patterns in 80 VLBW infants that were repeatedly assessed over the first 6 days of life: grade 0: steady flow, constant perfusion speed; grade 1: fluctuating flow, minimum speed never less than half maximum speed; grade 2: fluctuating flow, minimum speed less than half maximum speed; grade 3: fluctuating flow, speed eventually dropping to 0 cm/s. They showed that higher grades mainly occur between days 2–4 of life which duplicates the postnatal time window of IVH occurrence; they gradually disappear beyond 4 days of life for reasons not clearly identified. Thus, the minor flow fluctuations in our recordings (grade 0 and 1 only) underline the low risk of IVH in our cohort of infants. Increased flow fluctuations in the GCV have been also described in growth retarded fetuses and are associated with an increased risk of perinatal morbidity, especially if combined with a reduction in cerebral vascular resistance and an overall increment in brain blood flow (Figueroa-Diesel et al., 2008).

The perception of head-turning related increase in intracranial pressure (ICP) and reduced cerebral perfusion by a hampered venous drainage was pursued as early as the 70th of the last century using techniques being replaced nowadays. Watson (1974) demonstrated in 1974 the complete obstruction of the ipsilateral internal jugular vein following turn of the head by 90° in anesthetized and non-anesthetized children using a contrast medium directly injected into the jugular vein. Goldberg et al. (1983) then were first to study position-related changes in ICP in preterm infants applying a Ladd monitor probe attached to the anterior fontanelle. They described a reduction [from 10.0 ± 1.2 (SEM) cm H_2O to 6.9 ± 1.2, ns] after switching the head from a right lateral to a midline position; this effect, however, was mildly augmented in a subgroup of infants starting with a higher baseline level ICP (i.e., ≥7 cm H_2O; from 11.9 ± 1.5 cm H_2O to 10.0 ± 1.6, $p < 0.01$). Using the same ICP measurement technique Emery and Peabody (1983) also observed an increase in ICP by head turning [from 13.8 ± 2.5 (SEM) cm H_2O to 17.2 ± 2.1, $p < 0.01$] along with unchanged PI (blood flow velocity parameters not provided), as was described by Urlesberger et al. (1991) in preterm infants with posthemorrhagic hydrocephalus following cancelation of head/body elevation to a horizontal position. It remains questionable whether position-related changes in ICP present a valid risk parameter for IVH as ICP depends on a manifold of factors such as cardiac output, blood pressure, cerebral perfusion, compliance of the infant skull, cerebrospinal fluid drainage, carbon dioxide level, state of vigilance, body position, stress, and gestational age (to name a few). An emerging topic is the vulnerability of the blood-brain barrier in the preterm infant following perinatal perfusion disturbances with the consequences of a delayed enwrapping of astrocytes in the germinal matrix and a reduced expression of platelet-derived growth factor beta as a key player in angiogenesis (Lai et al., 2017).

As a quality control, we compared our arterial blood flow velocity data with data from Forster et al. (2018) assessing term neonates within their first 3 days of life and found an overall consistency: ACA PSV 36.3 ± 6.6 cm/s (our data: 29.6 ± 6.2 at t0/36.8 ± 8.5 at t1); ACA EDV 12.4 ± 3.9 cm/s (9.3 ± 2.8 at t0/8.9 ± 3.3 at t1); RI 0.67 ± 0.06 (0.66 ± 0.09 at t0/0.68 ± 0.08 at t1). GCV data had to be compared to the data from Figueroa-Diesel et al. (2008) studying growth restricted fetuses: maximum flow 8.2 ± 5.5 cm/s (our data: sagittal 4.0 ± 0.8, coronal 4.1 ± 1.0 at t0). For the comparison of $cStO_2$ data Fuchs et al. (2011) demonstrated a rapid rise in regional cerebral oxygenation values in preterm infants, starting at values of 35% immediately after birth and peaking within 7–10 min at 75% (our data: 83 ± 7% at t0, 76 ± 10 at t1). The slightly lower data measured in term infants may occur due to a lower oxygen extraction in the brain, a different compartment of the arterial and the venous compartment, and the registration of more central parts of the brain in preterm infants (Almaazmi et al., 2013). In addition, different devices use different types of probes to be attached to the infant's forehead and use different algorithms for data computation. Lower $cStO_2$ values of the t1 recordings may also have occurred secondary to an improved oxygen delivery to the brain parenchyma and an increased systemic blood flow (cardiac output) typically seen in neonatal transition (Vrancken et al., 2018).

There are limitations to this study concerning the small number of study patients included, the high percentage of patients excluded because of incomplete data acquisition, and the small number of extremely low birth weight infants (i.e., birthweight <1000 g, 6/21 = 28%). Around 90% of the infants received antenatal steroids, a rate in line with international publications describing large cohorts (Stichtenoth et al., 2012; Schindler et al., 2017). Major IVH is clearly linked with low gestational age, birth asphyxia, and missed administration of prenatal steroids. Indeed, our cohort of infants does not represent this subgroup of infants at highest risk for IVH.

Taken together, our data demonstrate that the change from supine with the head in a midline position to prone with turn of the head by 90° position does not affect arterial or venous cerebral blood flow velocities or regional cerebral oxygenation in stable preterm infants $\leq$32 weeks gestational age on day 2 or day 9 of life. Cerebral blood flow and regional oxygenation are not correlated probably due to transitional hemodynamic changes, however, blood flow and regional oxygenation show strong maturational changes. Our data do not support the widespread clinical practice to nurse preterm infants in supine position with midline head position solely. Even though our findings must not be generalized for infants at high risk of IVH, a growing number of premature infants may profit by less invasive treatment protocols requiring changes in body and head position.

AUTHOR CONTRIBUTIONS

DS and EL performed all Doppler ultrasound examinations and supervised each other. EL collected the clinical data and performed the statistics. DS and MK designed the study. MK wrote the first draft of the manuscript. All authors approved the final manuscript.

REFERENCES

Al-Abdi, S. Y., Nojoom, M. S., Alshaalan, H. M., and Al-Aamri, M. A. (2011). Pilot-randomized study on intraventricular hemorrhage with midline versus lateral head positions. *Saudi Med. J.* 32, 420–421.

Almaazmi, M., Schmid, M. B., Havers, S., Reister, F., Lindner, W., Mayer, B., et al. (2013). Cerebral near-infrared spectroscopy during transition of healthy term newborns. *Neonatology* 103, 246–251. doi: 10.1159/000345926

Ancora, G., Maranella, E., Aceti, A., Pierantoni, L., Grandi, S., Corvaglia, L., et al. (2010). Effect of posture on brain hemodynamics in preterm newborns not mechanically ventilated. *Neonatology* 97, 212–217. doi: 10.1159/000253149

Anstrom, J. A., Thore, C. R., Moody, D. M., and Brown, W. R. (2007). Immunolocalization of tight junction proteins in blood vessels in human germinal matrix and cortex. *Histochem. Cell Biol.* 127, 205–213. doi: 10.1007/s00418-006-0232-z

Baburamani, A. A., Ek, C. J., Walker, D. W., and Castillo-Melendez, M. (2012). Vulnerability of the developing brain to hypoxic-ischemic damage: contribution of the cerebral vasculature to injury and repair? *Front. Physiol.* 3:424. doi: 10.3389/fphys.2012.00424

Ballabh, P., Hu, F., Kumarasiri, M., Braun, A., and Nedergaard, M. (2005). Development of tight junction molecules in blood vessels of germinal matrix, cerebral cortex, and white matter. *Pediatr. Res.* 58, 791–798. doi: 10.1203/01.PDR.0000180535.14093.FB

Bhat, R. Y., Hannam, S., Pressler, R., Rafferty, G. F., Peacock, J. L., and Greenough, A. (2006). Effect of prone and supine position on sleep, apneas, and arousal in preterm infants. *Pediatrics* 118, 101–107. doi: 10.1542/peds.2005-1873

Bhat, R. Y., Leipälä, J. A., Singh, N. R.-P., Rafferty, G. F., Hannam, S., and Greenough, A. (2003). Effect of posture on oxygenation, lung volume, and respiratory mechanics in premature infants studied before discharge. *Pediatrics* 112, 29–32. doi: 10.1542/peds.112.1.29

Buckley, E. M., Cook, N. M., Durduran, T., Kim, M. N., Zhou, C., Choe, R., et al. (2009). Cerebral hemodynamics in preterm infants during positional intervention measured with diffuse correlation spectroscopy and transcranial Doppler ultrasound. *Opt. Express* 17, 12571–12581. doi: 10.1364/OE.17.012571

Cioni, G., and Prechtl, H. F. (1990). Preterm and early postterm motor behaviour in low-risk premature infants. *Early Hum. Dev.* 23, 159–191. doi: 10.1016/0378-3782(90)90012-8

de Bijl-Marcus, K. A., Brouwer, A. J., de Vries, L. S., and van Wezel-Meijler, G. (2017). The effect of head positioning and head tilting on the incidence of hemorrhage in very preterm infants: a systematic review. *Neonatology* 111, 267–279. doi: 10.1159/000449240

Elser, H. E., Holditch-Davis, D., Levy, J., and Brandon, D. H. (2012). The effects of environmental noise and infant position on cerebral oxygenation. *Adv. Neonatal Care* 12, S18–S27. doi: 10.1097/ANC.0b013e31826853fe

Emery, J. R., and Peabody, J. L. (1983). Head position affects intracranial pressure in newborn infants. *J. Pediatr.* 103, 950–953. doi: 10.1016/S0022-3476(83)80728-8

Figueroa-Diesel, H., Hernandez-Andrade, E., Benavides-Serralde, A., Crispi, F., Acosta-Rojas, R., Cabero, L., et al. (2008). Cerebral venous blood flow in growth restricted fetuses with an abnormal blood flow in the umbilical artery before 32 weeks of gestation. *Eur. J. Obstet. Gynecol. Reprod. Biol.* 140, 201–205. doi: 10.1016/j.ejogrb.2008.04.006

Forster, D. E., Koumoundouros, E., Saxton, V., Fedai, G., and Holberton, J. (2018). Cerebral blood flow velocities and cerebrovascular resistance in normal-term neonates in the first 72 hours. *J. Paediatr. Child Health* 54, 61–68. doi: 10.1111/jpc.13663

Francois, M., Elmaleh, M., Garel, C., and Narcy, P. (1992). Dimensions of the pharynx in function of the posture in neonates and infants. *Arch. Fr. Pediatr.* 49, 23–26.

Fuchs, H., Lindner, W., Buschko, A., Trischberger, T., Schmid, M., and Hummler, H. D. (2011). Cerebral oxygenation in very low birth weight infants supported with sustained lung inflations after birth. *Pediatr. Res.* 70, 176–180. doi: 10.1203/PDR.0b013e318220c1e0

Goldberg, R. N., Joshi, A., Moscoso, P., and Castillo, T. (1983). The effect of head position on intracranial pressure in the neonate. *Crit. Care Med.* 11, 428–430. doi: 10.1097/00003246-198306000-00006

Heimann, K., Vaeßen, P., Peschgens, T., Stanzel, S., Wenzl, T. G., and Orlikowsky, T. (2010). Impact of skin to skin care, prone and supine positioning on cardiorespiratory parameters and thermoregulation in premature infants. *Neonatology* 97, 311–317. doi: 10.1159/000255163

Humberg, A., Härtel, C., Paul, P., Hanke, K., Bossung, V., Hartz, A., et al. (2017). Delivery mode and intraventricular hemorrhage risk in very-low-birth-weight infants: observational data of the german neonatal network. *Eur. J. Obstet. Gynecol. Reprod. Biol.* 212, 144–149. doi: 10.1016/j.ejogrb.2017.03.032

Ikeda, T., Amizuka, T., Ito, Y., Mikami, R., Matsuo, K., Kawamura, N., et al. (2015). Changes in the perfusion waveform of the internal cerebral vein and intraventricular hemorrhage in the acute management of extremely low-birth-weight infants. *Eur. J. Pediatr.* 174, 331–338. doi: 10.1007/s00431-014-2396-1

Inder, T. E., Perlman, J. M., and Volpe, J. J. (2018). "Preterm intraventricular hemorrhage / posthemorrhagic hydrocephalus," in *Volpe's Neurology of the Newborn*, ed. J. J. Volpe (Philadelphia, PA: Elsevier), 637–698.

Lai, J. C. Y., Rocha-Ferreira, E., Ek, C. J., Wang, X., Hagberg, H., and Mallard, C. (2017). Immune responses in perinatal brain injury. *Brain Behav. Immun.* 63, 210–223. doi: 10.1016/j.bbi.2016.10.022

Lawson, B., Anday, E., Guillet, R., Wagerle, L. C., Chance, B., and Delivoria-Papadopoulos, M. (1987). Brain oxidative phosphorylation following alteration in head position in preterm and term neonates. *Pediatr. Res.* 22, 302–305. doi: 10.1203/00006450-198709000-00013

Liao, S. M.-C., Rao, R., and Mathur, A. M. (2015). Head position change is not associated with acute changes in bilateral cerebral oxygenation in stable preterm infants during the first three days of life. *Am. J. Perinatol.* 32, 645–652. doi: 10.1055/s-0034-1390348

Pickens, D. L., Schefft, G. L., and Thach, B. T. (1989). Pharyngeal fluid clearence and aspiration preventive mechanisms in sleeping infants. *J. Appl. Physiol.* 66, 1164–1171. doi: 10.1152/jappl.1989.66.3.1164

Rao, V. T., Ludwin, S. K., Fuh, S. C., Sawaya, R., Moore, C. S., Ho, M. K., et al. (2016). MicroRNA expression patterns in human astrocytes in relation to anatomical location and age. *J. Neuropathol. Exp. Neurol.* 75, 156–166. doi: 10.1093/jnen/nlv016

Romantsik, O., Calevo, M. G., and Bruschettini, M. (2017). Head midline position for preventing the occurrence or extension of germinal matrix-intraventricular hemorrhage in preterm infants. *Cochrane Database Syst. Rev.* 7:CD012362. doi: 10.1002/14651858.CD012362

Schindler, T., Koller-Smith, L., Lui, K., Bajuk, B., Bolisetty, S., and New South Wales and Australia Capital Territory Neonatal Intensive Care Units's Data Collection (2017). Causes of death in very preterm infants cared for in neonatal intensive care units: a population-based retrospective cohort study. *BMC Pediatr.* 17:59. doi: 10.1186/s12887-017-0810-3

Sherlock, R. L., Anderson, P. J., Doyle, L. W., and Victorian Infant Collaborative Study Group (2005). Neurodevelopmental sequelae of intraventricular haemorrhage at 8 years of age in a regional cohort of ELBW/very preterm infants. *Early Hum. Dev.* 81, 909–916. doi: 10.1016/j.earlhumdev.2005.07.007

Skinner, J. (2000). "Ductal shunting," in *Echocardiography for the Neonatologist*, eds J. Skinner, D. Alverson, and S. Hunter (London: Churchill Livingstone), 151–170.

Stichtenoth, G., Demmert, M., Bohnhorst, B., Stein, A., Ehlers, S., Heitmann, F., et al. (2012). Major contributors to hospital mortality in very-low-birth-weight infants: data of the birth year 2010 cohort of the german neonatal network. *Klin. Padiatr.* 224, 276–281. doi: 10.1055/s-0032-1306344

Urlesberger, B., Müller, W., Ritschl, E., and Reiterer, F. (1991). The influence of head position on the intracranial pressure in preterm infants with posthemorrhagic hydrocephalus. *Child's Nerv. Syst.* 7, 85–87. doi: 10.1007/BF00247862

Vrancken, S. L., van Heijst, A. F., and de Boode, W. P. (2018). Neonatal hemodynamics: from developmental physiology to comprehensive monitoring. *Front. Pediatr.* 6:87. doi: 10.3389/fped.2018.00087

Waisman, D. (2006). Non-traumatic nasopharyngeal suction in premature newborn infants with upper airway obstruction from secretions following nasal CPAP. *J. Pediatr.* 149:279. doi: 10.1016/j.jpeds.2006.02.044

Watson, G. H. (1974). Effect of head rotation on jugular vein blood flow. *Arch. Dis. Child.* 49, 237–239. doi: 10.1136/adc.49.3.237

Zubrow, A. B., Hulman, S., Kushner, H., and Falkner, B. (1995). Determinants of blood pressure in infants admitted to neonatal intensive care units: a prospective multicenter study. Philadelphia neonatal blood pressure study group. *J. Perinatol.* 15, 470–479.

3

Ketamine Reduces Inflammation Pathways in the Hypothalamus and Hippocampus Following Transient Hypoxia in the Late-Gestation Fetal Sheep

Eileen I. Chang[1], *Miguel A. Zarate*[1], *Thomas J. Arndt*[1], *Elaine M. Richards*[2], *Maria B. Rabaglino*[3], *Maureen Keller-Wood*[2] *and Charles E. Wood*[1]*

[1] Department of Physiology and Functional Genomics, University of Florida College of Medicine, Gainesville, FL, United States, [2] Department of Pharmacodynamics, University of Florida College of Pharmacy, Gainesville, FL, United States, [3] CEPROCOR, National Scientific and Technical Research Council (CONICET), Córdoba, Argentina

***Correspondence:**
Charles E. Wood
woodc@ufl.edu

The physiological response to hypoxia in the fetus has been extensively studied with regard to redistribution of fetal combined ventricular output and sparing of oxygen delivery to fetal brain and heart. Previously, we have shown that the fetal brain is capable of mounting changes in gene expression that are consistent with tissue inflammation. The present study was designed to use transcriptomics and systems biology modeling to test the hypothesis that ketamine reduces or prevents the upregulation of inflammation-related pathways in hypothalamus and hippocampus after transient hypoxic hypoxia. Chronically catheterized fetal sheep (122 $\pm$ 5 days gestation) were subjected to 30 min hypoxia (relative reduction in $P_aO_2 \sim 50\%$) caused by infusion of nitrogen into the inspired gas of the pregnant ewe. RNA was isolated from fetal hypothalamus and hippocampus collected 24 h after hypoxia, and was analyzed for gene expression using the Agilent 15.5 k ovine microarray. Ketamine, injected 10 min prior to hypoxia, reduced the cerebral immune response activation to the hypoxia in both brain regions. Genes both upregulated by hypoxia and downregulated by ketamine after hypoxia were significantly associated with gene ontology terms and KEGG pathways that are, themselves, associated with the tissue response to exposure to bacteria. We conclude that the results are consistent with interruption of the cellular response to bacteria by ketamine.

Keywords: fetal hypoxia, ketamine, fetal brain, inflammation, transcriptomics

Abbreviations: CASP8, caspase8; CD14, CD14 molecule; CXCL10, chemokine (C-X-C motif) ligand 10; ERK, extracellular signal-regulated kinase; HC, hypoxic control; HK, hypoxia + ketamine; IL1β, interleukin 1 beta; JAK/STAT, janus kinase/signal transducers and activators of transcription; KEGG, Kyoto Encyclopedia of Genes and Genomes; LPS, lipopolysaccharides; MAPK, mitogen-activated protein kinases; MYD88, myeloid differentiation primary response 88; NC, normoxic control; NFκB, nuclear factor kappa-light-chain-enhancer of activated B cells; NK, normoxia + ketamine; NMDA, *N*-Methyl-D-aspartate; PTGS2, prostaglandin-endoperoxide synthase 2; TLR, toll-like receptor; TNFα, tumor necrosis factor-alpha.

INTRODUCTION

Transient fetal hypoxia is a common homeostatic disturbance during fetal life. Any compromise of maternal oxygen supply, for example, high altitude or maternal hypoventilation secondary to any cause, decreases partial pressure of oxygen in the fetal blood (Assali et al., 1962; Makowski et al., 1968). Physiologists commonly view the fetal response to hypoxia through the lens of homeostatic cardiovascular responses that spare brain and heart viability (Dawes et al., 1969; Cohn et al., 1974). Cardiovascular and neuroendocrine reflex responses to hypoxia redirect blood flow such that a larger proportion of the combined ventricular output flows toward the brain, heart, and adrenal glands (Cohn et al., 1974).

We have recently reported that 30 min of transient hypoxia of the mother and fetus (caused by reducing the oxygen content of the mother's inspired gas) results in increased abundance of live bacteria in the fetal brain 24 h after the hypoxic episode (Zarate et al., 2017). Whole genome sequencing of bacteria recovered from the fetal cerebral cortex revealed that the bacteria isolated from the fetal brain were identical to those isolated from the placenta (Zarate et al., 2017). This suggested a route of transfer from placenta to fetal brain with hypoxia. Concomitant with appearance of bacteria in fetal brain is upregulation of molecular pathways that subserve inflammation (Chang et al., 2016a; Zarate et al., 2017). As we have previously reported, the pattern of activation of genes within inflammation-related pathways is consistent with the response to bacterial entry into the fetal brain after hypoxia (Zarate et al., 2017).

We have previously reported that ketamine, an FDA-approved agent used in Neonatal Intensive Care Units (Anand, 2007), attenuated the activation of inflammation-related pathways in fetal cerebral cortex and kidney (Chang et al., 2016a,b). Since the discovery of hypoxia-induced bacterial invasion of the fetus, we have concluded that the increase in abundance of bacteria was causative of the increased inflammation-like response in the fetal brain (Zarate et al., 2017). The mechanism of the effect of ketamine – originally hypothesized to reduce inflammation by blockade of NMDA-mediated glutamate signaling – was therefore unclear (Powers and Wood, 2007; Knutson and Wood, 2010). In this report we test the hypothesis that the effect of ketamine will be reflected by changes in inflammation-related genes in the hypothalamus and hippocampus. Furthermore, we test the hypothesis that ketamine reduces the influx of bacteria into the fetal brain, thereby blocking the stimulus to inflammation. We have reported, from these experiments, upregulated inflammation pathways in cerebral cortex, hypothalamus and hippocampus, as well as kidney cortex in response to hypoxic hypoxia. We have also reported the transfer of bacteria into the brains of these fetuses. This report specifically addresses the effect of ketamine on the inflammation response in hypothalamus and hippocampus, and addresses the question of whether ketamine reduces or prevents the appearance of bacteria in these brain regions.

MATERIALS AND METHODS

Ethics Statement

All experiments were approved by the University of Florida Animal Care and Use Committee and were performed in accordance with the Guiding Principles for Use of Animals of the American Physiological Society.

Fetal Ovine Surgery

The surgical procedures for fetal and maternal chronic femoral arterial and venous catheterizations were described previously (Chang and Wood, 2015; Chang et al., 2016b). Briefly, ewes were fasted 24 h before surgery, and received 750 mg ampicillin (Polyflex®, Boehringer Ingelheim VetMedica, Inc., St. Joseph, MO, United States) before the induction of anesthesia with 0.5–2% isoflurane with oxygen and intubation. The fetal hindlimbs were catheterized with a set of femoral arterial, venous, and amniotic catheters. Ampicillin (500 mg) was injected into the amniotic fluid before the uterus was sutured closed. The ewe also received a set of femoral arterial and venous vascular catheters. In addition, a non-occlusive catheter was implanted in the maternal trachea for the infusion of nitrogen gas as previously described

TABLE 1 | Primers and probes used for qPCR analysis (all sequences 5′–3′).

Gene	Forward primer	Reverse primer	Probe
ACTB	TTCCTTCCTGGG CATGGA	GACGTCACACTT CATGATGGAATT	TCCTGCGGCA TTCACGAAACT ACCTT
CASP8	TGGCTGCCCTCA AGTTCCT	GGAATAGCATCA AGGCATCCTT	SYBR Green
CD14	CCTAAAGGAC TGCCGACCAA	GCGGCTCCCTG CTTAGCT	SYBR Green
CRH	TCCCATTTC CCTGGATCTCA	GAGCTTGCTGCG CTAACTGA	TTCCACCTCCT CCGAGAAGTCTT GGAAAT
CXCL10	TTGAACTGATTC CTGCAAGTCA	TTCCTTTTCATT GTGGCAATAATCT	SYBR Green
IL1B	CGTGGCCAT GGAGAAGCT	GGTCATCATCACG GAAGACATGT	SYBR Green
MYD88	GCCTGAGTATTT TGATGCCTTCA	GCTGCCGGATC ATCTCATG	SYBR Green
NFKB1	TCCCACAGATGT TCACAAACAGT	GACGCTCAATCTT CATCTTGTGAT	SYBR Green
NFKBIA	CTACACCTTGCC TGTGAGCA	AGACACGTGTGG CCATTGTA	SYBR Green
OAS1	GAGGAAAGAGG GCGAGTTCT	GGATGAGGCTCT TCAGCTTG	SYBR Green
PTGS2	GCACAAATCTGA TGTTTGCATTCT	CTGGTCCTCGTT CATATCTGCTT	TGCCCAGCACTT CACCCATCAATTTT
PTX3	GCACCTGGGATT CAAAGAAA	TGTTTCATCAAA GCCACCAA	SYBR Green
TLR2	GATTCTGCTGGA GCCCATTG	TCATGATCTTCCG CAGCTTACA	SYBR Green
TLR4	ACTCGCTCCGG ATCCTAGACT	CCTTGGCAAATT CCGTAGTTCT	SYBR Green
TNF	CCCTTCCACCCC CTTGTT	ATGTTGACCTTG GTCTGGTAGGA	SYBR Green

(Chang and Wood, 2015). Post-operative care was provided to the ewe for a minimum of 5 days, including prophylactic administration of ampicillin (15–20 mg/kg, IM, bid), wound care, and monitoring of rectal temperature, food consumption and signs of infection or distress.

In vivo Transient Hypoxia

Studies were performed on chronically catheterized singleton (n = 1) and twin (n = 15) ovine fetuses at gestational age 122 ± 5 days (full term = 145–147 days), while the ewes were conscious and freestanding in their pens with access to food. Each pregnancy was randomly assigned to the experimental protocol of normoxia or hypoxia, therefore producing the four groups: normoxia control (NC), normoxia+ketamine (NK), HC, and hypoxia+ketamine (HK). For groups treated with ketamine, the fetuses received 3 mg/kg of ketamine intravenously through the femoral venous catheter 10 min prior to normoxic or hypoxic stimuli (30 min). Transient hypoxia was produced by infusing nitrogen gas into the maternal tracheostomy tube, resulting in a 50% decrease in arterial partial pressures of oxygen (P_aO_2) for both the ewe and the fetus. Changes in blood gas compositions (ABL80 Radiometer, Copenhagen, Denmark) were closely monitored by anaerobically drawing arterial blood (1 mL) at regular intervals. Fetal physiological responses (hemodynamics, blood gasses, and neuroendocrine values) to hypoxia, ketamine, and the combination of hypoxia and ketamine have been reported previously (Chang and Wood, 2015). Fetuses were euthanized 24 h post initial stimulation of normoxia or

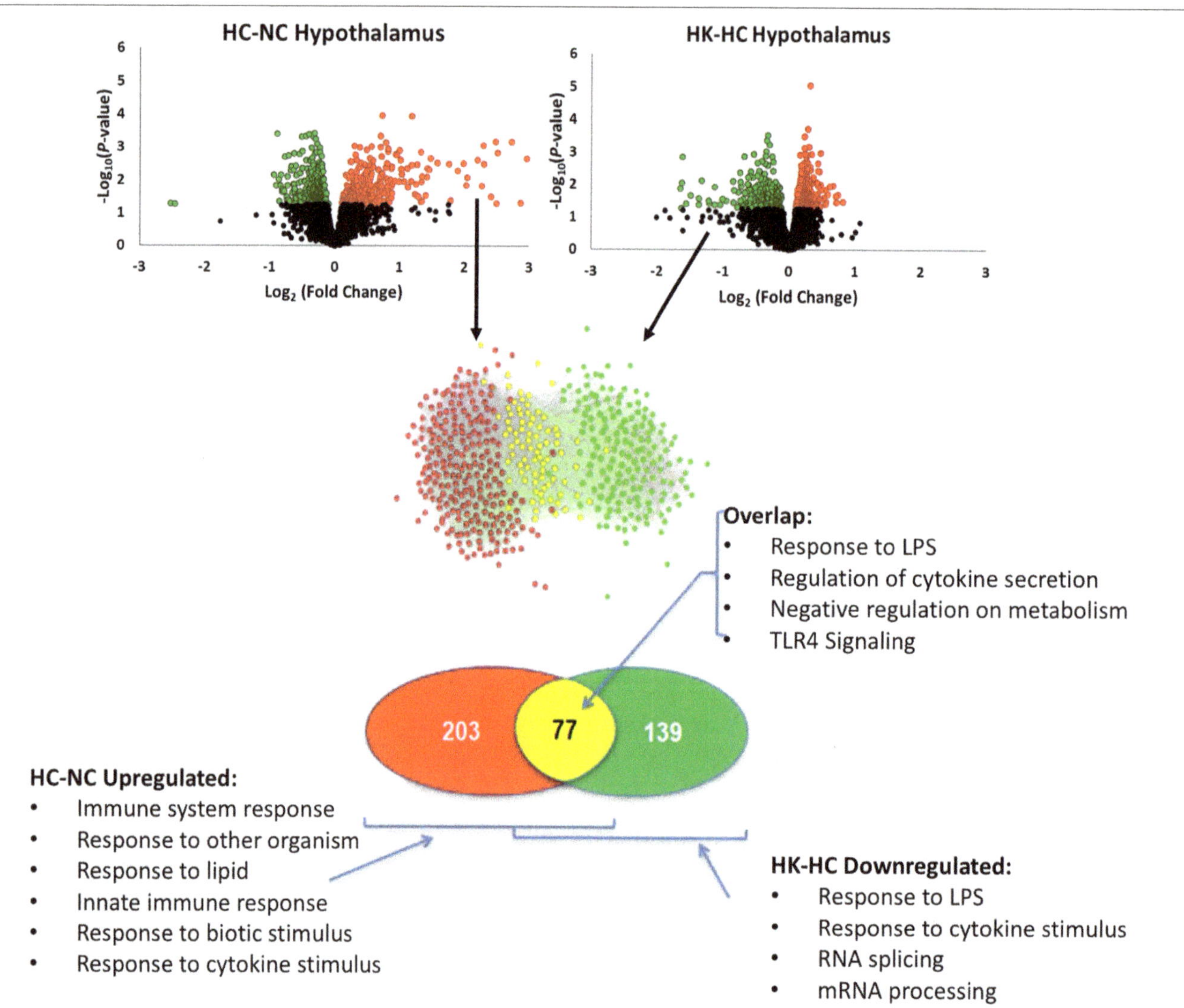

FIGURE 1 | As shown in top panels, analysis of gene expression using Agilent ovine 15.5 k array revealed significant up- and down-regulation of gene expression by hypoxia compared to normoxia [HC-NC, previously reported (Zarate et al., 2017)], as well as significant up- and down-regulation of gene expression in hypoxic animals by ketamine (HK-HC). Network inference and statistical modeling of gene ontology terms revealed that hypoxia upregulated pathways related to inflammation, and that ketamine was effective at decreasing the gene expression in those pathways in the hypoxic animals. Transcriptomic modeling indicated a high likelihood of the entire inflammation pathway from TLR2 and TLR4 being involved in the response. HC-NC plots were previously published under a Creative Commons Attribution 4.0 International License in Zarate et al. (2017).

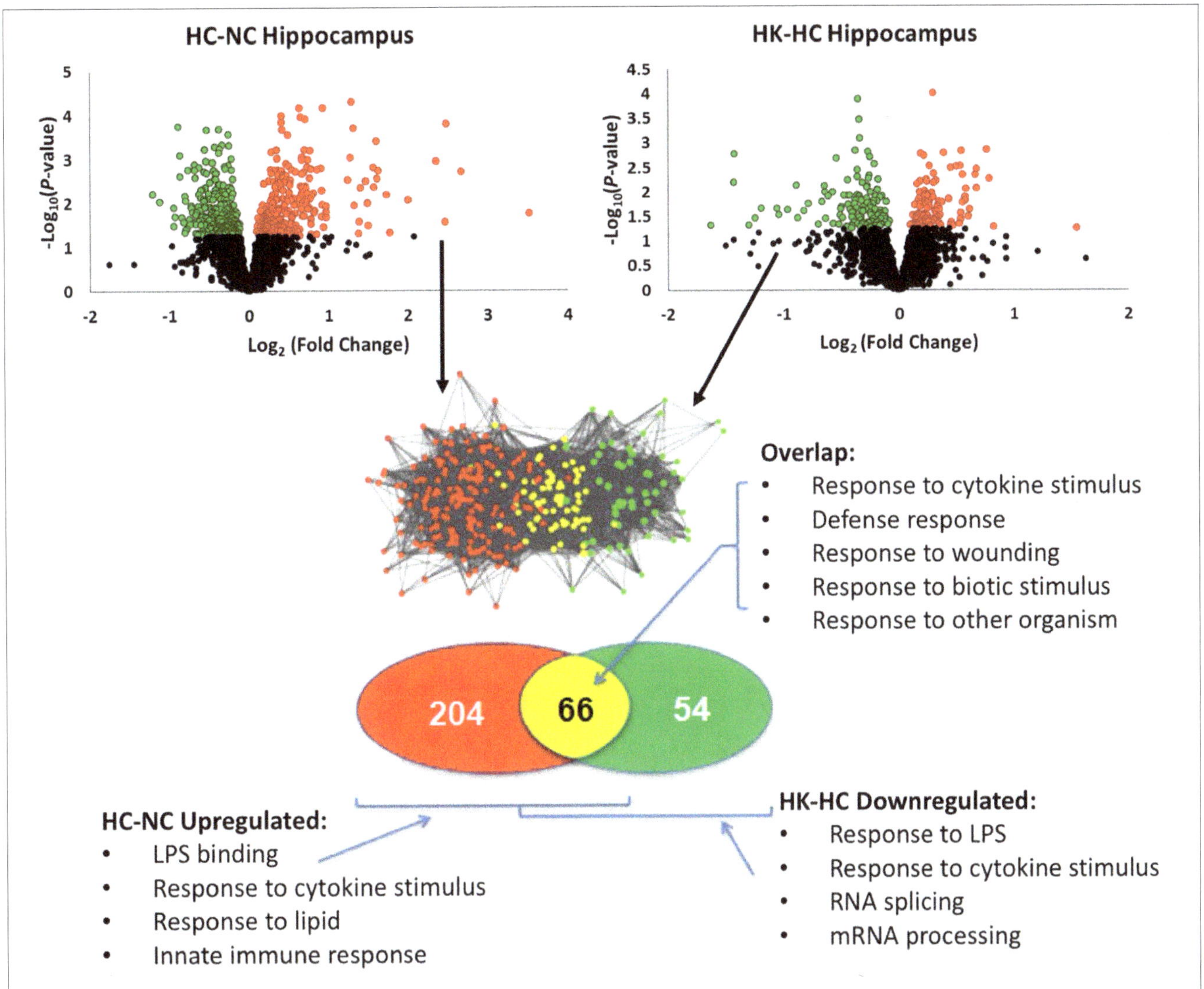

FIGURE 2 | Top panels, significant up- and down-regulation of gene expression in hippocampus by hypoxia compared to normoxia [HC-NC, previously reported (Zarate et al., 2017)], as well as significant up- and down-regulation of gene expression in hypoxic animals by ketamine (HK-HC). Network inference and statistical modeling of gene ontology terms were as described in legend to **Figure 1**. HC-NC plots were previously published under a Creative Commons Attribution 4.0 International License in Zarate et al. (2017).

transient hypoxia. The fetal brain was hemisected, with one half reserved for fixation and histological analysis and with the other half dissected for molecular analysis. Hypothalamus was removed as a single block of tissue, bounded on the rostral edge by the rostral edge of the optic chiasm, on the caudal side by the caudal edge of the median eminence, and on the side by the edges of the median eminence (Gersting et al., 2009). Hippocampus was dissected as the entire hippocampus (Gersting et al., 2009). Medulla oblongata was defined as the area between the obex and the caudal medulla-rostral spinal cord border (Gersting et al., 2009).

Microarray Procedures

Total mRNA was extracted from snap frozen fetal hypothalamus tissues using Trizol extraction followed by RNeasy Plus Mini Kit (Qiagen, Valencia, CA, United States), with on-column DNase digestion. RNA integrity number (RIN) values ranged between 8.0 and 9.0, RNA was labeled with cyanine 3 CTP with the Quick Amp Labeling Kit (Cat# 5190-0442, Agilent Technologies, Santa Clara, CA, United States), according to the manufacturer's protocol. The specific activities of the labeled cRNAs ranged from 11.6 to 15.2 pmol Cy3/μg RNA and yielded 8.9 to 10.96 μg. The cRNA samples were hybridized and processed for one-channel Sheep Gene Expression Microarray (8 × 15 K slide) – 8 arrays with 15208 oligomers each (Cat# G4813A-019921, Agilent Technologies, Santa Clara, CA, United States) as described (Rabaglino et al., 2014). The slides were scanned with Microarray Scanner System (G2505-90021, Agilent) and the measured fluorescence was detected and converted using Agilent Feature Extraction 9.1 software at the Genomics Division of the University of Florida's Interdisciplinary Center for Biotechnology Research. All microarray data have been uploaded to the Gene

TABLE 2 | Top 10 gene ontology biological processes and enriched KEGG pathways associated with genes that were significantly up regulated in the hypothalamus during acute hypoxic stress, but were down regulated with ketamine.

Analysis	Pathways, processes, functions, components	# Genes involved	Adjusted *P*-values
Biological Process	Defense response	30	1.93E-11
	Response to stress	45	2.09E-10
	Immune response	26	7.72E-09
	Immune system process	33	7.72E-09
	Regulation of defense response	16	1.67E-07
	Response to lipopolysaccharide	12	2.05E-07
	Response to other organism	18	2.05E-07
	Response to wounding	24	2.30E-07
	Innate immune response	17	2.85E-07
	Response to molecule of bacterial origin	12	2.85E-07
KEGG Pathways	MAPK signaling pathway	9	1.05E-07
	Osteoclast differentiation	7	1.17E-07
	Cytokine-cytokine receptor interaction	8	6.45E-07
	Hematopoietic cell lineage	5	8.36E-06
	Toll-like receptor signaling pathway	5	1.28E-05
	Chemokine signaling pathway	6	1.28E-05
	Pathways in cancer	7	1.94E-05
	Toxoplasmosis	5	2.96E-05
	Hepatitis C	5	3.96E-05
	Adipokine signaling pathway	4	4.60E-05

TABLE 3 | Top 10 gene ontology biological processes and enriched KEGG pathways associated with genes that were significantly up regulated in the hippocampus during acute hypoxic stress, but were down regulated with ketamine.

Analysis	Pathways, processes, functions, components	# Genes involved	Adjusted *P*-values
Biological Process	Response to lipid	18	4.49E-08
	Response to cytokine stimulus	15	1.49E-06
	Response to organic substance	27	1.49E-06
	Response to biotic stimulus	16	1.53E-06
	Response to chemical stimulus	33	1.53E-06
	Response to other organism	15	4.53E-06
	Response to lipopolysaccharide	10	4.53E-06
	Response to molecule of bacterial origin	10	6.95E-06
	Response to external stimulus	21	1.54E-05
	Response to stress	32	1.61E-05
KEGG Pathways	Cytokine-cytokine receptor interaction	7	8.15E-06
	Malaria	4	2.32E-05
	Toll-like receptor signaling pathway	4	2.00E-04
	MAPK signaling pathway	5	6.00E-04
	Adipocytokine signaling pathway	3	1.20E-03
	Chemokine signaling pathway	4	1.50E-03
	Amoebiasis	3	3.10E-03
	Osteoclast differentiation	3	4.60E-03
	African trypanosomiasis	2	5.20E-03
	Jak-STAT signaling pathway	3	6.50E-03

Expression Omnibus of the National Center for Biotechnology Information (accession numbers GSE82016 and GSE97916). We performed array analyses in the hippocampus and the hypothalamus for the following groups: NC (n = 3), NK (n = 4), HC (n = 5), and HK (n = 4).

Network Inference and Analysis, and Functional Annotation of Gene Ontology

Gene networks were inferred using the GeneMania (Montojo et al., 2010) plugin of Cytoscape (Shannon et al., 2003). The functional annotation of gene ontology for groups or networks of genes was analyzed using WEB-based GEne SeT AnaLysis Toolkit (WebGestalt) (Zhang et al., 2005; Wang et al., 2013).

Immunohistochemistry

Fetal brain tissues (n = 4 per group) were fixed in 4% buffered paraformaldehyde overnight, and stored in 70% reagent alcohol until embedded in paraffin wax. All tissue samples were sectioned with a microtome (5 μm) and counterstained with methyl green. To identify the presence of microglia or macrophages, the hypothalamus, hippocampus, and medulla were stained for Iba-1 (ionized calcium binding adaptor protein-1) antibody (Cat.# 019-19741, Waco Pure Chemical Industries, Richmond, VA, United States; 1:500 dilution) and peroxidase-PAP sandwich technique (Vectastain, Vector Labs, Burlingame, CA, United States). For each animal, five (hypothalamus and medulla) and ten (hippocampus) images (40× magnification) were randomly selected for quantification. Vascular integrity was assessed using immunostaining of ovine albumin (anti-Sheep Serum Albumin Polyclonal Antibody MBS715170, MyBiosource Inc., San Diego, CA, United States, dilution 1:200) with peroxidase-PAP sandwich visualization. The number of broken and leaky blood vessels were counted using seven (hypothalamus), ten (cerebral cortex), and five (medulla) random images (10× magnification) per animal. All microscopic quantification was done using a blinded protocol.

Real-Time PCR (qPCR)

The same set of mRNA used for the microarray was also used for qPCR validations. The primers were designed based on the known *Ovis aries* and *Bos taurus* genomes (**Table 1**) for SYBR green or TaqMan chemistry. Chemistries used for this analysis were Applied Biosystems Fast SYBR Green master mix, and Taqman Fast Advanced master mix (Cat. # 4385612, 4444558, respectively; Thermo-Fisher Scientific, Waltham, MA, United States). The ovine β-actin primers and probe were used as the house keeping gene control, as described previously (Chang et al., 2016b). Bacterial 16S rRNA was measured using universal 16S primers as described by Nadkarni and coworkers (Nadkarni et al., 2002). For each sample, the relative mRNA

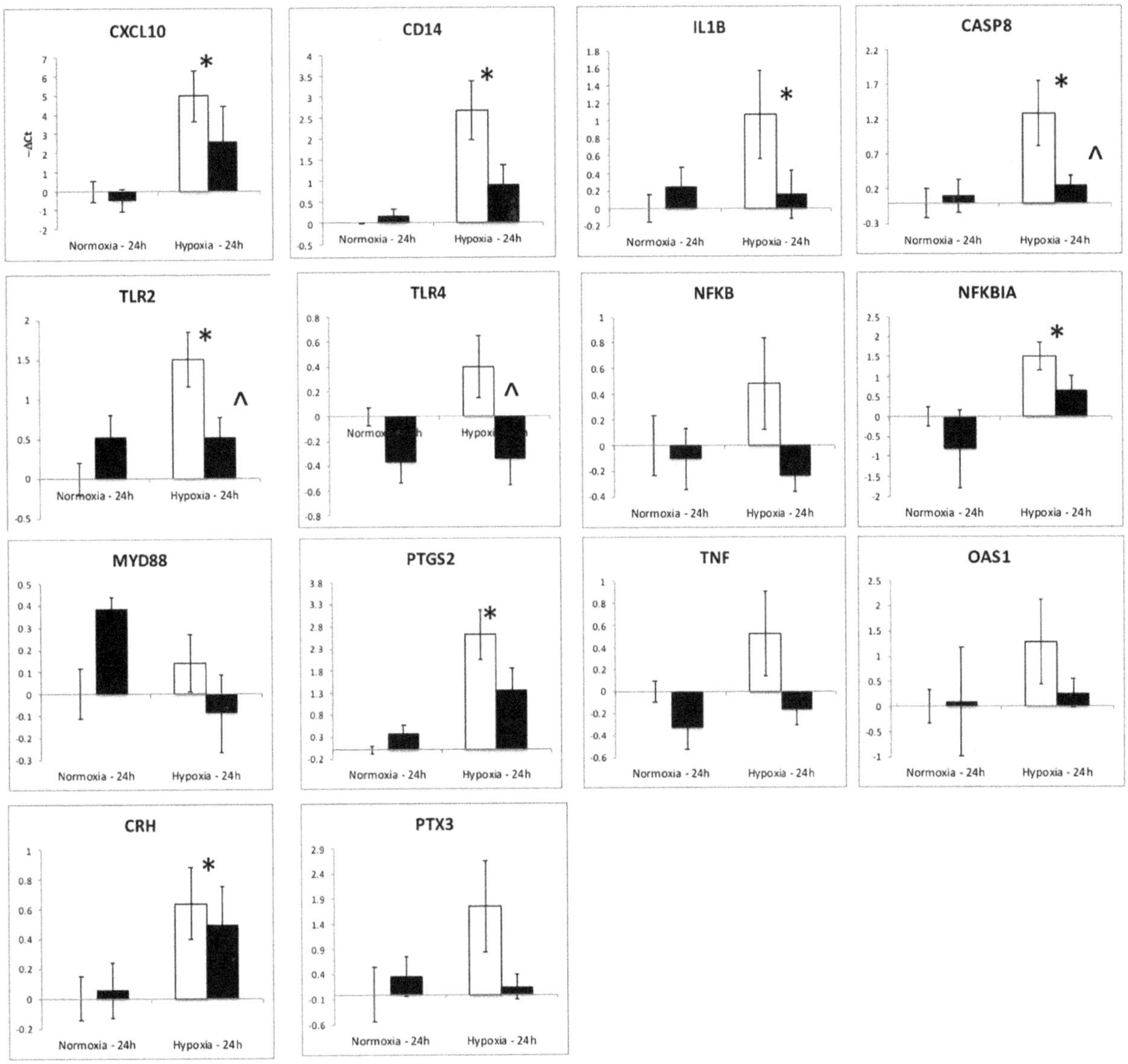

FIGURE 3 | Gene expression (mRNA abundance) in fetal hypothalamus measured by real-time qPCR for genes in the toll-like receptor inflammation pathway. Values are represented as negative delta cycle threshold ($-\Delta C_t$) compared to the NC group. Open bars represent experiments in which ketamine was not administered. Filled bars represent experiments in which ketamine was administered before normoxia or hypoxia. The criterion for statistical significance was $P < 0.05$ (Student's *t*-test). Data are presented as means ± SEM, and the y-axis scale varies between plots. *Statistically significant difference of hypoxia group compared to normoxia control. ^Statistically significant difference of hypoxia control group compared to hypoxia + ketamine group.

expression was calculated by the difference in threshold cycle (ΔC_t) between the triplicate mean C_t for each gene and for β-actin.

Statistics

As previously described, statistical analysis for Agilent 15.5 k array was performed with Bioconductor's Limma package for R software v.2.15.1, which utilized moderated *t*-test and empirical Bayes method for small sample size per group ($p < 0.05$) (Chang et al., 2016b). The qPCR data were analyzed by Student's *t*-test (Zar, 1984). Two-way nested ANOVA design was applied for immunohistochemistry data analysis, using the Genmod Procedure of SAS/STAT® 9.3 (SAS Institute Inc., Cary, NC, United States). Data are presented as mean values ± standard error of the mean (SEM), and the criterion for statistical significance was $p < 0.05$.

RESULTS

The blood gas and cardiovascular responses to hypoxia and normoxia, and the effect of ketamine on these variables in a larger cohort of experiments have been previously reported (Chang and Wood, 2015).

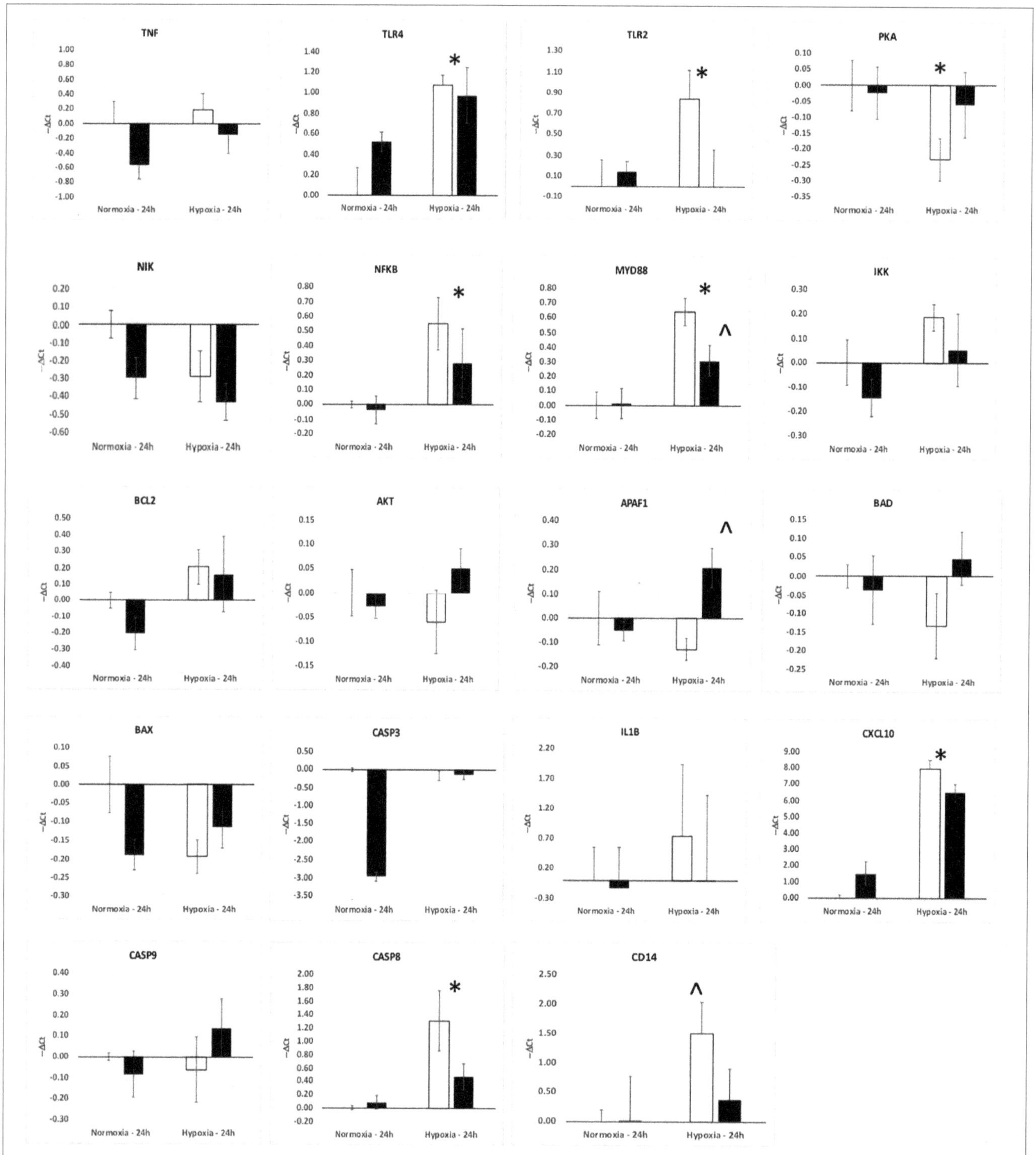

FIGURE 4 | Gene expression (mRNA abundance) in fetal hippocampus measured by real-time qPCR for genes in the toll-like receptor inflammation pathway. Values are represented as negative delta cycle threshold ($-\Delta C_t$) compared to the NC group. Open bars represent experiments in which ketamine was administered before normoxia or hypoxia. The criterion for statistical significance was $P < 0.05$ (Student's *t*-test). Data are presented as means ± SEM, and the y-axis scale varies between plots. *Statistically significant difference of hypoxia group compared to normoxia control. ∧Statistically significant difference of hypoxia control group compared to hypoxia + ketamine group.

Twenty-four hours after the onset of a 30 min period of hypoxia, 280 genes were upregulated and 357 genes were downregulated in hypothalamus compared to fetuses subjected to normoxia alone. In hippocampus, 270 genes were upregulated

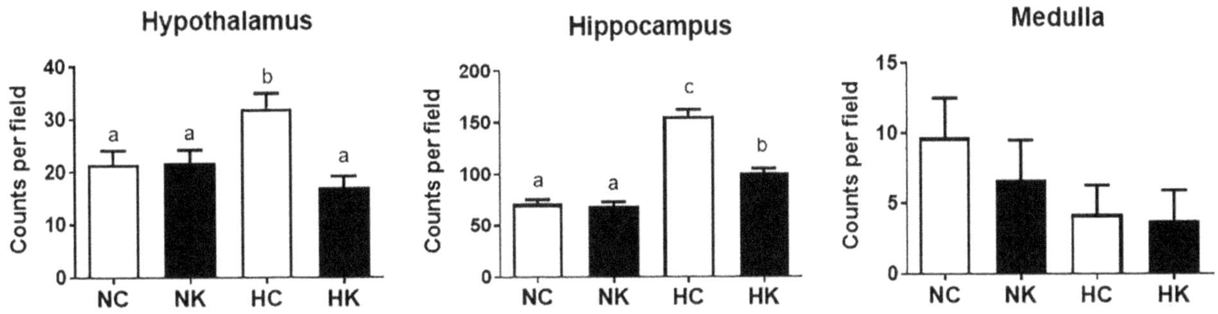

FIGURE 5 | Ketamine reduces the number of microglia and macrophages in the hypothalamus and hippocampus 24 h after transient hypoxia. For each brain region, the Iba-1 positive cells counted per 40X field (average of 7 fields analyzed for each animal) were averaged from 4 animals per group. Data from hippocampus are average measurements from regions CA1, CA2, CA3, CA4, and Dentate Gyrus. Data are expressed as mean ± SEM. Different letters indicate statistically significant difference ($P < 0.05$). NC, normoxia control; NK, normoxia + ketamine; HC, hypoxia control; HK, hypoxia + ketamine.

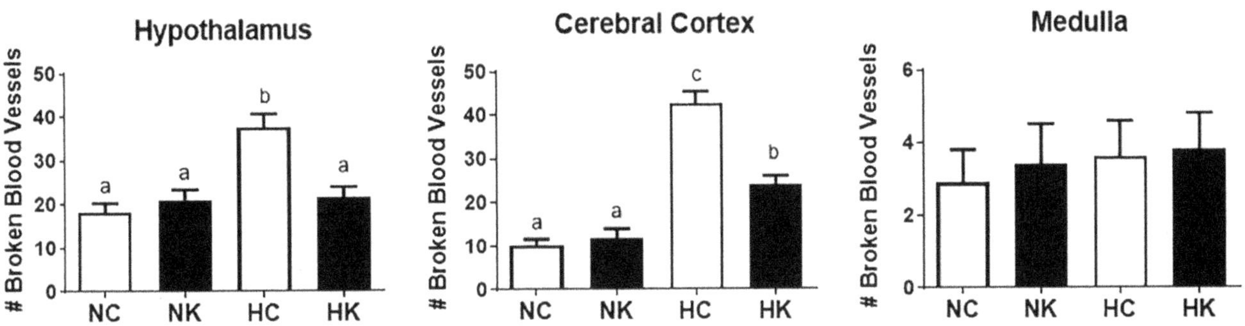

FIGURE 6 | Ketamine reduces the number of broken or leaky blood vessels in the fetal hypothalamus and cerebral cortex 24 h after transient hypoxia. Number of broken blood vessels were counted in 10X field images and averaged for each animal per brain region: hypothalamus, cerebral cortex, and medulla. Data are expressed as means ± SEM ($n = 4$/group). Different letters indicate statistically significant difference ($P < 0.05$). NC, normoxia control; NK, normoxia + ketamine; HC, hypoxia control; HK, hypoxia + ketamine.

and 240 were downregulated. We have previously reported these changes in gene expression as well as statistically significant over-represented gene ontology terms and KEGG pathways activation for these differentially regulated genes elsewhere (Zarate et al., 2017). Inflammation- and infection-related pathways were significantly upregulated in both brain regions (Zarate et al., 2017).

Ketamine alone (in normoxic fetuses) upregulated 15 genes and downregulated 21 genes in hypothalamus and upregulated 22 and downregulated 29 genes in hippocampus. Gene ontology analysis of the upregulated genes revealed significant association with extracellular matrix binding and collagen binding in hypothalamus, but the downregulated genes did not reveal any significant biological processes in hypothalamus. In the hippocampus, there was no significant biological processes revealed by gene ontology analysis that were associated with either the upregulated or the downregulated genes.

Ketamine had a substantial effect on the transcriptomic response to hypoxia. In hypothalamus, ketamine decreased the expression of 293 genes in and increased the expression of 238 genes in the fetuses subjected to hypoxia (**Figure 1**). In hippocampus, ketamine upregulated 125 and downregulated 130 genes when compared to hypoxia alone (**Figure 2**).

Comparison of the genes upregulated by hypoxia but downregulated by ketamine after hypoxia, allows identification of those pathways that are activated by hypoxia but whose activation is reversed by ketamine pretreatment. This analysis in hypothalamus revealed 77 genes with this pattern (**Figure 1**). Gene ontology analysis revealed that these genes were significantly associated with immune response, cellular response to lipopolysaccharide, response to other organism, innate immune response, and response to molecule of bacterial origin (**Table 2**). KEGG pathways significantly associated with these genes include MAPK signaling pathway, cytokine-cytokine receptor interaction, hematopoietic cell lineage, chemokine signaling, and TLR signaling pathway (**Table 2**).

The same analysis strategy in hippocampus revealed 66 genes that were upregulated by hypoxia but downregulated by ketamine (**Figure 2**). Significantly associated biological process terms of these genes included response to cytokine stimulus, response to lipopolysaccharide, response to molecule of bacterial origin, response to external stimulus, and response to stress (**Table 3**). KEGG pathways significantly overrepresented in this gene set were cytokine-cytokine receptor interaction, TLR signaling pathway, MAPK signaling pathway, adipocytokine signaling pathway, chemokine signaling pathway, osteoclast differentiation, and JAK/STAT signaling pathway (**Table 3**).

There were 57 genes in hypothalamus and 31 in hippocampus that were downregulated by hypoxia but increased in the fetuses subjected to hypoxia and ketamine. In both brain regions, these genes were not significantly associated with gene ontology terms. KEGG analysis of the hypothalamic genes revealed a significant association with metabolic pathways, vitamin digestion and absorption, fructose/mannose metabolism, endocytosis, and spliceosome, while a similar analysis in hippocampus did not yield any significantly associated KEGG pathways.

The upregulation of inflammation-related genes (MYD88, NFKB, etc.) and the subsequent modeling of the transcriptome led us to further explore the relationship between hypoxia and inflammation, and the modification of this relationship by ketamine at both the RNA and histological levels. We chose to probe, at the mRNA expression level, the TLR pathway and the apoptosis pathway. Hypoxia increased the abundance of mRNA for multiple inflammation-related genes in hypothalamus (**Figure 3**) and hippocampus (**Figure 4**), including TLR2, CD14, NFKBIA, IL1B, CXCL10, PTGS2, and CASP8 (previously reported in Zarate et al., 2017). Ketamine reduced the CD14, TLR2, TLR4, MYD88, NFKB, and CASP8 mRNA abundance in one or both of these brain regions compared to fetuses that were subjected to hypoxia but not to ketamine treatment (**Figures 3, 4**).

The gene ontology analysis and the qPCR analysis indicated that a major component of the response 24 h after hypoxia is inflammation, and more specifically genes related to the toll-like receptor (TLR2 and TLR4) inflammation pathway. We have reported, previously, that hypoxia increases microglia/macrophage abundance in cerebral cortex (Chang et al., 2016a), renal cortex (Chang et al., 2016b), and in hypothalamus and hippocampus (Zarate et al., 2017). We have also previously reported that anti-inflammatory actions of ketamine pretreatment were accompanied by reductions in microglia/macrophages in both fetal cerebral (Chang et al., 2016a) and renal (Chang et al., 2016b) cortex. In this report, we extend this effect of ketamine to hypothalamus and hippocampus (**Figure 5**).

We have previously demonstrated that hypoxia resulted in an increase in the abundance of bacterial 16S rRNA gene expression and vascular permeability in fetal cerebral cortex, hypothalamus, and hippocampus (Zarate et al., 2017). Ketamine significantly reduced the effect of hypoxia on vascular integrity in hypothalamus and cerebral cortex (**Figure 6**) and decreased the macrophage/microglia infiltration of hypothalamus and hippocampus (**Figure 5**). Likewise, ventilatory hypoxic hypoxia produced an increase in bacterial load though an upregulation of 16S gene; however, ketamine did not significantly reduce or block the hypoxia-induced increase in qPCR-detectable 16S bacterial rRNA (**Figure 7**). While not specifically the topic of this analysis, medulla was analyzed for Iba-1 and albumin immunostaining: neither hypoxia nor ketamine had any effect on either of these measured variables in medulla (**Figures 5, 6**).

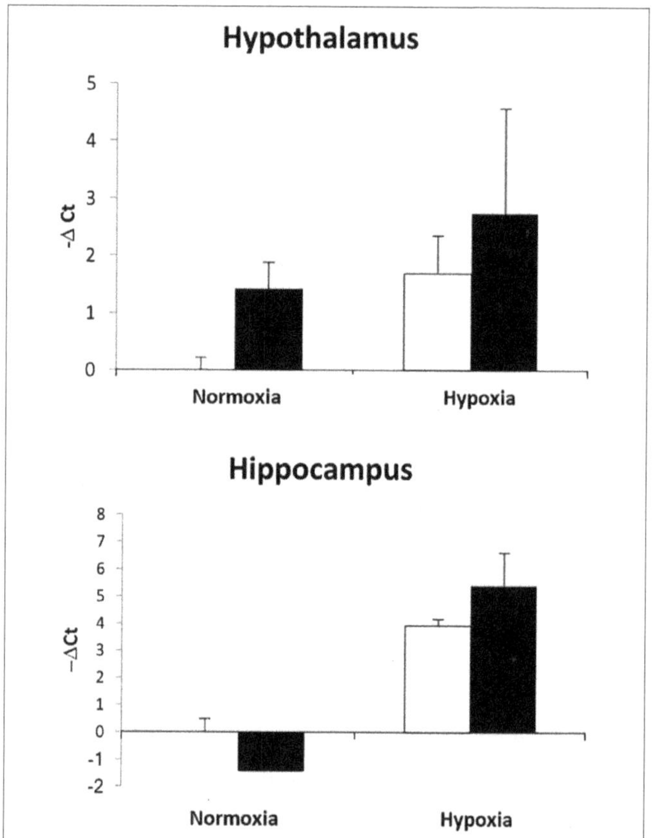

FIGURE 7 | Effect of ketamine on the expression of 16S bacterial rRNA in hypothalamus and hippocampus 24 h after transient hypoxia. Data are presented as $-\Delta C_t$ values relative to the NC group for each brain region (n = 4 animals per group). Data are expressed as mean ± SEM.

DISCUSSION

We hypothesized that ketamine would reduce hypothalamic inflammation secondary to its action to block NMDA receptor activity, thereby reducing the damaging effects of intense glutamate neurotransmission. Our original concept was that glutamate neurotransmission, followed by calcium influx into neurons, would increase apoptosis and cell death, ultimately initiating inflammation. Calcium is also released from macrophages into the extracellular space. It is possible that cell death and the associated release of cellular contents into the extracellular space could cause or contribute to the inflammation and increase in macrophage/microglia in hypothalamus and hippocampus. While the results of the present study do not reveal the ultimate cause of the inflammation, they do demonstrate that the entire inflammation cascade at a gene transcript level is activated, similar to the response to infection. Ketamine attenuates the activation of genes in inflammation-related pathways.

Although, we designed this experiment on the assumption that the mechanism of action of ketamine was the blockade of NMDA receptors, we propose that the anti-inflammatory action of the drug in the context of the present experiments is likely to involve other mechanisms. For example, the results could be explained by an action of ketamine to block macrophage activation or translocation. Shimaoka and colleagues reported that ketamine, but not other NMDA receptor antagonists, reduced nitrate production and TNFα production by J774 cells (a murine macrophage-like cell line) (Shimaoka et al., 1996). Ketamine reduces NFkB activation in A172 human glioblastoma cells exposed to LPS (Sakai et al., 2000) and reduces TNFα and IL6 production by LPS-stimulated RAW 267.4 (transformed mouse macrophage) cells (Wu et al., 2008). The mechanism of action may involve a reduction in ERK1/2 phosphorylation (Chang et al., 2010) and may, in cases of gram negative bacterial infection, interfere with LPS binding protein binding to LPS (Chen et al., 2009). The majority of bacteria appearing in fetal brain in the present experiments are gram positive (*Staphylococcus*), as reported previously (Zarate et al., 2017). Ketamine is known to reduce TLR2-mediated activation of ERK1/2 and NFKB by lipoteichoic acid, the principal component of cell wall in gram positive bacteria (Chang et al., 2010). However, in this study, ketamine did not produce any significant effects on bacterial load in the fetal hippocampus or hypothalamus. We believe that ketamine failed to have any affects on bacterial 16S gene expression because it has neither antibiotic properties nor any obstructive effects on the bacterial movement from maternal to fetal circulation. Histological data also indicates that hypoxia negatively affects the integrity of the blood vessels, and ketamine administration reduced the number of broken vessels. We have previously reported (Chang and Wood, 2015) that ventilatory hypoxia produces hemodynamic modifications in the fetus, and this response was attenuated by ketamine. Alterations in hemodynamics during acute episodes of hypoxia have been reported to affect the microvascular system, especially in the brain (Mark and Davis, 2002; Luo et al., 2012; Baburamani et al., 2013). These previous findings strongly supports our data and together they provide new insights on the therapeutical effects of ketamine in episodes of hypoxia-induced cerebral edema (Shu et al., 2012). The exact mehanisms on how blood vessels integrity are affected by hypoxia are not fully elucidated.

It is perhaps tempting to assume that inflammation in the fetal hypothalamus is damaging, or that inflammation might "program" an increased propensity for adult disease. The results of the present study do not, however, address the question of whether inflammation and the increase in tissue macrophages/microglia is damaging or whether the changes that we observe are reparative. Indeed, it is not clear from the present experiments that the inflammation reflects damage or cell death in any of the brain regions. Microglia and macrophages are important participants in tissue development and maturation. For example, microglia appear to be important in the turnover of neuronal progenitor cells in the developing brain. Arno and colleagues have proposed that microglia are a critical part of maintaining the balance between cell division and cell death in the developing brain (Arno et al., 2014). Loss of microglial function might be causative with regard to known conditions involving cellular overgrowth (Arno et al., 2014). Unknown variables important to fetal brain inflammation may have great relevance to the ultimate outcome of the offspring. Knowing, for example, that fetal brain response to transient hypoxic hypoxia involves several heretofore unrecognized variables - including bacteria after, for example, maternal antibiotic treatment or prophylactic indomethacin treatment during pregnancy or labor/delivery, or the use of ketamine for analgesia in the Neonatal Intensive Care Unit.

We conclude that the action of ketamine in the fetal brain (or, perhaps in the premature neonatal brain when ketamine is used in the Neonatal Intensive Care Unit) reflects a reduction in the inflammatory response to bacteria or to other pathogen-associated molecular patterns to which the brain is exposed. Future work should perhaps be focused on the programming effects of maternal ventilatory hypoxia as well as elucidating possible sex effects differences induced by hypoxic episodes in late gestation.

AUTHOR CONTRIBUTIONS

EC and CW conceived and designed the experiments, collected, analyzed, and interpreted the data, drafted the article, and critically revised the article for important intellectual content. MZ, TA, and MR collected, analyzed and interpreted the data, and critically revised the article for important intellectual content. ER and MK-W interpreted the data and critically revised article for important intellectual content. All authors approved the final version submitted for publication.

FUNDING

This research was supported by the National Institutes of Health (NIH) grant HD33053 (CW), and by the NIH Training in Endocrine, Metabolic, and Prenatal Basis of Chronic Kidney Disease Predoctoral Fellowship T32DK076541 (EC and CW).

ACKNOWLEDGMENTS

We thank Ms. Xiaoying (Lisa) Fang, Ms. Kristina Steinfeldt, and Ms. Heidi Straub for their expert technical assistance. We also thank the Genomics Division of the University of Florida's Interdisciplinary Center for Biotech Research for the use of the Agilent Bioanalyzer and Agilent scanner.

REFERENCES

Anand, K. J. (2007). Pharmacological approaches to the management of pain in the neonatal intensive care unit. *J. Perinatol.* 27(Suppl. 1), S4–S11. doi: 10.1038/sj.jp.7211712

Arno, B., Grassivaro, F., Rossi, C., Bergamaschi, A., Castiglioni, V., Furlan, R., et al. (2014). Neural progenitor cells orchestrate microglia migration and positioning into the developing cortex. *Nat. Commun.* 5:5611. doi: 10.1038/ncomms6611

Assali, N. S., Holm, L. W., and Sehgal, N. (1962). Hemodynamic changes in fetal lamb in uteroin response to asphyxia, hypoxia, and hypercapnia. *Circ. Res.* 11, 423–430. doi: 10.1161/01.RES.11.3.423

Baburamani, A. A., Castillo-Melendez, M., and Walker, D. W. (2013). VEGF expression and microvascular responses to severe transient hypoxia in the fetal sheep brain. *Pediatr. Res.* 73, 310–316. doi: 10.1038/pr.2012.191

Chang, E. I., and Wood, C. E. (2015). Ketamine attenuates the ACTH response to hypoxia in late-gestation ovine fetus. *Neonatology* 107, 249–255. doi: 10.1159/000369374

Chang, E. I., Zarate, M. A., Rabaglino, M. B., Richards, E. M., Arndt, T. J., Keller-Wood, M., et al. (2016a). Ketamine decreases inflammatory and immune pathways after transient hypoxia in late gestation fetal cerebral cortex. *Physiol. Rep.* 4:e12741. doi: 10.14814/phy2.12741

Chang, E. I., Zarate, M. A., Rabaglino, M. B., Richards, E. M., Keller-Wood, M., and Wood, C. E. (2016b). Ketamine suppresses hypoxia-induced inflammatory responses in the late-gestation ovine fetal kidney cortex. *J. Physiol.* 594, 1295–1310. doi: 10.1113/JP271066

Chang, H. C., Lin, K. H., Tai, Y. T., Chen, J. T., and Chen, R. M. (2010). Lipoteichoic acid-induced TNF-alpha and IL-6 gene expressions and oxidative stress production in macrophages are suppressed by ketamine through downregulating Toll-like receptor 2-mediated activation oF ERK1/2 and NFkappaB. *Shock* 33, 485–492. doi: 10.1097/SHK.0b013e3181c3cea5

Chen, T. L., Chang, C. C., Lin, Y. L., Ueng, Y. F., and Chen, R. M. (2009). Signal-transducing mechanisms of ketamine-caused inhibition of interleukin-1 beta gene expression in lipopolysaccharide-stimulated murine macrophage-like Raw 264.7 cells. *Toxicol. Appl. Pharmacol.* 240, 15–25. doi: 10.1016/j.taap.2009.06.013

Cohn, H. E., Sacks, E. J., Heymann, M. A., and Rudolph, A. M. (1974). Cardiovascular responses to hypoxemia and acidemia in fetal lambs. *Am. J. Obstet. Gynecol.* 120, 817–824. doi: 10.1016/0002-9378(74)90587-0

Dawes, G. S., Duncan, S. L., Lewis, B. V., Merlet, C. L., Owen-Thomas, J. B., and Reeves, J. T. (1969). Hypoxaemia and aortic chemoreceptor function in foetal lambs. *J. Physiol.* 201, 105–116. doi: 10.1113/jphysiol.1969.sp008745

Gersting, J. A., Schaub, C. E., and Wood, C. E. (2009). Development of prostaglandin endoperoxide synthase expression in the ovine fetal central nervous system and pituitary. *Gene Expr. Patterns* 9, 603–611. doi: 10.1016/j.gep.2009.08.003

Knutson, N., and Wood, C. E. (2010). Interaction of PGHS-2 and glutamatergic mechanisms controlling the ovine fetal hypothalamus-pituitary-adrenal axis. *Am. J. Physiol. Regul. Integr. Comp. Physiol.* 299, R365–R370. doi: 10.1152/ajpregu.00163.2010

Luo, J., Martinez, J., Yin, X., Sanchez, A., Tripathy, D., and Grammas, P. (2012). Hypoxia induces angiogenic factors in brain microvascular endothelial cells. *Microvasc. Res.* 83, 138–145. doi: 10.1016/j.mvr.2011.11.004

Makowski, E. L., Battaglia, F. C., Meschia, G., Behrman, R. E., Schruefer, J., Seeds, A. E., et al. (1968). Effect of maternal exposure to high altitude upon fetal oxygenation. *Am. J. Obstet. Gynecol.* 100, 852–861. doi: 10.1016/S0002-9378(15)33590-0

Mark, K. S., and Davis, T. P. (2002). Cerebral microvascular changes in permeability and tight junctions induced by hypoxia-reoxygenation. *Am. J. Physiol. Heart Circ. Physiol.* 282, H1485–H1494. doi: 10.1152/ajpheart.00645.2001

Montojo, J., Zuberi, K., Rodriguez, H., Kazi, F., Wright, G., Donaldson, S. L., et al. (2010). GeneMANIA Cytoscape plugin: fast gene function predictions on the desktop. *Bioinformatics* 26, 2927–2928. doi: 10.1093/bioinformatics/btq562

Nadkarni, M. A., Martin, F. E., Jacques, N. A., and Hunter, N. (2002). Determination of bacterial load by real-time PCR using a broad-range (universal) probe and primers set. *Microbiology* 148, 257–266. doi: 10.1099/00221287-148-1-257

Powers, M. J., and Wood, C. E. (2007). Ketamine inhibits fetal ACTH responses to cerebral hypoperfusion. *Am. J. Physiol. Regul. Integr. Comp. Physiol.* 292, R1542–R1549. doi: 10.1152/ajpregu.00300.2006

Rabaglino, M. B., Keller-Wood, M., and Wood, C. E. (2014). Transcriptomics of the late gestation ovine fetal brain: modeling the co-expression of immune marker genes. *BMC Genomics* 15:1001. doi: 10.1186/1471-2164-15-1001

Sakai, T., Ichiyama, T., Whitten, C. W., Giesecke, A. H., and Lipton, J. M. (2000). Ketamine suppresses endotoxin-induced NF-kappaB expression. *Can. J. Anaesth.* 47, 1019–1024. doi: 10.1007/BF03024876

Shannon, P., Markiel, A., Ozier, O., Baliga, N. S., Wang, J. T., Ramage, D., et al. (2003). Cytoscape: a software environment for integrated models of biomolecular interaction networks. *Genome Res.* 13, 2498–2504. doi: 10.1101/gr.1239303

Shimaoka, M., Iida, T., Ohara, A., Taenaka, N., Mashimo, T., Honda, T., et al. (1996). Ketamine inhibits nitric oxide production in mouse-activated macrophage-like cells. *Br. J. Anaesth.* 77, 238–242. doi: 10.1093/bja/77.2.238

Shu, L., Li, T., Han, S., Ji, F., Pan, C., Zhang, B., et al. (2012). Inhibition of neuron-specific CREB dephosphorylation is involved in propofol and ketamine-induced neuroprotection against cerebral ischemic injuries of mice. *Neurochem. Res.* 37, 49–58. doi: 10.1007/s11064-011-0582-3

Wang, J., Duncan, D., Shi, Z., and Zhang, B. (2013). WEB-based GEne SeT AnaLysis Toolkit (WebGestalt): update 2013. *Nucleic Acids Res.* 41, W77–W83. doi: 10.1093/nar/gkt439

Wu, G. J., Chen, T. L., Ueng, Y. F., and Chen, R. M. (2008). Ketamine inhibits tumor necrosis factor-alpha and interleukin-6 gene expressions in lipopolysaccharide-stimulated macrophages through suppression of toll-like receptor 4-mediated c-Jun N-terminal kinase phosphorylation and activator protein-1 activation. *Toxicol. Appl. Pharmacol.* 228, 105–113. doi: 10.1016/j.taap.2007.11.027

Zar, J. H. (1984). *Biostatistical Analysis*, Vol. 2. Englewood Cliffs, NJ: Prentice-Hall.

Zarate, M. A., Rodriguez, M. D., Chang, E. I., Russell, J. T., Arndt, T. J., Richards, E. M., et al. (2017). Post-hypoxia Invasion of the fetal brain by multidrug resistant Staphylococcus. *Sci. Rep.* 7:6458. doi: 10.1038/s41598-017-06789-6

Zhang, B., Kirov, S., and Snoddy, J. (2005). WebGestalt: an integrated system for exploring gene sets in various biological contexts. *Nucleic Acids Res.* 33, W741–W748. doi: 10.1093/nar/gki475

4

Measurement of Neurovascular Coupling in Neonates

*Dries Hendrikx[1,2], Anne Smits[3,4], Mario Lavanga[1,2], Ofelie De Wel[1,2], Liesbeth Thewissen[3,4], Katrien Jansen[3,4,5], Alexander Caicedo[6], Sabine Van Huffel[1,2] and Gunnar Naulaers[3,4]**

[1] *Department of Electrical Engineering, KU Leuven, Leuven, Belgium,* [2] *imec, Leuven, Belgium,* [3] *Department of Development and Regeneration, KU Leuven, Leuven, Belgium,* [4] *Neonatal Intensive Care Unit, University Hospitals Leuven, Leuven, Belgium,* [5] *Child Neurology, University Hospitals Leuven, Leuven, Belgium,* [6] *Facultad de Ciencias Naturales y Matemáticas, Universidad del Rosario, Bogotá, Colombia*

***Correspondence:**
Gunnar Naulaers
gunnar.naulaers@uzleuven.be

Neurovascular coupling refers to the mechanism that links the transient neural activity to the subsequent change in cerebral blood flow, which is regulated by both chemical signals and mechanical effects. Recent studies suggest that neurovascular coupling in neonates and preterm born infants is different compared to adults. The hemodynamic response after a stimulus is later and less pronounced and the stimulus might even result in a negative (hypoxic) signal. In addition, studies both in animals and neonates confirm the presence of a short hypoxic period after a stimulus in preterm infants. In clinical practice, different methodologies exist to study neurovascular coupling. The combination of functional magnetic resonance imaging or functional near-infrared spectroscopy (brain hemodynamics) with EEG (brain function) is most commonly used in neonates. Especially near-infrared spectroscopy is of interest, since it is a non-invasive method that can be integrated easily in clinical care and is able to provide results concerning longer periods of time. Therefore, near-infrared spectroscopy can be used to develop a continuous non-invasive measurement system, that could be used to study neonates in different clinical settings, or neonates with different pathologies. The main challenge for the development of a continuous marker for neurovascular coupling is how the coupling between the signals can be described. In practice, a wide range of signal interaction measures exist. Moreover, biomedical signals often operate on different time scales. In a more general setting, other variables also have to be taken into account, such as oxygen saturation, carbon dioxide and blood pressure in order to describe neurovascular coupling in a concise manner. Recently, new mathematical techniques were developed to give an answer to these questions. This review discusses these recent developments.

Keywords: neurovascular coupling, neonates, cerebral blood flow, EEG, NIRS, graph theory

INTRODUCTION

Neurovascular coupling refers to the regulation mechanism that links the transient neural activity to the subsequent change in cerebral blood flow. The first reports on this regulation mechanism date from more than 100 years ago (Donders, 1851). Neurovascular coupling can be studied from different points of view, including a macroscopic and microscopic perspective. At the macroscopic level, the extremely high vascularization and tight regulation of the cerebral blood flow provides the brain with adequate blood flow for a given metabolic demand. There is a close temporal and regional link between neuronal activity and cerebral blood flow, brain regions with high activity receive an increased amount of blood flow. At the microscopic level, the neurovascular unit is comprised of the vascular smooth muscle, the neuron and the astrocyte glial cell. Glutamate is released upon neuronal activation, which causes both neurons and astrocytes to transmit signals in order to regulate cerebral blood flow. Although it was assumed for a long time that these signals were only associated with a vasodilatory effect, recent studies show a more complex balance of vasodilation and vasoconstriction, in which both chemical and mechanical effects play an important role. Known chemical signals include prostaglandins, nitric oxide and adenosine, secreted by both neurons and astrocytes, which cause a vasodilation of the smooth muscle cell (**Figure 1**). In addition, astrocytes also secrete other vasodilators like potassium and epoxyeicosatrienoic acids. Besides these vasodilators, astrocytes are also known to secrete arachidonic acid, which has a vasoconstrictive effect. All these mediators have a direct impact on the smooth muscle of the arterioles and therefore control cerebral blood flow in a direct way. In addition to these mechanisms present in the neurovascular unit, a second mechanism was recently described by which also pericytes around the capillaries cause vasodilation, probably also playing a role in the local flow distribution. For further description of these mechanisms, we refer to recent reviews (Huneau et al., 2015; Phillips et al., 2016). As a concluding remark, it is also important to mention that most of the studies on neurovascular coupling are done in the adult population; currently, we do not know whether these mechanisms are present in preterm neonates, and if they work in the same way as described in adults.

In general, there are two main categories of studies to describe and investigate neurovascular coupling. First of all, there are *spatiotemporal* studies, which link changes in local blood flow to an artificially applied stimulus. Second, *general* studies are available that investigate resting-state neurovascular coupling using spontaneous electrical activity of the brain.

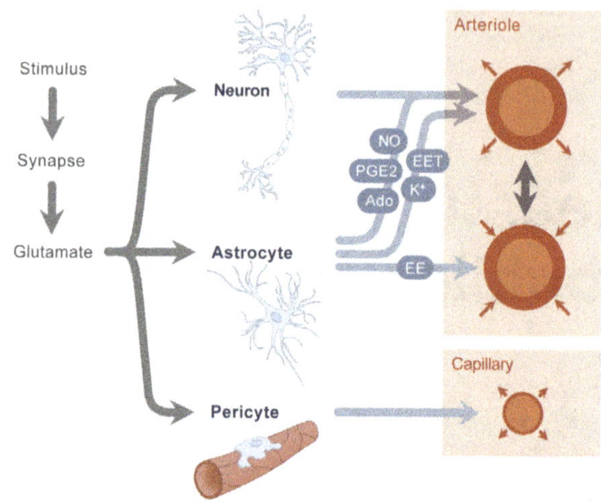

FIGURE 1 | A stimulus causes the secretion of glutamate. Glutamate stimulates neurons and astrocytes, which results in the secretion of nitric oxide (NO), potassium (K^+), adenosine (Ado), epoxyeicosatrienoic acids (EET) and prostaglandins (PGE2), which in turn results in arteriolar vasodilation. Astrocytes also secrete arachidonic acid (AA), which causes vasoconstriction. A second mechanism is the stimulation of pericytes, resulting in capillary vasodilation.

SPATIOTEMPORAL STUDIES

In order to test neurovascular coupling hypotheses in adults, spatiotemporal studies are standard of practice. In such studies, a standardized motor, visual, auditive, or cognitive task is given and simultaneously, the flow and/or activity in the brain is measured. There are different recommendations regarding optimal stimulus and assessment methods for adult research (Huneau et al., 2015). The most widely used stimulus in adults is finger tapping, which is known to cause an increase in blood flow at the contralateral motor cortex (Dettmers et al., 1996). In (preterm) neonates, spatiotemporal studies are also of interest, but they are inherently more difficult to perform. The majority the spatiotemporal studies in neonates makes use of visual stimuli, which includes the projection of checkerboard patterns on LCD displays (Meek et al., 1998; Liao et al., 2010), or flashing LEDs (Karen et al., 2008). The latter has the advantage that the neonates can be kept asleep throughout the measurements. Other less frequently used stimuli in preterm neonates include auditory (Sakatani et al., 1999; Zaramella et al., 2001) and somatosensory stimuli (Erberich et al., 2006; Arichi et al., 2010, 2012). To the best of our knowledge, guidelines regarding optimal stimulus selection for newborns are not available.

The classical response to the stimulus described in adults is a sudden increase in cerebral blood flow and cerebral oxygenation with a secondary, less pronounced decrease (Heekeren et al., 1997). This type of response is typically called 'functional hyperemia,' and is generally referred to as a *positive* response. A *negative* response, on the other hand, occurs when the increase in blood flow to the brain is insufficient to meet the metabolic demand. In this setting, however, the relation of functional hyperemia to neuronal metabolisms is unclear (Hillman, 2014). Since functional hyperemia is observed in hyperoxic, hypoglycemic and hyperglycemic states, it is clear that the blood flow increases are not simply triggered by local sensing of depleted nutrients (Powers et al., 1996; Wolf et al., 1997; Lindauer et al., 2010). The relative delay in the peak of increased blood flow further confirms that neurons do not rely upon functional hyperemia to meet their initial needs for increased oxygen and glucose, since neuronal firing may have ended prior to measurable changes in blood flow (Hillman, 2014).

In practice, different techniques are used to test neurovascular coupling in humans. In *spatiotemporal* studies, functional magnetic resonance imaging (fMRI) and functional near-infrared spectroscopy (fNIRS) are the most frequently used methods. The fMRI studies investigate the response of the blood oxygen level dependent (BOLD) signal. According to the definition, fMRI and fNIRS studies only measure blood flow changes and thus not neural activity. However, since the change in blood flow occurs mainly at the part of the brain responsible for the imposed activity (verbal, motor, visual), the measured response can be a good surrogate measurement for neurovascular coupling. In addition to the sign of the underlying mechanism (*positive* versus *negative* response), fMRI studies are also used to determine the location of brain activity after a specific stimulus. In healthy humans, cognitive, verbal, and motor tasks will on average lead to a 10–20% increase in cerebral blood flow in the posterior cerebral artery and a 5–8% increase in the middle cerebral artery (Huneau et al., 2015). In fNIRS studies, a positive response is comprised of an increase in oxyhemoglobin and total hemoglobin, together with a slight decrease in deoxygenated hemoglobin, which overall leads to an increase in tissue oxygenation. In adults, impaired neurovascular coupling has been described in different pathological conditions like stroke, hypertension, hypotension, autonomic dysfunction, Alzheimer's disease, diabetes, and traumatic brain injury (Duschek and Schandry, 2004; Girouard and Iadecola, 2006; Azevedo et al., 2011; Vetri et al., 2012; Phillips et al., 2014; Jang et al., 2017). In addition, also smoking and healthy aging are associated with a negative effect on neurovascular coupling (Boms et al., 2010; Tarantini et al., 2017; Nowak-Fluck et al., 2018).

Besides the use of fMRI and fNIRS, other techniques can also be used to carry out spatiotemporal studies. These techniques are however less frequently used – and, to the best of our knowledge – not yet employed in studies on neurovascular coupling in preterm neonates. fMRI BOLD imaging depends on specific coupling relations between cerebral metabolic rate of oxygen, cerebral blood flow and cerebral blood volume, which are not unambiguously described in preterm neonates to date (Muramoto et al., 2002; Kusaka et al., 2004). Furthermore, these relations are altered in case of brain injury (Lin et al., 2016). Perfusion-MRI techniques, such as arterial spin labeling (ASL) MRI, can be used to overcome these limits (Tortora et al., 2017). In addition, oxygen based techniques such as BOLD fMRI and fNIRS only perform indirect measures of functional hyperemia (Hyder, 2009). More precise, direct measurements of cerebral blood flow can be obtained using laser Doppler flowmetry (Dyson et al., 2014) or laser speckle imaging (Farraro et al., 2016). A disadvantage of these techniques is the sensitivity of the probe, which results in signals that are prone to artifacts, and which impedes continuous measurements – typically, laser imaging measurements are taken at discrete points in time. A new promising technique is functional ultrasound imaging, where fast ultrasound sonography is coupled with EEG (Demene et al., 2017).

Recent studies suggest that neurovascular coupling in neonates and preterm born infants can differ compared to adults. This is typically attributed to the fact that many of the components involved in actuating and propagating the hemodynamic response are still in further development, including perivascular cells such as astrocytes and pericytes (Kozberg and Hillman, 2016a). Neural and vascular networks develop, expand and are then selectively pruned over the first year of human life. In addition, the metabolic demands of the newborn brain are still evolving and are vastly different compared to the adult brain. On the first day after birth, very low values of brain oxygenation are observed, in combination with high values of cerebral oxygen extraction (Brew et al., 2014). Brain oxygenation increases during the first days of life, while cerebral oxygen extraction decreases. In extremely preterm infants, there is no correlation between cerebral blood flow and spontaneous changes in the cerebral metabolic rate of oxygen during the first 2 days after birth (Kissack et al., 2005; Wong et al., 2009). Instead, changes in cerebral oxygen extraction rather than cerebral blood flow meet changes in oxygen requirements arising from variations of the cerebral metabolic rate of oxygen. The vast differences in both neural and vascular network structure, as well as substantially different metabolic needs of the preterm brain are highly likely to affect early postnatal neurovascular coupling.

The differences in neurovascular coupling hypotheses in neonates versus adults are confirmed in fMRI studies, which are discussed in this paragraph, and in fNIRS studies, which are summarized in the next paragraph. Heep et al. (2009) described a negative response in preterm infants after stimulation, which was also confirmed by others (Yamada et al., 1997; Born et al., 1998; Erberich et al., 2006). Arichi et al. (2012) found a positive BOLD response in adults, term infants and preterm infants. Furthermore, they identified a systematic maturational trend in terms of decreasing time-to-peak and increasing positive peak amplitude. These findings suggest that in young infants the increase in cerebral oxygen consumption may be relatively greater than the corresponding increase in cerebral blood flow during functional activation. The age-dependency of the neurovascular coupling was also confirmed in a rodent model by Kozberg et al. (2013). The development of the neurovascular coupling alongside neuronal development in the postnatal brain suggests that in the developmental period the brain may be experiencing differences in energy supply and demand dynamics compared to the adult brain (Kozberg and Hillman, 2016a).

Another approach to study the neurovascular coupling is by means of fNIRS. Again, the results and conclusions of the different studies available in literature are not unambiguous. Liao et al. (2010) described a normal hyperemic signal using NIRS in the visual cortex after visual stimulation in a cohort of term neonates in the first weeks of life. Furthermore, no simultaneous reaction was observed at the motor cortex, indicating that the observed response was a local reaction. On the other hand, however, an increase in brain deoxygenation was observed in awake infants in another study (Meek et al., 1998). Verriotis et al. (2016) described the response on noxious (heel lance prick) and innoxious stimuli (tactile cutaneous stimulation) in 30 term infants. In general, noxious stimulation was found to elicit a more pronounced hemodynamic response than innoxious stimulation. However, the hemodynamic pattern after stimulation was observed to be characterized by pronounced inter-patient differences, which might suggest that increased oxygen consumption does not always lead to regional overperfusion, likely due to the immature vascular regulation or to greater metabolic demands of neurotransmission in unmyelinated white matter.

In addition to the fNIRS studies on neonates, other authors have used this technique on animals. Nakamura et al. (2017) studied the neurovascular coupling in newborn lambs. They found subjects with a positive response, i.e., an increase in oxygenated hemoglobin, but also subjects with a negative response after a motor stimulation. Furthermore, blood pressure at the start of the investigation did not seem to have any influence, but the negative response became positive in hypercapnia (Nakamura et al., 2017). Kozberg et al. (2016) studied the neurovascular coupling in rats of different ages. They described a less positive response in rats of postnatal age P10–P13, and even a negative response in rats of postnatal age P7–P8. In order to compare these results to the human population, it is common to assume that the newborn full-term and 1 year old human brain are developmentally equivalent to the postnatal days 7 and 14 in rats, respectively, based on the codevelopment of factors such as eye opening and myelination (Quinn, 2005).

In addition to the uncertainty regarding the sign of the hemodynamic response (*positive* versus *negative*) in neonates, more questions arise when we focus on specific pathologic conditions like bronchopulmonary dysplasia, congenital heart disease and pulmonary hypertension, where a lower oxygen saturation is present (Rosengarten et al., 2006). Furthermore, the effect of anesthetic and sedative drugs, which are frequently used in fMRI studies, needs to be investigated (Franceschini et al., 2010). From a broader perspective, also the effect of other drugs, such as anti-epileptic drugs on neurovascular coupling in neonates is not properly defined to date (Schwartz, 2007). Since an elaborate discussion on these topics is out of the scope of this text, we will not go into further detail.

It is important to mention that studies both in animals and neonates confirm the presence of a short hypoxic period in the brain after a stimulus in preterm infants. These short hypoxic moments are hypothesized to cause an increase in vascular endothelial growth factor and oligodendrocyte-encoded hypoxia-inducible factor function, resulting in new angiogenesis and neurogenesis in the brain (Kozberg and Hillman, 2016b). This hypothesis could explain the mechanisms of the positive effect of sensitive stimulation and the negative effect of overstimulation in newborns (Kozberg and Hillman, 2016a).

Despite the fact that the fMRI and fNIRS studies listed above aim to investigate neurovascular coupling, they actually only describe the hemodynamic changes observed in the brain after applying a stimulus. These studies can be used to describe these hemodynamic changes after a particular stimulus and how these hemodynamic patterns change with age, from preterm neonates to adults. Precise studies on neurovascular coupling are based on concomitant measurements of brain hemodynamics and brain function (electrical activity of the brain). This can be done by combining EEG measurements with fMRI measurements (Mullinger and Bowtell, 2011), with fNIRS measurements (Shin et al., 2018) or with positron emission tomography measurements (Juhász et al., 2000), although such studies are challenging from a technical point of view due to for example electrode heating (Vanhatalo et al., 2014) and the presence of numerous artifacts (Galderisi et al., 2016; Abrue et al., 2018). Therefore, such studies are very scarce, especially in (preterm) neonates. Singh et al. (2014) explored the use of concomitant multichannel EEG-fNIRS measurements during epileptic seizures in neonates and found a hemodynamic response to seizure activity which consists of an initial increase in cortical blood volume prior to a large and extended decrease typically lasting several minutes.

GENERAL STUDIES

Another approach to investigate the neurovascular coupling is to study the relation between the general metabolism of the brain and cerebral blood flow. Obviously, EEG is the most commonly used non-invasive method to assess the electrical activity of the brain, although it remains limited to the cortical activity. Cerebral blood flow can be measured at the bedside in a non-invasive way using transcranial Doppler ultrasound or near-infrared spectroscopy (NIRS). Therefore, these two modalities are generally used in *general* studies on neurovascular coupling. Both technologies are safe, relatively cheap and easy to use, however, ultrasound imaging has the disadvantage of being investigator dependent.

Roche-Labarbe et al. (2007) used NIRS in combination with EEG and found a decrease in oxygenation during bursts (high EEG activity in very preterm infants), followed by an important overflow (increase in cerebral oxygenation), suggesting a neurovascular signal that differs from the pattern commonly observed in adults. Tataranno et al. (2015) investigated functional brain activity and found an increase in oxygen extraction in preterm infants with increased electro-cerebral activity. In another study, Mahmoudzadeh et al. (2018) compared the neurovascular coupling in preterm neonates with versus without intraventricular hemorrhage. They reported that in neonates with brain injury the cerebral vascular network was unable to compensate for the increased metabolism resulting from neuronal activation in response to external stimulation. Pfurtscheller et al. (2008) investigated the behavior of the heart rate (HR) variability during the preterm EEG transients and found that EEG burst are associated with increases in HR. In addition, this positive variation of HR was found to disappear over age with the emergence of a continuous EEG trace.

The most recent advancements in signal processing allow an investigation of the neurovascular coupling in a non-invasive way focusing on "resting-state" conditions. In such a setting, the clinical goal is to develop a non-invasive and continuous measurement of the neurovascular coupling, which can be used as bedside monitoring without evoking a potential, i.e., inducing an artificial response via a stimulus. In the past decades, one of the most commonly studied neuronal couplings has been the scalp EEG connectivity, for which a large variety of methodologies has been developed (Pereda et al., 2005). In general, the methods can be classified in *functional methods* on the one hand, if only statistical correlations among the time series are taken into account, versus *effective methods* on the other hand, if the directionality of the coupling is considered as well (Friston, 2011). An overview of these methodologies is presented in **Table 1**.

Based on the EEG connectivity literature, further coupling methodologies have been developed to assess the interaction

TABLE 1 | Overview of the signal processing techniques used to assess neurovascular coupling by integrating NIRS and EEG measurements.

	Linear techniques	Non-linear techniques
Functional methods	► Time domain • Correlation • Time delay stability ► Frequency domain • Coherency ► Time-frequency domain • Wavelet coherency	► Information theory • Mutual information ► Dynamic time warping ► Phase locking value
Effective methods	► Transfer function ► Granger causality	► Information theory • Transfer entropy ► Evolutionary map approach (directionality index)

among signals with different origins or sources. These methodologies can consequently be used to assess regulation mechanisms like neurovascular coupling. Clinical examples on neurovascular coupling are the studies of Pfurtscheller et al. (2008) and Roche-Labarbe et al. (2008). Although these studies investigate the interaction of signals of different nature, these studies do not assess the concise nature of their interaction. The main difficulty to tackle in studies on multimodal integration is the fact that the different time series operate on different time scale, while simultaneously interacting with each other with a certain linear or non-linear degree.

In order to overcome this limitation, the new field of Network Physiology has the scope to describe how the time series of multiple origins interact, either linearly or non-linearly at a specific scale, in a graph or lattice structure (Bashan et al., 2012; Bartsch et al., 2015). Based on a Network Physiology framework, this review will explain new mathematical models to assess the neurovascular coupling, with a specific focus on:

(1) The necessary preprocessing steps that are required to match the temporal scales at which neuronal and vascular activities interact,
(2) The variety of methods to assess the coupling itself, which includes linear and non-linear approaches,
(3) The graph theory approach to describe the multiple simultaneous interactions and manage them in a statistically compact way.

Preprocessing Steps

In order to measure the neurovascular coupling in a correct and robust way, it is very important that the dynamics of the various signals are represented and matched in a careful way. In general, biomedical signals arise from a variety of sources, including movements, breathing, electrical activity of neurons (EEG) and optical absorption of light (NIRS), among others (Clemenson and Lancaster, 2016). Due to the different sources, biomedical time series are typically associated with different time scales of operation. An EEG signal, for example, changes rapidly due to the (de)synchronization of numerous neurons, while a NIRS signal only changes very slowly, due to the fact that the hemodynamic effects that it captures work on a slow time scale. When one wants to compute the interaction between two signals, it is important to define on which time scale the coupling is ought to be computed (the signals are interacting), and the signals have to be matched correspondingly. Although biological systems are extremely complex, it is possible to decompose their macroscopic behavior using mathematical techniques (**Table 1**).

One of the concepts that is frequently used is the notion of frequency, which gives an indication about the dynamics of a signal. By looking at the frequency content of a signal, we can make conclusions on how fast (slow) the signal changes over time. Information about the frequency content of a signal can be deduced from its frequency spectrum, which can be computed using a mathematical transformation (Challis and Kitney, 1991). Some signals change very rapidly, and are therefore mainly associated with high-frequency components. Other signals change very slowly; the frequency spectrum of such signal is mainly comprised of a very narrow band of low frequency components. Examples of the former and the latter include EEG and cerebral hemodynamics, measured by NIRS, respectively. In addition, one can also describe the biological oscillations at different time scales via a time-frequency representation. The extraction of the oscillatory components is not only useful to reduce the complexity of the system, but can also be used to describe the underlying physiology. In the world of neurovascular coupling, the brain heart interaction takes place at long-term scale (low frequency activity), since the NIRS reflects the cardiovascular oscillations which develop in a timeframe of seconds. The speed of fluctuations of NIRS is then much lower compared to EEG oscillations. In addition, however, a NIRS signal can also contain frequency components which are faster, which are caused interference from cardiac pulsations. These frequency components are typically not considered in EEG-NIRS neurovascular coupling studies.

In addition, the recent literature on EEG-NIRS integration also focuses on the low-frequency activity of the EEG, i.e., the delta oscillations. According to Knyazev, the delta oscillation belongs to the "old brain," which phylogenetically traces back to lizards (Knyazev, 2012). This explains why delta brushes dominate the preterm and the neonatal EEG activity. During the development, the scalp electrical activity tends to be discontinuous and is centered around a frequency between 1 and 2 Hz, which defines the periodicity of the bursts in the cortical trace (Andre et al., 2010). Consequently, delta oscillations are of primary importance in the preterm brain. An additional reason is the implication that delta oscillations regulate basic homeostatic needs, such as the blood flow circulation and normotension enforcement. The slow-wave EEG is considered as the expression of the regulation of the brainstem (which is in charge of cerebral hemodynamics) or, at least, as a projection of the subcortical activity to the cortical areas.

Finally, when comparing biomedical signals of different origin, it is very important that the time scales of the various signals are synchronized. In the setting of neurovascular coupling, this means that a rapidly changing neuronal signal (EEG) has to be matched with a very slowly varying cerebral hemodynamics signal (NIRS). In general, there are multiple approaches to overcome this problem. However, it is common practice to use a running estimate of the power of the slow wave activity, i.e., the delta oscillations. There are mainly three methods to extract such a running measure from the EEG. The most commonly used methodology is the use of the wavelet transform and average the power in the frequency band of interest, as reported by Clemenson and Lancaster (2016). A second option is to extract the delta band from an estimate of the power spectral density that is computed in running windows (Faes et al., 2015). The last option, which is very simple, but also very effective, is the use of the running root mean square (RMS) value, where the window length is chosen large enough to cut off the high frequency components, as reported by Caicedo et al. (2016).

Methodologies to Assess Coupling

Despite the fact that research on bedside markers of neurovascular coupling is a very new domain, there are some studies available that have investigated how different signal processing techniques can be used to quantify the neurovascular coupling based on spontaneous cerebral and vascular activities. As mentioned before, these studies mainly focus on the quantification of interaction between EEG and NIRS as surrogates for brain function and brain hemodynamics, respectively.

In signal processing terms, this interaction can be regarded as a pairwise similarity, which denotes the degree to which a given time series resembles another one. Therefore, pairwise similarity measures can be used to evaluate a regulation mechanism such as neurovascular coupling. As mentioned before, the pairwise similarity belongs to the *functional connectivity* field, which focuses (only) on the statistical correlation among the investigated signals (**Table 1**).

The most commonly used linear similarity methods are the cross-correlation function (CCF) and magnitude squared coherence (MSC), which quantify the linear correlation between two signals at different lags or frequencies, respectively. In the world of neurovascular coupling, the former has been applied by Bari et al. (2011) to study the regulation mechanism in adults during a divided attention cognitive task. In summary, the CCF was able to reveal the presence of a cascade of responses, which was observed to be strongly influenced by the task performed by the patient. Govindan et al. (2016) used the MSC to obtain a measure for the degree of coupling between EEG and NIRS data in premature neonates and identified more signal interaction (higher MSC values) in infants without brain injury compared to other patients that died of brain injury during the course of the study.

A well-known extension of these linear methods is the wavelet coherence, which is a time-variant representation of the neurovascular coupling dynamics, as performed by Musizza et al. (2007) and Chalak et al. (2017). The main advantage of using a wavelet coherence approach is the fact that this technique is able to deal with the non-stationary nature of NIRS and EEG signals. Chalak et al. (2017) performed the time-frequency coherence analysis on the raw data of amplitude-integrated EEG and brain oxygenation signals, while Musizza applied the continuous wavelet transform to extract the oscillation of interest (with frequency below 0.05 Hz). In both studies, the authors emphasize the importance of phase coupling, which defines at which time delay the oscillations lock in.

A further development consists in the usage of the *effective connectivity*, which takes into account the directionality of the neurovascular coupling (**Table 1**). Caicedo et al. (2016) have applied the linear transfer entropy in neonates to quantify the directionality between NIRS signals and the RMS of the EEG (where the window length was chosen large enough to capture only the delta oscillations). In general, transfer entropy assesses whether the current transient of a signal can be explained by the past trajectory of another signal (Lee et al., 2012). More specifically, Caicedo et al. (2016) found that the cortical activity is caused by the hemodynamic and metabolic course of the brain. Remarkably, however, the directionality was found to be reversed when, in addition to the linear interactions, also the non-linear interactions were taken into account (Hendrikx et al., 2018a).

Another mathematical technique to study directionality is the use of parametric transfer function models, as applied by Talukdar et al. (2015). In this study, multiple sets of gamma transfer functions were used. Using such sets, the authors were able to predict NIRS hemodynamics from EEG spectral envelopes, indicating that the gamma transfer function approach can be used to study neurovascular coupling. In addition, the resulting parameters of the model could provide additional insights into the neurovascular coupling mechanism.

To the best of our knowledge, there are currently no studies available that have investigated non-linear signal processing techniques, except for the preliminary results reported by Hendrikx et al. (2018a). In addition to the methods discussed in this section, other methodologies can be considered for the computation of neurovascular coupling markers, based on studies of the brain heart connectivity literature:

(1) The first option is to assess the interaction delays among signals via the cross-correlation landscape [time delay stability (TDS)].
(2) One can extend the transfer entropy to a model-free approach, in order to capture any possible type of interaction, i.e., linear and non-linear interactions.
(3) The combination of the previous two points can be regarded as a general type of phase coupling, which looks only at the phase of the signal and their non-linear interaction.

Graph Theory

Including More Signal Modalities in the Assessment of Neurovascular Coupling

In the previous section, several techniques were introduced to compute parameters for neurovascular coupling, based on multimodal processing of NIRS and EEG signals. From a broader perspective, however, there are in fact multiple regulation mechanisms that are working simultaneously in order to provide and maintain an adequate brain perfusion (Banaji et al., 2005). On a very general level, two major regulation mechanisms can be distinguished in addition to the neurovascular coupling: cerebral autoregulation and cerebral oxygen balance (Smits et al., 2017).

The former ensures that cerebral blood flow is kept more or less constant, despite variations in cerebral perfusion pressure, while the latter determines the relation between oxygen delivery and metabolic demand of the brain.

A concise study on brain perfusion thus has to take into account that multiple regulation mechanisms are working at the same time. Therefore, such an analysis requires the incorporation of other signal modalities besides EEG and NIRS, such as arterial blood pressure (ABP) and fractional tissue oxygen extraction (FTOE). The former is needed to compute a marker for cerebral autoregulation, while the latter can be used to get insight into the cerebral oxygen balance (Naulaers et al., 2007). A simultaneous analysis of EEG, NIRS, ABP, and FTOE measurements leads to the definition of three markers, each indicating and assessing the status of one of the regulation mechanisms that are essential in providing the brain with a proper amount of energy in order to support its function.

Once all of these signals are available, recent studies indicate that it is also useful to compare the interaction between the remaining pairs of signals. Indeed, Semenova et al. (2017) compared the dynamics of EEG and ABP signals in preterm neonates and found that a higher degree of EEG-ABP interaction is associated with a worse clinical outcome, assessed using clinical risk index for babies II scores. Furthermore, if we add other signals like HR, which is known to have a key influence on cerebral hemodynamics in preterm infants, simultaneous markers on HR passivity can be obtained (Mitra et al., 2014). Such markers were found to be of diagnostic value in identifying impaired cerebrovascular reactivity, leading to adverse clinical outcome. In summary, it is important to incorporate a wide variety of signal modalities in order to enable an adequate study on brain perfusion, since the pairwise interactions between the different modalities can be used as physiological markers.

One of the first studies that investigated the simultaneous interactions in a multimodal dataset, is a study by Pfurtscheller et al. (2008). More specifically, in this study, NIRS, EEG, ABP, respiration and HR were combined with cross spectral and sliding cross correlation calculations, which are both linear, functional methods (**Table 1**). Results indicate that slow precentral (de)oxyhemoglobin concentration oscillations during awake rest can be temporarily coupled with EEG fluctuations in sensorimotor areas and modulate the excitability level in the brains' motor areas, respectively. Therefore, this study provides support for the idea that resting state networks fluctuate with frequencies between 0.01 and 0.1 Hz (Mantini et al., 2007).

Graph Theory for Functional Connectivity

The main limitation of the methodology outlined above is the combinatorial number of couplings based on the variables involved. If one starts with five variables (e.g., HR, ABP, SpO_2, NIRS, and EEG), one gets 10 couples of interaction. The complexity of the interaction problem thus increases exponentially, which is difficult to manage statistically (Pavlopoulos et al., 2011). Furthermore, it is often of interest to study the interaction among systems, rather than the interaction between single signals (e.g., the interaction between the cerebral system and the cardiovascular system). A possible solution is the description of the couplings among variables as a graph of a network, whose activity can be compactly represented using graph theory.

Formally, a graph is defined by a non-zero number of nodes (vertices) and a number of links (edges) between these nodes. In general, graphs can be used to describe a great variety of real-world situations, which explains the extensive use of these mathematical objects in many different fields. A good introduction on graph theory mathematics and an overview of the numerous applications of graph theory is presented in Pavlopoulos et al. (2011). Using graph structures has some advantages:

(1) It is a straightforward methodology to deal with the exponentially increasing number of interaction pairs when adding signals to the analysis.
(2) It allows for a clear and visual representation.
(3) It allows to study clusters of signals in a straightforward way. This is especially useful when the interaction between different subsystems is of interest, rather than the interaction between the signals themselves.
(4) The behavior of the network as a whole can easily be studied, using the extensive methods on connectivity that are available in literature.

Despite the fact that graph theory was only recently introduced in the field of Network Physiology, it has been used extensively in studies on functional connectivity of the brain, as outlined by Fallani et al. (2010). Naturally, the brain is modeled by a graph in these studies, which allows to study the interactions between different brain regions. Depending on the number of nodes, it can even be possible to study the interactions in one particular brain region. However, in such case, the number of nodes has to be large enough, which is mainly limited by the data at hand, i.e., the number of channels in the multichannel EEG recording. In general, studies on functional connectivity of the brain build graph models using one signal or imaging modality, mostly EEG (Hata et al., 2016; Tokariev et al., 2016) or fMRI (Wang et al., 2010; Smitha et al., 2017).

Gao et al. (2011) constructed graph models from fMRI BOLD data recorded in a large cohort of normal pediatric subjects. Using sequential measurements, they observed a remarkable improvement in whole brain wiring from 3 weeks up to 2 years after birth, which is a critical time period for brain development. Lavanga et al. (2018) investigated the use of graph models constructed from multichannel EEG measurements in order to construct a brain-age model for preterm neonates (**Figure 3**). Using 8-channel EEG measurements, they observed a decrease in functional connectivity with post-menstrual age (PMA). In addition, the functional connectivity was found to be an accurate predictor for the age of neonates.

Graph Theory in Network Physiology

In the field of Network Physiology, graph models are constructed from a multimodal dataset (Bashan et al., 2012; Bartsch et al., 2015). Before constructing such graphs, one has to make sure that the time scales of the signals are synchronized, as

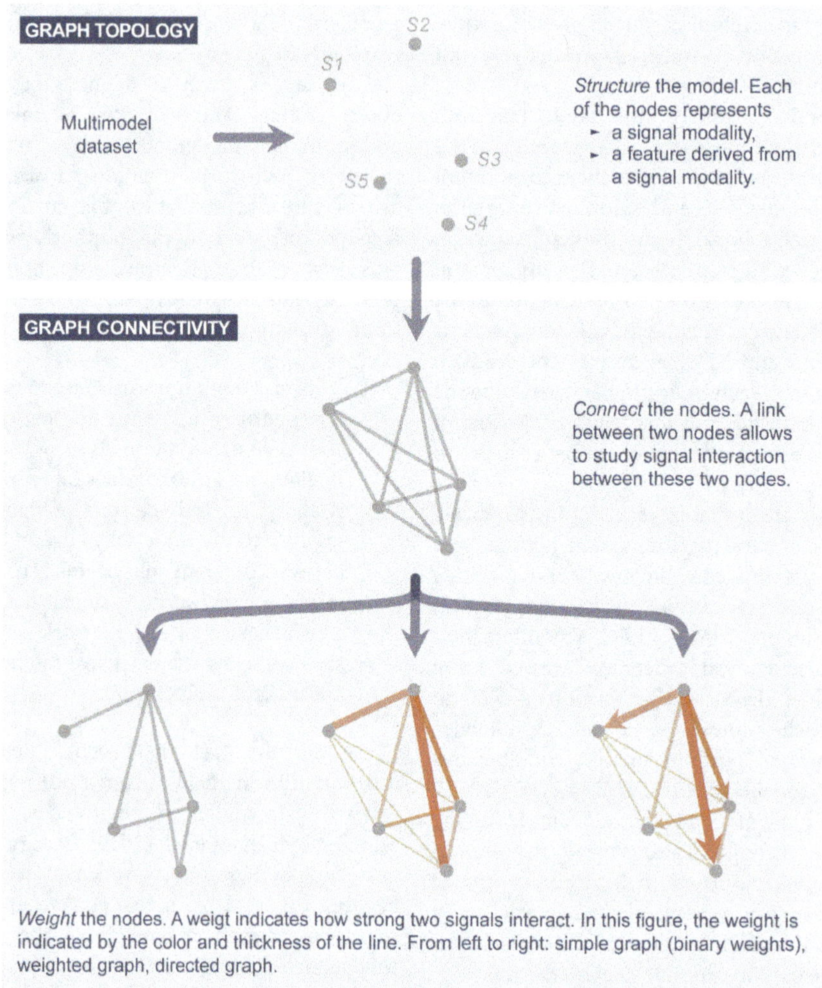

FIGURE 2 | A systematic approach to construct graph models.

explained in subsection G1. Afterward, a signal interaction graph is constructed as follows (**Figure 2**).

Graph topology

The structure of the graph is defined by the nodes. In a signal interaction graph, a node corresponds to one particular signal modality of the analysis, or a feature extracted from a signal (e.g., the power in the delta frequency band of the EEG).

Graph connectivity

(a) Define a link between each two nodes for which the signal coupling is of interest.
(b) Associate each link with a weight value, which indicates the strength of the signal interaction (coupling) and/or the directionality.

Regarding the *graph topology*, there is an endless amount of possibilities to define the structure of signal interaction graphs. Some networks to model physiological function can be quite simple (Bashan et al., 2012), while other networks are more detailed, and thus, more complex (Bartsch et al., 2015). To illustrate the variety of applications in the field of biomedical signal processing, some examples are presented in **Figure 3**, based on studies by Hendrikx et al. (2018b) and Lavanga et al. (2018). For each application, a graph with a specific topology can be constructed, based on the research question(s) of the analysis. The structure of the graph is limited by the signal modalities available in the dataset and/or the features derived from these signals.

Regarding the *graph connectivity*, there is again a wide variety of design choices on how to connect the nodes and how to define the weights associated with the links. First of all, one has to define which nodes are connected and which nodes lack a connection. Second, one has to specify how the weights associated with the links are computed. This is equivalent to the choice of one particular signal processing technique, since the weights denote signal interaction (coupling). Which signal processing technique to use has to be defined by the researcher, based on the characteristics of the research. In particular, one has to think about the nature of the interactions that needs to be captured: *linear* versus *non-linear* interactions and similarity (*functional*

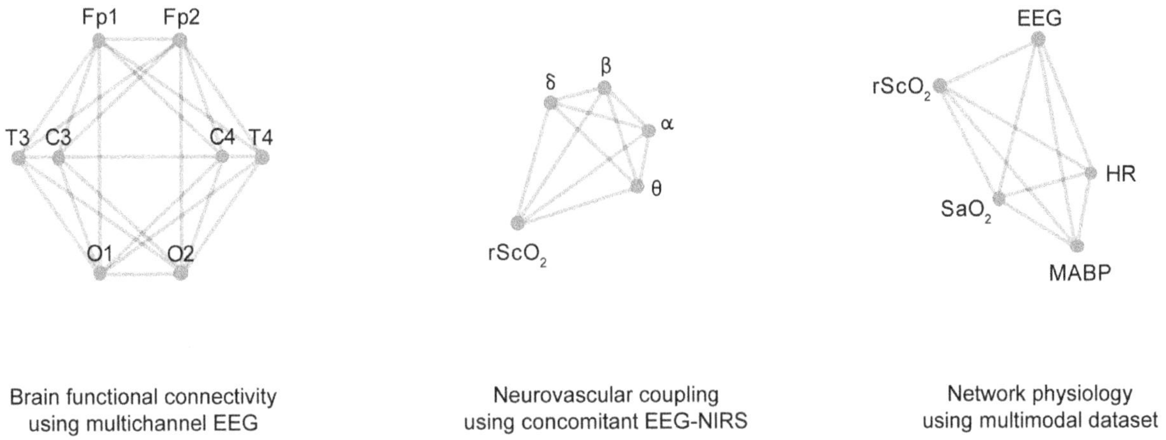

FIGURE 3 | Examples of graph models in biomedical data processing, from left to right: a graph model used for functional connectivity using 8-channel EEG; a graph model to quantify neurovascular coupling by incorporating different frequency bands of the EEG and a NIRS signal; and a graph model to study network physiology, which includes five different signal modalities.

methods) versus directionality (*effective* methods). The most commonly used signal processing techniques are summarized in **Table 1**. In the setting of graph connectivity, two additional remarks need to be taken into account.

As a first remark, it is important to note that the graphs depicted in **Figure 3** are characterized by the presence of a link between every pair of nodes. Formally, this type of graph is referred to as a *complete* graph. Such graphs are the most general type of graphs, since they allow to investigate the interaction between every possible pair of signals. It is important to note that in general it is always a good strategy to consider a link between every pair of signals, even when the signals are not expected to interact. Indeed, the weights of such links could be used as a validation for signal processing technique used to define the signal interaction: can the method detect that these signals are not interacting?

As a second remark, it is also possible to determine the presence (or absence) of a link automatically. In such an analysis, the weights are generally chosen binary. Graphs which only include the presence and absence of links (and no specific weight value), are formally referred to as *simple* graphs. An example: one could assign a '1' (presence of a link) if there is a significant correlation between two signals, while a '0' (absence of a link) denotes the lack of a significant correlation. In this setting, it is thus not necessary to manually define the presence of the links, since this is automatically detected by the signal processing technique.

The first study on the use of graph models in the field of Network Physiology is a study by Bashan et al. (2012). This study demonstrated that each physiological state is characterized by a specific network structure, demonstrating a robust interplay between network topology and function. Furthermore, high network flexibility in response to perturbations was observed, since the network was observed to be able to reorganize on time scales of a few minutes. A follow-up study on graph models in Network Physiology, is a study by Bartsch et al. (2015), who used the TDS framework in order to define the strength of the signal interactions. In short, TDS is based on linear correlations and is therefore only able of capturing linear signal interactions. The results of this study again demonstrated a direct association between network topology and physiologic function. In addition, the graph models were found to be useful in understanding how health and distinct physiologic states emerge from networked interactions among non-linear multi-component complex systems.

A second study on graph models in the field of Network Physiology is a study by our own group (Hendrikx et al., 2018b). In this study, graph models were used to investigate the interaction between cerebral hemodynamics, brain function and systemic variables. The graph models were constructed using the RBF kernel function, which is a non-linear similarity measure. Therefore, the methodological framework is able to capture non-linear signal interactions. The study showed that graph theory can be used to capture changes in signal interaction accurately and that the resulting graph models can be used to study the difference between distinct physiological states (Hendrikx et al., 2018b).

Graph models do not only provide a compact, efficient, and statistically well-defined framework to study simultaneous signal interaction, but they are in fact an entirely new way of thinking, which has been shown to produce an added value in multiple studies already (Bashan et al., 2012; Bartsch et al., 2015; Hendrikx et al., 2018b). The usage of interaction and coupling techniques provides an in-depth view of the interaction among physiological systems, moving from sectorial or univariate medicine to a more holistic approach. The latter is well-suited in case of continuous monitoring of critical states (e.g., in cases where it's likely to have multiple organ failures), and the well-being and mental status of a person, which is known to rely on the interaction between multiple systems (Chaparro-Vargas et al., 2016). Moreover, the necessity to improve the sleep quality and the developmental and cognitive abilities of neonates in the near future (which interact differently in neonates compared to adults) will require the summarized view of a graph approach instead of long recordings of multiple apparently unrelated variables. In this perspective, Network Physiology gives a broader view on the body activity (Bashan et al., 2012), comparable to the broader view on the cortical status given by the brain connectivity at its discovery (Friston, 1994).

In general, the overall purpose of the signal processing techniques (such as computational graph models) is to obtain physiological markers starting from raw measurements that are routinely obtained in neonatal intensive care units. These physiological markers could in turn be used in clinical practice to make neonatal intensive care more patient-specific. In addition, signal processing advancements are also of high importance in neonatal pharmacological studies, since the effect of medication on the neurovascular coupling in neonates is yet unclear (Smits et al., 2017). Neonates are exposed to a large number of medications, most of which are used off-label in infants because clinical trials for safety, dosing, and efficacy of drugs are lacking in this population (Hsieh et al., 2014; Ku and Smith, 2015). In this setting, signal processing techniques could thus be used to identify neonates at risk for neurodevelopmental disabilities and could assist clinicians in making a timely diagnosis, which enables to start appropriate personalized therapies early. Therefore, this patient-centered neonatal intensive care can help to reduce the occurrence of neurodevelopmental disabilities in the preterm population (Molteno et al., 1999; Cioni et al., 2016).

CONCLUSION

We suggest that further research in the field of physiology is required in order to gain more insight into the exact working principle of the neurovascular coupling in neonates (*spatiotemporal* studies). In addition, further studies on the use of signal processing in EEG-NIRS integration are also required (*general* studies). Such studies enable to construct new software, based on algorithms that describe the relation between cerebral metabolism and oxygen delivery. Graph models in particular can be of special interest in future studies, since these models allow to study the simultaneous action of different regulation mechanisms, which is essential in studies on brain perfusion. These new measurements will provide a better understanding of the coupling mechanisms in the neonatal brain, and will eventually lead to an improvement of the neonatal intensive care in general.

AUTHOR CONTRIBUTIONS

DH, ML, and GN wrote the review together. AS, ODW, LT, KJ, AC, and SVH reviewed and corrected the text.

FUNDING

The authors acknowledge the financial support of Bijzonder Onderzoeksfonds KU Leuven (BOF): SPARKLE – Sensor-based Platform for the Accurate and Remote monitoring of Kinematics Linked to E-health #: IDO-13-0358, The effect of perinatal stress on the later outcome in preterm babies #: C24/15/036, and TARGID – Development of a novel diagnostic medical device to assess gastric motility #: C32-16-00364; Fonds voor Wetenschappelijk Onderzoek-Vlaanderen (FWO): Hercules Foundation (AKUL 043) 'Flanders BCI Lab - High-End, Modular EEG Equipment for Brain Computer Interfacing'; Agentschap Innoveren en Ondernemen (VLAIO): 150466: OSA+, and O&O HBC 2016 0184 eWatch; imec funds 2017; imec ICON projects: ICON HBC.2016.0167, 'SeizeIT'; Belgian Foreign Affairs-Development Cooperation: VLIR UOS programs (2013–2019); EU: European Union's Seventh Framework Program (FP7/2007–2013) The HIP Trial: #260777, EU H2020 FETOPEN 'AMPHORA' #766456, EU EFRO Interreg: Nano4Sports, EU H2020 MSCA-ITN-2018: 'INtegrating Magnetic Resonance SPectroscopy and Multimodal Imaging for Research and Education in MEDicine (INSPiRE-MED)', funded by the European Commission under Grant Agreement #813120, and EU H2020 MSCA-ITN-2018: 'INtegrating Functional Assessment measures for Neonatal Safeguard (INFANS)', funded by the European Commission under Grant Agreement #813483. ERASMUS+: INGDIVS 2016-1-SE01-KA203-022114; European Research Council: The research leading to these results has received funding from the European Research Council under the European Union's Seventh Framework Program (FP7/2007–2013)/ERC Advanced Grant: BIOTENSORS (n° 339804). This paper reflects only the authors' views and the Union is not liable for any use that may be made of the contained information. Dries Hendrikx and Mario Lavanga are SB Ph.D. fellows at Fonds voor Wetenschappelijk Onderzoek (FWO), Vlaanderen, supported by the Flemish government. The research activities of AS are supported by the Clinical Research and Education Council of the University Hospitals Leuven.

REFERENCES

Abrue, R., Leal, A., and Figueirdo, P. (2018). EEG-informed fMRI: a review of data analysis methods. *Front. Hum. Neurosci.* 12:29. doi: 10.3389/fnhum.2018.00029

Andre, M., Lamblin, M. D., d'Allest, A. M., Curzi-Dascalova, L., Moussalli-Salefranque, F., Tich, S. N. T., et al. (2010). Electroencephalography in premature and full-term infants. developmental features and glossary. *Neurophysiol. Clin.* 40, 59–124. doi: 10.1016/j.neucli.2010.02.002

Arichi, T., Fagiolo, G., Varela, M., Melendez-Calderon, A., Allievi, A., Merchant, N., et al. (2012). Development of BOLD signal hemodynamic responses in the human brain. *Neuroimage* 63, 663–673. doi: 10.1016/j.neuroimage.2012.06.054

Arichi, T., Moraux, A., Melendez, A., Doria, V., Groppo, M., Mechant, N., et al. (2010). Somatosensory cortical activation identified by functional MRI in preterm and term infants. *NeuroImage* 49, 2063–2071. doi: 10.1016/j.neuroimage.2009.10.038

Azevedo, E., Castro, P., Santos, R., Freitas, J., Coelho, T., Rosengarten, B., et al. (2011). Autonomic dysfunction affects cerebral neurovascular coupling. *Clin. Auton. Res.* 21, 395–403. doi: 10.1007/s10286-011-0129-3

Banaji, M., Tachtsidis, I., Delpy, D., and Baigent, S. (2005). A physiological model of cerebral blood flow control. *Math. Biosci.* 194, 125–173. doi: 10.1016/j.mbs.2004.10.005

Bari, V., Calcagnile, P., Molteni, E., Re, R., Contini, D., Spinelli, L., et al. (2011). Study of neurovascular and autonomic response in a divided attention test by means of EEG, ECG and NIRS signals. *Conf. Proc. IEEE Eng. Med. Biol. Soc.* 2011, 1403–1406. doi: 10.1109/IEMBS.2011.6090330

Bartsch, R. P., Liu, K. K., Bashan, A., and Ivanov, P. (2015). Network physiology: how organ systems dynamically interact. *PLoS One* 10:e0142143. doi: 10.1371/journal.pone.0142143

Bashan, A., Bartsch, R. P., Kantelhardt, J. W., Havlin, S., and Ch Ivanov, P. (2012). Netwrok physiology reveals relations between network topology and physiological function. *Nat. Commun.* 28:702. doi: 10.1038/ncomms1705

Boms, N., Yonai, Y., Molnar, S., Rosengarten, B., Bornstein, N. M., Csiba, L., et al. (2010). Effect of smoking cessation on visually evoked cerebral blood flow response in healthy volunteers. *J. Vasc. Res.* 47, 214–220. doi: 10.1159/000255964

Born, P., Leth, H., Miranda, M. J., Rostrup, E., Stensgaard, A., Peitersen, B., et al. (1998). Visual activation in infants and young children studied by functional magnetic resonance imaging. *Pediatr. Res.* 44, 578–583. doi: 10.1203/00006450-199810000-00018

Brew, N., Walker, D., and Wong, F. (2014). Cerebral vascular regulation and brain injury in preterm infants. *Am. J. Physiol. Regul. Integr. Comp. Physiol.* 206, R773–R786. doi: 10.1152/ajpregu.00487.2013

Caicedo, A., Thewissen, L., Smits, A., Naulaers, G., Allegaert, K., and Van Huffel, S. (2016). Changes in oxygenation levels precede changes in amplitude of the EEG in premature infants. *Adv. Exp. Med. Biol.* 923, 143–149. doi: 10.1007/978-3-319-38810-6_19

Chalak, L. F., Tian, F., Adams-Huet, B., Vasil, D., Laptook, A., Tarumi, T., et al. (2017). Novel wavelet real time analysis of neurovascular coupling in neonatal encephalopathy. *Sci. Rep.* 7:45958. doi: 10.1038/srep45958

Challis, R. E., and Kitney, R. I. (1991). Biomedical signal processing (in four parts). Part 3. The power spectrum and coherence function. *Med. Biol. Eng. Comput.* 29, 225–242. doi: 10.1007/BF02446704

Chaparro-Vargas, R., Schilling, C., Schredl, M., and Cvetkovic, D. (2016). Sleep electroencephalography and heart rate variability interdependence among health subjects and insomnia/schizophrenia patients. *Med. Biol. Eng. Comput.* 54, 77–91. doi: 10.1007/s11517-015-1297-4

Cioni, G., Inguaggiato, E., and Sgandurra, G. (2016). Early intervention in neurodevelopmental disorders: underlying neural mechanisms. *Dev. Med. Child Neurol.* 58, 61–66. doi: 10.1111/dmcn.13050

Clemenson, P., and Lancaster, G. (2016). Reconstructing time-dependent dynamics. *Proc. IEEE* 104:18.

Demene, C., Baranger, J., Bernal, M., Delanoe, C., Auvin, S., Biran, V., et al. (2017). Functional ultrasound imaging of brain activity in human newborns. *Sci. Transl. Med.* 9:411. doi: 10.1126/scitranslmed.aah6756

Dettmers, C., Connelly, A., Stephan, K. M., Turner, R., Friston, K. J., Frackowiak, R. S., et al. (1996). Quantitative comparison of functional magnetic resonance imaging with positron emission tomography using a force-related paradigm. *Neuroimage* 4(3 Pt 1), 201–209. doi: 10.1006/nimg.1996.0071

Donders, F. C. (1851). Bewegungen des gehirns und die veränderungen der gefässfüllung der pia mater. *Schmid's Fahrbucher* 69:5.

Duschek, S., and Schandry, R. (2004). Cognitive performance and cerebral blood flow in essential hypotension. *Psychophysiology* 41, 905–913. doi: 10.1111/j.0048-5772.2004.00249.x

Dyson, R. M., Palliser, H. K., Lakkundi, A., de Waal, K., Latter, J. L., Clifton, V. L., et al. (2014). Early miscrovascular changes in the preterm neonate: a comparative study of the human and guinea pig. *Physiol. Rep.* 2:e12145. doi: 10.14814/phy2.12145

Erberich, S. G., Panigraphy, A., Friedlich, P., Seri, I., Nelson, M. D., and Gilles, F. (2006). Somatosensory lateralization in the newborn brain. *NeuroImage* 29, 155–161. doi: 10.1016/j.neuroimage.2005.07.024

Faes, L., Marinazzo, D., Jurysta, F., and Nollo, G. (2015). Linear and non-linear brain-heart and brain-brain interactions during sleep. *Physiol. Meas.* 36, 683–698. doi: 10.1088/0967-3334/36/4/683

Fallani, F. D. V., da Fontoura Costa, L., Rodriguez, F. A., Astolfi, L., Vecchiato, G., Toppi, J., et al. (2010). A graph-theoretical approach in brain functional networks. Possible implications in EEG studies. *Nonlin. Biomed. Phys.* 4:S8. doi: 10.1186/1753-4631-4-S1-S8

Farraro, R., Fathi, O., and Choi, B. (2016). Handheld, point-of-care laser speckle imaging. *J. Biomed. Opt.* 21:094001. doi: 10.1117/1/JBO.21.9.094001

Franceschini, M. A., Radhakrishnan, H., Thakur, K., Wu, W., Ruvinskaya, S., Carp, S., et al. (2010). The effect of different anesthetics on neurovascular coupling. *Neuroimage* 51, 1367–1377. doi: 10.1016/j.neuroimage.2010.03.060

Friston, K. J. (1994). Functional and effective connectivity in neuroimaging: a synthesis. *Hum. Brain Mapp.* 2, 56–78. doi: 10.1002/hbm.460020107

Friston, K. J. (2011). Functional and effective connectivity: a review. *Brain Connect* 1, 13–36. doi: 10.1089/brain.2011.0008

Galderisi, A., Brigadoi, S., Cutini, S., Moro, S. B., Lolli, E., Meconi, F., et al. (2016). Long-term continuous monitoring of the preterm brain with diffuse optical tomography and electroencephalography: a technical note on cap manufacturing. *Neurophoton* 3:045009. doi: 10.1117/1.NPh.3.4.045009

Gao, W., Gilmore, J. H., Giovanello, K. S., Smith, J. K., Shen, D., Zhu, H., et al. (2011). Temporal and spatial evolution of brain network topology during the first two years of life. *PLoS One* 6:e25278. doi: 10.1371/journal.pone.0025278

Girouard, H., and Iadecola, C. (2006). Neurovascular coupling in the normal brain and in hypertension, stroke, and Alzheimer disease. *J. Appl. Physiol.* 100, 328–335. doi: 10.1152/japplphysiol.00966.2005

Govindan, R. B., Massaro, A., Chang, T., Gilbert, V., and du Plessis, A. (2016). A novel technique for quantitative bedside monitoring of neurovascular coupling. *J. Neurosci. Meth.* 259:7. doi: 10.1016/j.jneumeth.2015.11.025

Hata, M., Kazui, H., Tanaka, T., Ishii, R., Canuet, L., Pascual-Marqui, R. D., et al. (2016). Functional connectivity assessed by resting state EEG correlates with cognitive decline of Alzheimer's disease – An eLORETA study. *Clin. Neurophys.* 127, 1269–1278. doi: 10.1016/j.clinph.2015.10.030

Heekeren, H. R., Obrig, H., Wenzel, R., Eberle, K., Ruben, J., Villringer, K., et al. (1997). Cerebral haemoglobin oxygenation during sustained visual stimulation – a near-infrared spectroscopy study. *Philos. Trans. R. Soc. Lond. B Biol. Sci.* 352, 743–750. doi: 10.1098/rstb.1997.0057

Heep, A., Scheef, L., Jankowski, J., Born, M., Zimmermann, N., Sival, D., et al. (2009). Functional magnetic resonance imaging of the sensorimotor system in preterm infants. *Pediatrics* 123, 294–300. doi: 10.1542/peds.2007-3475

Hendrikx, D., Thewissen, L., Smits, A., Naulaers, G., Allegaert, K., Van Huffel, S., et al. (2018a). Nonlinear transfer entropy to assess the neurovascular coupling in premature infants. *Adv. Exp. Med. Biol.*

Hendrikx, D., Thewissen, L., Smits, A., Naulaers, G., Allegaert, K., Van Huffel, S., et al. (2018b). Using graph theory to assess the interaction between cerebral function, brain hemodynamics, and systemic variables in premature infants. *Complexity* 2018:6504039. doi: 10.1155/2018/6504039

Hillman, E. M. C. (2014). Coupling mechanism and significance of the BOLD signal: a status report. *Annu. Rev. Neurosci.* 37, 161–181. doi: 10.1146/annurev-neuro-071013-014111

Hsieh, E. M., Hornik, C. P., Clark, R. H., Laughon, M. M., Benjamin, D. K., Smith, P. B., et al. (2014). Medication use in the neonatal intensive care unit. *Am. J. Perinatol.* 31, 811–822. doi: 10.1055/s-0033-1361933

Huneau, C., Benali, H., and Chabriat, H. (2015). Investigating human neurovascular coupling using functional neuroimaging: a critical review of dynamic models. *Front. Neurosci.* 9:467. doi: 10.3389/fnins.2015.00467

Hyder, F. (2009). Dynamic imaging of brain function. *Methods Mol. Biol.* 489, 3–21. doi: 10.1007/978-1-59745-543-5_1

Jang, H., Huang, S., Hammer, D. X., Wang, L., Rafi, H., Ye, M., et al. (2017). Alterations in neurovascular coupling following acute traumatic brain injury. *Neurophotonics* 4:045007. doi: 10.1117/1.NPh.4.4.045007

Juhász, C., Chugani, D. C., Muzik, O., Watson, C., Shah, J., Shah, A., et al. (2000). Relationship between EEG and positron emission tomography abnormalities in clinical epilepsy. *J. Clin. Neurophysiol.* 17, 29–42. doi: 10.1097/00004691-200001000-00004

Karen, T., Morren, G., Haensse, E., Bauschatz, A. S., Bucher, H. U., and Wolf, M. (2008). Hemodynamic response to visual stimulation in newborn infants using functional near-infrared spectroscopy. *Hum. Brain Mapp.* 29, 453–460. doi: 10.1002/hbm.20411

Kissack, C. M., Garr, R., Wardle, S. P., and Weindling, A. M. (2005). Cerebral fractional oxygen extraction is inversely correlated with oxygen delivery in the sick, newborn, preterm infant. *J. Cereb. Blood Flow Metab.* 25, 545–553. doi: 10.1038/sj.jcbfm.9600046

Knyazev, G. G. (2012). EEG delta oscillations as a correlate of basic homeostatic and motivational processes. *Neurosci. Biobehav. Rev.* 36, 677–695. doi: 10.1016/j.neubiorev.2011.10.002

Kozberg, M., and Hillman, E. (2016a). Neurovascular coupling and energy metabolism in the developing brain. *Prog. Brain Res.* 225, 213–242. doi: 10.1016/bs.pbr.2016.02.002

Kozberg, M. G., Chen, B. R., DeLeo, S. E., Bouchard, M. B., and Hillman, E. M. (2013). Resolving the transition from negative to positive blood oxygen level-dependent responses in the developing brain. *Proc. Natl. Acad. Sci. U.S.A.* 110, 4380–4385. doi: 10.1073/pnas.1212785110

Kozberg, M. G., and Hillman, E. M. (2016b). Neurovascular coupling develops alongside neural circuits in the postnatal brain. *Neurogenesis* 3:e1244439. doi: 10.1080/23262133.2016.1244439

Kozberg, M. G., Ma, Y., Shaik, M. A., Kim, S. H., and Hillman, E. M. (2016). Rapid postnatal expansion of neural networks occurs in an environment of altered neurovascular and neurometabolic coupling. *J. Neurosci.* 36, 6704–6717. doi: 10.1523/JNEUROSCI.2363-15.2016

Ku, L. C., and Smith, B. (2015). Dosing in neonates: special considerations in physiology and trial design. *Pediatr. Res.* 77, 2–9. doi: 10.1038/pr.2014.143

Kusaka, T., Kawada, K., Okubo, K., Namba, M., Okada, H., Imai, T., et al. (2004). Noninvasice optical imaging in the visual cortex in young infants. *Hum. Brain Mapp.* 22, 122–132. doi: 10.1002/hbm.20020

Lavanga, M., De Wel, O., Caicedo, A., Jansen, K., Dereymaeker, A., Naulaers, G., et al. (2018). A brain-age model for preterm infants based on functional connectivity. *Physiol. Meas.* 39:044006. doi: 10.1088/1361-6579/aabac4

Lee, J., Nemati, S., Silva, I., Edwards, B. A., Butler, J. P., and Malhotra, A. (2012). Transfer entropy estimation and directional coupling change detection in biomedical time series. *Biomed. Eng. Online* 11:19. doi: 10.1186/1475-925X-11-19

Liao, S. M., Gregg, N. M., White, B. R., Zeff, B. W., Bjerkaas, K. A., Inder, T. E., et al. (2010). Neonatal hemodynamic response to visual cortex activity: high-density near-infrared spectroscopy study. *J. Biomed. Opt.* 15:026010. doi: 10.1117/1.3369809

Lin, P.-Y., Hagan, K., Fenoglio, A., Grant, P. E., and Franceschini, M. A. (2016). Reduced cerebral blood flow and oxygen metabolism in extremely preterm neonates with low-grade germinal matrix- intraventricular hemorrhage. *Sci. Rep.* 6:25903. doi: 10.1038/srep25903

Lindauer, U., Leithner, C., Kaasch, H., Rohrer, B., Foddis, M., Füchtemeier, M., et al. (2010). Neurovascular coupling in rat brain operates independent of hemoglobin deoxygenation. *J. Cereb. Blood Flow Metab.* 30, 757–768. doi: 10.1038/jcbfm.2009.259

Mahmoudzadeh, M., Dehaene-Lamberts, G., Kongolo, G., Fournier, M., Goudjil, S., and Wallois, F. (2018). Conseuqnece of intraventricular hemorrhage on neurovascular coupling evoked by speech syllables in preterm neonates. *Dev. Cogn. Neurosci.* 30, 60–69. doi: 10.1016/j.dcn.2018.01.001

Mantini, D., Perrucci, M. G., Del Gratta, C., Romani, G. L., and Corbetta, M. (2007). Electrophysiological signatures of resting state networks in the human brain. *Proc. Natl. Acad. Sci. U.S.A.* 104, 13170–13175. doi: 10.1073/pnas.0700668104

Meek, J. H., Firbank, M., Elwell, C. E., Atkinson, J., Braddick, O., and Wyatt, J. S. (1998). Regional hemodynamic reponses to visual stimulation in awake infants. *Pediatr. Res.* 43, 840–843. doi: 10.1203/00006450-199806000-00019

Mitra, S., Czosnyka, M., Smielewski, P., O'Reilly, H., Brady, K., and Austin, T. (2014). Heart rate passivity of cerebral tissue oxygenation is associated with predictors of poor outcome in preterm infants. *Acta Paediatr.* 103, e374–e382. doi: 10.1111/apa.12696

Molteno, C. D., Thompson, M. C., Buccimazza, S. S., Magasiner, V., and Hann, F. M. (1999). Evaluation of the infant at risk for neurovelopmental disability. *S. Afr. Med. J.* 89, 1084–1087.

Mullinger, K., and Bowtell, R. (2011). Combining EEG and fMRI. *Methods Mol. Biol.* 711, 303–326. doi: 10.1007/978-1-61737-992-5_15

Muramoto, S., Yamada, H., Sadato, N., Kimura, H., Konishi, Y., Kimura, K., et al. (2002). Age-dependent change in metabolic response to photic stimulation of the primary visual cortex in infants: functional magnetic resonance imaging study. *J. Comput. Assist. Tomogr.* 26, 894–901. doi: 10.1097/00004728-200211000-00007

Musizza, B., Stefanovska, A., McClintock, P. V., Palus, M., Petrovcic, J., Ribaric, S., et al. (2007). Interactions between cardiac, respiratory and EEG-delta oscillations in rats during anaesthesia. *J. Physiol.* 580(Pt 1), 315–326. doi: 10.1113/jphysiol.2006.126748

Nakamura, S., Walker, D. W., and Wong, F. Y. (2017). Cerebral haemodynamic response to somatosensory stimulation in near-term fetal sheep. *J. Physiol.* 595, 1289–1303. doi: 10.1113/JP273163

Naulaers, G., Meyns, B., Miserez, M., Leunens, V., Van Huffel, S., Casaer, P., et al. (2007). Use of tissue oxygenation index and fractional tissue oxygen extraction as non-invasive parameters for cerebral oxygenation. A validation study in piglets. *Neonatology* 92, 120–126. doi: 10.1159/000101063

Nowak-Fluck, D., Ainslie, P. N., Bain, A. R., Ahmed, A., Wildfong, K. W., Morris, L. E., et al. (2018). Effect of healthy ageing on cerebral blood flow, CO2 reactivity and neurovascular coupling during exercise. *J. Appl. Physiol.* 125, 1917–1930. doi: 10.1152/japplphysiol.00050.2018

Pavlopoulos, G. A., Secrier, M., Moschopoulos, C. N., Soldator, T. G., Kossida, S., Aerts, J., et al. (2011). Using graph theory to analyze biological networks. *Biodata Min.* 4:10. doi: 10.1186/1756-0381-4-10

Pereda, E., Quiroga, R. Q., and Bhattacharya, J. (2005). Nonlinear multivariate analysis of neurophysiological signals. *Prog. Neurobiol.* 77, 1–37. doi: 10.1016/j.pneurobio.2005.10.003

Pfurtscheller, K., Bauernfeind, G., Muller-Putz, G. R., Urlesberger, B., Muller, W., and Pfurtscheller, G. (2008). Correlation between EEG burst-to-burst intervals and HR acceleration in preterm infants. *Neurosci. Lett.* 437, 103–106. doi: 10.1016/j.neulet.2008.03.079

Phillips, A. A., Chan, F. H., Zheng, M. M., Krassioukov, A. V., and Ainslie, P. N. (2016). Neurovascular coupling in humans: physiology, methodological advances and clinical implications. *J. Cereb. Blood Flow Metab.* 36, 647–664. doi: 10.1177/0271678X15617954

Phillips, A. A., Warburton, D. E., Ainslie, P. N., and Krassioukov, A. V. (2014). Regional neurovascular coupling and cognitive performance in those with low blood pressure secondary to high-level spinal cord injury: improved by alpha-1 agonist midodrine hydrochloride. *J. Cereb. Blood Flow Metab.* 34, 794–801. doi: 10.1038/jcbfm.2014.3

Powers, W. J., Hirsch, I. B., and Cryer, P. E. (1996). Effect of stepped hypoglycemia on regional cerebral blood flow response to physioloigcal brain activation. *Am. J. Physiol.* 270, H554–H559. doi: 10.1152/ajpheart.1996.270.2.H554

Quinn, R. (2005). Comparing rat's to human's age: how old is my rat in people years? *Nutrition* 21, 775–777. doi: 10.1016/j.nut.2005.04.002

Roche-Labarbe, N., Wallois, F., Ponchel, E., Kongolo, G., and Grebe, R. (2007). Coupled oxygenation oscillation measured by NIRS and intermittent cerebral activation on EEG in premature infants. *Neuroimage* 36, 718–727. doi: 10.1016/j.neuroimage.2007.04.002

Roche-Labarbe, N., Zaaimi, B., Berquin, P., Nehlig, A., Grebe, R., and Wallois, F. (2008). NIRS-measured oxy- and deoxyhemoglobin changes associated with EEG spike-and-wave discharges in children. *Epilepsia* 49, 1871–1880. doi: 10.1111/j.1528-1167.2008.01711.x

Rosengarten, B., Schermuly, R. T., Voswinckel, R., Kohstall, M. G., Olschewski, H., Weissmann, N., et al. (2006). Sildenafil improves dynamic vascular function in the brain: studies in patients with pulmonary hypertension. *Cerebrovasc. Dis.* 21, 194–200. doi: 10.1159/000090555

Sakatani, K., Chen, S., Lichty, W., Zuo, H., and Wang, Y. P. (1999). Cerebral blood oxygenation changes induced by auditory stimulation in newbord infants measured by near infrared spectroscopy. *Early Hum. Dev.* 55, 229–236. doi: 10.1016/S0378-3782(99)00019-5

Schwartz, T. H. (2007). Neurovascular coupling and epilepsy: hemodynamic markers for localizing and predicting seizure onset. *Epilepsy. Curr.* 7, 91–94. doi: 10.1111/j.1535-7511.2007.00183.x

Semenova, O., Lightbody, G., O'Toole, J. M., Boylan, G., Dempsey, E., and Temko, A. (2017). Modelling interactions between blood pressure and brain activity in preterm neonates. *Conf. Proc. IEEE Eng. Med. Biol. Soc.* 2017:3972. doi: 10.1109/EMBC.2017.8037725

Shin, J., van Lühmann, A., Kim, D.-W., Mehnert, J., Hwang, H.-J., and Müller, K.-R. (2018). Simultaneous acquisition of EEG and NIRS during cognitive tasks for an open accedd dataset. *Sci. Data* 5:180003. doi: 10.1038/sdata.2018.3

Singh, H., Cooper, R. J., Lee, C. W., Dempsey, L., Edwards, A., Brigadoi, S., et al. (2014). Mapping cortical haemodynamics during neonatal seizures using diffuse optical tomography: a case study. *NeuroImage Clin.* 5, 256–265. doi: 10.1016/j.nicl.2014.06.012

Smitha, K. A., Raja, K. A., and Arun, K. M. (2017). Resting state fMRI: a review on methods in resting state connectivity analysis and resting state networks. *Neuroradiol. J.* 30, 305–317. doi: 10.1177/1971400917697342

Smits, A., Thewissen, L., Dereymaeker, A., Dempsey, E., Caicedo, A., and Naulaers, G. (2017). The use of hemodynamic and cerebral monitoring to study pharmacodynamics in neonates. *Curr. Pharm. Des.* 23, 5955–5963. doi: 10.2174/1381612823666170918124419

Talukdar, M. T., Frost, H. R., and Diamong, S. G. (2015). Modeling neurovascular coupling from clustered parameter sets for multimodal EEG-NIRS. *Comp. Math. Meth. Med.* 2015:830849. doi: 10.1155/2015/830849

Tarantini, S., Tran, C. H. T., Gordon, G. R., Ungvari, Z., and Csiszar, A. (2017). Impaired neurovascular coupling in aging and Alzheimer's disease: contribution of astrocyte dysfunction and endothelial impairment to cognitive decline. *Exp. Gerontol.* 94, 52–58. doi: 10.1016/j.exger.2016.11.004

Tataranno, M. L., Alderliesten, T., de Vries, L., Groenendaal, F., Toet, M. C., Lemmers, P. M. A., et al. (2015). Early oxygen-utilization and brain activity in preterm infants. *PLoS One* 10:e0124623. doi: 10.1371/journal.pone.0124623

Tokariev, A., Videman, M., Palva, J. M., and Vanhatalo, S. (2016). Functional brain connectivity develops rapidly around term age and changes between vigilance states in the human newborn. *Cereb. Cortex* 26, 4540–4550. doi: 10.1093/cercor/bhv219

Tortora, D., Mattei, P. A., Navarra, R., Panara, V., Salomone, R., Rossi, A., et al. (2017). Prematurity and brain perfusion: arterial spin labeling MRI. *NeuroImage Clin.* 15, 401–407. doi: 10.1016/j.nicl.2017.05.023

Vanhatalo, S., Alnaijar, A., Nguyen, V. T., Colditz, P., and Fransson, P. (2014). Safety of EEG-fMRI recodrings in newborn infants at 3T: a study using baby-size phantom. *Clin. Neurophysiol.* 125, 941–946. doi: 10.1016/j.clinph.2013.09.041

Verriotis, M., Fabrizi, L., Lee, A., Cooper, R. J., Fitzgerald, M., and Meek, J. (2016). Mapping cortical responses to somatosensory stimuli in human infants with simultaneous near-infrared spectroscopy and event-related potential recording. *eNeuro* 3:ENEURO.0026-16.2016. doi: 10.1523/ENEURO.0026-16.2016

Vetri, F., Xu, H., Paisansathan, C., and Pelligrino, D. A. (2012). Impairment of neurovascular coupling in type 1 diabetes mellitus in rats is linked to PKC modulation of BK(Ca) and Kir channels. *Am. J. Physiol. Heart Circ. Physiol.* 302, H1274–H1284. doi: 10.1152/ajpheart.01067.2011

Wang, J., Zuo, X., and He, Y. (2010). Graph-based network analysis of resting-state functional MRI. *Front. Syst. Neurosci.* 4:16. doi: 10.3389/fnsys.2010.00016

Wolf, T., Lindauer, U., Villringer, A., and Dirnagl, U. (1997). Excessive oxygen or glucose supply does not alter the blood flow response to somatosensory stimulation or spreading depression in rats. *Brain Res.* 761, 290–299. doi: 10.1016/S0006-8993(97)00354-5

Wong, F. Y., Barfield, C. P., Horne, R. S., and Walker, A. M. (2009). Dopamine theray promotes cerebral flow-metabolism coupling in preterm infants. *Intens. Care Med.* 35, 1777–1782. doi: 10.1007/s00134-009-1602-5

Yamada, H., Sadato, N., Konishi, Y., Kimura, K., Tanaka, M., Yonekura, Y., et al. (1997). A rapid brain metabolic change in infants detected by fMRI. *Neuroreport* 8, 3775–3778. doi: 10.1097/00001756-199712010-00024

Zaramella, P., Freato, F., Amigoni, A., Salvadori, S., Marangoni, P., Suppjei, A., et al. (2001). Brain auditory activation measured by near-infrared spectroscopy (NIRS) in neonates. *Pediatr. Res.* 49, 213–219. doi: 10.1203/00006450-200102000-00014

5

Chorioamnionitis is a Risk Factor for Intraventricular Hemorrhage in Preterm Infants

*Eduardo Villamor-Martinez[1], Monica Fumagalli[2], Owais Mohammed Rahim[1], Sofia Passera[2], Giacomo Cavallaro[2], Pieter Degraeuwe[1], Fabio Mosca[2] and Eduardo Villamor[1]**

[1] Department of Pediatrics, School for Oncology and Developmental Biology (GROW), Maastricht University Medical Center, Maastricht, Netherlands, [2] Neonatal Intensive Care Unit, Department of Clinical Sciences and Community Health, Fondazione IRCCS Cà Granda Ospedale Maggiore Policlinico, Università degli Studi di Milano, Milan, Italy

***Correspondence:**
Eduardo Villamor
e.villamor@mumc.nl

Although chorioamnionitis (CA) is a well-known risk factor for white matter disease of prematurity, the association with intraventricular hemorrhage (IVH) is controversial and has not been yet systematically reviewed. We performed a systematic review and meta-analysis of studies exploring the association between CA and IVH. A comprehensive literature search was conducted using PubMed/MEDLINE and EMBASE, from their inception to 1 July 2017. Studies were included if they examined preterm infants and reported primary data that could be used to measure the association between exposure to CA and the presence of IVH. A random-effects model was used to calculate odds ratios (OR) and 95% confidence intervals (CI). We found 1,284 potentially relevant studies, of which 85 met the inclusion criteria (46,244 infants, 13,432 CA cases). Meta-analysis showed that CA exposure was significantly associated with all grades IVH (OR 1.88, 95% CI 1.61–2.19), with grades 1–2 IVH (OR 1.69, 95% CI 1.22–2.34), and with grades 3–4 IVH (OR 1.62, 95% CI 1.42–1.85). Both clinical and histological CA were associated with an increased risk for developing IVH in very preterm infants. In contrast, the presence of funisitis did not increase IVH risk when compared to CA in the absence of funisitis (OR 1.22, 95% CI 0.89–1.67). Further meta-analyses confirmed earlier findings that CA-exposed infants have significantly lower gestational age (GA; mean difference [MD] −1.20 weeks) and lower birth weight (BW; MD −55 g) than the infants not exposed to CA. However, meta-regression and subgroup analysis could not demonstrate an association between the lower GA and BW and the risk of IVH in the CA-exposed infants. In conclusion, our data show that CA is a risk factor for IVH, but also a risk factor for greater prematurity and more clinical instability. In contrast to other complications of prematurity, such as patent ductus arteriosus, retinopathy of prematurity, or bronchopulmonary dysplasia, the effect of CA on IVH appears to be independent of CA as causative factor for very preterm birth.

Keywords: chorioamnionitis, intraventricular hemorrhage, very preterm infant, systematic review, meta-analysis

INTRODUCTION

Germinal matrix hemorrhage–intraventricular hemorrhage (GMH-IVH) is one of the most common complications of prematurity (Ballabh, 2010; Volpe, 2015; Inder et al., 2018). IVH typically initiates in the germinal matrix, which is a richly vascularized collection of neuronal-glial precursor cells in the developing brain and may disrupt the ependymal lining and extend into the lateral ventricle (Ballabh, 2010; Volpe, 2015; Inder et al., 2018). Severe IVH (grade 3–4) is associated with increased mortality as well as short- and long-term neurological morbidity, whilst the short-term and long-term outcomes of milder forms of IVH (grade 1–2) are less established, and they remain a significant research area (Volpe, 2015; Tortora et al., 2017; Inder et al., 2018).

As extensively reviewed by Inder et al. (2018) the pathogenesis of IVH is multifactorial and may involve intravascular, vascular, and extravascular factors. Intravascular factors relate to the regulation of blood flow, pressure, and volume in the microvascular bed of the germinal matrix as well as to platelet-capillary function and blood clotting capability (Inder et al., 2018). Vascular factors refer to the intrinsic fragility and vulnerability of germinal matrix blood vessels (Inder et al., 2018). Extravascular factors include the poor support of the extravascular space surrounding the germinal matrix capillaries, the postnatal decrease in extravascular tissue pressure, and an excessive fibrinolytic activity (Inder et al., 2018). As assessed by Inder et al. (2018) not all the pathogenetic factors are present in every IVH and the clinical circumstances determine which factors are most relevant in each infant. Among these clinical circumstances, very preterm birth, generally defined as birth before 32 completed weeks of gestation, is the most consistently associated with the development of IVH. However, a number of risk factors including, among others, absent antenatal corticosteroid (ACS) treatment, vaginal delivery, peri- and postnatal hypoxic-ischemic events, severe respiratory distress syndrome (RDS), pneumothorax, hypercapnia, hemodynamic disturbances (either systemic hypertension or hypotension), rapid volume expansion, decreased hematocrit, glucose and/or electrolyte disturbances, seizures, patent ductus arteriosus (PDA), thrombocytopenia, inherited thrombophilia, and infection may predispose to the development of IVH (Ballabh, 2010; Ramenghi et al., 2011; Volpe, 2015; Bermick et al., 2016; Romantsik et al., 2017; Inder et al., 2018; Poryo et al., 2018).

Several studies suggest that IVH is unequally distributed among the different leading causes of very preterm delivery (DiSalvo, 1998; Chevallier et al., 2017). An estimated 40% of very preterm births are associated with placental inflammation, which is often subclinical. This inflammation may be localized to the maternal placenta or membrane (chorioamnionitis) or may extend to the fetus, inducing an inflammatory response, which is evidenced by funisitis (Cornette, 2004; Gantert et al., 2010; Tita and Andrews, 2010; Thomas and Speer, 2011; Pugni et al., 2016; Jackson et al., 2017). Chorioamnionitis (CA) is not only a major risk factor for (very) preterm birth, but it is also considered a major risk factor for the morbidity and mortality associated with prematurity (Cornette, 2004; Gantert et al., 2010; Tita and Andrews, 2010; Thomas and Speer, 2011; Pugni et al., 2016; Jackson et al., 2017). The pathogenetic role of CA in the development of complications of prematurity, such as necrotizing enterocolitis (NEC), bronchopulmonary dysplasia (BPD), PDA, retinopathy of prematurity (ROP), or cerebral palsy has been addressed in several systematic reviews (Wu and Colford, 2000; Hartling et al., 2012; Been et al., 2013; Mitra et al., 2014; Park et al., 2015; Behbodi et al., 2016; Villamor-Martinez et al., 2018a). Although intrauterine inflammation is a well-known risk factor for white matter disease of prematurity (Strunk et al., 2014), the association with IVH is controversial and has not been yet systematically reviewed. Moreover, a consideration with any analysis of CA as a risk factor for preterm morbidity, is accounting for the role of GA, birth weight (BW) and other baseline characteristics which differ between CA-exposed and CA-unexposed infants (Hartling et al., 2012; Mitra et al., 2014; Behbodi et al., 2016; Villamor-Martinez et al., 2018a). With this in mind, we aimed to perform a systematic review and meta-analysis of studies exploring the association between CA and IVH, as well as the role of potential confounding factors.

METHODS

The methodology followed the same structure as earlier meta-analyses on CA and ROP (Villamor-Martinez et al., 2018a), and CA and PDA (Behbodi et al., 2016). We developed a protocol a priori, which specified the objectives, inclusion criteria, method for evaluating study quality, included outcomes and covariates, and statistical methodology. We report the study according to the guidelines for Preferred Reporting Items for Systematic Reviews and Meta-Analysis (PRISMA) (Moher et al., 2009).

Sources and Search Strategy

We performed a comprehensive literature search in the PubMed/MEDLINE and EMBASE databases from their inception to July 1, 2017. The search strategy involved combining the following keywords in various ways: "chorioamnionitis," "intrauterine infection," "intrauterine inflammation," "antenatal infection," "antenatal inflammation," "intraventricular hemorrhage," "risk factors," "outcome," "cohort," and "case-control." No studies were excluded based on language. In addition, we used the following strategies to identify additional studies: review of reference lists of previous systematic reviews on CA, and of articles included in the present review, and the use of the "cited by" tool in Web of Science and Google Scholar.

Study Selection

We included studies which evaluated infants who were preterm (<37 weeks) or low BW (<2,500g), as well as studies which used stricter inclusion criteria. Studies were included if they reported primary data on the association between CA-exposure and IVH. We included studies which reported the rate of IVH in infants with and without CA, and studies which reported the rate of CA in infants with and without IVH. The results of the total search were screened independently by two reviewers (O.M.R, E.V.), in several rounds: first by title only, second by title and abstract, and thirdly by consulting the full text. The reviewers resolved discrepancies in inclusion through discussion and by consulting a third reviewer (P.D).

Data Extraction

Using a predetermined worksheet, two researchers (E.V.-M., O.M.R.) extracted data from the studies included. Another two investigators (P.D., E.V.) checked the extracted data for accuracy and completeness. We resolved discrepancies by discussion and through checking the primary report. The following data were extracted from each study: citation information, location of study, primary objective, criteria for inclusion/exclusion of infants, definitions used for CA and for IVH, infant baseline characteristics in the total group and the CA-exposed and CA-unexposed groups, and reported results on the outcomes of interest (including raw numbers, summary statistics and adjusted analyses on CA and IVH where available).

Quality Assessment

We used the Newcastle-Ottawa Scale (NOS) for cohort or case-control studies to assess the methodological quality of included studies. Three aspects of a study are evaluated by the NOS: selection, comparability and exposure/outcome, and these are scored individually and tallied up to a total of 9 points. Two researchers (E.V.-M. and E.V.) independently used the NOS to evaluate the quality of each study, and discrepancies were discussed and resolved by consensus.

Statistical Analysis

We combined and analyzed studies using COMPREHENSIVE META-ANALYSIS V 3.0 software (CMA, RRID:SCR_012779, Biostat Inc., Englewood, NJ, USA). We calculated the odds ratio (OR) and 95% confidence intervals (CI) for dichotomous outcomes from the data extracted from the studies. We calculated the mean difference (MD) and 95% CI for continuous outcomes. We used the method of Wan et al. (2014) to estimate the mean and standard deviation, when continuous variables were reported as median and range/interquartile range in studies. We used a random-effects model to calculate summary statistics, due to anticipated heterogeneity. This method accounts for both intra-study and inter-study variability.

A mixed-effects model was used for subgroup analyses (Borenstein et al., 2009a). This model is characterized by a random-effects model that combines studies within subgroups, and a fixed-effects model that combines subgroups together to create an overall effect. This model does not assume that study-to-study variance (tau-squared) is the same in all subgroups. We assessed statistical heterogeneity using the Cochran's Q statistic, which reflects the degree of variance, and the I^2-statistic, which describes the proportion of observed variance that is due to variance in true effect sizes rather than sampling error (Borenstein et al., 2009b). Visual inspection of funnel plots and Egger's regression test were used to evaluate evidence of publication bias.

We used univariate random-effects meta-regression (method of moments) to evaluate covariates which may affect the effect size (Borenstein et al., 2009c). We defined the following covariates a priori as potential sources of variability: CA type (clinical or histological), funisitis, differences in GA and BW between the infants with and without CA, use of ACS, mode of delivery, rate of preeclampsia, rate of small for gestational age (SGA), rate of premature rupture of membranes (PROM), rate of RDS, rate of PDA, rate of early onset sepsis (EOS), rate of late onset sepsis (LOS) and mortality. We considered probability values under 0.05 (0.10 for heterogeneity) as statistically significant.

RESULTS

Description of Studies

After removing duplicates, we found 1,284 potentially relevant studies, of which 85 (Morales, 1987; Yoon et al., 1995; Gray et al., 1997; Alexander et al., 1998; Watterberg et al., 1999; Dexter et al., 2000; Elimian et al., 2000; Kosuge et al., 2000; Hitti et al., 2001; Suarez et al., 2001; González-Luis et al., 2002; Ohyama et al., 2002; Fung et al., 2003; Holcroft et al., 2003; Linder et al., 2003; Ogunyemi et al., 2003; Vergani et al., 2004; Dempsey et al., 2005; Lau et al., 2005; Osmanagaoglu et al., 2005; Polam et al., 2005; Sarkar et al., 2005; Babnik et al., 2006; Kaukola et al., 2006; Mehta et al., 2006; Richardson et al., 2006; Rocha et al., 2006; Yanowitz et al., 2006; Kirchner et al., 2007; Baumert et al., 2008; Mu et al., 2008; Zanardo et al., 2008; Been et al., 2009; Soraisham et al., 2009, 2013; Suppiej et al., 2009; Austeng et al., 2010; Botet et al., 2010; Kallankari et al., 2010; Lee et al., 2010, 2011; Mestan et al., 2010; Alfiero Bordigato et al., 2011; Barrera-Reyes et al., 2011; Hendson et al., 2011; Lim et al., 2011; Ryckman et al., 2011; Sato et al., 2011; Wirbelauer et al., 2011; Ahn et al., 2012; Klebermass-Schrehof et al., 2012; Perrone et al., 2012; Poralla et al., 2012; Rong et al., 2012; Vaihinger et al., 2012; van Vliet et al., 2012; Xu et al., 2012; Adén et al., 2013; Erdemir et al., 2013; Gawade et al., 2013; Logan et al., 2013; Nasef et al., 2013; Salas et al., 2013; Seliga-Siwecka and Kornacka, 2013; Trevisanuto et al., 2013; Tsiartas et al., 2013; Arayici et al., 2014; Ecevit et al., 2014; Gagliardi et al., 2014; García-Muñoz Rodrigo et al., 2014; Kidokoro et al., 2014; Liu et al., 2014; Pappas et al., 2014; Shankaran et al., 2014; Bry et al., 2015; Dalton et al., 2015; Kim et al., 2015; Oh et al., 2015, 2018; Smit et al., 2015; Yamada et al., 2015; Bermick et al., 2016; Lu et al., 2016; Miyazaki et al., 2016; Rodríguez-Trujillo et al., 2016) met the inclusion criteria. **Figure 1** depicts the PRISMA flow diagram of the search. The included studies evaluated 46,244 infants, including 13,432 cases of CA. The characteristics of the included studies are summarized in **Supplementary Table 1**. Fifty-eight studies examined the outcomes of maternal CA and included IVH as one of the outcomes. Twenty-four studies evaluated risk factors for developing IVH and included maternal CA as of the risk factors. Five studies studied the association between CA and IVH as their primary outcome (De Felice et al., 2001; Sarkar et al., 2005; Babnik et al., 2006; Mehta et al., 2006; Zanardo et al., 2008). Fifty-four studies used a histological definition of CA and 24 studies used a clinical definition of CA. Only two studies (Hitti et al., 2001; Kirchner et al., 2007) examined microbiological CA and IVH. One study (Nasef et al., 2013) provided data on IVH and its association with histological and clinical CA separately.

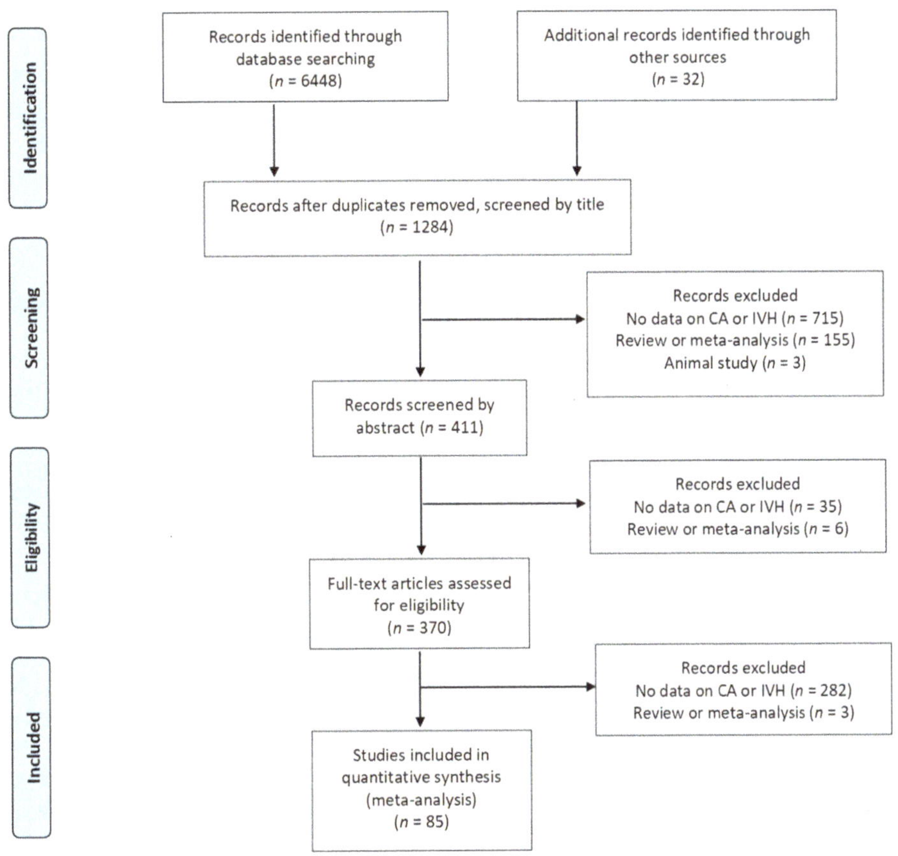

FIGURE 1 | Flow diagram of search process (Moher et al., 2009).

In four studies (Gray et al., 1997; Fung et al., 2003; Klebermass-Schrehof et al., 2012; Xu et al., 2012) infants were assigned to the CA group if they presented histological and/or clinical CA.

Quality Assessment

A summary of the quality assessment of each study using the NOS is shown in **Supplementary Table 2**. One study received a quality score of 5 points, 19 studies achieved a quality score of six points, 43 studies achieved a quality score of seven points, 11 studies achieved a quality score of eight, and 11 studies achieved the maximum score of 9 points. Studies were downgraded in quality for not adjusting the risk of IVH for confounders ($k = 62$), for not defining IVH clearly ($k = 9$), for only adjusting the risk of IVH for one confounding factor ($k = 7$), for not defining CA clearly ($k = 6$), and for losing a substantial portion of infants to follow-up ($k = 4$).

Analysis Based on Unadjusted Data

Meta-analysis showed that CA exposure was significantly associated with all grades IVH (**Figure 2A**), with grades 2–4 IVH (**Figure 2B**), with grades 1–2 IVH (**Figure 2C**), and with grades 3–4 IVH (**Figure 2D**). When the type of CA was analyzed separately, histological CA remained significantly associated with all grades IVH (**Figure 3**), with grades 2–4 IVH (**Figure 2B**), with grades 1–2 IVH (**Figure 2C**), and with grades 3–4 IVH (**Figure 4**). Clinical CA was significantly associated with all grades IVH (**Figure 5**) and with grades 3–4 IVH (**Figure 6**), but not with grades 1–2 IVH (**Figure 2C**). There was only one study providing data on the association of clinical CA and IVH grades 2–4 (**Figure 2B**). We could not find significant evidence of publication bias through visual inspection of the funnel plot (**Figure 7**), or through Egger's regression test.

Analysis of Covariates

To confirm findings from earlier reports (Behbodi et al., 2016; Villamor-Martinez et al., 2018a) on the differences in baseline and clinical characteristics between infants with and without CA, we carried out further meta-analyses. Infants exposed to CA had significantly lower GA and BW, as shown in **Table 1**. Moreover, infants with CA had significantly higher rates of exposure to ACS, significantly higher rates of PROM, significantly higher rates of EOS, significantly higher rates of LOS, and significantly higher rates of PDA (**Table 1**). Infants with CA also had significantly lower rates of cesarean delivery, significantly lower rates of small for gestational age (SGA) and significantly lower rates of preeclampsia (**Table 1**).

We carried out meta-regression analysis to determine the possible influence of GA and BW on the association between CA

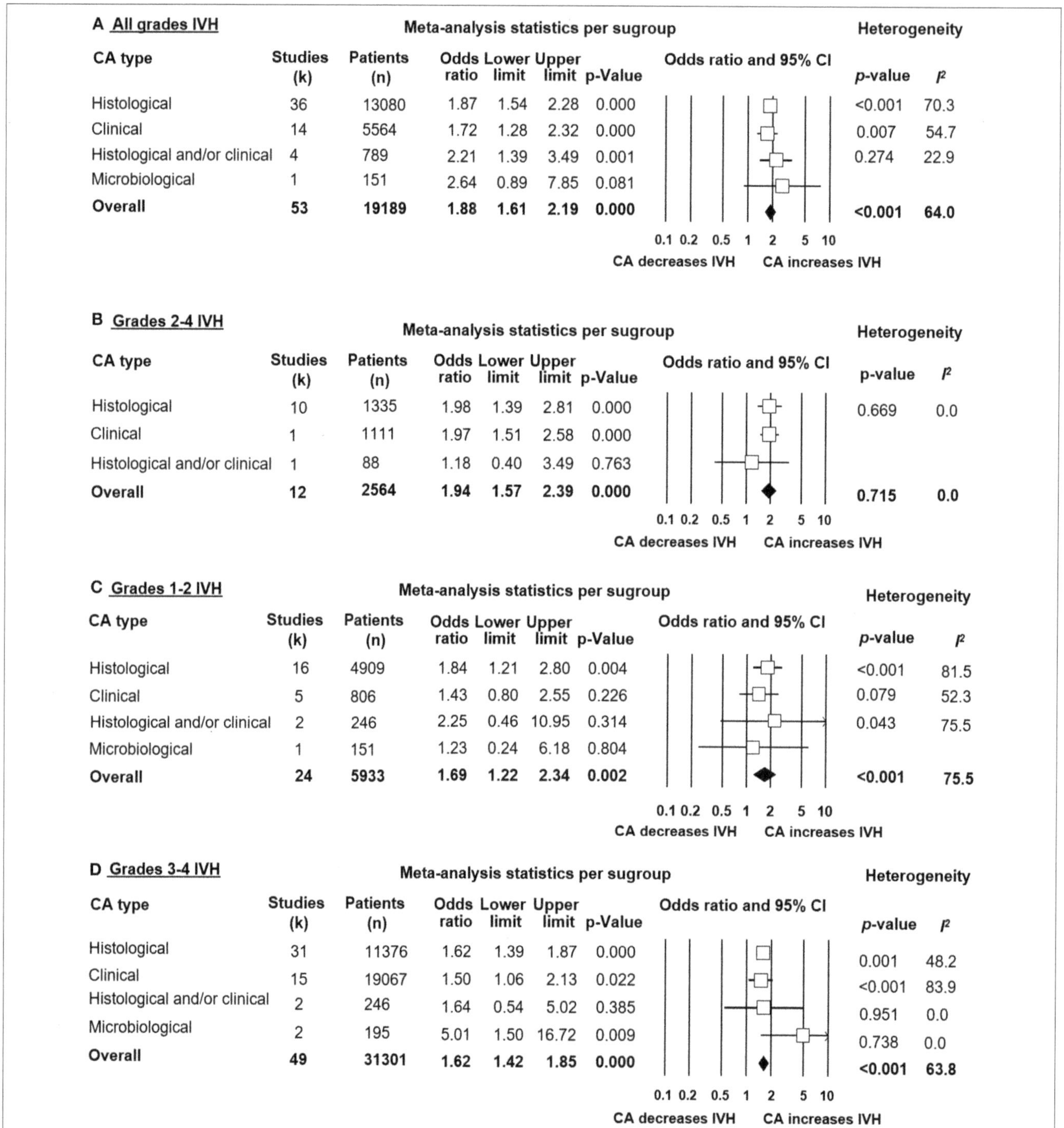

A All grades IVH — Meta-analysis statistics per sugroup

CA type	Studies (k)	Patients (n)	Odds ratio	Lower limit	Upper limit	p-Value	Heterogeneity *p*-value	I^2
Histological	36	13080	1.87	1.54	2.28	0.000	<0.001	70.3
Clinical	14	5564	1.72	1.28	2.32	0.000	0.007	54.7
Histological and/or clinical	4	789	2.21	1.39	3.49	0.001	0.274	22.9
Microbiological	1	151	2.64	0.89	7.85	0.081		
Overall	**53**	**19189**	**1.88**	**1.61**	**2.19**	**0.000**	**<0.001**	**64.0**

B Grades 2-4 IVH — Meta-analysis statistics per sugroup

CA type	Studies (k)	Patients (n)	Odds ratio	Lower limit	Upper limit	p-Value	Heterogeneity p-value	I^2
Histological	10	1335	1.98	1.39	2.81	0.000	0.669	0.0
Clinical	1	1111	1.97	1.51	2.58	0.000		
Histological and/or clinical	1	88	1.18	0.40	3.49	0.763		
Overall	**12**	**2564**	**1.94**	**1.57**	**2.39**	**0.000**	**0.715**	**0.0**

C Grades 1-2 IVH — Meta-analysis statistics per sugroup

CA type	Studies (k)	Patients (n)	Odds ratio	Lower limit	Upper limit	p-Value	Heterogeneity *p*-value	I^2
Histological	16	4909	1.84	1.21	2.80	0.004	<0.001	81.5
Clinical	5	806	1.43	0.80	2.55	0.226	0.079	52.3
Histological and/or clinical	2	246	2.25	0.46	10.95	0.314	0.043	75.5
Microbiological	1	151	1.23	0.24	6.18	0.804		
Overall	**24**	**5933**	**1.69**	**1.22**	**2.34**	**0.002**	**<0.001**	**75.5**

D Grades 3-4 IVH — Meta-analysis statistics per sugroup

CA type	Studies (k)	Patients (n)	Odds ratio	Lower limit	Upper limit	p-Value	Heterogeneity *p*-value	I^2
Histological	31	11376	1.62	1.39	1.87	0.000	0.001	48.2
Clinical	15	19067	1.50	1.06	2.13	0.022	<0.001	83.9
Histological and/or clinical	2	246	1.64	0.54	5.02	0.385	0.951	0.0
Microbiological	2	195	5.01	1.50	16.72	0.009	0.738	0.0
Overall	**49**	**31301**	**1.62**	**1.42**	**1.85**	**0.000**	**<0.001**	**63.8**

FIGURE 2 | Meta-analyses of the association between chorioamnionitis (CA) and intraventricular hemorrhage (IVH), according to definition of IVH. CI, confidence interval. **(A)** CA and all grades IVH; **(B)** CA and grades 2-4 IVH; **(C)** CA and grades 1–2 IVH; **(D)** CA and grades 3–4 IVH.

and IVH. As **Table 2** shows, meta-regression did not find that differences in GA or BW had a significant effect on the association between CA and IVH.

To further analyze the effect of GA on the risk of IVH, we carried out subgroup analyses. We found that in the group of studies where the CA-group did not differ significantly ($p > 0.05$) in GA from the control group, CA was a risk factor for all grades IVH but not for grades 3–4 IVH (**Table 3**). We analyzed a subgroup of studies where the CA-group had a MD in GA of $\leq$0.5 weeks, and we found that CA was a risk factor for all grades IVH

Study name	ALL IVH-Yes / Total CA-Yes	CA-No	Statistics for each study Odds ratio	Lower limit	Upper limit	p-Value	Relative Weight (%)
Sarkar 2005	3 / 29	6 / 33	0.52	0.12	2.30	0.388	1.31
Kosuge 2000	4 / 44	5 / 37	0.64	0.16	2.58	0.531	1.44
Seong-Hee 2015			0.72	0.23	2.18	0.555	1.95
Dempsey 2005	11 / 130	21 / 200	0.79	0.37	1.69	0.542	2.90
Watterberg 1999	8 / 22	7 / 18	0.90	0.25	3.25	0.870	1.61
Ecevit 2014	4 / 21	3 / 15	0.94	0.18	5.00	0.943	1.10
Suppiej 2009	5 / 41	8 / 63	0.95	0.29	3.15	0.940	1.78
Richardson 2006	66 / 292	78 / 368	1.09	0.75	1.57	0.665	4.36
Mu 2008	15 / 64	11 / 55	1.22	0.51	2.95	0.651	2.55
Tsiartas 2013	31 / 142	16 / 89	1.27	0.65	2.49	0.480	3.22
Liu 2014	23 / 49	18 / 46	1.38	0.61	3.11	0.443	2.74
Elimian 2000	169 / 527	170 / 733	1.56	1.22	2.01	0.000	4.75
Zanardo 2008	11 / 68	22 / 219	1.73	0.79	3.78	0.170	2.85
Logan 2013	26 / 335	27 / 586	1.74	1.00	3.04	0.050	3.65
Miyazaki 2016	243 / 1235	350 / 2843	1.74	1.46	2.09	0.000	4.94
Lee. Hyun Ju 2011	33 / 71	25 / 76	1.77	0.91	3.46	0.093	3.24
Rocha 2006	31 / 125	50 / 327	1.83	1.10	3.03	0.019	3.85
Been 2009	24 / 121	21 / 180	1.87	0.99	3.54	0.054	3.35
Mehta 2006	30 / 64	31 / 100	1.96	1.03	3.76	0.041	3.31
Dexter 2000	60 / 157	28 / 118	1.99	1.17	3.39	0.011	3.74
Nasef 2013	26 / 95	23 / 146	2.02	1.07	3.80	0.030	3.36
Babnik 2006	23 / 49	23 / 76	2.04	0.97	4.29	0.061	2.97
Bermick 2016	58 / 88	62 / 128	2.06	1.17	3.61	0.012	3.64
Dalton 2015	58 / 88	62 / 128	2.06	1.17	3.61	0.012	3.64
Sato 2011	54 / 158	28 / 144	2.15	1.27	3.65	0.004	3.76
Yanowitz 2006	16 / 24	12 / 25	2.17	0.68	6.88	0.190	1.86
Soraisham 2013	55 / 197	27 / 187	2.30	1.37	3.83	0.002	3.82
van Vliet 2012	9 / 21	12 / 51	2.44	0.83	7.17	0.106	2.02
Lu 2016	21 / 60	12 / 77	2.92	1.29	6.57	0.010	2.75
Erdemir 2013	3 / 12	4 / 45	3.42	0.65	18.00	0.147	1.11
Polam 2005	36 / 102	10 / 75	3.55	1.63	7.73	0.001	2.85
Ohyama 2002	11 / 90	2 / 53	3.55	0.76	16.68	0.108	1.23
Perrone 2012	31 / 48	13 / 44	4.35	1.81	10.45	0.001	2.55
Bordigato 2010	6 / 14	2 / 15	4.88	0.78	30.29	0.089	0.95
Bry 2015	4 / 16	0 / 8	6.12	0.29	129.08	0.244	0.39
Ogunyemi 2003	181 / 254	120 / 520	8.26	5.88	11.61	0.000	4.47
HISTOLOGICAL OVERALL			**1.87**	**1.54**	**2.28**	**0.000**	

Heterogeneity: Q = 114; I^2 = 70.3%; $p < 0.00001$

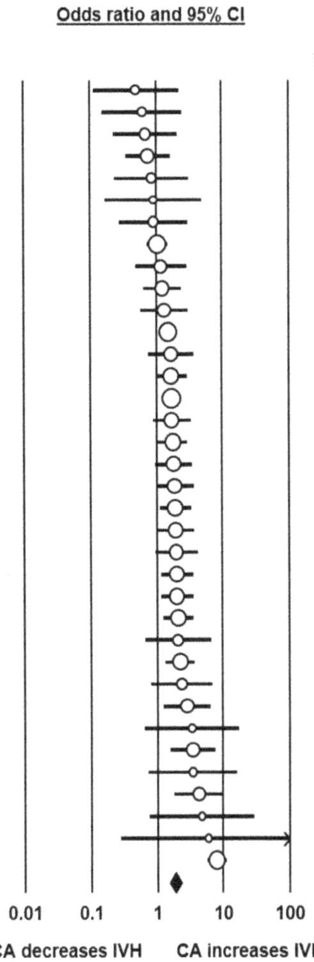

FIGURE 3 | Meta-analysis of the association between histological chorioamnionitis (CA) and all grades intraventricular hemorrhage (IVH). CI, confidence interval.

and for grades 3–4 IVH (**Table 3**). We also found that in studies where the CA-group had a MD in GA of less than 1 week, CA was a risk factor for all grades IVH and for grades 3–4 IVH (**Table 3**).

To evaluate the role of other prespecified covariates in the association between CA and IVH, we performed additional meta-regression analyses. Meta-regression could not find a significant difference in IVH risk between infants with clinical and infants with histological CA (**Table 4**). Meta-regression did find a significant association between the CA-associated risk of grades 3–4 IVH and the risk of preeclampsia (**Supplementary Figure 1**), mortality (**Supplementary Figure 2**), risk of LOS (**Supplementary Figure 3**) and risk of PDA (**Supplementary Figure 4**) Other meta-regressions could not find a significant association between the CA-associated risk of IVH and other covariates (**Table 4**).

Analysis of Funisitis

To evaluate the role of funisitis (i.e., fetal inflammatory response) in the development of IVH, we carried out further meta-analyses. Thirteen studies reported on IVH (Ohyama et al., 2002; Lau et al., 2005; Babnik et al., 2006; Richardson et al., 2006; Rocha et al., 2006; Been et al., 2009; Mestan et al., 2010; Logan et al., 2013; Trevisanuto et al., 2013; Tsiartas et al., 2013; Liu et al., 2014; Kim et al., 2015; Smit et al., 2015) in infants with histological CA with or without funisitis. As shown in **Figure 8**, meta-analysis could not show a significant difference in IVH risk between infants with funisitis and infants with CA without funisitis (OR all grades IVH: 1.22, 95% CI 0.89 to 1.67; grades 3-4 IVH: 1.17, 95% CI 0.74 to 1.85). Using meta-regression, we also found no significant difference in IVH risk between infants with funisitis, and infants with CA without funisitis (**Table 4**).

Analysis Based on Adjusted Data

Thirteen studies adjusted the association between CA and the risk of IVH for confounding factors. As shown in **Supplementary Tables 3, 4**, studies adjusted for different covariates. Meta-analysis pooling this adjusted data found that CA was significantly associated with a higher risk of all grades IVH (OR 1.25, 95% CI 1.02–1.53, **Supplementary Table 3**). This association became non-significant when only

Study name	Grades 3-4 IVH-Yes / Total CA-Yes	CA-No	Odds ratio	Lower limit	Upper limit	p-Value	Relative Weight (%)
Wirbelauer 2011	0 / 17	6 / 54	0.21	0.01	3.98	0.301	0.25
Nasef HC 2013	0 / 95	3 / 146	0.21	0.01	4.20	0.311	0.24
Zanardo 2008	0 / 68	3 / 219	0.45	0.02	8.85	0.600	0.24
Trevisanuto 2013	2 / 71	4 / 71	0.49	0.09	2.74	0.413	0.71
Smit 2015	5 / 135	8 / 165	0.75	0.24	2.36	0.629	1.59
Been 2009	5 / 121	8 / 180	0.93	0.30	2.90	0.896	1.59
Mu 2008	11 / 64	9 / 55	1.06	0.40	2.79	0.905	2.18
Rodríguez-Trujillo 2016	11 / 111	5 / 54	1.08	0.35	3.27	0.895	1.67
Lee. Ju Young 2010	18 / 79	21 / 98	1.08	0.53	2.21	0.829	3.81
Sarkar 2005	2 / 29	2 / 33	1.15	0.15	8.71	0.894	0.52
Pappas 2014	259 / 1063	179 / 855	1.22	0.98	1.51	0.073	20.39
Tsiartas 2013	2 / 142	1 / 89	1.26	0.11	14.07	0.853	0.37
Seliga-Siwecka 2013	69 / 141	103 / 242	1.29	0.85	1.96	0.227	9.28
Liu 2014	5 / 49	3 / 46	1.63	0.37	7.24	0.522	0.95
Watterberg 1999	2 / 22	1 / 18	1.70	0.14	20.42	0.676	0.35
Ogunyemi 2003	17 / 254	21 / 520	1.70	0.88	3.29	0.112	4.40
Elimian 2000	79 / 527	66 / 733	1.78	1.26	2.52	0.001	11.99
Hendson 2011	58 / 298	38 / 319	1.79	1.15	2.79	0.010	8.44
Kim 2015	7 / 92	6 / 143	1.88	0.61	5.78	0.271	1.64
Dexter 2000	19 / 156	8 / 117	1.89	0.80	4.48	0.149	2.69
Arayici 2014	20 / 145	9 / 136	2.26	0.99	5.15	0.053	2.93
Salas 2013	35 / 148	24 / 199	2.27	1.28	4.02	0.005	5.61
Rocha 2006	18 / 125	22 / 327	2.33	1.20	4.52	0.012	4.36
Lau 2005	32 / 403	29 / 893	2.53	1.51	4.23	0.000	6.67
Soraisham 2013	20 / 197	8 / 187	2.53	1.09	5.89	0.032	2.79
Yamada 2015	18 / 73	4 / 39	2.86	0.89	9.17	0.076	1.53
Yanowitz 2006	1 / 24	0 / 25	3.26	0.13	83.90	0.476	0.20
Bordigato 2010	1 / 14	0 / 15	3.44	0.13	91.79	0.460	0.20
Mestan 2010	6 / 94	3 / 162	3.61	0.88	14.80	0.074	1.06
Polam 2005	11 / 102	2 / 75	4.41	0.95	20.54	0.059	0.89
Ahn 2012	5 / 89	1 / 168	9.94	1.14	86.45	0.037	0.46
HISTOLOGICAL OVERALL			**1.62**	**1.39**	**1.87**	**0.000**	

Heterogeneity: Q = 33; I^2 = 10.0%; p =0.308

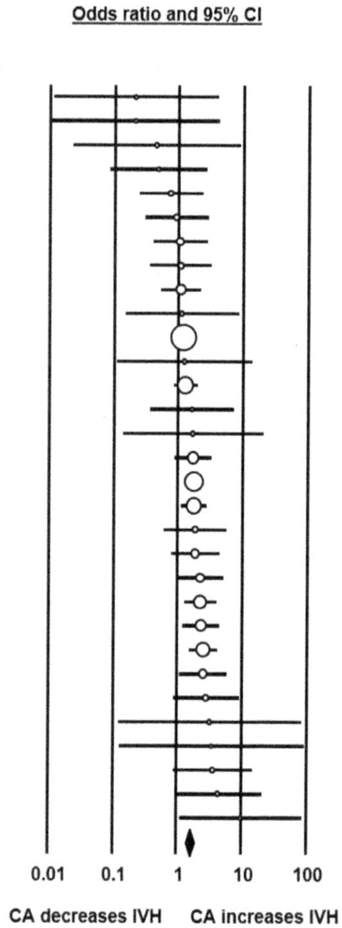

FIGURE 4 | Meta-analysis of the association between histological chorioamnionitis (CA) and grades 3–4 intraventricular hemorrhage (IVH). CI, confidence interval.

analyzing studies which used a histological definition of CA (**Supplementary Table 3**). Meta-analysis of adjusted data also found a significant association between CA and grades 3–4 IVH (OR 1.22, 95% CI 1.04–1.43, **Supplementary Table 4**). This association became non-significant when grouping studies by clinical or histological CA definition (**Supplementary Table 4**).

DISCUSSION

The current systematic review and meta-analysis demonstrates that both clinical and histological CA are associated with an increased risk for developing IVH in very preterm infants. In contrast, the presence of funisitis did not increase IVH risk when compared to CA in the absence of funisitis. We found through additional meta-analyses that CA-exposed infants had significantly lower GA and BW than infants not exposed to CA. However, meta-regression and subgroup analysis could not demonstrate an association between the lower GA and BW and the risk of IVH in the CA-exposed infants. This suggests that the effects of CA on IVH risk might be at least partially independent on the role of CA as an etiological factor for very preterm birth.

The association between CA and increased risk of IVH is biologically and clinically plausible. IVH generally occurs within the three first days of life and affects the infants with higher hemodynamic and respiratory instability, frequently associated with extreme prematurity and/or severe perinatal infections (Mohamed and Aly, 2010; Inder et al., 2018). Therefore, the clinical circumstances around birth and during the first days of life are critical for the development of IVH. Our study confirms previous reports showing that these clinical circumstances are different in CA-exposed and CA-unexposed very preterm infants (Hartling et al., 2012; Behbodi et al., 2016; Villamor-Martinez et al., 2018a). Thus, CA-exposed infants were born 1.2 weeks earlier, they were 55g lighter at birth, and they were more frequently exposed to ACS, PROM, vaginal delivery, early and late onset sepsis, and PDA. As mentioned in the introduction, some of these factors may have affected IVH risk.

The degree of prematurity is the most important predisposing factor for the occurrence of IVH (Ballabh, 2010; Volpe, 2015; Inder et al., 2018), as well as for other complications of prematurity such as BPD, ROP, NEC, or PDA (Hartling et al., 2012; Been et al., 2013; Mitra et al., 2014; Behbodi et al., 2016;

Study name	All IVH-Yes / Total CA-Yes	All IVH-Yes / Total CA-No	Odds ratio	Lower limit	Upper limit	p-Value	Relative Weight (%)
Ryckman 2011	6 / 33	41 / 186	0.79	0.30	2.03	0.619	5.74
Botet 2010	44 / 165	45 / 163	0.95	0.59	1.55	0.848	10.09
Holcroft 2003	16 / 45	61 / 168	0.97	0.49	1.92	0.926	7.96
Morales 1987	37 / 43	37 / 43	1.00	0.30	3.39	1.000	4.16
Rong 2012	16 / 44	63 / 188	1.13	0.57	2.25	0.719	7.98
Gawade 2013	6 / 12	28 / 66	1.36	0.40	4.65	0.627	4.10
Gonzalez-Luis 2002	11 / 45	16 / 90	1.50	0.63	3.57	0.363	6.35
Baumert 2008	21 / 101	371 / 2574	1.56	0.95	2.55	0.078	10.02
Vaihinger 2013	16 / 47	33 / 151	1.85	0.90	3.78	0.094	7.68
Poralla 2012	30 / 52	28 / 80	2.53	1.24	5.19	0.011	7.67
Barrera-Reyes 2011	11 / 23	19 / 81	2.99	1.14	7.86	0.026	5.62
Vergani 2004	12 / 73	33 / 580	3.26	1.60	6.64	0.001	7.72
Nasef 2013	13 / 33	23 / 146	3.48	1.52	7.96	0.003	6.68
Suarez 2001	22 / 52	34 / 228	4.18	2.16	8.09	0.000	8.23
CLINICAL OVERALL			**1.72**	**1.28**	**2.32**	**0.000**	

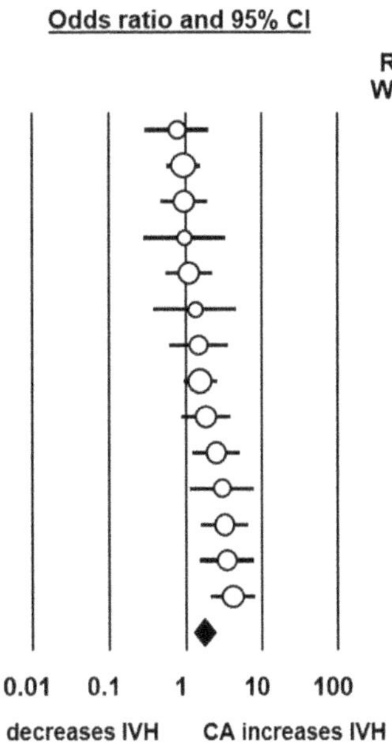

Heterogeneity: Q = 29; I^2 = 54.7%; p =0.007

FIGURE 5 | Meta-analysis of the association between clinical chorioamnionitis (CA) and all grades intraventricular hemorrhage (IVH). CI, confidence interval.

Study name	Grades 3-4 IVH-Yes / Total CA-Yes	Grades 3-4 IVH-Yes / Total CA-No	Odds ratio	Lower limit	Upper limit	p-Value	Relative weight
Kidokoro 2014			0.51	0.11	2.43	0.398	3.16
Linder 2003	6 / 25	30 / 80	0.53	0.19	1.46	0.219	5.24
Nasef CC 2013	0 / 33	3 / 146	0.61	0.03	12.13	0.747	1.11
Aden 2013	69 / 223	154 / 389	0.68	0.48	0.97	0.033	9.35
Lim 2011	4 / 9	32 / 63	0.78	0.19	3.16	0.722	3.64
Botet 2010	17 / 165	21 / 163	0.78	0.39	1.53	0.466	7.26
Morales 1987	12 / 43	12 / 43	1.00	0.39	2.57	1.000	5.67
De Felice CC 2001	11 / 81	43 / 402	1.31	0.65	2.67	0.454	7.06
Gonzalez-Luis 2002	4 / 45	6 / 90	1.37	0.37	5.11	0.643	3.95
Austeng 2010			1.40	0.71	2.75	0.329	7.29
Garcia-Muñoz 2014	215 / 1480	575 / 6850	1.85	1.57	2.19	0.000	10.15
Soraisham 2009	105 / 477	311 / 2617	2.09	1.63	2.67	0.000	9.86
Alexander 1998	23 / 95	145 / 1272	2.48	1.51	4.09	0.000	8.43
Gawade 2013	3 / 12	6 / 66	3.33	0.71	15.75	0.129	3.18
Gagliardi 2014	274 / 1510	120 / 2096	3.65	2.91	4.58	0.000	9.95
Osmanagaoglu 2005	6 / 31	8 / 223	6.45	2.07	20.10	0.001	4.70
CLINICAL OVERALL			**1.49**	**1.07**	**2.08**	**0.019**	

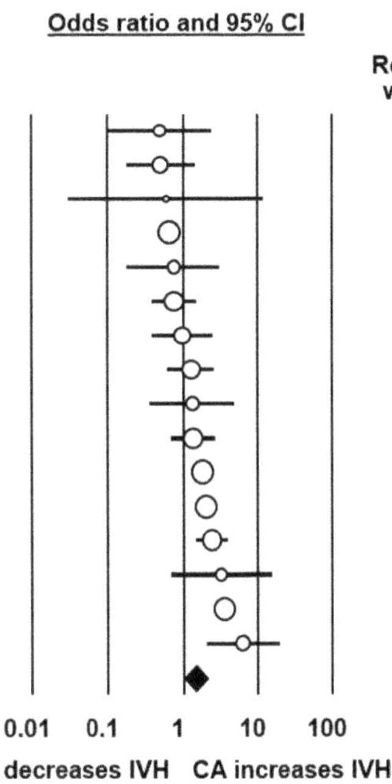

Heterogeneity: Q = 93; I^2 = 83.9%; $p < 0.001$

FIGURE 6 | Meta-analysis of the association between clinical chorioamnionitis (CA) and grades 3–4 intraventricular hemorrhage (IVH). CI, confidence interval.

Villamor-Martinez et al., 2018a). Nevertheless, very preterm birth is always a pathological event and very preterm infants have a morbidity and mortality risk associated with whichever condition led to their early delivery (McElrath et al., 2008; Wilcox et al., 2011; Gagliardi et al., 2013; Barros et al., 2015). Therefore, CA may affect infant morbidity through inducing very preterm birth or through the deleterious effects of infection/inflammation. Interestingly, previous meta-analyses showed an association between the lower gestational age of the CA-exposed group and the CA-associated risk of BPD (Hartling et al., 2012), PDA (Behbodi et al., 2016), and ROP (Mitra et al., 2014; Villamor-Martinez et al., 2018a). In contrast, our meta-regression could not show that the difference in GA between CA-exposed and CA-unexposed infants significantly correlated with IVH risk.

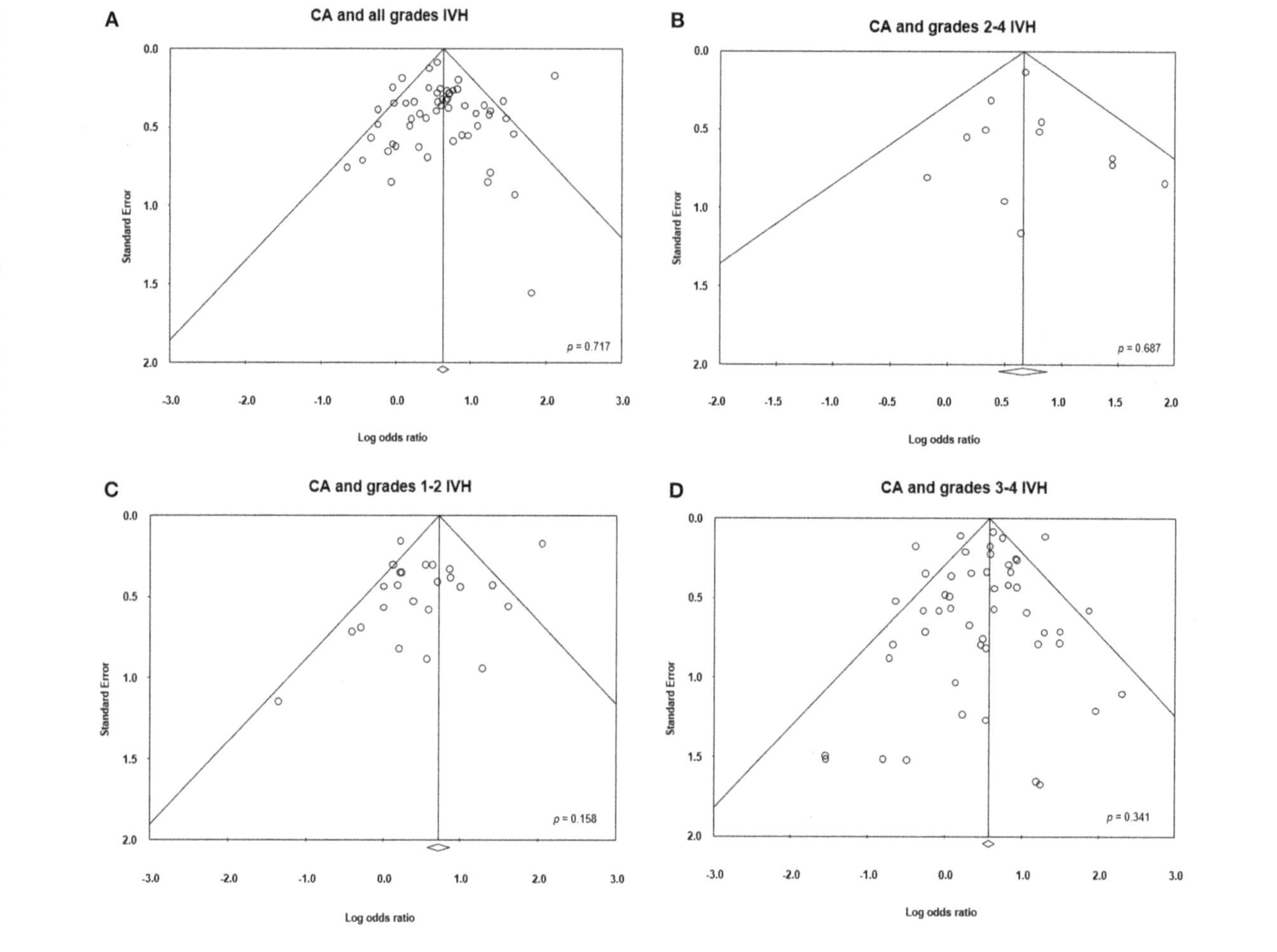

FIGURE 7 | Funnel plots assessing publication bias for the association between chorioamnionitis (CA) and intraventricular hemorrhage (IVH).

Moreover, we performed subgroup analyses in which we only included the studies showing small or no differences in GA between the CA-exposed and the control group and we observed that the significant IVH risk was maintained in this subgroup of studies. In contrast, this was not the case when the same subgroup analysis was performed for PDA (Behbodi et al., 2016) or ROP (Mitra et al., 2014; Villamor-Martinez et al., 2018a). Altogether this suggests that CA may increase complications such as PDA or ROP through GA-dependent mechanisms, whereas the effect on IVH may be mediated by GA-independent mechanisms.

Besides GA, several other factors potentially confound the association between CA and IVH. A number of studies provided data adjusted for confounding factors, but confounders accounted for in each model differed across studies. We performed separate analyses aggregating adjusted association measures. This reduced or made non-significant the association between CA and IVH (**Supplementary Tables 3, 4**). Earlier meta-analyses on the association between CA and cerebral palsy (Wu and Colford, 2000), BPD (Hartling et al., 2012), ROP (Villamor-Martinez et al., 2018a) also showed that the positive association found when unadjusted data were pooled, was reduced or became non-significant when only adjusted data were pooled. Moreover, in our previous meta-analysis on CA and PDA (Behbodi et al., 2016) we found that CA was risk factor for PDA when unadjusted data were pooled, and that CA was a protective factor for PDA when adjusted data were pooled.

Adjustment for potential confounders, particularly for GA and/or BW, is a common strategy used in observational studies analyzing predictors of outcomes of prematurity (Gagliardi et al., 2013). Quality assessment tools such as the NOS even downgrade studies for not adjusting for confounding factors. However, adjustment for GA and BW is controversial and can arguably lead to biased conclusions (Wilcox et al., 2011; Gagliardi et al., 2013). Preterm infants are at risk of adverse outcomes both due to their immaturity and due to the pathological conditions that led to their preterm birth (McElrath et al., 2008; Basso and Wilcox, 2010; Wilcox et al., 2011; Gagliardi et al., 2013). Very low GA is therefore both a risk factor for adverse outcomes, as well as a mediator in the causal pathway that links preterm birth to adverse outcomes (Wilcox et al., 2011; Gagliardi et al., 2013). The problem with adjusting for intermediate variables, such as GA, is that it may introduce bias unless each confounder is accounted

TABLE 1 | Meta-analysis of the association between chorioamnionitis and covariates.

Meta-analysis	Chorioamnionitis	*k*	Effect size	95% CI	*Z*	*p*	Heterogeneity		
							Q	*p*	I^2
Gestational age (weeks)	Clinical	11	MD −0.73	−1.16 to −0.30	−3.35	0.001	140	<0.001	92.9
	Histological	42	MD −1.27	−1.49 to −1.05	−11.42	<0.001	495	<0.001	91.7
	Any type	56	MD −1.20	−1.40 to −1.00	−11.66	<0.001	839	<0.001	93.4
Birth weight (g)	Clinical	11	MD −29.14	−77.66 to 19.39	−1.18	0.239	107	<0.001	90.6
	Histological	41	MD −70.21	−96.71 to −43.72	−5.19	<0.001	362	<0.001	89.0
	Any type	55	MD −55.00	−74.89 to −35.12	−5.42	<0.001	474	<0.001	88.6
Antenatal corticosteroids	Clinical	5	OR 1.10	0.76 to 1.60	0.52	0.605	55	<0.001	92.8
	Histological	31	OR 1.20	1.01 to 1.42	2.03	0.043	95	<0.001	68.3
	Any type	38	OR 1.19	1.02 to 1.38	2.28	0.023	155	<0.001	76.1
Cesarean section	Clinical	8	OR 0.53	0.30 to 0.93	−2.23	0.026	316	<0.001	97.8
	Histological	28	OR 0.33	0.25 to 0.45	−7.32	<0.001	177	<0.001	84.8
	Any type	36	OR 0.37	0.29 to 0.47	−8.06	<0.001	495	<0.001	92.9
SGA	Histological	15	OR 0.33	0.23 to 0.49	−5.53	<0.001	79	<0.001	82.3
	Any type	16	OR 0.34	0.23 to 0.50	−5.64	<0.001	80	<0.001	81.2
Preeclampsia	Clinical	3	OR 0.16	0.09 to 0.29	−5.98	<0.001	2	0.369	<0.001
	Histological	23	OR 0.15	0.11 to 0.20	−13.09	<0.001	65	<0.001	66.2
	Any type	27	OR 0.15	0.12 to 0.20	−15.25	<0.001	69	<0.001	62.2
PROM	Clinical	3	OR 5.02	2.71 to 9.31	5.12	<0.001	2	<0.001	18
	Histological	27	OR 3.14	2.54 to 3.87	10.63	<0.001	149	<0.001	82.6
	Any type	30	OR 3.29	2.70 to 4.02	11.76	<0.001	155	<0.001	81.3
Male sex	Clinical	8	OR 1.10	0.80 to 1.53	0.58	0.560	80	<0.001	91.2
	Histological	35	OR 0.99	0.89 to 1.11	−0.15	0.881	91	<0.001	62.8
	Any type	46	OR 1.00	0.90 to 1.12	0.07	0.941	193	<0.001	76.7
Maternal diabetes	Any type	9	OR 0.81	0.65 to 1.01	−1.92	0.055	5	0.725	0.0
EOS	Clinical	7	OR 4.41	3.58 to 5.42	14.08	<0.001	9	0.197	30.3
	Histological	18	OR 2.62	1.88 to 3.65	5.68	<0.001	48	<0.001	64.9
	Any type	25	OR 3.81	3.20 to 4.54	14.96	<0.001	87	<0.001	72.4
LOS	Clinical	5	OR 1.41	1.10 to 1.81	2.68	0.007	17	0.002	76.8
	Histological	30	OR 1.53	1.27 to 1.84	4.45	<0.001	134	<0.001	78.3
	Any type	37	OR 1.55	1.34 to 1.80	5.82	<0.001	174	<0.001	79.3
PDA	Clinical	4	OR 1.30	1.04 to 1.64	2.27	0.023	7	0.062	59.0
	Histological	26	OR 1.41	1.15 to 1.72	3.35	0.001	144	<0.001	82.6
	Any type	31	OR 1.60	1.35 to 1.80	6.00	<0.001	195	<0.001	84.6
RDS	Clinical	3	OR 2.01	0.48 to 8.41	0.95	0.341	11	0.004	82.0
	Histological	15	OR 1.09	0.81 to 1.45	0.55	0.582	89	<0.001	84.3
	Any type	21	OR 1.00	0.78 to 1.29	0.01	0.990	149	<0.001	86.6

CI, confidence interval; MD, mean difference; OR, odds ratio; SGA, small for gestational age; PROM, premature rupture of membranes; EOS, early-onset sepsis; LOS, late-onset sepsis; PDA, patent ductus arteriosus; RDS, respiratory distress syndrome.

for in the model (Hernández-Díaz et al., 2006; Basso and Wilcox, 2010; Wilcox et al., 2011; Gagliardi et al., 2013). As discussed by Gagliardi et al., "the difficulty of achieving—at least at the current level of knowledge of etiology of preterm birth—full control of all mediator-outcome confounders limits the possibility of causal interpretation of the associations found but not their descriptive

TABLE 2 | Random effects meta-regression of IVH risk in the chorioamnionitis group, and mean difference in gestational age and birth weight.

IVH grade	Meta-regression	k	CC	95% CI	Z	p	R^2
All grades IVH	Mean difference gestational age (per week)	35	−0.02	−0.19 to 0.16	−0.17	0.863	0.00
	Mean difference birth weight (per 100 g)	35	0.00	−0.001 to 0.001	0.07	0.942	0.00
Grades 1–2 IVH	Mean difference gestational age (per week)	20	0.05	−0.15 to 0.25	0.51	0.613	0.00
	Mean difference birth weight (per 100 g)	20	0.13	−0.07 to 0.33	1.27	0.203	0.54
Grades 3–4 IVH	Mean difference gestational age (per week)	37	−0.19	−0.43 to 0.04	−1.62	0.105	0.29
	Mean difference birth weight (per 100 g)	37	−0.10	−0.30 to 0.10	−1.01	0.312	0.00

IVH, intraventricular hemorrhage; k, number of included studies; CC, coefficient; CI, confidence interval.

TABLE 3 | Subgroup meta-analyses based on difference in gestational age (GA).

Subgroup of studies	IVH definition	k	OR	95% CI	p
Studies where CA-group did not differ significantly in GA from control ($p > 0.05$)	All grades IVH	15	1.59	1.20 to 2.10	0.001
	Grades 3–4 IVH	14	1.54	0.99 to 2.39	0.055
Studies where CA-group did differ significantly in GA from control ($p < 0.05$)	All grades IVH	20	1.71	1.46 to 2.01	< 0.001
	Grades 3–4 IVH	23	1.90	1.56 to 2.33	0.000
Studies where CA-group had a MD in GA of ≤0.5 weeks compared to control	All grades IVH	11	1.66	1.25 to 2.22	< 0.001
	Grades 3–4 IVH	13	1.36	1.03 to 1.80	0.028
Studies where CA-group had a MD in GA of >0.5 weeks compared to control	All grades IVH	24	1.68	1.43 to 1.98	< 0.001
	Grades 3–4 IVH	23	1.99	1.64 to 2.41	< 0.001
Studies where CA-group had a MD in GA of <1 weeks compared to control	All grades IVH	16	1.72	1.37 to 2.15	< 0.001
	Grades 3–4 IVH	18	1.52	1.21 to 1.92	< 0.001
Studies where CA-group had a MD in GA of ≥1 weeks compared to control	All grades IVH	19	1.65	1.37 to 1.97	< 0.001
	Grades 3–4 IVH	18	2.00	1.60 to 2.50	< 0.001

CA, chorioamnionitis; GA, gestational age; IVH, intraventricular hemorrhage; k, number of studies included; CI, confidence interval; MD, mean difference.

value" (121, p. 798). In this sense, by providing analysis of both the unadjusted and adjusted data, our study may be a valuable contribution to the understanding of CA as etiopathogenic factor of both prematurity and IVH.

Our data suggest that CA-exposed infants are not only younger but also more clinically unstable than the non-exposed infants. This is reflected in the higher mortality and the higher rate of sepsis and PDA in CA-exposed infants (**Table 1**). Of note, meta-regression showed a correlation between the effect size of the association between CA and grade 3-4 IVH and the effect sizes of the association between CA and PDA. As mentioned elsewhere, the presence of a hemodynamically relevant PDA has been correlated with the occurrence of IVH and the proposed mechanism is the disturbance of cerebral blood flow (Ballabh, 2010, 2014; Inder et al., 2018; Poryo et al., 2018). Our data support this association between IVH and PDA in CA-exposed infants.

The biological plausibility of the association between CA and IVH is supported by the direct and indirect effects of inflammatory mediators. Hemodynamic disturbances in preterm infants with CA have been correlated with elevated cord blood concentrations of proinflammatory cytokines such as IL-6, IL-1beta and TNF-alpha (Yanowitz et al., 2002). Cytokines can act directly on the vascular smooth muscle, producing vascular relaxation and hypotension or indirectly by increasing the production of endothelium-derived vasoactive mediators (Yanowitz et al., 2002). In addition, cytokines can eventually promote a neuro-inflammatory cascade in the fetal brain penetrating across the blood brain barrier or activating specific receptors such as CD14 and TLR4 which are constitutively expressed in the circumventricular organs, choroid plexus and leptomeninges (Rivest, 2003; McAdams and Juul, 2012). Inflamed glial or endothelial cells, challenged by external stimuli, enhance the release/expression of various chemoattractants and adhesion molecules which may promote the platelet and neutrophil activation and adhesion determining possible endothelial cell damage and changes in blood rheology and flow (Stanimirovic and Satoh, 2000; Molina-Holgado and Molina-Holgado, 2010). These changes, occurring inside the fragile germinal matrix capillaries or within the vascular connection between germinal matrix and the subependymal venous network, may increase the likelihood of IVH in preterm infants with CA.

TABLE 4 | Random effects meta-regression of IVH risk in the chorioamnionitis group, and predefined covariates.

IVH grade	Meta-regression	*k*	CC	95% CI	*Z*	*P*	R^2
All grades IVH	Chorioamnionitis type (histological/clinical)	49	−0.08	−0.45 to 0.29	−0.42	0.673	0.00
	Funisitis (CA+F+ vs. CA+F−)	9	−0.12	−0.62 to 0.38	−0.49	0.627	0.00
	ACS (log OR)	25	0.01	−0.46 to 0.49	0.05	0.964	0.00
	Cesarean section (log OR)	22	−0.07	−0.47 to 0.32	−0.36	0.717	0.00
	Maternal age (MD)	17	−0.08	−0.24 to 0.07	−1.09	0.276	0.00
	SGA (log OR)	11	0.39	−0.09 to 0.88	1.59	0.111	0.54
	PROM (log OR)	20	−0.40	−1.06 to 0.26	−1.19	0.233	0.08
	Preeclampsia (log OR)	16	0.03	−0.40 to 0.45	0.13	0.897	0.00
	Mortality (log OR)	26	0.18	−0.15 to 0.50	1.07	0.285	0.07
	Early onset sepsis (log OR)	14	0.13	−0.47 to 0.73	0.42	0.672	0.00
	Late onset sepsis (log OR)	24	−0.04	−0.39 to 0.32	−0.19	0.846	0.00
	PDA (log OR)	22	0.13	−0.21 to 0.48	0.75	0.453	0.00
	RDS (log OR)	21	0.02	−0.22 to 0.27	0.22	0.827	0.00
Grades 3–4 IVH	Chorioamnionitis type (histological/clinical)	46	−0.07	−0.44 to 0.30	−0.37	0.708	0.00
	Funisitis (CA+F+ vs. CA+F−)	8	0.07	−0.29 to 0.44	0.40	0.691	0.00
	ACS (log OR)	28	−0.11	−0.60 to 0.38	0.42	0.672	0.00
	Cesarean section (log OR)	27	0.08	−0.09 to 0.26	0.92	0.358	0.06
	Maternal age (MD)	18	−0.01	−0.25 to 0.22	−0.11	0.911	0.00
	SGA (log OR)	12	0.24	−0.19 to 0.67	1.08	0.280	0.22
	PROM (log OR)	22	−0.09	−0.35 to 0.17	−0.65	0.515	0.00
	Preeclampsia (log OR)	18	0.41	0.20 to 0.63	3.74	0.0004	1.00
	Mortality (log OR)	30	0.42	0.17 to 0.67	3.33	0.001	0.58
	Early onset sepsis (log OR)	20	0.11	−0.32 to 0.54	0.51	0.613	0.00
	Late onset sepsis (log OR)	26	0.35	0.01 to 0.70	1.99	0.047	0.22
	PDA (log OR)	21	0.40	0.04 to 0.76	2.18	0.029	0.48
	RDS (log OR)	27	−0.06	−0.34 to 0.21	−0.49	0.627	0.14

k, number of studies included; CA, chorioamnionitis; F, funisitis; CC, coefficient; CI, confidence interval; MD, mean difference; OR, odds ratio; ACS, antenatal corticosteroids; SGA, small for gestational age; PROM, premature rupture of membranes; PDA, patent ductus arteriosus; RDS, respiratory distress syndrome.

We have discussed the role of funisitis in earlier meta-analyses on CA and ROP (Villamor-Martinez et al., 2018a) and CA and PDA (Behbodi et al., 2016). It is worth noting that not all intraamniotic infections will induce an inflammatory response in the fetus (Revello et al., 2015). Funisitis is generally considered the histologic counterpart to fetal inflammatory response syndrome (Gantert et al., 2010; Revello et al., 2015). We found that exposure to funisitis did not significantly increase the risk of IVH, when compared to exposure to CA without funisitis. This is an argument against role of the fetal inflammatory response in the etiopathogenesis of IVH. We have previously reported that funisitis is not an additional risk factor for developing PDA (Behbodi et al., 2016) but the presence of funisitis significantly increased the risk of developing severe ROP (Villamor-Martinez et al., 2018a).

Our meta-analysis has several limitations that should be considered. Firstly, there was substantial heterogeneity in how CA was defined in studies. The definitions of clinical CA in particular varied substantially, and recent recommendations propose restricting the term CA to pathologic diagnosis (Higgins et al., 2016). Secondly, only 5 out of 85 included studies studied the association between CA and IVH as their main objective. However, this could also have reduced the effect of publication bias. Thirdly, only 13 out of the 85 included studies provided adjusted data, and they used different models and adjusted for different confounders. Finally, in this study and earlier studies on ROP (Villamor-Martinez et al., 2018a) and PDA (Behbodi et al., 2016), we had a much more limited number of studies to draw from for analyzing funisitis than when analyzing CA. The strengths of our study include: the use of a comprehensive search, duplication of screening, inclusion and data extraction to reduce bias, a large number of included studies, and an extensive analysis of confounding factors, through meta-analysis, meta-regression and the inclusion of adjusted data.

A significant limitation in any meta-analysis on IVH is the potential for heterogeneity in defining the condition. The grading system most commonly used for neonatal IVH was first reported by Papile et al. and later modified by Volpe and is based on the presence and amount of blood in the germinal matrix, lateral ventricles, and periventricular white matter (Volpe, 2015). Grade 1 represents germinal matrix hemorrhage only with no or minimal IVH (<10% of ventricular area on parasagittal view). When IVH occupies 10–50% of ventricular area on parasagittal view, it is defined as grade 2 (Volpe, 2015). Grade 3 is IVH with blood occupying more than 50%

	Study name	IVH-Yes / Total CA-Yes. Fun-Yes	IVH-Yes / Total CA-Yes. Fun-No	Odds ratio	Lower limit	Upper limit	p-Value
All gardes IVH	Ohyama 2002	0 / 8	11 / 82	0.37	0.02	6.78	0.499
	Logan 2013	9 / 147	17 / 188	0.66	0.28	1.52	0.324
	Rocha 2006	10 / 44	21 / 81	0.84	0.35	1.99	0.693
	Tsiartas 2013	11 / 45	20 / 97	1.25	0.54	2.88	0.608
	Richardson 2006	43 / 178	23 / 114	1.26	0.71	2.23	0.428
	Babnik 2006	14 / 27	9 / 22	1.56	0.50	4.85	0.446
	Been 2009	17 / 68	7 / 53	2.19	0.83	5.76	0.112
	Liu 2014	15 / 26	8 / 23	2.56	0.80	8.14	0.112
	All IVH			**1.22**	**0.89**	**1.67**	**0.226**
	Heteregeneity: Q = 7; I^2 = 0.0%; p = 0.467						
Grades 3-4 IVH	Trevisanuto 2013	1 / 44	1 / 27	0.60	0.04	10.09	0.726
	Rocha 2006	10 / 44	21 / 81	0.84	0.35	1.99	0.693
	Smit 2015	2 / 55	3 / 80	0.97	0.16	6.00	0.973
	Lau 2005	20 / 250	12 / 153	1.02	0.48	2.15	0.955
	Been 2009	3 / 68	2 / 53	1.18	0.19	7.31	0.861
	Kim 2015	3 / 31	4 / 61	1.53	0.32	7.29	0.596
	Mestan 2010	5 / 54	1 / 40	3.98	0.45	35.48	0.216
	Liu 2014	4 / 26	1 / 23	4.00	0.41	38.70	0.231
	Tsiartas 2013	2 / 45	0 / 97	11.21	0.53	238.38	0.121
	Severe IVH			**1.17**	**0.74**	**1.85**	**0.490**
	Heteregeneity: Q = 5; I^2 = 0.0%; p = 0.705						

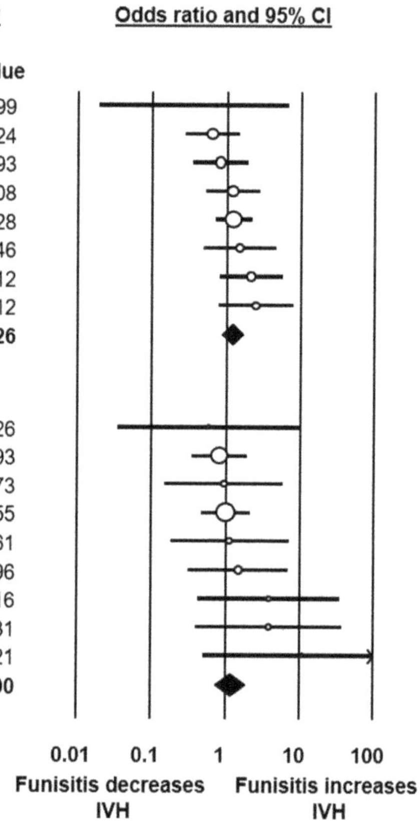

FIGURE 8 | Meta-analysis of the association between funisitis and intraventricular hemorrhage (IVH). Fun, funisitis; CI, confidence interval.

of the ventricular area on parasagittal view. Grade 4 represents severe IVH with associated periventricular echodensity (Volpe, 2015). Although grade 4 IVH is a periventricular hemorrhagic infarction rather than an extension of IVH *per se*, the 1–4 grading system remains pervasive in the literature and clinical setting despite debate regarding appropriate nomenclature (Leviton et al., 2007). In addition grade 3 and 4 IVHs are frequently grouped together as severe or high grade IVH (Leviton et al., 2007). Nevertheless, our meta-analysis shows a significant increased risk of both severe and less severe (grade 1–2) IVH in CA-exposed infants. Therefore, potential differences in IVH classification may not have affected the results.

CONCLUSION

IVH is a multifactorial complication that is more common in more preterm and more clinically unstable infants. We established for the first time through meta-analysis that CA is a risk factor for IVH. We also confirmed earlier findings that CA is a risk factor for being born more preterm and presenting more clinical instability. However, in contrast to other complications of prematurity, such as PDA, ROP, or BPD (Hartling et al., 2012; Mitra et al., 2014; Behbodi et al., 2016; Villamor-Martinez et al., 2018a), the effect of CA on IVH appears to be independent of CA as a causative factor for very preterm birth.

AUTHOR CONTRIBUTIONS

EV-M carried out data collection, carried out statistical analyses, assessed methodological quality, contributed to interpretation of results, drafted the initial manuscript, and reviewed and revised the manuscript. MF contributed to the design of the study, the statistical analysis and interpretation of results and reviewed and revised the manuscript. OM selected studies for inclusion, carried out data collection and carried out statistical analyses. SP contributed to interpretation of results and reviewed and revised the manuscript. GC contributed to interpretation of results and reviewed and revised the manuscript. PD carried out and supervised data collection and contributed to interpretation of results. FM contributed to interpretation of results and reviewed and revised the manuscript. EV conceptualized and designed the study, carried out the search and selected studies for inclusion, supervised data collection, contributed to statistical analyses and interpretation of results, and reviewed and revised the manuscript. All authors approved the final manuscript as submitted.

REFERENCES

Adén, U., Lin, A., Carlo, W., Leviton, A., Murray, J. C., Hallman, M., et al. (2013). Candidate gene analysis: severe intraventricular hemorrhage in inborn preterm neonates. *J. Pediatr.* 163:1503-6. e1. doi: 10.1016/j.jpeds.2013.06.025

Ahn, H. M., Park, E. A., Cho, S. J., Kim, Y.-J., and Park, H.-S. (2012). The association of histological chorioamnionitis and antenatal steroids on neonatal outcome in preterm infants born at less than thirty-four weeks' gestation. *Neonatology* 102, 259–264. doi: 10.1159/000339577

Alexander, J. M., Gilstrap, L. C., Cox, S. M., McIntire, D. M., and Leveno, K. J. (1998). Clinical chorioamnionitis and the prognosis for very low birth weight infants. *Obstet. Gynecol.* 91(5 Part 1), 725–729.

Alfiero Bordigato, M., Piva, D., Di Gangi, I. M., Giordano, G., Chiandetti, L., and Filippone, M. (2011). Asymmetric dimethylarginine in ELBW newborns exposed to chorioamnionitis. *Early Hum. Dev.* 87, 143–145. doi: 10.1016/j.earlhumdev.2010.11.004

Arayici, S., Kadioglu Simsek, G., Oncel, M. Y., Eras, Z., Canpolat, F. E., Oguz, S. S., et al. (2014). The effect of histological chorioamnionitis on the short-term outcome of preterm infants≤ 32 weeks: a single-center study. *J. Matern. Fetal Neonatal Med.* 27, 1129–1133. doi: 10.3109/14767058.2013.850668

Austeng, D., Blennow, M., Ewald, U., Fellman, V., Fritz, T., Hellstrom-Westas, L., et al. (2010). Incidence of and risk factors for neonatal morbidity after active perinatal care: extremely preterm infants study in Sweden (EXPRESS). *Acta Paediatr.* 99, 978–992. doi: 10.1111/j.1651-2227.2010.01846.x

Babnik, J., Stucin-Gantar, I., Kornhauser-Cerar, L., Sinkovec, J., Wraber, B., and Derganc, M. (2006). Intrauterine inflammation and the onset of peri-intraventricular hemorrhage in premature infants. *Neonatology* 90, 113–121. doi: 10.1159/000092070

Ballabh, P. (2010). Intraventricular hemorrhage in premature infants: mechanism of disease. *Pediatr. Res.* 67, 1–8. doi: 10.1203/PDR.0b013e3181c1b176

Ballabh, P. (2014). Pathogenesis and prevention of intraventricular hemorrhage. *Clin. Perinatol.* 41, 47–67. doi: 10.1016/j.clp.2013.09.007

Barrera-Reyes, R., Ruiz-Macias, H., and Segura-Cervantes, E. (2011). [Neurodevelopment at one year of age (corrected) in preterm newborns with history of maternal chorioamnionitis]. *Ginecol. Obstet. Mex.* 79, 31–37.

Barros, F. C., Papageorghiou, A. T., Victora, C. G., Noble, J. A., Pang, R., Iams, J., et al. (2015). The distribution of clinical phenotypes of preterm birth syndrome: implications for prevention. *JAMA Pediatr.* 169, 220–229. doi: 10.1001/jamapediatrics.2014.3040

Basso, O., and Wilcox, A. (2010). Mortality risk among preterm babies: immaturity vs. underlying pathology. *Epidemiology* 21, 521–527. doi: 10.1097/EDE.0b013e3181debe5e

Baumert, M., Brozek, G., Paprotny, M., Walencka, Z., Sodowska, H., Cnota, W., et al. (2008). Epidemiology of peri/intraventricular haemorrhage in newborns at term. *J. Physiol. Pharmacol.* 59(Suppl. 4), 67–75.

Been, J. V., Lievense, S., Zimmermann, L. J., Kramer, B. W., and Wolfs, T. G. (2013). Chorioamnionitis as a risk factor for necrotizing enterocolitis: a systematic review and meta-analysis. *J. Pediatr.* 162, 236-42 e2. doi: 10.1016/j.jpeds.2012.07.012

Been, J. V., Rours, I. G., Kornelisse, R. F., Lima Passos, V., Kramer, B. W., Schneider, T. A., et al. (2009). Histologic chorioamnionitis, fetal involvement, and antenatal steroids: effects on neonatal outcome in preterm infants. *Am. Obstet. Gynecol.* 201, 587. e1-e8. doi: 10.1016/j.ajog.2009.06.025

Behbodi, E., Villamor-Martínez, E., Degraeuwe, P. L., and Villamor, E. (2016). Chorioamnionitis appears not to be a risk factor for patent ductus arteriosus in preterm infants: a systematic review and meta-analysis. *Sci. Rep.* 6:37967. doi: 10.1038/srep37967

Bermick, J., Dechert, R. E., and Sarkar, S. (2016). Does hyperglycemia in hypernatremic preterm infants increase the risk of intraventricular hemorrhage? *J. Perinatol.* 36, 729–732. doi: 10.1038/jp.2016.86

Borenstein, M., Hedges, L. V., Higgins, J., and Rothstein, H. R. (2009a). *Subgroup Analyses. Introduction to Meta-Analysis.* Chichester, UK: John Wiley & Sons.

Borenstein, M., Hedges, L. V., Higgins, J., and Rothstein, H. R. (2009b). *Identifying and Quantifying Heterogeneity. Introduction to Meta-Analysis.* Chichester, UK: John Wiley & Sons.

Borenstein, M., Hedges, L. V., Higgins, J., and Rothstein, H. R. (2009c). *Meta-Regression. Introduction to Meta-Analysis.* Chichester, UK: John Wiley & Sons.

Botet, F., Figueras, J., Carbonell-Estrany, X., Arca, G., and Group, C. S. (2010). Effect of maternal clinical chorioamnionitis on neonatal morbidity in very-low birthweight infants: a case-control study. *J. Perinat. Med.* 38, 269–273. doi: 10.1515/jpm.2010.029

Bry, K. J., Jacobsson, B., Nilsson, S., and Bry, K. (2015). Gastric fluid cytokines are associated with chorioamnionitis and white blood cell counts in preterm infants. *Acta Paediatr.* 104, 575–580. doi: 10.1111/apa.12947

Chevallier, M., Debillon, T., Pierrat, V., Delorme, P., Kayem, G., Durox, M., et al. (2017). Leading causes of preterm delivery as risk factors for intraventricular hemorrhage in very preterm infants: results of the EPIPAGE 2 cohort study. *Am. J. Obstet. Gynecol.* 216, 518. e1-. e12. doi: 10.1016/j.ajog.2017.01.002

Cornette, L. (2004). Fetal and neonatal inflammatory response and adverse outcome. *Semin. Fetal Neonatal Med.* 9, 459–470. doi: 10.1016/j.siny.2004.08.004

Dalton, J., Dechert, R. E., and Sarkar, S. (2015). Assessment of association between rapid fluctuations in serum sodium and intraventricular hemorrhage in hypernatremic preterm infants. *Am. J. Perinatol.* 32, 795–802. doi: 10.1055/s-0034-1396691

De Felice, C., Toti, P., Laurini, R. N., Stumpo, M., Picciolini, E., Todros, T., et al. (2001). Early neonatal brain injury in histologic chorioamnionitis. *J. Pediatr.* 138, 101–104. doi: 10.1067/mpd.2001.109605

Dempsey, E., Chen, M.-F., Kokottis, T., Vallerand, D., and Usher, R. (2005). Outcome of neonates less than 30 weeks gestation with histologic chorioamnionitis. *Am. J. Perinatol.* 22, 155–159. doi: 10.1055/s-2005-865020

Dexter, S. C., Pinar, H., Malee, M. P., Hogan, J., Carpenter, M. W., and Vohr, B. R. (2000). Outcome of very low birth weight infants with histopathologic chorioamnionitis. *Obstet. Gynecol.* 96, 172–177. doi: 10.1016/S0029-7844(00)00886-3

DiSalvo, D. (1998). The correlation between placental pathology and intraventricular hemorrhage in the preterm infant. The developmental epidemiology network investigators. *Pediatr. Res.* 43, 15–19.

Ecevit, A., Anuk-Ince, D., Yapak,çi, E., Kupana-Ayva, S., Kurt, A., Yanik, F. F., et al. (2014). Association of respiratory distress syndrome and perinatal hypoxia with histologic chorioamnionitis in preterm infants. *Turk. J. Pediatr.* 56, 56–61.

Elimian, A., Verma, U., Beneck, D., Cipriano, R., Visintainer, P., and Tejani, N. (2000). Histologic chorioamnionitis, antenatal steroids, and perinatal outcomes. *Obstet. Gynecol.* 96, 333–336. doi: 10.1016/S0029-7844(00)00928-5

Erdemir, G., Kultursay, N., Calkavur, S., Zekioglu, O., Koroglu, O. A., Cakmak, B., et al. (2013). Histological chorioamnionitis: effects on premature delivery and neonatal prognosis. *Pediatr. Neonatol.* 54, 267–274. doi: 10.1016/j.pedneo.2013.03.012

Fung, G., Bawden, K., Chow, P., and Yu, V. (2003). Long-term outcome of extremely preterm infants following chorioamnionitis 絨毛膜羊膜炎對極早早產兒的長影響. *HK J Paediatr (new series)* 8, 87–92.

Gagliardi, L., Rusconi, F., Bell,ù, R., Zanini, R., and Network, I. N. (2014). Association of maternal hypertension and chorioamnionitis with preterm outcomes. *Pediatrics* 134, e154–e61. doi: 10.1542/peds.2013-3898

Gagliardi, L., Rusconi, F., Da Fr,è, M., Mello, G., Carnielli, V., Di Lallo, D., et al. (2013). Pregnancy disorders leading to very preterm birth influence neonatal outcomes: results of the population-based ACTION cohort study. *Pediatr. Res.* 73, 794–801. doi: 10.1038/pr.2013.52

Gantert, M., Been, J. V., Gavilanes, A. W., Garnier, Y., Zimmermann, L. J., and Kramer, B. W. (2010). Chorioamnionitis: a multiorgan disease of the fetus? *J Perinatol* 30(Suppl.), S21–S30. doi: 10.1038/jp.2010.96

García-Muñoz Rodrigo, F., Galan Henriquez, G., Figueras Aloy, J., Garcia-Alix Perez, A., and Network, S. (2014). Outcomes of very-low-birth-weight infants exposed to maternal clinical chorioamnionitis: a multicentre study. *Neonatology* 106, 229–234. doi: 10.1159/000363127

Gawade, P. L., Whitcomb, B. W., Chasan-Taber, L., Pekow, P. S., Ronnenberg, A. G., Shah, B., et al. (2013). Second stage of labor and intraventricular hemorrhage in early preterm infants in the vertex presentation. *J. Matern. Fetal Neonatal Med.* 26, 1292–1298. doi: 10.3109/14767058.2013.783804

González-Luis, G., García, I. J., Rodríguez-Miguélez, J., Mussons, F. B., and Aloy, J. F. (2002). Patología neonatal en los menores de 1.500 gramos con relación al antecedente de corioamnionitis. *Anal. Pediatr.* 56, 551–555. doi: 10.1016/S1695-4033(02)77863-6

Gray, P. H., Hurley, T. M., Rogers, Y. M., O'Callaghan, M. J., Tudehope, D. I., Burns, Y. R., et al. (1997). Survival and neonatal and neurodevelopmental outcome of 24–29 week gestation infants according to primary cause of preterm delivery. *Austr. N. Z. J. Obstet. Gynaecol.* 37, 161–168. doi: 10.1111/j.1479-828X.1997.tb02245.x

Hartling, L., Liang, Y., and Lacaze-Masmonteil, T. (2012). Chorioamnionitis as a risk factor for bronchopulmonary dysplasia: a systematic review and meta-analysis. *Arch. Dis. Child. Fetal Neonatal Ed.* 97, F8–F17. . doi: 10.1136/adc.2010.210187

Harvard Dataverse (2018). *Chorioamnionitis and Intraventricular, Hemorrhage, Studies Included in Systematic Review [Internet]*. Available online at: doi: 10.7910/DVN/J9RHUF

Hendson, L., Russell, L., Robertson, C. M., Liang, Y., Chen, Y., Abdalla, A., et al. (2011). Neonatal and neurodevelopmental outcomes of very low birth weight infants with histologic chorioamnionitis. *J. Pediatr.* 158, 397–402. doi: 10.1016/j.jpeds.2010.09.010

Hernández-Díaz, S., Schisterman, E. F., and Hernán, M. A. (2006). The birth weight "paradox" uncovered? *Am. J. Epidemiol.* 164, 1115–1120. doi: 10.1093/aje/kwj275

Higgins, R. D., Saade, G., Polin, R. A., Grobman, W. A., Buhimschi, I. A., Watterberg, K., et al. (2016). Evaluation and management of women and newborns with a maternal diagnosis of chorioamnionitis: summary of a workshop. *Obstet. Gynecol.* 127, 426–436. doi: 10.1097/AOG.0000000000001246

Hitti, J., Tarczy-Hornoch, P., Murphy, J., Hillier, S. L., Aura, J., and Eschenbach, D. A. (2001). Amniotic fluid infection, cytokines, and adverse outcome among infants at 34 weeks' gestation or less. *Obstet. Gynecol.* 98, 1080–1088. doi: 10.1016/S0029-7844(01)01567-8

Holcroft, C. J., Blakemore, K. J., Allen, M., and Graham, E. M. (2003). Association of prematurity and neonatal infection with neurologic morbidity in very low birth weight infants. *Obstet. Gynecol.* 101, 1249–1253. doi: 10.1016/S0029-7844(03)00354-5

Inder, T. E., Perlman, J. M., and Volpe, J. J. (2018). *Preterm Intraventricular Hemorrhage/Posthemorrhagic Hydrocephalus Volpe's Neurology of the Newborn, 6th Edn.* Elsevier. Available online at: https://www.sciencedirect.com/book/9780323428767/volpes-neurology-of-the-newborn

Jackson, C. M., Wells, C. B., Tabangin, M. E., Meinzen-Derr, J., Jobe, A. H., and Chougnet, C. A. (2017). Pro-inflammatory immune responses in leukocytes of premature infants exposed to maternal chorioamnionitis or funisitis. *Pediatr. Res.* 81, 384–390. doi: 10.1038/pr.2016.232

Kallankari, H., Kaukola, T., Ojaniemi, M., Herva, R., Perhomaa, M., Vuolteenaho, R., et al. (2010). Chemokine CCL18 predicts intraventricular hemorrhage in very preterm infants. *Ann. Med.* 42, 416–425. doi: 10.3109/07853890.2010.481085

Kaukola, T., Herva, R., Perhomaa, M., Pääkkö, E., Kingsmore, S., Vainionpää, L., et al. (2006). Population cohort associating chorioamnionitis, cord inflammatory cytokines and neurologic outcome in very preterm, extremely low birth weight infants. *Pediatr. Res.* 59, 478–483. doi: 10.1203/01.pdr.0000182596.66175.ee

Kidokoro, H., Anderson, P. J., Doyle, L. W., Woodward, L. J., Neil, J. J., and Inder, T. E. (2014). Brain injury and altered brain growth in preterm infants: predictors and prognosis. *Pediatrics* 134, e444–e453. doi: 10.1542/peds.2013-2336

Kim, S. Y., Choi, C. W., Jung, E., Lee, J., Lee, J. A., Kim, H., et al. (2015). Neonatal morbidities associated with histologic chorioamnionitis defined based on the site and extent of inflammation in very low birth weight infants. *J. Korean Med. Sci.* 30, 1476–1482. doi: 10.3346/jkms.2015.30.10.1476

Kirchner, L., Helmer, H., Heinze, G., Wald, M., Brunbauer, M., Weninger, M. et al. (2007). Amnionitis with ureaplasma urealyticum or other microbes leads to increased morbidity and prolonged hospitalization in very low birth weight infants. *Eur. J. Obstet. Gynecol. Reprod. Biol.* 134, 44–50. doi: 10.1016/j.ejogrb.2006.09.013

Klebermass-Schrehof, K., Czaba, C., Olischar, M., Fuiko, R., Waldhoer, T., Rona, Z., et al. (2012). Impact of low-grade intraventricular hemorrhage on long-term neurodevelopmental outcome in preterm infants. *Childs Nerv. Syst.* 28, 2085–2092. doi: 10.1007/s00381-012-1897-3

Kosuge, S., Ohkuchi, A., Minakami, H., Matsubara, S., Uchida, A., Eguchi, Y., et al. (2000). Influence of chorioamnionitis on survival and morbidity in singletons live-born at< 32 weeks of gestation. *Acta Obstet. Gynecol. Scand.* 79, 861–865. doi: 10.1034/j.1600-0412.2000.079010861.x

Lau, J., Magee, F., Qiu, Z., Houb,é, J., Von Dadelszen, P., and Lee, S. K. (2005). Chorioamnionitis with a fetal inflammatory response is associated with higher neonatal mortality, morbidity, and resource use than chorioamnionitis displaying a maternal inflammatory response only. *Am. J. Obstet. Gynecol.* 193, 708–713. doi: 10.1016/j.ajog.2005.01.017

Lee, H. J., Kim, E.-K., Kim, H.-S., Choi, C. W., Kim, B. I., and Choi, J.-H. (2011). Chorioamnionitis, respiratory distress syndrome and bronchopulmonary dysplasia in extremely low birth weight infants. *J. Perinatol.* 31, 166–170. doi: 10.1038/jp.2010.113

Lee, J. Y., Kim, H. S., Jung, E., Kim, E. S., Shim, G. H., Lee, H. J., et al. (2010). Risk factors for periventricular-intraventricular hemorrhage in premature infants. *J. Korean Med. Sci.* 25, 418–424. doi: 10.3346/jkms.2010.25.3.418

Leviton, A., Kuban, K., and Paneth, N. (2007). Intraventricular haemorrhage grading scheme: time to abandon? *Acta Paediatr.* 96, 1254–1256. doi: 10.1111/j.1651-2227.2007.00379.x

Lim, W., Lien, R., Chiang, M., Fu, R., Lin, J., Chu, S., et al. (2011). Hypernatremia and grade III/IV intraventricular hemorrhage among extremely low birth weight infants. *J. Perinatol.* 31, 193–198. doi: 10.1038/jp.2010.86

Linder, N., Haskin, O., Levit, O., Klinger, G., Prince, T., Naor, N., et al. (2003). Risk factors for intraventricular hemorrhage in very low birth weight premature infants: a retrospective case-control study. *Pediatrics* 111, e590–e5. doi: 10.1542/peds.111.5.e590

Liu, Z., Tang, Z., Li, J., and Yang, Y. (2014). Effects of placental inflammation on neonatal outcome in preterm infants. *Pediatr. Neonatol.* 55, 35–40. doi: 10.1016/j.pedneo.2013.05.007

Logan, J. W., Westra, S. J., Allred, E. N., O'Shea, T. M., Kuban, K., and Paneth, N., et al. (2013). Antecedents of perinatal cerebral white matter damage with and without intraventricular hemorrhage in very preterm newborns. *Pediatr. Neurol.* 49, 88–96. doi: 10.1016/j.pediatrneurol.2013.03.018

Lu, H., Wang, Q., Lu, J., Zhang, Q., and Kumar, P. (2016). Risk factors for intraventricular hemorrhage in preterm infants born at 34 weeks of gestation or less following preterm premature rupture of membranes. *J. Stroke Cerebrovasc. Dis.* 25, 807–812. doi: 10.1016/j.jstrokecerebrovasdis.2015.12.011

McAdams, R. M., and Juul, S. E. (2012). The role of cytokines and inflammatory cells in perinatal brain injury. *Neurol. Res. Int.* 2012:561494. doi: 10.1155/2012/561494

McElrath, T. F., Hecht, J. L., Dammann, O., Boggess, K., Onderdonk, A., Markenson, G., et al. (2008). Pregnancy disorders that lead to delivery before the 28th week of gestation: an epidemiologic approach to classification. *Am. J. Epidemiol.* 168, 980–989. doi: 10.1093/aje/kwn202

Mehta, R., Nanjundaswamy, S., Shen-Schwarz, S., and Petrova, A. (2006). Neonatal morbidity and placental pathology. *Indian J. Pediatr.* 73, 25–28. doi: 10.1007/BF02758255

Mestan, K., Yu, Y., Matoba, N., Cerda, S., Demmin, B., Pearson, C., et al. (2010). Placental inflammatory response is associated with poor neonatal growth: preterm birth cohort study. *Pediatrics* 125, e891–e98. doi: 10.1542/peds.2009-0313

Mitra, S., Aune, D., Speer, C. P., and Saugstad, O. D. (2014). Chorioamnionitis as a risk factor for retinopathy of prematurity: a systematic review and meta-analysis. *Neonatology* 105, 189–199. doi: 10.1159/000357556

Miyazaki, K., Furuhashi, M., Ishikawa, K., Tamakoshi, K., Hayashi, K., Kai, A., et al. (2016). Impact of chorioamnionitis on short-and long-term outcomes in very low birth weight preterm infants: the neonatal research network Japan. *J. Matern. Fetal Neonatal Med.* 29, 331–337. doi: 10.3109/14767058.2014.1000852

Mohamed, M. A., and Aly, H. (2010). Transport of premature infants is associated with increased risk for intraventricular haemorrhage. *Arch. Dis. Child Fetal Neonatal Ed.* 95, F403– F407. doi: 10.1136/adc.2010.183236

Moher, D., Liberati, A., Tetzlaff, J., Altman, D. G., and Group, P. (2009). Preferred reporting items for systematic reviews and meta-analyses: the PRISMA statement. *PLoS Med.* 6:e1000097. doi: 10.1371/journal.pmed.1000097

Molina-Holgado, E., and Molina-Holgado, F. (2010). Mending the broken brain: neuroimmune interactions in neurogenesis. *J. Neurochem.* 114, 1277–1290. doi: 10.1111/j.1471-4159.2010.06849.x

Morales, W. J. (1987). The effect of chorioamnionitis on the developmental outcome of preterm infants at one year. *Obstet. Gynecol.* 70, 183–186.

Mu, S.-C., Lin, C.-H., Chen, Y.-L., Ma, H.-J., Lee, J.-S., Lin, M.-I., et al. (2008). Impact on neonatal outcome and anthropometric growth in very low birth weight infants with histological chorioamnionitis. *J. Formos. Med. Assoc.* 107, 304–310. doi: 10.1016/S0929-6646(08)60091-1

Nasef, N., Shabaan, A. E., Schurr, P., Iaboni, D., Choudhury, J., Church, P., et al. (2013). Effect of clinical and histological chorioamnionitis on the outcome of preterm infants. *Am. J. Perinatol.* 30, 059–68. doi: 10.1055/s-0032-1321501

Ogunyemi, D., Murillo, M., Jackson, U., Hunter, N., and Alperson, B. (2003). The relationship between placental histopathology findings and perinatal outcome in preterm infants. *J. Matern. Fetal Neonatal Med.* 13, 102–109. doi: 10.1080/jmf.13.2.102.109

Oh, K. J., Park, J. Y., Lee, J., Hong, J.-S., Romero, R., and Yoon, B. H. (2018). The combined exposure to intra-amniotic inflammation and neonatal respiratory distress syndrome increases the risk of intraventricular hemorrhage in preterm neonates. *J. Perinat. Med.* 46, 9–20. doi: 10.1515/jpm-2016-0348

Oh, S.-H., Kim, J.-,j, Do, H.-,j, Lee, B. S., Kim, K.-S., and Kim, E. A.-R. (2015). Preliminary study on neurodevelopmental outcome and placental pathology among extremely low birth weight infants. *Korean J. Perinatol.* 26, 67–77. doi: 10.14734/kjp.2015.26.1.67

Ohyama, M., Itani, Y., Yamanaka, M., Goto, A., Kato, K., Ijiri, R., et al. (2002). Re-evaluation of chorioamnionitis and funisitis with a special reference to subacute chorioamnionitis. *Hum. Pathol.* 33, 183–190. doi: 10.1053/hupa.2002.31291

Osmanagaoglu, M. A., Ünal, S., and Bozkaya, H. (2005). Chorioamnionitis risk and neonatal outcome in preterm premature rupture of membranes. *Arch. Gynecol. Obstet.* 271, 33–39. doi: 10.1007/s00404-004-0644-8

Pappas, A., Kendrick, D. E., Shankaran, S., Stoll, B. J., Bell, E. F., Laptook, A. R., et al. (2014). Chorioamnionitis and early childhood outcomes among extremely low-gestational-age neonates. *JAMA Pediatr.* 168, 137–147. doi: 10.1001/jamapediatrics.2013.4248

Park, H. W., Choi, Y. S., Kim, K. S., and Kim, S. N. (2015). Chorioamnionitis and patent ductus arteriosus: a systematic review and meta-analysis. *PLoS ONE* 10:e0138114. doi: 10.1371/journal.pone.0138114

Perrone, S., Toti, P., Toti, M. S., Badii, S., Becucci, E., Gatti, M. G., et al. (2012). Perinatal outcome and placental histological characteristics: a single-center study. *J. Matern. Fetal Neonatal Med.* 25(Supp. 1), 110–113. doi: 10.3109/14767058.2012.664344

Polam, S., Koons, A., Anwar, M., Shen-Schwarz, S., Hegyi, T. (2005). Effect of chorioamnionitis on neurodevelopmental outcome in preterm infants. *Arch. Pediatr. Adolesc. Med.* 159, 1032–1035. doi: 10.1001/archpedi.159.11.1032

Poralla, C., Hertfelder, H.-J., Oldenburg, J., Müller, A., and Bartmann, P., Heep, A. (2012). Elevated interleukin-6 concentration and alterations of the coagulation system are associated with the development of intraventricular hemorrhage in extremely preterm infants. *Neonatology* 102, 270–275. doi: 10.1159/000341266

Poryo, M., Boeckh, J. C., Gortner, L., Zemlin, M., Duppr,é, P., Ebrahimi-Fakhari, D., et al. (2018). Ante-, peri-and postnatal factors associated with intraventricular hemorrhage in very premature infants. *Early Hum. Dev.* 116, 1–8. doi: 10.1016/j.earlhumdev.2017.08.010

Pugni, L., Pietrasanta, C., Acaia, B., Merlo, D., Ronchi, A., Ossola, M. W., et al. (2016). Chorioamnionitis and neonatal outcome in preterm infants: a clinical overview. *J. Matern. Fetal Neonatal Med.* 29, 1525–1529. doi: 10.3109/14767058.2015.1053862

Ramenghi, L. A., Fumagalli, M., Groppo, M., Consonni, D., Gatti, L., Bertazzi, P. A., et al. (2011). Germinal matrix hemorrhage: intraventricular hemorrhage in very-low-birth-weight infants: the independent role of inherited thrombophilia. *Stroke* 42, 1889–1893. doi: 10.1161/STROKEAHA.110.590455

Revello, R., Alcaide, M. J., Dudzik, D., Abehsera, D., and Bartha, J. L. (2015). Differential amniotic fluid cytokine profile in women with chorioamnionitis with and without funisitis. *J. Matern. Fetal Neonatal Med.* 29, 2161–2165. doi: 10.3109/14767058.2015.1077512

Richardson, B. S., Wakim, E., and Walton, J. (2006). Preterm histologic chorioamnionitis: impact on cord gas and pH values and neonatal outcome. *Am. J. Obstet. Gynecol.* 195, 1357–1365. doi: 10.1016/j.ajog.2006.03.053

Rivest, S. (2003). Molecular insights on the cerebral innate immune system. *Brain Behav. Immun.* 17, 13–19. doi: 10.1016/S0889-1591(02)00055-7

Rocha, G., Proença, E., Quintas, C., Rodrigues, T., and Guimarães, H. (2006). Chorioamnionitis and neonatal morbidity. *Acta Med. Port.* 19, 207–212.

Rodríguez-Trujillo, A., Cobo, T., Vives, I., Bosch, J., Kacerovsky, M., Posadas, D. E., et al. (2016). Gestational age is more important for short-term neonatal outcome than microbial invasion of the amniotic cavity or intra-amniotic inflammation in preterm prelabor rupture of membranes. *Acta Obstet. Gynecol. Scand.* 95, 926–933. doi: 10.1111/aogs.12905

Romantsik, O., Bruschettini, M., Calevo, M. G., Banzi, R., and Ley, D. (2017). Pharmacological pain and sedation interventions for the prevention of intraventricular hemorrhage in preterm infants on assisted ventilation - an overview of systematic reviews. *Cochrane Libr.* CD012706. doi: 10.1002/14651858.CD012706

Rong, Z., Liu, H., Xia, S., and Chang, L. (2012). Risk and protective factors of intraventricular hemorrhage in preterm babies in Wuhan, China. *Childs Nerv. Syst.* 28, 2077–2084. doi: 10.1007/s00381-012-1875-9

Ryckman, K. K., Dagle, J. M., Kelsey, K., Momany, A. M., and Murray, J. C. (2011). Replication of genetic associations in the inflammation, complement, and coagulation pathways with intraventricular hemorrhage in LBW preterm neonates. *Pediatr. Res.* 70, 90–95. doi: 10.1203/PDR.0b013e31821ceb63

Salas, A. A., Faye-Petersen, O. M., Sims, B., Peralta-Carcelen, M., Reilly, S. D., McGwin, G., et al. (2013). Histological characteristics of the fetal inflammatory response associated with neurodevelopmental impairment and death in extremely preterm infants. *J. Pediatr.* 163, 652-7. e2. doi: 10.1016/j.jpeds.2013.03.081

Sarkar, S., Kaplan, C., Wiswell, T. E., Spitzer, A. R. (2005). Histological chorioamnionitis and the risk of early intraventricular hemorrhage in infants born≤ 28 weeks gestation. *J. Perinatol.* 25, 749–752. doi: 10.1038/sj.jp.7211399

Sato, M., Nishimaki, S., Yokota, S., Seki, K., Horiguchi, H., An, H., et al. (2011). Severity of chorioamnionitis and neonatal outcome. *J. Obstet. Gynaecol. Res.* 37, 1313–1319. doi: 10.1111/j.1447-0756.2010.01519.x

Seliga-Siwecka, J. P., and Kornacka, M. K. (2013). Neonatal outcome of preterm infants born to mothers with abnormal genital tract colonisation and chorioamnionitis: a cohort study. *Early Hum. Dev.* 89, 271–275. doi: 10.1016/j.earlhumdev.2012.10.003

Shankaran, S., Lin, A., Maller-Kesselman, J., Zhang, H., O'shea, T. M., Bada, H. S., et al. (2014). Maternal race, demography, and health care disparities impact risk for intraventricular hemorrhage in preterm neonates. *J. Pediatr.* 164, 1005-11. e3. doi: 10.1016/j.jpeds.2014.01.036

Smit, A. L., Been, J. V., Zimmermann, L. J., Kornelisse, R. F., Andriessen, P., Vanterpool, S. F., et al. (2015). Automated auditory brainstem response in preterm newborns with histological chorioamnionitis. *J. Matern. Fetal Neonatal Med.* 28, 1864–1869. doi: 10.3109/14767058.2014.971747

Soraisham, A., Trevenen, C., Wood, S., Singhal, N., and Sauve, R. (2013). Histological chorioamnionitis and neurodevelopmental outcome in preterm infants. *J. Perinatol.* 33, 70–75. doi: 10.1038/jp.2012.49

Soraisham, A. S., Singhal, N., McMillan, D. D., Sauve, R. S., Lee, S. K., and Network, C. N. (2009). A multicenter study on the clinical outcome of chorioamnionitis in preterm infants. *Am. J. Obstet. Gynecol.* 200, 372 e1–e6. doi: 10.1016/j.ajog.2008.11.034

Stanimirovic, D., and Satoh, K. (2000). Inflammatory mediators of cerebral endothelium: a role in ischemic brain inflammation. *Brain Pathol.* 10, 113–126. doi: 10.1111/j.1750-3639.2000.tb00248.x

Strunk, T., Inder, T., Wang, X., Burgner, D., Mallard, C., and Levy, O. (2014). Infection-induced inflammation and cerebral injury in preterm infants. *Lancet Infect. Dis.* 14, 751–762. doi: 10.1016/S1473-3099(14)70710-8

Suarez, R. D., Grobman, W. A., and Parilla, B. V. (2001). Indomethacin tocolysis and intraventricular hemorrhage. *Obstet. Gynecol.* 97, 921–925.

Suppiej, A., Franzoi, M., Vedovato, S., Marucco, A., Chiarelli, S., and Zanardo, V. (2009). Neurodevelopmental outcome in preterm histological chorioamnionitis. *Early Hum. Dev.* 85, 187–189. doi: 10.1016/j.earlhumdev.2008.09.410

Thomas, W., and Speer, C. P. (2011). Chorioamnionitis: important risk factor or innocent bystander for neonatal outcome? *Neonatology* 99, 177–187. doi: 10.1159/000320170

Tita, A. T., and Andrews, W. W. (2010). Diagnosis and management of clinical chorioamnionitis. *Clin. Perinatol.* 37, 339–354. doi: 10.1016/j.clp.2010.02.003

Tortora, D., Severino, M., Malova, M., Parodi, A., Morana, G., Sedlacik, J., et al. (2017). Differences in subependymal vein anatomy may predispose preterm infants to GMH-IVH. *Arch. Dis. Child Fetal Neonatal Ed.* 103,F59–F65. doi: 10.1136/archdischild-2017-312710

Trevisanuto, D., Peruzzetto, C., Cavallin, F., Vedovato, S., Cosmi, E., Visentin, S., et al. (2013). Fetal placental inflammation is associated with poor neonatal growth of preterm infants: a case-control study. *J. Matern. Fetal Neonatal Med.* 26, 1484–1490. doi: 10.3109/14767058.2013.789849

Tsiartas, P., Kacerovsky, M., Musilova, I., Hornychova, H., Cobo, T., Sävman, K., et al. (2013). The association between histological chorioamnionitis, funisitis and neonatal outcome in women with preterm prelabor rupture of membranes. *J. Matern. Fetal Neonatal Med.* 26, 1332–1336. doi: 10.3109/14767058.2013.784741

Vaihinger, M., Mazzitelli, N., Balanian, N., and Grandi, C. (2012). The relationship between placental lesions and early hemorrhagic-ischemic cerebral injury in very low birth weight infants. *Rev. Fac. Cienc. Med. Cordoba* 70, 123–133.

van Vliet, E. O., de Kieviet, J. F., van der Voorn, J. P., Been, J. V., Oosterlaan, J., and van Elburg, R. M. (2012). Placental pathology and long-term neurodevelopment of very preterm infants. *Am. J. Obstet. Gynecol.* 206, 489. e1-e7. doi: 10.1016/j.ajog.2012.03.024

Vergani, P., Locatelli, A., Doria, V., Assi, F., Paterlini, G., Pezzullo, J. C., et al. (2004). Intraventricular hemorrhage and periventricular leukomalacia in preterm infants. *Obstet. Gynecol.* 104, 225–231. doi: 10.1097/01.AOG.0000130838.02410.b7

Villamor-Martinez, E., Cavallaro, G., Raffaeli, G., Rahim, O. M. M., Gulden, S., Ghazi, A. M., et al. (2018a). Chorioamnionitis as a risk factor for retinopathy of prematurity: an updated systematic review and meta-analysis. *bioRxiv* [Preprint]. doi: 10.1101/291476

Villamor-Martinez, E., Fumagalli, M., Mohammed Rahim, O. M. M., Passera, S., Cavallaro, G., Degraeuwe, P., et al. (2018b). Chorioamnionitis is a risk factor for intraventricular hemorrhage in preterm infants: a systematic review and meta-analysis. *bioRxiv*. 1–30. doi: 10.1101/334375

Volpe, J. J. (2015). Impaired neurodevelopmental outcome after mild germinal matrix-intraventricular hemorrhage. *Pediatrics* 136, 1185–1187. doi: 10.1542/peds.2015-3553

Wan, X., Wang, W., Liu, J., and Tong, T. (2014). Estimating the sample mean and standard deviation from the sample size, median, range and/or interquartile range. *BMC Med. Res. Methodol.* 14:135. doi: 10.1186/1471-2288-14-135

Watterberg, K. L., Gerdes, J. S., Gifford, K. L., and Lin, H.-M. (1999). Prophylaxis against early adrenal insufficiency to prevent chronic lung disease in premature infants. *Pediatrics* 104, 1258–1263. doi: 10.1542/peds.104.6.1258

Wilcox, A. J., Weinberg, C. R., and Basso, O. (2011). On the pitfalls of adjusting for gestational age at birth. *Am. J. Epidemiol.* 174, 1062–1068. doi: 10.1093/aje/kwr230

Wirbelauer, J., Thomas, W., and Speer, C. P. (2011). Response of leukocytes and nucleated red blood cells in very low-birth weight preterm infants after exposure to intrauterine inflammation. *J. Matern. Fetal Neonatal Med.* 24, 348–353. doi: 10.3109/14767058.2010.497568

Wu, Y. W., and Colford, J. M. Jr. (2000). Chorioamnionitis as a risk factor for cerebral palsy: a meta-analysis. *JAMA* 284, 1417–1424. doi: 10.1001/jama.284.11.1417

Xu, L. P., Ren, R., Zhu, S., Zhuang, H., Huang, Z., and Yang, H. (2012). Effect of chorioamnionitis on brain injury in preterm infants. *Zhongguo Dang Dai Er Ke Za Zhi* 14, 661–663.

Yamada, N., Sato, Y., Moriguchi-Goto, S., Yamashita, A., Kodama, Y., Sameshima, H., et al. (2015). Histological severity of fetal inflammation is useful in predicting neonatal outcome. *Placenta* 36, 1490–1493. doi: 10.1016/j.placenta.2015.10.021

Yanowitz, T. D., Jordan, J. A., Gilmour, C. H., Towbin, R., Bowen, A. D., Roberts, J. M., et al. (2002). Hemodynamic disturbances in premature infants born after chorioamnionitis: association with cord blood cytokine concentrations. *Pediatr. Res.* 51, 310–316. doi: 10.1203/00006450-200203000-00008

Yanowitz, T. D., Potter, D. M., Bowen, A. D., Baker, R. W., and Roberts, J. M. (2006). Variability in cerebral oxygen delivery is reduced in premature neonates exposed to chorioamnionitis. *Pediatr. Res.* 59, 299–304. doi: 10.1203/01.pdr.0000196738.03171.f1

Yoon, B. H., Romero, R., Kim, C. J., Jun, J. K., Gomez, R., Choi, J. -H., et al. (1995). Amniotic fluid interleukin-6: a sensitive test for antenatal diagnosis of acute inflammatory lesions of preterm placenta and prediction of perinatal morbidity. *Am. J. Obstet. Gynecol.* 172, 960–970. doi: 10.1016/0002-9378(95)90028-4

Zanardo, V., Vedovato, S., Suppiej, A., Trevisanuto, D., Migliore, M., Di Venosa, B., et al. (2008). Histological inflammatory responses in the placenta and early neonatal brain injury. *Pediatr. Dev. Pathol.* 11, 350–354. doi: 10.2350/07-08-0324.1

6

Prevention, Reduction and Repair of Brain Injury of the Preterm Infant

Frank van Bel[1]*, Josine Vaes[2] and Floris Groenendaal[1]

[1]Department of Neonatology, Wilhelmina Children's Hospital and Brain Center Rudolf Magnus, University Medical Center Utrecht, Utrecht University, Utrecht, Netherlands, [2]Laboratory of Neuroimmunology and Developmental Origins of Disease, University Medical Center Utrecht, Utrecht University, Utrecht, Netherlands

*Correspondence:
Frank van Bel
f.vanBel@umcutrecht.nl

Periventricular-intraventricular hemorrhages (PIVH) and (diffuse) white matter injury (WMI) are the most important acquired brain lesions of the very and extremely prematurely born neonate. Both carry a high risk for death or adverse neurodevelopmental outcome. The first part of the review discusses the standard of care and latest insights with respect to prevention and/or reduction of PIVH and WMI, taking into account their etiopathogenesis which is tightly linked to (functional) immaturity of the cerebral vascular bed and nervous system and commonly encountered inflammation. The second part discusses repair of hemorrhagic- ischemic and post-inflammatory brain lesions as it is an increasingly important topic in newborn medicine. In the near future trials of trophic and (autologous or allogenic) cell-therapy in infants at risk of or demonstrating established PIVH and WMI will be started. The focus of these potential trials will be discussed.

Keywords: prematurity, brain hemorrhage, white matter injury in the preterm infant, neuroprotection, neuroregeneration

INTRODUCTION

The most important acquired brain injuries in very and extremely preterm infants born in developed countries are periventricular-intraventricular hemorrhages (PIVH) and diffuse white matter injury (dWMI, **Figure 1**; Stoll et al., 2010; Hamilton et al., 2013; Pierrat et al., 2017). This brain injury may lead to cerebral palsy and learning difficulties, and can have major impact on the quality of life (Stoll et al., 2010; Pierrat et al., 2017).

The first aim of this review is to link the etiopathogenesis of PIVH and dWMI to the standard of care and its latest insights with respect to prevention and reduction of these complications.

The second aim is to focus on repair of the sequelae of PIVH and dWMI. There is increasing evidence that repair of perinatal brain injury with trophic and/or stem cell therapy is currently becoming a realistic and exciting option (Fleiss et al., 2014; Fischer et al., 2017; Wagenaar et al., 2017). We discuss this development in relation with repair of the sequelae of severe PIVH and dWMI.

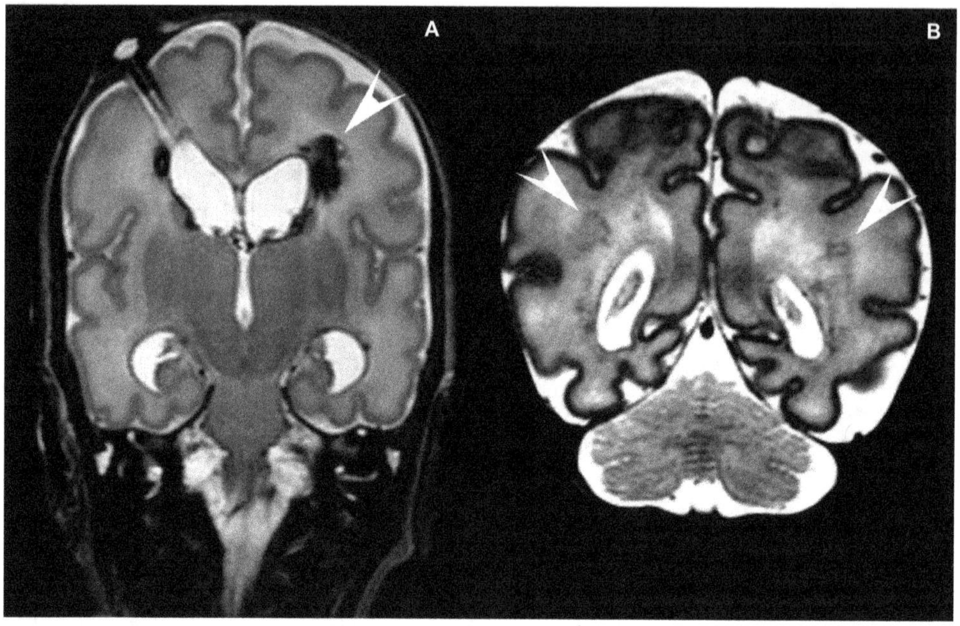

FIGURE 1 | (A) MRI of a preterm infant (gestational age 26 2/7 weeks, birthweight 965 g) with a large IVH and a large left-sided (arrowhead) and small right-sided venous infarct. Post-hemorrhagic ventricular dilatation was treated with CSF removal from a subcutaneous reservoir. T2 weighted coronal image at the age of 8 weeks after birth. **(B)** MRI of a preterm infant (gestational age 32 2/7 weeks, birthweight 1,670 g) with several lesions in the periventricular white matter (arrowheads). T2 weighted coronal image at the age of 6 days after birth.

PERIVENTRICULAR-INTRAVENTRICULAR HEMORRHAGE

PIVH has still a high incidence in the developed world: 25–35% of preterm infants born before 30 weeks of gestation or a birth weight less than 1,500 g develop PIVH. PIVH develops from the fragile vascular network of the germinal matrix mostly within the first 3 days after birth with the highest incidence in extremely low birth weight infants being up to 45% (Jain et al., 2009; Stoll et al., 2010; Mukerji et al., 2015). Although a minority of these infants develop severe PIVH grade III (intraventricular blood in dilated lateral cerebral ventricles) or IV (intraventricular blood with extension into the adjacent parenchymal region, more recently described as venous infarction) according to the Papile grading (Papile et al., 1978), up to 75% develop mild to severe PIVH-related sequelae in later life (Sherlock et al., 2005; Luu et al., 2009). PIVH remains therefore a major health concern.

Although multifactorial, the pathogenesis of PIVH and its extension to more severe stages is firmly linked to pulmonary immaturity. This is clinically represented by the idiopathic respiratory distress syndrome (IRDS), and (functional) immaturity of the cerebral vascular bed (Ozdemir et al., 1997; Krediet et al., 2006; Ballabh, 2014). IRDS may lead to hypoxia and hypercapnia, lack of cerebral autoregulation and the need for blood pressure support often causing fluctuations and hyperperfusion of the immature brain of the extremely and very preterm infant (Perlman et al., 1985; van Bel et al., 1987), although this mechanism may also be operative in the moderate and late preterm neonate with IRDS (Thygesen et al., 2016). Cerebral hemodynamic instability often leads to PIVH, mostly originating in the germinal matrix, which has a dense but fragile vasculature (Ballabh, 2014). Moreover, IRDS has been associated with inflammatory processes and oxidative stress in the immature lung. Several studies showed elevated pro-inflammatory cytokines, chemokines and indicators of oxidative stress in broncho-alveolar lavage fluid and blood in very preterm neonates with IRDS (Beresford and Shaw, 2002; Gitto et al., 2004). A recent study showed that intra-amniotic inflammation and postnatal IRDS markedly increased the risk for PIVH (Oh et al., 2018). PIVHs, which develop within 12 hours of age, inflammation may play an important role as indicated by the strong association between early PIVH and pro-inflammatory cytokines and oxidative stress (Krediet et al., 2006; Chisholm et al., 2016; Chevallier et al., 2017; Villamor-Martinez et al., 2018). Finally genetic factors can be related to the occurrence of PIVH, but this issue is beyond the scope of this review (Bilguvar et al., 2009; Harteman et al., 2011; Ballabh, 2014).

Prevention and Reduction of PIVH: Standard of Care

Prevention and reduction of PIVH starts already in the womb: *maternal corticosteroids* during imminent preterm birth have shown to reduce the occurrence of PIVH and is common practice during preterm labor and imminent preterm birth in most high income countries since the late eighties of the last century (Ment et al., 1995; Ballabh, 2014; Roberts et al., 2017). A recent population study (EPICE Cohort) showed even a risk reduction of up to 50% of severe neonatal injury after antenatal corticosteroids administered shortly before birth (Norman et al., 2017). Mostly betamethasone or dexamethasone are used although there is an ongoing debate about their superiority (Brownfoot et al., 2013). Besides the well proven effect of antenatal steroids on lung maturation with a positive effect on respiratory and hemodynamic systems (Roberts et al., 2017), a maturational effect of steroids on the germinal matrix microvasculature has been postulated (Xu et al., 2008). This will establish a decrease in permeability of the cerebral vasculature and stabilization of the endothelial basement membrane (Hedley-Whyte and Hsu, 1986; Tokida et al., 1990).

As antenatally administered corticosteroids induce lung maturation and pulmonary stabilization, *exogenous surfactant application via* the trachea does so postnatally (McPherson and Wambach, 2018). Surfactant may add therefore to a hemodynamic stabilization of the systemic and cerebral circulation leading to less disturbances of cerebral autoregulatory ability of the vascular bed (Lemmers et al., 2006).

Several studies indicated a decrease in the incidence in PIVH after the introduction of surfactant therapy, especially regarding more severe PIVHs (Walti et al., 1995; Greenough and Ahmed, 2013). An older meta-analysis, however, showed no clear benefits of surfactant therapy on the incidence of PIVH, although there was a tendency for a reduction of severe PIVH (Rojas-Reyes et al., 2012). A recent systematic review and meta-analysis investigating the use of early surfactant, defined as surfactant administration within one hour after birth, with noninvasive ventilation and stress reduction found a decrease in severe PIVH with this strategy (Anand et al., 1999; Isayama et al., 2015; Ng et al., 2017).

Pharmacologic interventions aiming to prevent or reduce PIVH are numerous. Muscle paralysis was used in order to minimize swings in cerebral perfusion to influence the incidence of PIVH in artificially ventilated preterm infants. PIVH incidence indeed decreased sharply after muscle paralysis (Perlman et al., 1985). More sophisticated ventilation modalities nowadays, including non-invasive ventilation makes muscle paralysis obsolete (McPherson and Inder, 2017). Phenobarbital sedation did not decrease PIVH incidence (Donn et al., 1981; Bedard et al., 1984). Vitamin E, a potent anti-oxidative agent, reduced the incidence of PIVH but routine use was not encouraged because of serious side effects (Brion et al., 2003). Ethamsylate, which has a stabilizing effect on the vascular basement membrane, was widely investigated in the 1980s, but had no positive effect on the PIVH incidence (Benson et al., 1986).

Only prophylactic indomethacin made its way to the clinic. Indomethacin is a (nonselective) cyclo-oxygenase inhibitor which showed a positive effect on PIVH incidence and induced (early) patent ductus arteriosus closure (Vohr and Ment, 1996). Especially in the United States prophylactic indomethacin administration (low dose indomethacin starting within 6 h after birth up to day 3–5) has been utilized in many centers (Nelin et al., 2017). Although, in 2001 the TIPP trial suggested that despite a decreased incidence of (severe) PIVH, long-term developmental outcome did not improve (Schmidt et al., 2001). A recent large study did show improved survival after indomethacin prophylaxis in especially the extremely preterm infants (Nelin et al., 2017). This seemed to be confirmed by a recent meta-analysis which showed a positive effect on mortality of a prophylactic indomethacin regime (Jensen et al., 2018). It has been suggested that indomethacin promotes maturation of the cerebral vasculature (Ment et al., 1992; Ballabh, 2014). We suggest that also an indomethacin-induced stabilization of cerebral perfusion and improvement of cerebral vascular autoregulation plays a role with respect to reduction of PIVH. Earlier studies of our group in preterm fetal and neonatal lambs showed that indomethacin improved the autoregulatory ability of the cerebrovascular bed, probably due to its vasoconstrictive action,

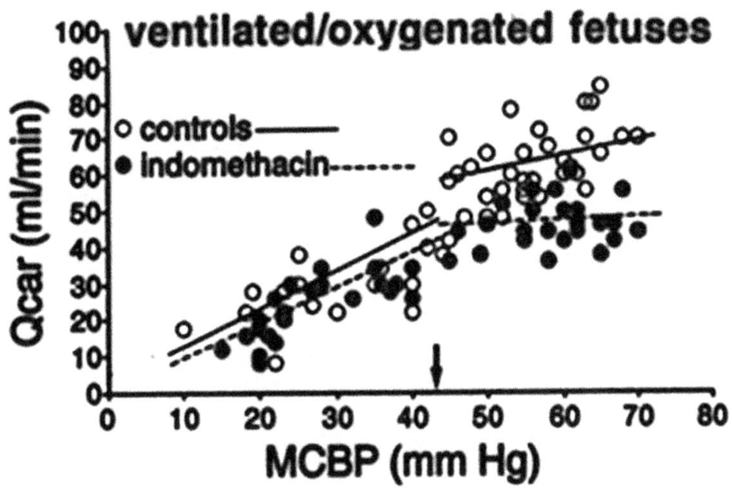

FIGURE 2 | Individual values of Carotid blood flow [Qcar (ml/min)], representing global cerebral blood flow, as a function of (mean) carotid blood pressure (MCBP; mm Hg), representing cerebral perfusion pressure, in pretreated with indomethacin (filled circles) and non-treated ventilated preterm sheep fetuses, representing a perinatal lamb model (van Bel et al., 1993,1994,1995). Note the lower Qcar values and better autoregulatory curve in the indomethacin-treated animals. The small black arrow indicates the lower limit of MCBP where cerebral autoregulation is still operative.

preventing cerebral hyperperfusion as compared to placebo-treated controls (**Figure 2**; van Bel et al., 1993, 1994, 1995).

Head position and especially left or right deviation of the head of very and extremely preterm infants may affect venous drainage by partial occlusion of the jugular vein. This can induce a temporary increase in intracranial pressure. It has been postulated that this may contribute to the occurrence of PIVH (Goldberg et al., 1983).

However, a meta-analysis of relevant studies where the infant was kept supine with the head in the midline position and the bed tilted in 30° to reduce PIVH incidence failed to show a decrease in PIVH incidence as compared to their control counterparts (Romantsik et al., 2017). Additional studies are ongoing.

Prevention and Reduction of PIVH: Emerging Interventions

Suboptimal blood gas values and hypoxia due to pulmonary immaturity and IRDS play a role in the pathogenesis of PIVH (Ballabh, 2014). Experimental studies and clinical studies using near infrared spectroscopy (NIRS) showed that prolonged episodes of cerebral oxygen saturation lower than 40–45% were related to damage in the developing brain (Dent et al., 2005; Hou et al., 2007). With NIRS-derived monitoring of cerebral oxygenation and perfusion it is possible to timely identify and intervene during episodes of suboptimal oxygenation and perfusion of the immature brain (Skov et al., 1991; van Bel et al., 2008; Wintermark et al., 2014; Alderliesten et al., 2016; van Bel and Mintzer, 2018). Recently, a European randomized controlled multicenter intervention trial (the SafeboosC study) focusing on the reduction of hypoxia and/or hyperoxia, provided evidence that *monitoring cerebral oxygenation* with NIRS lowered the hypoxic burden in extremely preterm neonates in the first days after birth (Hyttel-Sorensen et al., 2015), the episode in which most PIVH occur and/or extend. A follow-up study from this SafeboosC cohort showed that the (early) burden of hypoxia was associated with the occurrence of severe PIVH (Plomgaard et al., 2017). To confirm that interventions on basis of NIRS-monitored cerebral oxygenation can decrease PIVH incidence a contemporary randomized controlled trial with adequate patient inclusions is mandatory. In this respect it is also important to emphasize that clinical application of NIRS in the neonatal intensive care unit, to assess (in) adequacy of cerebral oxygenation, requires international consensus with respect to normative values and understanding of cerebral oxygen utilization patterns (van Bel and Mintzer, 2018).

A potentially promising intervention to lower PIVH incidence is *delayed cord clamping or DCC*. The underlying mechanism may be that a greater neonatal blood volume due to DCC gives rise to an improved cardiac preload leading to a stable cardiac output, stable blood pressure and intact cerebral autoregulation with less need for inotropic therapy (Hooper et al., 2015; Perlman et al., 2015; Wyllie et al., 2015). Consequently the stable hemodynamics may ensure an appropriate cerebral perfusion (Baenziger et al., 2007; Ersdal et al., 2014). Especially lack of cerebral autoregulation and use of positive inotropes seem to be related to a higher incidence and extension of PIVH (Alderliesten et al., 2013). Several studies suggest a positive effect of DCC on PIVH incidence (Rabe et al., 2008, 2012). However, a recent meta-analysis did not yet confirm this although there was a strong tendency for a reducing effect of DCC on PIVH incidence (Fogarty et al., 2018). A key issue with respect to the beneficial effects of DCC on PIVH incidence in very and extremely preterm infants to be solved, is the optimal time of DCC. The delay time in the 27 studies included in the meta-analysis of Fogarty et al was very variable, from 30-up to-more than 120 s (Fogarty et al., 2018). It has been suggested by others that an optimal delay time should be 180 s which may optimize the beneficial effects of DCC (Yao et al., 1969).

Preventive treatment with *trophic factors* and especially *Erythropoietin (EPO)* and *Insulin Growth Factor-1 (IGF-1)* and its *binding protein 3 (IGF-1-BP3)* are increasingly recognized to have neuroprotection and PIVH-reducing properties (Juul and Pet, 2015; Hellstrom et al., 2016).

EPO stimulates red cell production, cell survival and differentiation and EPO receptors are detected on endothelial, glial and neuronal cells (van der Kooij et al., 2008; Chateauvieux et al., 2011; Koulnis et al., 2014; Rangarajan and Juul, 2014). EPO has also a modulating effect on glutamate toxicity, stimulating effect on antioxidative ability and anti-inflammatory effect protecting endothelial cells from apoptotic death (Yamaji et al., 1996; Bernaudin et al., 1999; Kawakami et al., 2001). These latter properties of EPO may imply that recombinant human (rh) EPO can also have a positive impact on the PIVH incidence in premature neonates. An older study from Neubauer et al showed indeed a decrease in the incidence of severe PIVH after early rhEPO (Neubauer et al., 2010), although later studies showed conflicting results with respect to PIVH incidence after rhEPO (Ohls et al., 2014; Fauchere et al., 2015). A recent meta-analysis including 3,643 extremely and very preterm infants receiving early EPO therapy reported a reducing effect on PIVH incidence (Fischer et al., 2017; Ohlsson and Aher, 2017).

IGF-1 is an endogenous protein which exerts several actions: its positive effect on proper vascularization (Hellstrom et al., 2001; Bach, 2015) and brain development are important for a normal neurodevelopment (Hellstrom et al., 2016). Following extremely preterm birth, serum IGF-1 levels are much lower than in utero serum concentrations at corresponding gestational ages. Inadequate endogenous postnatal IGF-1 production is regarded to be the result of preterm birth related events such as hypoxia, inflammation and reduced nutrient availability (Hellstrom et al., 2016). The fact that extremely preterm born infants have deficient serum IGF-1 and IGF-1-BP3 concentrations stimulated researchers and clinicians to perform studies in which suppletion of IGF-1 and its IGF-1 bounding protein BP3 were expected to have maturational effects on vascularization of the extremely preterm neonate (Ley et al., 2013). Intranasal IGF-1 reduced germinal matrix hemorrhages in a preterm rat pup model (Lekic et al., 2016). A clinical study of Hellstrom et al on the effects of IGF-1 on ROP, PIVH and bronchopulmonary dysplasia is ongoing (ClinicalTrials.gov: NCT01096784).

In summary, antenatal corticosteroids and the introduction of exogenous surfactant substantially reduced the PIVH incidence

TABLE 1 | Summary of standard care and emerging therapies respectively, for the prevention and reduction of periventricular-intraventricular hemorrhage (PIVH) and (diffuse) white matter injury (dWMI).

PIVH and (d)WMI
Standard care
– Antenatal corticosteroids
– Exogenous surfactant instillation
– Non-invasive ventilation techniques/stress reduction
– Prophylactic early (<6 h) indomethacin
Emerging therapies
– Delayed cord clamping
– Trophic factors i.e. erythropoietin (rhEPO) insulin growth factor-1 and its binding protein 3 (IGF-1/IGF-1BP3)

of the preterm born infant in high income countries. Better and non-invasive ventilation techniques together with exogenous surfactant treatment and stress reduction during patient care had a further reducing effect on PIVH incidence, as did prophylactic indomethacin treatment.

Promising future therapies for PIVH prevention and/or reduction of severity are delayed cord clamping and early and adequate treatment with trophic factors such as erythropoietin and IGF-1. However, further research is mandatory here. **Table 1** shows schematically the above discussed therapeutic considerations.

WHITE MATTER INJURY IN THE VERY AND EXTREMELY PRETERM INFANT

Extremely preterm born infants (or ELGANs) carry a substantial risk of diffuse white matter injury or abnormal white matter development (Volpe, 2009; Chau et al., 2013). In the early days of neonatal intensive care, white matter injury (WMI; or periventricular leukomalacia) was encountered in the form of cystic periventricular leukomalacia (cPVL), as described by Banker and Larroche (1962). cPVL was hard to detect using CT, but could be detected with the use of cranial ultrasound (cUS), in particular when used longitudinally after the first week after birth (de Vries et al., 2004). The cysts of cPVL appear 10–20 days after an insult, and disappear around term equivalent age. Remaining injury can be seen as widening and irregularity of the ventricles on cUS, and loss of white matter and delayed myelination on cranial MRI (Chau et al., 2013; Martinez-Biarge et al., 2016). Later in life gliosis can be seen in the affected areas. The cysts of cPVL occur alongside the ventricles in preterm infants, whereas subcortical cysts are more common in term infants.

Several causes of cPVL have been suggested, including hypoxia-ischemia and inflammation. Fetal inflammation has been reported to be common in preterm birth (reviewed by Hagberg et al., 2015). Furthermore, preterm CSF appears to show a neuroinflammatory response compared to term infants. Although many have reported white matter injury after maternal chorioamnionitis with infection (reviewed by Paton et al., 2017) (O'Shea et al., 2012; Strunk et al., 2014; Paton et al., 2017), a recent study failed to show a detrimental effect of chorioamnionitis (Bierstone et al., 2018). Reactive oxygen species are considered to play a role in the injury of the cerebral white matter of the preterm infant (Hagberg et al., 2015).

Occurrence of cPVL has been demonstrated after severe hypocapnia and subsequent cerebral vasoconstriction (Groenendaal and de Vries, 2001). The incidence of cPVL is decreasing in modern neonatal intensive care to 1.3% of a NICU cohort of very preterm infants (van Haastert et al., 2011). Probably multiple factors may have contributed to the decrease of cPVL, such as monitoring of blood pressure, low carbon dioxide levels, blood glucose, and cerebral oxygenation using NIRS. The role of maternal antibiotics is still unresolved (Shepherd et al., 2017).

Nowadays, diffuse white matter injury (dWMI), and 'punctate white matter lesions' are more commonly seen in extremely preterm infants (Kersbergen et al., 2014a) (**Figure 1**). Diffuse WMI might even be present in more than 50% of extremely and very preterm infants (Hinojosa-Rodríguez et al., 2017).

A recent review by our group (van Tilborg et al., 2018b), summarizing a substantial amount of preclinical studies, suggested that an arrest in maturation of oligodendrocyte precursors is responsible for hypomyelination as seen in experimental models of dWMI (van de Looij et al., 2012; van Tilborg et al., 2018a). As reviewed by Hagberg et al. (2015) pro-inflammatory cytokines, including IL-6, and TNF-alpha will lead to increased activation of microglia with adverse effects on developing oligodendrocyte precursors. Systemic inflammation in common in extremely and very preterm infants. Although beyond the aim of this review it is important to state that also in moderate and late preterm infants inflammation can lead to brain damage and adverse outcome (Gisslen et al., 2016; Musilova et al., 2018).

Preterm white matter can be studied in far more detail using MRI, and longitudinal scans can visualize brain growth, including growth of specific brain regions, cortical folding and white matter development (Kersbergen et al., 2014b), but identification of tissue microstructure is still challenging (Stolp et al., 2018). Scoring systems have been developed to quantify the abnormalities seen at term equivalent age in this population, and the predictive power for neurodevelopment is under investigation (Inder et al., 2005; Kidokoro et al., 2013). At present, MRI might be more informative in hospitals that are dedicated for neonatal MRI than in general.

Prevention and Reduction of (Diffuse) White Matter Injury

Antenatal and perinatal strategies are very important in the prevention of dWMI. *Magnesium sulphate given antenatally* to women at risk of preterm birth substantially reduced the risk of cerebral palsy of the infant (Crowther et al., 2017). The mechanism of this neuroprotection is still unknown. Improved uterine perfusion through vasodilation, and a reduction of neonatal IVH have been proposed mechanisms. Although magnesium reduces EEG activity and the number of seizures in an animal model of preterm asphyxia (Galinsky et al., 2017; Bennet et al., 2018b), blockade of NMDA receptors or other excitotoxic pathways is unlikely. Although plasma concentrations achieved in mothers and fetuses are increased after maternal administration of magnesium, extracellular magnesium concentrations in the brain are probably lower than those needed for neuroprotection after experimental hypoxia-ischemia. (Crowther et al., 2017; Galinsky et al., 2017).

A recent trial (NCT00724594) tested the pharmacokinetics of maternal and neonatal N-Acetylcysteine. Interestingly, umbilical cord concentrations frequently exceeded maternal concentrations (Wiest et al., 2014). Future studies may aim at the use of N-Acetylcysteine to reduce free radical injury in preterm infants.

Delayed umbilical cord clamping has been advised in 'vigorous' preterm infants. It is associated with significant neonatal benefits, including improved transitional circulation, better establishment of red blood cell volume, decreased need for blood transfusion, and lower incidence of necrotizing enterocolitis, leading to massive systemic inflammation and subsequent white matter injury, and intraventricular hemorrhage (as already discussed above; (Practice, 2017). Thereby it may have an indirect beneficial effect on white matter injury (see also above: emerging therapies for prevention of PIVH (Mercer et al., 2016)).

Reduction of severe IRDS not only reduces IVH (see above), but it may also important in the reduction of severe white matter injury. As through a reduction of severe respiratory illness large fluctuations in oxygen and carbon dioxide levels are avoided, production of reactive oxygen species may be reduced. Furthermore, *stabilization of blood pressure* reduces major swings in cerebral perfusion.

Postnatal pharmacologic interventions for reduction or prevention of dWMI are increasingly recognized as being potentially neuroprotective. Although early *postnatal administration of the corticosteroid dexamethasone* has been reported to be associated with cerebral palsy (Doyle et al., 2017), this may be not the case for *hydrocortisone* (Karemaker et al., 2006). Recently a trial was finished comparing hydrocortisone versus placebo in ventilated preterm infants to reduce chronic lung disease (Onland et al., 2011). Neurodevelopment of these infants will provide information on the benefits (or risks) of postnatal hydrocortisone. Postnatal use of *caffeine* resulted in improved neurodevelopmental outcome (Schmidt et al., 2007). Neonatal caffeine therapy for apnea of prematurity improved visuomotor, visuoperceptual, and visuospatial abilities at age 11 years (Murner-Lavanchy et al., 2018).

It has been suggested that improvement of preterm *nutrition* may contribute to optimizing brain development. In particular the so-called microbiome-gut-brain-*Axis axis* is a proposed mechanism of interaction, including neural, endocrine, and immunological pathways (Cryan and Dinan, 2012). Nutritional components such as fatty acids and protein may stimulate brain growth and neurodevelopment (Uauy and Mena, 2015; Coviello et al., 2018). Also probiotics might be beneficial in reducing the incidence of necrotizing enterocolitis and thereby reduce white matter injury.

Monitoring of cerebral oxygenation with NIRS (as already discussed above in relation with prevention of PIVH) and *of brain function* (amplitude EEG [aEEG]), may also play an important preventing role with relation to dWMI.

Since very low arterial CO_2 levels may contribute to cerebral hypoperfusion and white matter injury (Greisen and Vannucci, 2001). Tools to monitor the neonatal brain oxygenation and function with NIRS and aEEG may contribute to optimize cerebral oxygenation (Hyttel-Sorensen et al., 2015; Plomgaard et al., 2017), and early recognition and treatment of subclinical seizure activity (Glass et al., 2017). Further studies are needed to describe the association with long-term neurodevelopment (Hyttel-Sorensen et al., 2017; Thewissen et al., 2018).

Pain and stress are shown to have negative effects on brain development (Duerden et al., 2018). Avoidance of pain appears to be useful. In very preterm infants on mechanical ventilation, continuous fentanyl infusion might protect the developing brain by relieving pain during the first 72 h of mechanical ventilation (Qiu et al., 2018). In contrast others have demonstrated impaired cerebellar growth in the neonatal period and poorer neurodevelopmental outcomes in early childhood of preterm infants after morphine use (Zwicker et al., 2016).

To find an optimal balance between pain and stress reduction and use of opioids may aid in the reduction of white matter injury. Alternative strategies for stress and pain reduction, such as sucrose, use of pacifiers, or non-sedative analgetics need to be explored further.

Inflammation

Extremely preterm birth is commonly associated with fetal and postnatal systemic inflammation which is likely to contribute to dWMI through adverse effects on oligodendrocyte precursors (Strunk et al., 2014; Hagberg et al., 2015). Novel strategies are explored to counteract these inflammatory pathways to counteract the deleterious effects on preterm white matter (see below).

Prevention and Reduction of (d)WMI: Emerging Pharmacologic Interventions

Many anti-inflammatory interventions have been suggested as a result from animal experiments (reviewed by Hagberg et al., 2015). Almost none of these have been tested in human infants.

Erythropoietin or EPO has been suggested to inhibit glutamate release, reduce accumulation of intracellular calcium, to induce antiapoptotic factors, to reduce inflammation and nitric oxide-mediated injury, and to contribute to regeneration (van der Kooij et al., 2008; Chateauvieux et al., 2011; Rangarajan and Juul, 2014).

In the EpoKids study in Switzerland very preterm infants were randomized to 3 doses of rhEPO (one before birth, 2 after birth) versus placebo. The secondary outcome of MRI at term equivalent age showed less white matter injury in the EPO group compared with the placebo group (Leuchter et al., 2014). A meta-analysis of administration of rhEPO showed an improved the cognitive development of very preterm infants, as assessed by the MDI at a corrected age of 18–24 months, without affecting other neurodevelopmental outcomes (Fischer et al., 2017). Several trials are still ongoing to study neuroprotection by EPO in preterm infants (Juul and Pet, 2015). Given its positive effect on neurogenesis and angiogenesis a more prolonged course of appropriately (high) dosed rhEPO (up to 2,500 IU/kg daily) may further optimize clinical outcome of the preterm infant (van der Kooij et al., 2008; Chateauvieux et al., 2011; Rangarajan and Juul, 2014).

In animal models *melatonin* has antioxidant properties by influencing several pathways, and reduces (neuro-) inflammation. Through reduction of proinflammatory cytokines pro-oligodendrocyte maturation could be preserved. Administration of *melatonin* to pregnant women with fetal growth restriction or pre-eclampsia is under investigation (NCT02395783 and NCT01695070). Neonatal administration of *melatonin* has been used in preterm newborns with sepsis, surgical procedures or chronic lung disease (Marseglia et al., 2015). However, no beneficial effect on MRI parameters of the preterm brain at term equivalent age could be demonstrated in the relatively low dose administered in this study (Merchant et al., 2014).

IGF-1 plays a crucial role in fetal and postnatal brain development: IGF-1 is shown to stimulate neurogenesis and proliferation, differentiation and survival of brain cells. Regarding white matter development, IGF-1 also stimulates oligodendrocyte maturation and subsequent myelination (Cao et al., 2003; Pang et al., 2010; Cai et al., 2011; Hansen-Pupp et al., 2011; O'Kusky and Ye, 2012). Moreover, genetic studies in mice display lower total brain volumes and severe hypomyelination following IGF-1 knockout (O'Kusky and Ye, 2012). Human studies relating serum IGF-1 levels to brain development show a positive association between postnatal serum IGF-1 concentrations and head circumference, brain volume measures and developmental scores at 2 years of age (Hansen-Pupp et al., 2011). Main focus of previous studies with IGF-1 and its IGF-1- binding protein 3 was the prevention of retinopathy of prematurity, but the incidence of PIVH will be studied in addition (*ClinicalTrials.gov: NCT01096784*). Further studies are needed to explore potential neuroprotective effects of IGF-1 with respect to dWMI.

In summary, Injury to and subnormal development of the periventricular white matter is still very common in extremely preterm born infants. Although improved neonatal intensive care may contribute to improved outcomes, additional strategies to counteract (d) WMI may add to an improved neurodevelopmental outcome.

REPAIR OF SEQUELAE OF PIVH AND dWMI

Increasing experimental evidence shows that regeneration of the injured immature brain with stem cell-based therapies is promising and may serve as an effective treatment strategy. Stem cells have an intrinsic potential for self-renewal and can differentiate into several cellular phenotypes (Fleiss et al., 2014). Given their pluripotent capacity, embryonic stem cells seem the most obvious choice for repair of brain injury, but can induce formation of teratoma after transplantation. Their clinical application raises therefore considerable ethical concerns. This is also true for multipotent neural stem cells: although very attractive given their possibility to derive all neural lineages, their accessibility in humans is limited because they carry also a substantial risk for tumor formation (Comi et al., 2008). Among all progenitor cells, the mesenchymal stem (or stromal) cell (MSC) is at this moment the most optimal choice for near-future use in (preterm) neonates because of the evident neuroregenerative properties and favorable immunological profile and, not for the least, of its favorable safety profile (Uccelli et al., 2008; Fleiss et al., 2014). MSCs are considered to adapt their secretome, after which paracrine signaling results in endogenous brain repair rather than direct cell replacement through MSC differentiation (Qu et al., 2007; van Velthoven et al., 2011). Paracrine effects of MSCs include many growth factors such as insulin-like growth factor (IGF-1), brain-derived neurotrophic factor (BDNF), glial-derived neurotrophic factor (GDNF), and vascular endothelial growth factors (VEGF) (Kizil et al., 2015; Ophelders et al., 2016; Bennet et al., 2018a). These factors can promote endogenous repair through brain cell formation in the sub ventricular zone as well as boost neuronal and glial cell proliferation, maturation and survival on other regions, Moreover, MSCs are shown to secrete anti-inflammatory cytokines, involved in reduction of neuroinflammation (**Figure 3**). Upregulation of neoneurogenesis and downregulation of genes involved in inflammation after MSC transplantation has been reported in a review (Wagenaar et al., 2017).

MSCs can be administered to the brain *via* several routes: intravenously, intracranially/intrathecally and nasally. The nasal route is non-invasive and seems more effective without loss of MSCs in other organ systems as compared to intravenous administration (Fischer et al., 2009; Wagenaar et al., 2017). In a neonatal stroke model in mice pups substantial beneficial effects on infarction size, motor function and cognition were demonstrated (Wagenaar et al., 2017). The nasally administered MSC cells were no longer detectable 3 days after the implantation, minimizing the risk for Graft-versus Host Disease and tumor growth (Donega et al., 2014). This is confirmed by a long-term safety study of our group (Donega et al., 2015). Moreover

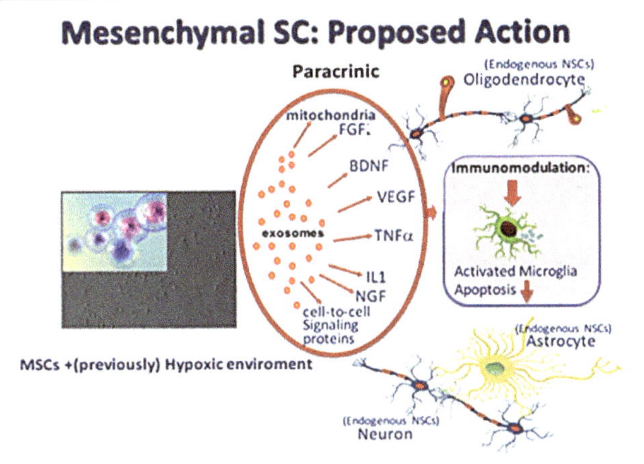

FIGURE 3 | Proposed actions of mesenchymal stem cells (MSC) when present in a (previously) hypoxic–ischemic environment: production of vesicles (exosomes) of various growth factors, (anti-inflammatory) cytokines, signaling proteins and mitochondria which give rise to recovery of affected neurons and to proliferation of endogenous paraventricular-situated neural stem cells to form oligodendrocytes, astrocytes and neurons.

human trials on MSC therapy in adults and children did not provide evidence for serious long-term effects (Lalu et al., 2012). An important advantage of MSC-based cell therapy is that autologous as well as allogeneic transplantation can be applied. Autologous intravenous MSC-transplantations, mostly derived and cultured from MSC-rich umbilical cord tissue or cord blood, as well as allogeneic MSCs (see below) are already reported for clinical use in neonatal medicine (Chang et al., 2014; Cotten et al., 2014). A detailed review concerning stem cell-based therapy in neonatology is beyond the scope of this review but is summarized in several recent reviews (Wagenaar et al., 2017; Gronbach et al., 2018; Niimi and Levison, 2018; Vaes et al., in preparation).

Stem Cell-Therapy and PIVH

Experimental studies reported that cord-derived MSCs substantially attenuated reactive gliosis and cell death which went along with an increase of brain-derived neurotrophic factor (BDNF) (Mukai et al., 2017). Further study showed that MSC-derived BDNF secretion was indeed a critical paracrine factor playing a central role in the attenuation of PIVH-induced brain injury (Ahn et al., 2017). Preclinical data pointed to a repairing effect of MSCs on the sequelae of severe PIVH (Park et al., 2017). Ahn et al showed that in preterm rat pups (P4), in which severe IVH was induced, intraventricularly transplanted human umbilical cord-derived MSCs attenuated posthemorrhagic ventricular dilatation and the area of brain injury (Ahn et al., 2013). They also showed that the window of effective treatment was at least up to 2 days after induction of brain damage (Park et al., 2016).

Clinical experience is still scarce. Some investigators consider DCC as a form of autologous cord blood transplantation since the number of nucleated cord cells in the newborn which also contain pluripotent stem cells increase (Bayer, 2016). A recent small study from Poland in which very preterm infants were given autologous umbilical cord blood showed significantly higher concentrations of growth factors (among them insulin growth factor, epidermal growth factor and stem cell factor), whereas (severe) PIVH incidence seemed lower in the transplanted group as compared to a control group (Kotowski et al., 2017). Although not directly related to the immature brain, a Korean safety and feasibility study in extremely preterm infants to lower the risk of bronchopulmonary dysplasia with allogeneic cord-derived MSCs (endotracheal administration) reported that allogeneic MSC transplantation seemed safe and well-tolerated by the infants (Chang et al., 2014). A safety and efficacy study of the same group is currently including patients with PIVH (*ClinicalTrial.gov: NCT02673788*).

Although MSC transplantation seems very promising, it may be clear that further clinical research is mandatory to proof its efficacy to attenuate the consequences of (severe) PIVH. In particular, optimization of dosing of MSCs, the preferred type of MSCs (cord-derived vs bone marrow-derived; (Chen et al., 2009)) and most optimal route of administration are important pending questions, which have to be elucidated.

Stem Cell-Therapy and Diffuse WMI

Treatment with MSCs in preterm neonates with or at risk for dWMI provides us with an exciting and potentially powerful therapy to reduce or even prevent damage to the vulnerable white matter of the preterm neonate. Experimental studies in which perinatal insults as inflammation and hypoxia-ischemia are used separately or in combination showed us already that the paracrine factors secreted by the MSCs promote oligodendrocyte lineage specification, myelination and maturation (Chen et al., 2010; Jadasz et al., 2013; Jellema et al., 2013; Li et al., 2016; Drommelschmidt et al., 2017). It remains to be proven whether MSC-induced endogenous repair mechanisms also lead to substantial positive effects in diffuse WMI of the preterm infant in whom the interplay of inflammation and hypoxia-ischemia appears to be most relevant. Further research is emerging and mandatory.

AUTHOR CONTRIBUTIONS

All authors listed have made a substantial, direct and intellectual contribution to the work, and approved it for publication.

REFERENCES

Ahn, S. Y., Chang, Y. S., Sung, D. K., Sung, S. I., Yoo, H. S., Lee, J. H., et al. (2013). Mesenchymal stem cells prevent hydrocephalus after severe intraventricular hemorrhage. *Stroke* 44, 497–504. doi: 10.1161/STROKEAHA.112.679092

Ahn, S. Y., Chang, Y. S., Sung, D. K., Sung, S. I., Ahn, J. Y., and Park, W. S. (2017). Pivotal role of brain-derived neurotrophic factor secreted by mesenchymal stem cells in severe intraventricular hemorrhage in newborn rats. *Cell Transplant.* 26, 145–156. doi: 10.3727/096368916X692861

Alderliesten, T., Lemmers, P. M., Smarius, J. J., van de Vosse, R. E., Baerts, W., and van Bel, F. (2013). Cerebral oxygenation, extraction, and autoregulation in very preterm infants who develop peri-intraventricular hemorrhage. *J. Pediatr.* 162, 698–704.e692. doi: 10.1016/j.jpeds.2012.09.038

Alderliesten, T., De Vis, J. B., Lemmers, P. M. A., van Bel, F., Benders, M., Hendrikse, J., et al. (2016). T2-prepared velocity selective labelling: a novel idea for full-brain mapping of oxygen saturation. *NeuroImage* 139, 65–73. doi: 10.1016/j.neuroimage.2016.06.012

Anand, K. J., Barton, B. A., McIntosh, N., Lagercrantz, H., Pelausa, E., Young, T. E., et al. (1999). Analgesia and sedation in preterm neonates who require ventilatory support: results from the NOPAIN trial. Neonatal outcome and prolonged analgesia in neonates. *Arch. Pediatr. Adolesc. Med.* 153, 331–338.

Bach, L. A. (2015). Endothelial cells and the IGF system. *J. Mol. Endocrinol.* 54, R1–R13. doi: 10.1530/JME-14-0215

Baenziger, O., Stolkin, F., Keel, M., von Siebenthal, K., Fauchere, J. C., Das Kundu, S., et al. (2007). The influence of the timing of cord clamping on postnatal cerebral oxygenation in preterm neonates: a randomized, controlled trial. *Pediatrics* 119, 455–459. doi: 10.1542/peds.2006-2725

Ballabh, P. (2014). Pathogenesis and prevention of intraventricular hemorrhage. *Clin. Perinatol.* 41, 47–67. doi: 10.1016/j.clp.2013.09.007

Banker, B. Q., and Larroche, J. C. (1962). Periventricular leukomalacia of infancy. A form of neonatal anoxic encephalopathy. *Arch. Neurol.* 7, 386–410. doi: 10.1001/archneur.1962.04210050022004

Bayer, K. (2016). Delayed umbilical cord clamping in the 21st century: indications for Practice. *Adv. Neonatal Care* 16, 68–73. doi: 10.1097/ANC.0000000000000247

Bedard, M. P., Shankaran, S., Slovis, T. L., Pantoja, A., Dayal, B., and Poland, R. L. (1984). Effect of prophylactic phenobarbital on intraventricular hemorrhage in high-risk infants. *Pediatrics* 73, 435–439.

Bennet, L., Dhillon, S., Lear, C. A., van den Heuij, L., King, V., Dean, J. M., et al. (2018a). Chronic inflammation and impaired development of the preterm brain. *J. Reprod. Immunol.* 125, 45–55. doi: 10.1016/j.jri.2017.11.003

Bennet, L., Galinsky, R., Draghi, V., Lear, C. A., Davidson, J. O., Unsworth, C. P., et al. (2018b). Time and sex dependent effects of magnesium sulphate on post-asphyxial seizures in preterm fetal sheep. *J. Physiol.* 596, 6079–6092. doi: 10.1113/JP275627

Benson, J. W., Drayton, M. R., Hayward, C., Murphy, J. F., Osborne, J. P., Rennie, J. M., et al. (1986). Multicentre trial of ethamsylate for prevention of periventricular haemorrhage in very low birthweight infants. *Lancet* 2, 1297–1300. doi: 10.1016/S0140-6736(86)91432-7

Beresford, M. W., and Shaw, N. J. (2002). Detectable IL-8 and IL-10 in bronchoalveolar lavage fluid from preterm infants ventilated for respiratory distress syndrome. *Pediatr. Res.* 52, 973–978. doi: 10.1203/00006450-200212000-00025

Bernaudin, M., Marti, H. H., Roussel, S., Divoux, D., Nouvelot, A., MacKenzie, E. T., et al. (1999). A potential role for erythropoietin in focal permanent cerebral ischemia in mice. *J. Cereb. Blood Flow Metab.* 19, 643–651.

Bierstone, D., Wagenaar, N., Gano, D. L., Guo, T., Georgio, G., Groenendaal, F., et al. (2018). Association of histologic chorioamnionitis with perinatal brain injury and early childhood neurodevelopmental outcomes among preterm neonates. *JAMA Pediatr.* 172, 534–541. doi: 10.1001/jamapediatrics.2018.0102

Bilguvar, K., DiLuna, M. L., Bizzarro, M. J., Bayri, Y., Schneider, K. C., Lifton, R. P., et al. (2009). COL4A1 mutation in preterm intraventricular hemorrhage. *J. Pediatr.* 155, 743–745. doi: 10.1016/j.jpeds.2009.04.014

Brion, L. P., Bell, E. F., and Raghuveer, T. S. (2003). Vitamin E supplementation for prevention of morbidity and mortality in preterm infants. *Cochrane Database Syst. Rev.* Cd003665. doi: 10.1002/14651858.CD003665

Brownfoot, F. C., Gagliardi, D. I., Bain, E., Middleton, P., and Crowther, C. A. (2013). Different corticosteroids and regimens for accelerating fetal lung maturation for women at risk of preterm birth. *Cochrane Database Syst. Rev.* Cd006764. doi: 10.1002/14651858.CD006764.pub3

Cai, Z., Fan, L. W., Lin, S., Pang, Y., and Rhodes, P. G. (2011). Intranasal administration of insulin-like growth factor-1 protects against lipopolysaccharide-induced injury in the developing rat brain. *Neuroscience* 194, 195–207. doi: 10.1016/j.neuroscience.2011.08.003

Cao, Y., Gunn, A. J., Bennet, L., Wu, D., George, S., Gluckman, P. D., et al. (2003). Insulin-like growth factor (IGF)-1 suppresses oligodendrocyte caspase-3 activation and increases glial proliferation after ischemia in near-term fetal sheep. *J. Cereb. Blood Flow Metab.* 23, 739–747. doi: 10.1097/01.WCB.0000067720.12805.6F

Chang, Y. S., Ahn, S. Y., Yoo, H. S., Sung, S. I., Choi, S. J., Oh, W. I., et al. (2014). Mesenchymal stem cells for bronchopulmonary dysplasia: phase 1 dose-escalation clinical trial. *J. Pediatr.* 164, 966–972.e966. doi: 10.1016/j.jpeds.2013.12.011

Chateauvieux, S., Grigorakaki, C., Morceau, F., Dicato, M., and Diederich, M. (2011). Erythropoietin, erythropoiesis and beyond. *Biochem. Pharmacol.* 82, 1291–1303. doi: 10.1016/j.bcp.2011.06.045

Chau, V., Synnes, A., Grunau, R. E., Poskitt, K. J., Brant, R., and Miller, S. P. (2013). Abnormal brain maturation in preterm neonates associated with adverse developmental outcomes. *Neurology* 81, 2082–2089. doi: 10.1212/01.wnl.0000437298.43688.b9

Chen, M. Y., Lie, P. C., Li, Z. L., and Wei, X. (2009). Endothelial differentiation of Wharton's jelly-derived mesenchymal stem cells in comparison with bone marrow-derived mesenchymal stem cells. *Exp. Hematol.* 37, 629–640. doi: 10.1016/j.exphem.2009.02.003

Chen, A., Siow, B., Blamire, A. M., Lako, M., and Clowry, G. J. (2010). Transplantation of magnetically labeled mesenchymal stem cells in a model of perinatal brain injury. *Stem Cell Res.* 5, 255–266. doi: 10.1016/j.scr.2010.08.004

Chevallier, M., Debillon, T., Pierrat, V., Delorme, P., Kayem, G., Durox, M., et al. (2017). Leading causes of preterm delivery as risk factors for intraventricular hemorrhage in very preterm infants: results of the EPIPAGE 2 cohort study. *Am. J. Obstet. Gynecol.* 216, 518.e511–518.e512. doi: 10.1016/j.ajog.2017.01.002

Chisholm, K. M., Heerema-McKenney, A., Tian, L., Rajani, A. K., Saria, S., Koller, D., et al. (2016). Correlation of preterm infant illness severity with placental histology. *Placenta* 39, 61–69. doi: 10.1016/j.placenta.2016.01.012

Comi, A. M., Cho, E., Mulholland, J. D., Hooper, A., Li, Q., Qu, Y., et al. (2008). Neural stem cells reduce brain injury after unilateral carotid ligation. *Pediatr. Neurol.* 38, 86–92. doi: 10.1016/j.pediatrneurol.2007.10.007

Cotten, C. M., Murtha, A. P., Goldberg, R. N., Grotegut, C. A., Smith, P. B., Goldstein, R. F., et al. (2014). Feasibility of autologous cord blood cells for infants with hypoxic-ischemic encephalopathy. *J. Pediatr.* 164, 973–979.e971. doi: 10.1016/j.jpeds.2013.11.036

Coviello, C., Keunen, K., Kersbergen, K. J., Groenendaal, F., Leemans, A., Peels, B., et al. (2018). Effects of early nutrition and growth on brain volumes, white matter microstructure, and neurodevelopmental outcome in preterm newborns. *Pediatr. Res.* 83, 102–110. doi: 10.1038/pr.2017.227

Crowther, C. A., Middleton, P. F., Voysey, M., Askie, L., Duley, L., Pryde, P. G., et al. (2017). Assessing the neuroprotective benefits for babies of antenatal magnesium sulphate: an individual participant data meta-analysis. *PLoS Med.* 14:e1002398. doi: 10.1371/journal.pmed.1002398

Cryan, J. F., and Dinan, T. G. (2012). Mind-altering microorganisms: the impact of the gut microbiota on brain and behaviour. *Nat. Rev. Neurosci.* 13, 701–712. doi: 10.1038/nrn3346

de Vries, L. S., van Haastert, I. C., Rademaker, K. J., Koopman, C., and Groenendaal, F. (2004). Ultrasound abnormalities preceding cerebral palsy in high risk preterm infants. *J. Pediatr.* 144, 815–820. doi: 10.1016/j.jpeds.2004.03.034

Dent, C. L., Spaeth, J. P., Jones, B. V., Schwartz, S. M., Glauser, T. A., Hallinan, B.., et al. (2005). Brain magnetic resonance imaging abnormalities after the Norwood procedure using regional cerebral perfusion. *J. Thorac. Cardiovasc. Surg.* 130, 1523–1530. doi: 10.1016/j.jtcvs.2005.10.003

Donega, V., Nijboer, C. H., van Tilborg, G., Dijkhuizen, R. M., Kavelaars, A., and Heijnen, C. J. (2014). Intranasally administered mesenchymal stem cells promote a regenerative niche for repair of neonatal ischemic brain injury. *Exp. Neurol.* 261, 53–64. doi: 10.1016/j.expneurol.2014.06.009

Donega, V., Nijboer, C. H., van Velthoven, C. T., Youssef, S. A., de Bruin, A., van Bel, F., et al. (2015). Assessment of long-term safety and efficacy of intranasal mesenchymal stem cell treatment for neonatal brain injury in the mouse. *Pediatr. Res.* 78, 520–526. doi: 10.1038/pr.2015.145

Donn, S. M., Roloff, D. W., and Goldstein, G. W. (1981). Prevention of intraventricular haemorrhage in preterm infants by phenobarbitone. A controlled trial. *Lancet* 2, 215–217. doi: 10.1016/S0140-6736(81)90470-0

Doyle, L. W., Cheong, J. L., Ehrenkranz, R. A., and Halliday, H. L. (2017). Early (<8 days) systemic postnatal corticosteroids for prevention of bronchopulmonary dysplasia in preterm infants. *Cochrane Database Syst. Rev.* 10:Cd001146. doi: 10.1002/14651858.CD001145.pub4

Drommelschmidt, K., Serdar, M., Bendix, I., Herz, J., Bertling, F., Prager, S., et al. (2017). Mesenchymal stem cell-derived extracellular vesicles ameliorate inflammation-induced preterm brain injury. *Brain Behav. Immun.* 60, 220–232. doi: 10.1016/j.bbi.2016.11.011

Duerden, E. G., Grunau, R. E., Guo, T., Foong, J., Pearson, A., Au-Young, S., et al. (2018). Early procedural pain is associated with regionally-specific alterations in thalamic development in preterm neonates. *J. Neurosci.* 38, 878–886. doi: 10.1523/JNEUROSCI.0867-17.2017

Ersdal, H. L., Linde, J., Mduma, E., Auestad, B., and Perlman, J. (2014). Neonatal outcome following cord clamping after onset of spontaneous respiration. *Pediatrics* 134, 265–272. doi: 10.1542/peds.2014-0467

Fauchere, J. C., Koller, B. M., Tschopp, A., Dame, C., Ruegger, C., and Bucher, H. U. (2015). Safety of early high-dose recombinant erythropoietin for Neuroprotection in very preterm infants. *J. Pediatr.* 167, 52–57.e51-53. doi: 10.1016/j.jpeds.2015.02.052

Fischer, U. M., Harting, M. T., Jimenez, F., Monzon-Posadas, W. O., Xue, H., Savitz, S. I., et al. (2009). Pulmonary passage is a major obstacle for intravenous stem cell delivery: the pulmonary first-pass effect. *Stem Cells Dev.* 18, 683–692. doi: 10.1089/scd.2008.0253

Fischer, H. S., Reibel, N. J., Buhrer, C., and Dame, C. (2017). Prophylactic early erythropoietin for neuroprotection in preterm infants: a meta-analysis. *Pediatrics* 139:e20164317. doi: 10.1542/peds.2016-4317

Fleiss, B., Guillot, P. V., Titomanlio, L., Baud, O., Hagberg, H., and Gressens, P. (2014). Stem cell therapy for neonatal brain injury. *Clin. Perinatol.* 41, 133–148. doi: 10.1016/j.clp.2013.09.002

Fogarty, M., Osborn, D. A., Askie, L., Seidler, A. L., Hunter, K., Lui, K., et al. (2018). Delayed vs early umbilical cord clamping for preterm infants: a systematic review and meta-analysis. *Am. J. Obstet. Gynecol.* 218, 1–18. doi: 10.1016/j.ajog.2017.10.231

Galinsky, R., Draghi, V., Wassink, G., Davidson, J. O., Drury, P. P., Lear, C. A., et al. (2017). Magnesium sulfate reduces EEG activity but is not neuroprotective after asphyxia in preterm fetal sheep. *J. Cereb. Blood Flow Metab.* 37, 1362–1373. doi: 10.1177/0271678X16655548

Gisslen, T., Alvarez, M., Wells, C., Soo, M. T., Lambers, D. S., Knox, C. L., et al. (2016). Fetal inflammation associated with minimal acute morbidity in moderate/late preterm infants. *Arch. Dis. Child. Fetal Neonatal Ed.* 101, F513–F519. doi: 10.1136/archdischild-2015-308518

Gitto, E., Reiter, R. J., Cordaro, S. P., La Rosa, M., Chiurazzi, P., Trimarchi, G., et al. (2004). Oxidative and inflammatory parameters in respiratory distress syndrome of preterm newborns: beneficial effects of melatonin. *Am. J. Perinatol.* 21, 209–216. doi: 10.1055/s-2004-828610

Glass, H. C., Shellhaas, R. A., Tsuchida, T. N., Chang, T., Wusthoff, C. J., Chu, C. J., et al. (2017). Seizures in preterm neonates: a multicenter observational cohort study. *Pediatr. Neurol.* 72, 19–24. doi: 10.1016/j.pediatrneurol.2017.04.016

Goldberg, R. N., Joshi, A., Moscoso, P., and Castillo, T. (1983). The effect of head position on intracranial pressure in the neonate. *Crit. Care Med.* 11, 428–430. doi: 10.1097/00003246-198306000-00006

Greenough, A., and Ahmed, N. (2013). Perinatal prevention of bronchopulmonary dysplasia. *J. Perinat. Med.* 41, 119–126. doi: 10.1515/jpm-2012-0084

Greisen, G., and Vannucci, R. C. (2001). Is periventricular leucomalacia a result of hypoxic-ischaemic injury? hypocapnia and the preterm brain. *Biol. Neonate* 79, 194–200. doi: 10.1159/000047090

Groenendaal, F., and de Vries, L. S. (2001). Hypocarbia and white matter echolucencies in newborns < 28 weeks gestation [letter]. *Pediatr. Res.* 50, 772–773. doi: 10.1203/00006450-200112000-00024

Gronbach, J., Shahzad, T., Radajewski, S., Chao, C. M., Bellusci, S., Morty, R. E., et al. (2018). The potentials and caveats of mesenchymal stromal cell-based therapies in the preterm infant. *Stem Cells International.* 2018:9652897. doi: 10.1155/2018/9652897

Hagberg, H., Mallard, C., Ferriero, D. M., Vannucci, S. J., Levison, S. W., Vexler, Z. S., et al. (2015). The role of inflammation in perinatal brain injury. *Nat. Rev. Neurol.* 11, 192–208. doi: 10.1038/nrneurol.2015.13

Hamilton, B. E., Hoyert, D. L., Martin, J. A., Strobino, D. M., and Guyer, B. (2013). Annual summary of vital statistics: 2010-2011. *Pediatrics* 131, 548–558. doi: 10.1542/peds.2012-3769

Hansen-Pupp, I., Hovel, H., Hellstrom, A., Hellstrom-Westas, L., Lofqvist, C., Larsson, E. M., et al. (2011). Postnatal decrease in circulating insulin-like growth factor-I and low brain volumes in very preterm infants. *J. Clin. Endocrinol. Metab.* 96, 1129–1135. doi: 10.1210/jc.2010-2440

Harteman, J. C., Groenendaal, F., van, H. I., Liem, K. D., Stroink, H., Bierings, M. B., et al. (2011). A typical timing and presentation of periventricular haemorrhagic infarction in preterm infants: the role of thrombophilia. *Dev. Med. Child Neurol.* 54, 140–147. doi: 10.1111/j.1469-8749.2011.04135.x

Hedley-Whyte, E. T., and Hsu, D. W. (1986). Effect of dexamethasone on blood-brain barrier in the normal mouse. *Ann. Neurol.* 19, 373–377. doi: 10.1002/ana.410190411

Hellstrom, A., Perruzzi, C., Ju, M., Engstrom, E., Hard, A. L., Liu, J. L., et al. (2001). Low IGF-I suppresses VEGF-survival signaling in retinal endothelial cells: direct correlation with clinical retinopathy of prematurity. *Proc. Natl. Acad. Sci. U. S. A.* 98, 5804–5808. doi: 10.1073/pnas.101113998

Hellstrom, A., Ley, D., Hansen-Pupp, I., Hallberg, B., Ramenghi, L. A., Lofqvist, C., et al. (2016). Role of insulinlike growth factor 1 in fetal development and in the early postnatal life of premature infants. *Am. J. Perinatol.* 33, 1067–1071. doi: 10.1055/s-0036-1586109

Hinojosa-Rodríguez, M., Harmony, T., Carrillo-Prado, C., Van Horn, J. D., Irimia, A., Torgerson, C., et al. (2017). Clinical neuroimaging in the preterm infant: diagnosis and prognosis. *Neuroimage Clin.* 16, 355–368. doi: 10.1016/j.nicl.2017.08.015

Hooper, S. B., Te Pas, A. B., Lang, J., van Vonderen, J. J., Roehr, C. C., Kluckow, M., et al. (2015). Cardiovascular transition at birth: a physiological sequence. *Pediatr. Res.* 77, 608–614. doi: 10.1038/pr.2015.21

Hou, X., Ding, H., Teng, Y., Zhou, C., Tang, X., Li, S., et al. (2007). Research on the relationship between brain anoxia at different regional oxygen saturations and brain damage using near-infrared spectroscopy. *Physiol. Meas.* 28, 1251–1265. doi: 10.1088/0967-3334/28/10/010

Hyttel-Sorensen, S., Pellicer, A., Alderliesten, T., Austin, T., van Bel, F., Benders, M., et al. (2015). Cerebral near infrared spectroscopy oximetry in extremely preterm infants: phase II randomised clinical trial. *BMJ* 350:g7635. doi: 10.1136/bmj.g7635

Hyttel-Sorensen, S., Greisen, G., Als-Nielsen, B., and Gluud, C. (2017). Cerebral near-infrared spectroscopy monitoring for prevention of brain injury in very preterm infants. *Cochrane Database Syst. Rev.* 9:Cd011506. doi: 10.1002/14651858.CD011506.pub2

Inder, T. E., Warfield, S. K., Wang, H., Huppi, P. S., and Volpe, J. J. (2005). Abnormal cerebral structure is present at term in premature infants. *Pediatrics* 115, 286–294. doi: 10.1542/peds.2004-0326

Isayama, T., Chai-Adisaksopha, C., and McDonald, S. D. (2015). Noninvasive ventilation with vs without early surfactant to prevent chronic lung disease in preterm infants: a systematic review and meta-analysis. *JAMA Pediatr.* 169, 731–739. doi: 10.1001/jamapediatrics.2015.0510

Jadasz, J. J., Kremer, D., Gottle, P., Tzekova, N., Domke, J., Rivera, F. J., et al. (2013). Mesenchymal stem cell conditioning promotes rat oligodendroglial cell maturation. *PLoS One* 8:e71814. doi: 10.1371/journal.pone.0071814

Jain, N. J., Kruse, L. K., Demissie, K., and Khandelwal, M. (2009). Impact of mode of delivery on neonatal complications: trends between 1997 and 2005. *J. Matern. Fetal Neonatal Med.* 22, 491–500. doi: 10.1080/14767050902769982

Jellema, R. K., Wolfs, T. G., Lima Passos, V., Zwanenburg, A., Ophelders, D. R., Kuypers, E., et al. (2013). Mesenchymal stem cells induce T-cell tolerance and protect the preterm brain after global hypoxia-ischemia. *PLoS One* 8:e73031. doi: 10.1371/journal.pone.0073031

Jensen, E. A., Foglia, E. E., and Schmidt, B. (2018). Association between prophylactic indomethacin and death or bronchopulmonary dysplasia: a systematic review and meta-analysis of observational studies. *Semin. Perinatol.* 42, 228–234. doi: 10.1053/j.semperi.2018.05.005

Juul, S. E., and Pet, G. C. (2015). Erythropoietin and neonatal Neuroprotection. *Clin. Perinatol.* 42, 469–481. doi: 10.1016/j.clp.2015.04.004

Karemaker, R., Heijnen, C. J., Veen, S., Baerts, W., Samsom, J., Visser, G. H., et al. (2006). Differences in behavioral outcome and motor development at school age after neonatal treatment for chronic lung disease with dexamethasone versus hydrocortisone. *Pediatr. Res.* 60, 745–750. doi: 10.1203/01.pdr.0000246200.76860.de

Kawakami, M., Sekiguchi, M., Sato, K., Kozaki, S., and Takahashi, M. (2001). Erythropoietin receptor-mediated inhibition of exocytotic glutamate release confers neuroprotection during chemical ischemia. *J. Biol. Chem.* 276, 39469–39475. doi: 10.1074/jbc.M105832200

Kersbergen, K. J., Benders, M. J., Groenendaal, F., Koopman-Esseboom, C., Nievelstein, R. A., van Haastert, I. C., et al. (2014a). Different patterns of punctate white matter lesions in serially scanned preterm infants. *PLoS One* e108904. doi: 10.1371/journal.pone.0108904

Kersbergen, K. J., Leemans, A., Groenendaal, F., van der Aa, N. E., Viergever, M. A., de Vries, L. S., et al. (2014b). Microstructural brain development between 30 and 40 weeks corrected age in a longitudinal cohort of extremely preterm infants. *NeuroImage* 103, 214–224. doi: 10.1016/j.neuroimage.2014.09.039

Kidokoro, H., Neil, J. J., and Inder, T. E. (2013). New MR imaging assessment tool to define brain abnormalities in very preterm infants at term. *AJNR Am. J. Neuroradiol.* 34, 2208–2214. doi: 10.3174/ajnr.A3521

Kizil, C., Kyritsis, N., and Brand, M. (2015). Effects of inflammation on stem cells: together they strive? *EMBO Rep.* 16, 416–426. doi: 10.15252/embr.201439702

Kotowski, M., Litwinska, Z., Klos, P., Pius-Sadowska, E., Zagrodnik-Ulan, E., Ustianowski, P., et al. (2017). Autologous cord blood transfusion in preterm infants - could its humoral effect be the key to control prematurity-related complications? A preliminary study. *J. Physiol. Pharmacol.* 68, 921–927.

Koulnis, M., Porpiglia, E., Hidalgo, D., and Socolovsky, M. (2014). Erythropoiesis: from molecular pathways to system properties. *Adv. Exp. Med. Biol.* 844, 37–58. doi: 10.1007/978-1-4939-2095-2_3

Krediet, T. G., Kavelaars, A., Vreman, H. J., Heijnen, C. J., and van Bel, F. (2006). Respiratory distress syndrome-associated inflammation is related to early but not late peri/intraventricular hemorrhage in preterm infants. *J. Pediatr.* 148, 740–746. doi: 10.1016/j.jpeds.2006.01.037

Lalu, M. M., McIntyre, L., Pugliese, C., Fergusson, D., Winston, B. W., Marshall, J. C., et al. (2012). Safety of cell therapy with mesenchymal stromal cells (SafeCell): a systematic review and meta-analysis of clinical trials. *PLoS One* 7:e47559. doi: 10.1371/journal.pone.0047559

Lekic, T., Flores, J., Klebe, D., Doycheva, D., Rolland, W. B., Tang, J., et al. (2016). Intranasal IGF-1 reduced rat pup germinal matrix hemorrhage. *Acta Neurochir. Suppl.* 121, 209–212. doi: 10.1007/978-3-319-18497-5_38

Lemmers, P. M., Toet, M., van Schelven, L. J., and van Bel, F. (2006). Cerebral oxygenation and cerebral oxygen extraction in the preterm infant: the impact of respiratory distress syndrome. *Exp. Brain Res.* 173, 458–467. doi: 10.1007/s00221-006-0388-8

Leuchter, R. H., Gui, L., Poncet, A., Hagmann, C., Lodygensky, G. A., Martin, E., et al. (2014). Association between early administration of high-dose erythropoietin in preterm infants and brain MRI abnormality at term-equivalent age. *JAMA* 312, 817–824. doi: 10.1001/jama.2014.9645

Ley, D., Hansen-Pupp, I., Niklasson, A., Domellof, M., Friberg, L. E., Borg, J., et al. (2013). Longitudinal infusion of a complex of insulin-like growth factor-I and IGF-binding protein-3 in five preterm infants: pharmacokinetics and short-term safety. *Pediatr. Res.* 73, 68–74. doi: 10.1038/pr.2012.146

Li, J., Yawno, T., Sutherland, A., Loose, J., Nitsos, I., Bischof, R., et al. (2016). Preterm white matter brain injury is prevented by early administration of umbilical cord blood cells. *Exp. Neurol.* 283, 179–187. doi: 10.1016/j.expneurol.2016.06.017

Luu, T. M., Ment, L. R., Schneider, K. C., Katz, K. H., Allan, W. C., and Vohr, B. R. (2009). Lasting effects of preterm birth and neonatal brain hemorrhage at 12 years of age. *Pediatrics* 123, 1037–1044. doi: 10.1542/peds.2008-1162

Marseglia, L., D'Angelo, G., Manti, S., Aversa, S., Reiter, R. J., Antonuccio, P., et al. (2015). Oxidative stress-mediated damage in newborns with necrotizing enterocolitis: a possible role of melatonin. *Am. J. Perinatol.* 32, 905–909. doi: 10.1055/s-0035-1547328

Martinez-Biarge, M., Groenendaal, F., Kersbergen, K. J., Benders, M. J., Foti, F., Cowan, F. M., et al. (2016). MRI based preterm white matter injury classification: the importance of sequential imaging in determining severity of injury. *PLoS One* 11:e0156245. doi: 10.1371/journal.pone.0156245

McPherson, C., and Inder, T. (2017). Perinatal and neonatal use of sedation and analgesia. *Semin. Fetal Neonatal Med.* 22, 314–320. doi: 10.1016/j.siny.2017.07.007

McPherson, C., and Wambach, J. A. (2018). Prevention and treatment of respiratory distress syndrome in preterm neonates. *Neonatal Netw.* 37, 169–177. doi: 10.1891/0730-0832.37.3.169

Ment, L. R., Stewart, W. B., Ardito, T. A., Huang, E., and Madri, J. A. (1992). Indomethacin promotes germinal matrix microvessel maturation in the newborn beagle pup. *Stroke* 23, 1132–1137. doi: 10.1161/01.STR.23.8.1132

Ment, L. R., Oh, W., Ehrenkranz, R. A., Philip, A. G., Duncan, C. C., and Makuch, R. W. (1995). Antenatal steroids, delivery mode, and intraventricular hemorrhage in preterm infants. *Am. J. Obstet. Gynecol.* 172, 795–800. doi: 10.1016/0002-9378(95)90001-2

Mercer, J. S., Erickson-Owens, D. A., Vohr, B. R., Tucker, R. J., Parker, A. B., Oh, W., et al. (2016). Effects of placental transfusion on neonatal and 18 month outcomes in preterm infants: a randomized controlled trial. *J. Pediatr.* 168, 50–55.e51. doi: 10.1016/j.jpeds.2015.09.068

Merchant, N., Azzopardi, D., Counsell, S., Gressens, P., Dierl, A., Gozar, I., et al. (2014). Melatonin as a novel neuroprotectant in preterm infants – a double blinded randomised controlled trial (MINT study). *Arch. Dis. Child.* 99:A43.

Mukai, T., Mori, Y., Shimazu, T., Takahashi, A., Tsunoda, H., Yamaguchi, S., et al. (2017). Intravenous injection of umbilical cord-derived mesenchymal stromal cells attenuates reactive gliosis and hypomyelination in a neonatal intraventricular hemorrhage model. *Neuroscience* 355, 175–187. doi: 10.1016/j.neuroscience.2017.05.006

Mukerji, A., Shah, V., and Shah, P. S. (2015). Periventricular/intraventricular hemorrhage and neurodevelopmental outcomes: a meta-analysis. *Pediatrics* 136, 1132–1143. doi: 10.1542/peds.2015-0944

Murner-Lavanchy, I. M., Doyle, L. W., Schmidt, B., Roberts, R. S., Asztalos, E. V., Costantini, L., et al. (2018). Neurobehavioral outcomes 11 years after neonatal caffeine therapy for apnea of prematurity. *Pediatrics* 141:e20174047. doi: 10.1542/peds.2017-4047

Musilova, I., Andrys, C., Drahosova, M., Zednikova, B., Hornychova, H., Pliskova, L., et al. (2018). Late preterm prelabor rupture of fetal membranes: fetal inflammatory response and neonatal outcome. *Pediatr. Res.* 83, 630–637. doi: 10.1038/pr.2017.300

Nelin, T. D., Pena, E., Giacomazzi, T., Lee, S., Logan, J. W., Moallem, M., et al. (2017). Outcomes following indomethacin prophylaxis in extremely preterm infants in an all-referral NICU. *J. Perinatol.* 37, 932–937. doi: 10.1038/jp.2017.71

Neubauer, A. P., Voss, W., Wachtendorf, M., and Jungmann, T. (2010). Erythropoietin improves neurodevelopmental outcome of extremely preterm infants. *Ann. Neurol.* 67, 657–666. doi: 10.1002/ana.21977

Ng, E., Taddio, A., and Ohlsson, A. (2017). Intravenous midazolam infusion for sedation of infants in the neonatal intensive care unit. *Cochrane Database Syst. Rev.* 1:Cd002052. doi: 10.1002/14651858.CD002052.pub3

Niimi, Y., and Levison, S. W. (2018). Pediatric brain repair from endogenous neural stem cells of the subventricular zone. *Pediatr. Res.* 83, 385–396. doi: 10.1038/pr.2017.261

Norman, M., Piedvache, A., Borch, K., Huusom, L. D., Bonamy, A. E., Howell, E. A., et al. (2017). Association of short antenatal corticosteroid administration-to-birth intervals with survival and morbidity among very preterm infants: results from the EPICE cohort. *JAMA Pediatr.* 171, 678–686. doi: 10.1001/jamapediatrics.2017.0602

Oh, K. J., Park, J. Y., Lee, J., Hong, J. S., Romero, R., and Yoon, B. H. (2018). The combined exposure to intra-amniotic inflammation and neonatal respiratory distress syndrome increases the risk of intraventricular hemorrhage in preterm neonates. *J. Perinat. Med.* 46, 9–20. doi: 10.1515/jpm-2016-0348

Ohls, R. K., Kamath-Rayne, B. D., Christensen, R. D., Wiedmeier, S. E., Rosenberg, A., Fuller, J., et al. (2014). Cognitive outcomes of preterm infants randomized to darbepoetin, erythropoietin, or placebo. *Pediatrics* 133, 1023–1030. doi: 10.1542/peds.2013-4307

Ohlsson, A., and Aher, S. M. (2017). Early erythropoiesis-stimulating agents in preterm or low birth weight infants. *Cochrane Database Syst. Rev.* 11:Cd004863. doi: 10.1002/14651858.CD004863.pub5

O'Kusky, J., and Ye, P. (2012). Neurodevelopmental effects of insulin-like growth factor signaling. *Front. Neuroendocrinol.* 33, 230–251. doi: 10.1016/j.yfrne.2012.06.002

Onland, W., Offringa, M., Cools, F., De Jaegere, A. P., Rademaker, K., BlomH., et al. (2011). Systemic hydrocortisone to prevent bronchopulmonary dysplasia in preterm infants (the SToP-BPD study); a multicenter randomized placebo controlled trial. *BMC Pediatr.* 11:102. doi: 10.1186/1471-2431-11-102

Ophelders, D. R., Wolfs, T. G., Jellema, R. K., Zwanenburg, A., Andriessen, P., Delhaas, T., et al. (2016). Mesenchymal stromal cell-derived extracellular vesicles protect the fetal brain after hypoxia-ischemia. *Stem Cells Transl. Med.* 5, 754–763. doi: 10.5966/sctm.2015-0197

O'Shea, T. M., Allred, E. N., Kuban, K. C., Dammann, O., Paneth, N., Fichorova, R., et al. (2012). Elevated concentrations of inflammation-related proteins in postnatal blood predict severe developmental delay at 2 years of age in extremely preterm infants. *J. Pediatr.* 160, 395–401.e394. doi: 10.1016/j.jpeds.2011.08.069

Ozdemir, A., Brown, M. A., and Morgan, W. J. (1997). Markers and mediators of inflammation in neonatal lung disease. *Pediatr. Pulmonol.* 23, 292–306. doi: 10.1002/(SICI)1099-0496(199704)23:4<292::AID-PPUL7>3.0.CO;2-O

Pang, Y., Zheng, B., Campbell, L. R., Fan, L. W., Cai, Z., and Rhodes, P. G. (2010). IGF-1 can either protect against or increase LPS-induced damage in the developing rat brain. *Pediatr. Res.* 67, 579–584. doi: 10.1203/PDR.0b013e3181dc240f

Papile, L. A., Burstein, J., Burstein, R., and Koffler, H. (1978). Incidence and evolution of subependymal and intraventricular hemorrhage: a study of infants with birth weights less than 1,500 gm. *J. Pediatr.* 92, 529–534. doi: 10.1016/S0022-3476(78)80282-0

Park, W. S., Sung, S. I., Ahn, S. Y., Sung, D. K., Im, G. H., Yoo, H. S., et al. (2016). Optimal timing of mesenchymal stem cell therapy for neonatal intraventricular hemorrhage. *Cell Transplant.* 25, 1131–1144. doi: 10.3727/096368915X689640

Park, W. S., Ahn, S. Y., Sung, S. I., Ahn, J. Y., and Chang, Y. S. (2017). Mesenchymal stem cells: the magic cure for intraventricular hemorrhage? *Cell Transplant.* 26, 439–448. doi: 10.3727/096368916X694193

Paton, M. C. B., McDonald, C. A., Allison, B. J., Fahey, M. C., Jenkin, G., and Miller, S. L. (2017). Perinatal brain injury as a consequence of preterm birth and intrauterine inflammation: designing targeted stem cell therapies. *Front. Neurosci.* 11:200. doi: 10.3389/fnins.2017.00200

Perlman, J. M., Goodman, S., Kreusser, K. L., and Volpe, J. J. (1985). Reduction in intraventricular hemorrhage by elimination of fluctuating cerebral blood-flow velocity in preterm infants with respiratory distress syndrome. *N. Engl. J. Med.* 312, 1353–1357. doi: 10.1056/NEJM198505233122104

Perlman, J. M., Wyllie, J., Kattwinkel, J., Wyckoff, M. H., Aziz, K., Guinsburg, R., et al. (2015). Part 7: neonatal resuscitation: 2015 international consensus on cardiopulmonary resuscitation and emergency cardiovascular care science with treatment recommendations (reprint). *Pediatrics* 136(Suppl. 2), S120–S166. doi: 10.1542/peds.2015-3373D

Pierrat, V., Marchand-Martin, L., Arnaud, C., Kaminski, M., Resche-Rigon, M., Lebeaux, C., et al. (2017). Neurodevelopmental outcome at 2 years for preterm children born at 22 to 34 weeks' gestation in France in 2011: EPIPAGE-2 cohort study. *BMJ* 358:j3448. doi: 10.1136/bmj.j3448

Plomgaard, A. M., Alderliesten, T., Austin, T., van Bel, F., Benders, M., Claris, O., et al. (2017). Early biomarkers of brain injury and cerebral hypo- and hyperoxia in the SafeBoosC II trial. *PLoS One* 12:e0173440. doi: 10.1371/journal.pone.0173440

Practice, C. O. (2017). Committee opinion no. 684: delayed umbilical cord clamping after birth. *Obstet. Gynecol.* 129, e5–e10. doi: 10.1097/AOG.0000000000001860

Qiu, J., Zhao, L., Yang, Y., Zhang, J. H., Feng, Y., and Cheng, R. (2018). Effects of fentanyl for pain control and neuroprotection in very preterm newborns on mechanical ventilation. *J. Matern. Fetal Neonatal Med.* 15, 1–7. doi: 10.1080/14767058.2018.1471593

Qu, R., Li, Y., Gao, Q., Shen, L., Zhang, J., Liu, Z., et al. (2007). Neurotrophic and growth factor gene expression profiling of mouse bone marrow stromal cells induced by ischemic brain extracts. *Neuropathology* 27, 355–363. doi: 10.1111/j.1440-1789.2007.00792.x

Rabe, H., Reynolds, G., and Diaz-Rossello, J. (2008). A systematic review and meta-analysis of a brief delay in clamping the umbilical cord of preterm infants. *Neonatology* 93, 138–144. doi: 10.1159/000108764

Rabe, H., Diaz-Rossello, J. L., Duley, L., and Dowswell, T. (2012). Effect of timing of umbilical cord clamping and other strategies to influence placental transfusion at preterm birth on maternal and infant outcomes. *Cochrane Database Syst. Rev.* Cd003248. doi: 10.1002/14651858.CD003248.pub3

Rangarajan, V., and Juul, S. E. (2014). Erythropoietin: emerging role of erythropoietin in neonatal neuroprotection. *Pediatr. Neurol.* 51, 481–488. doi: 10.1016/j.pediatrneurol.2014.06.008

Roberts, D., Brown, J., Medley, N., and Dalziel, S. R. (2017). Antenatal corticosteroids for accelerating fetal lung maturation for women at risk of preterm birth. *Cochrane Database Syst. Rev.* 3:Cd004454. doi: 10.1002/14651858.CD004454.pub3

Rojas-Reyes, M. X., Morley, C. J., and Soll, R. (2012). Prophylactic versus selective use of surfactant in preventing morbidity and mortality in preterm infants. *Cochrane Database Syst. Rev.* 14:Cd000510. doi: 10.1002/14651858.CD000510.pub2

Romantsik, O., Calevo, M. G., and Bruschettini, M. (2017). Head midline position for preventing the occurrence or extension of germinal matrix-intraventricular hemorrhage in preterm infants. *Cochrane Database Syst. Rev.* 7:Cd012362. doi: 10.1002/14651858.CD012362.pub2

Schmidt, B., Davis, P., Moddemann, D., Ohlsson, A., Roberts, R. S., Saigal, S., et al. (2001). Long-term effects of indomethacin prophylaxis in extremely-low-birth-weight infants. *N. Engl. J. Med.* 344, 1966–1972. doi: 10.1056/NEJM200106283442602

Schmidt, B., Roberts, R. S., Davis, P., Doyle, L. W., Barrington, K. J., Ohlsson, A., et al. (2007). Long-term effects of caffeine therapy for apnea of prematurity. *N. Engl. J. Med.* 357, 1893–1902. doi: 10.1056/NEJMoa073679

Shepherd, E., Salam, R. A., Middleton, P., Makrides, M., McIntyre, S., Badawi, N., et al. (2017). Antenatal and intrapartum interventions for preventing cerebral palsy: an overview of Cochrane systematic reviews. *Cochrane Database Syst. Rev.* 8:Cd012077. doi: 10.1002/14651858.CD012077.pub2

Sherlock, R. L., Anderson, P. J., and Doyle, L. W. (2005). Neurodevelopmental sequelae of intraventricular haemorrhage at 8 years of age in a regional cohort of ELBW/very preterm infants. *Early Hum. Dev.* 81, 909–916. doi: 10.1016/j.earlhumdev.2005.07.007

Skov, L., Pryds, O., and Greisen, G. (1991). Estimating cerebral blood flow in newborn infants: comparison of near infrared spectroscopy and 133Xe clearance. *Pediatr. Res.* 30, 570–573. doi: 10.1203/00006450-199112000-00016

Stoll, B. J., Hansen, N. I., Bell, E. F., Shankaran, S., Laptook, A. R., Walsh, M. C., et al. (2010). Neonatal outcomes of extremely preterm infants from the NICHD neonatal research network. *Pediatrics* 126, 443–456. doi: 10.1542/peds.2009-2959

Stolp, H. B., Ball, G., So, P. W., Tournier, J. D., Jones, M., Thornton, C., et al. (2018). Voxel-wise comparisons of cellular microstructure and diffusion-MRI in mouse hippocampus using 3D bridging of optically-clear histology with neuroimaging data (3D-BOND). *Sci. Rep.* 8:4011. doi: 10.1038/s41598-018-22295-9

Strunk, T., Inder, T., Wang, X., Burgner, D., Mallard, C., and Levy, O. (2014). Infection-induced inflammation and cerebral injury in preterm infants. *Lancet Infect. Dis.* 14, 751–762. doi: 10.1016/S1473-3099(14)70710-8

Thewissen, L., Caicedo, A., Lemmers, P., van Bel, F., Van Huffel, S., and Naulaers, G. (2018). Measuring near-infrared spectroscopy derived cerebral autoregulation in neonates: from research tool toward bedside multimodal monitoring. *Front Pediatr.* 6:117. doi: 10.3389/fped.2018.00117

Thygesen, S. K., Olsen, M., Ostergaard, J. R., and Sorensen, H. T. (2016). Respiratory distress syndrome in moderately late and late preterm infants and risk of cerebral palsy: a population-based cohort study. *BMJ Open* 6:e011643. doi: 10.1136/bmjopen-2016-011643

Tokida, Y., Aratani, Y., Morita, A., and Kitagawa, Y. (1990). Production of two variant laminin forms by endothelial cells and shift of their relative levels by angiostatic steroids. *J. Biol. Chem.* 265, 18123–18129.

Uauy, R., and Mena, P. (2015). Long-chain polyunsaturated fatty acids supplementation in preterm infants. *Curr. Opin. Pediatr.* 27, 165–171. doi: 10.1097/MOP.0000000000000203

Uccelli, A., Moretta, L., and Pistoia, V. (2008). Mesenchymal stem cells in health and disease. *Nat. Rev. Immunol.* 8, 726–736. doi: 10.1038/nri2395

van Bel, F., and Mintzer, J. P. (2018). Monitoring cerebral oxygenation of the immature brain: a neuroprotective strategy? *Pediatr. Res.* 84, 159–164. doi: 10.1038/s41390-018-0026-8

van Bel, F., Van de Bor, M., Stijnen, T., Baan, J., and Ruys, J. H. (1987). Aetiological role of cerebral blood-flow alterations in development and extension of peri-intraventricular haemorrhage. *Dev. Med. Child Neurol.* 29, 601–614. doi: 10.1111/j.1469-8749.1987.tb08502.x

van Bel, F., Klautz, R. J., Steendijk, P., Schipper, I. B., Teitel, D. F., and Baan, J. (1993). The influence of indomethacin on the autoregulatory ability of the cerebral vascular bed in the newborn lamb. *Pediatr. Res.* 34, 178–181. doi: 10.1203/00006450-199308000-00015

van Bel, F., Roman, C., Klautz, R. J., Teitel, D. F., and Rudolph, A. M. (1994). Relationship between brain blood flow and carotid arterial flow in the sheep fetus. *Pediatr. Res.* 35, 329–333. doi: 10.1203/00006450-199403000-00011

van Bel, F., Bartelds, B., Teitel, D. F., and Rudolph, A. M. (1995). Effect of indomethacin on cerebral blood flow and oxygenation in the normal and ventilated fetal lamb. *Pediatr. Res.* 38, 243–250. doi: 10.1203/00006450-199508000-00018

van Bel, F., Lemmers, P., and Naulaers, G. (2008). Monitoring neonatal regional cerebral oxygenation saturation in clinical practice: value and pitfalls. *Neonatology* 94, 237–244. doi: 10.1159/000151642

van de Looij, Y., Lodygensky, G. A., Dean, J., Lazeyras, F., Hagberg, H., Kjellmer, I., et al. (2012). High-field diffusion tensor imaging characterization of cerebral white matter injury in lipopolysaccharide-exposed fetal sheep. *Pediatr. Res.* 72, 285–292. doi: 10.1038/pr.2012.72

van der Kooij, M. A., Groenendaal, F., Kavelaars, A., Heijnen, C. J., and van B. F. (2008). Neuroprotective properties and mechanisms of erythropoietin in in vitro and in vivo experimental models for hypoxia/ischemia. *Brain Res. Rev.* 59, 22–33. doi: 10.1016/j.brainresrev.2008.04.007

van Haastert, I. C., Groenendaal, F., Uiterwaal, C. S., Termote, J. U., van der Heide-Jalving, M., Eijsermans, M. J., et al. (2011). Decreasing incidence and severity of cerebral palsy in prematurely born children. *J. Pediatr.* 159, 86–91. doi: 10.1016/j.jpeds.2010.12.053

van Tilborg, E., Achterberg, E. J. M., van Kammen, C. M., van der Toorn, A., Groenendaal, F., Dijkhuizen, R. M., et al. (2018a). Combined fetal inflammation and postnatal hypoxia causes myelin deficits and autism-like behavior in a rat model of diffuse white matter injury. *Glia* 66, 78–93. doi: 10.1002/glia.23216

van Tilborg, E., de Theije, C. G. M., van Hal, M., Wagenaar, N., de Vries, L. S., Benders, M. J., et al. (2018b). Origin and dynamics of oligodendrocytes in the developing brain: implications for perinatal white matter injury. *Glia* 66, 221–238. doi: 10.1002/glia.23256

van Velthoven, C. T., Kavelaars, A., van Bel, F., and Heijnen, C. J. (2011). Mesenchymal stem cell transplantation changes the gene expression profile of the neonatal ischemic brain. *Brain Behav. Immun.* 25, 1342–1348. doi: 10.1016/j.bbi.2011.03.021

Villamor-Martinez, E., Fumagalli, M., Mohammed Rahim, O., Passera, S., Cavallaro, G., Degraeuwe, P., et al. (2018). Chorioamnionitis is a risk factor for intraventricular hemorrhage in preterm infants: a systematic review and meta-analysis. *Front. Physiol.* 9:1253. doi: 10.3389/fphys.2018.01253

Vohr, B., and Ment, L. R. (1996). Intraventricular hemorrhage in the preterm infant. *Early Hum. Dev.* 44, 1–16. doi: 10.1016/0378-3782(95)01692-9

Volpe, J. J. (2009). Brain injury in premature infants: a complex amalgam of destructive and developmental disturbances. *Lancet Neurol.* 8, 110–124. doi: 10.1016/S1474-4422(08)70294-1

Wagenaar, N., Nijboer, C. H., and van Bel, F. (2017). Repair of neonatal brain injury: bringing stem cell-based therapy into clinical practice. *Dev. Med. Child Neurol.* 59, 997–1003. doi: 10.1111/dmcn.13528

Walti, H., Paris-Llado, J., Breart, G., and Couchard, M. (1995). Porcine surfactant replacement therapy in newborns of 25-31 weeks' gestation: a randomized, multicentre trial of prophylaxis versus rescue with multiple low doses. The French collaborative multicentre study group. *Acta Paediatr.* 84, 913–921. doi: 10.1111/j.1651-2227.1995.tb13792.x

Wiest, D. B., Chang, E., Fanning, D., Garner, S., Cox, T., and Jenkins, D. D. (2014). Antenatal pharmacokinetics and placental transfer of N-acetylcysteine in chorioamnionitis for fetal neuroprotection. *J. Pediatr.* 165, 672–677.e672. doi: 10.1016/j.jpeds.2014.06.044

Wintermark, P., Hansen, A., Warfield, S. K., Dukhovny, D., and Soul, J. S. (2014). Near-infrared spectroscopy versus magnetic resonance imaging to study brain perfusion in newborns with hypoxic-ischemic encephalopathy treated with hypothermia. *NeuroImage* 85, 287–293. doi: 10.1016/j.neuroimage.2013.04.072

Wyllie, J., Bruinenberg, J., Roehr, C. C., Rudiger, M., Trevisanuto, D., and Urlesberger, B. (2015). European resuscitation council guidelines for resuscitation 2015: section 7. Resuscitation and support of transition of babies at birth. *Resuscitation* 95, 249–263. doi: 10.1016/j.resuscitation.2015.07.029

Xu, H., Hu, F., Sado, Y., Ninomiya, Y., Borza, D. B., Ungvari, Z., et al. (2008). Maturational changes in laminin, fibronectin, collagen IV, and perlecan in germinal matrix, cortex, and white matter and effect of betamethasone. *J. Neurosci. Res.* 86, 1482–1500. doi: 10.1002/jnr.21618

Yamaji, R., Okada, T., Moriya, M., Naito, M., Tsuruo, T., Miyatake, K., et al. (1996). Brain capillary endothelial cells express two forms of erythropoietin receptor mRNA. *Eur. J. Biochem.* 239, 494–500. doi: 10.1111/j.1432-1033.1996.0494u.x

Yao, A. C., Moinian, M., and Lind, J. (1969). Distribution of blood between infant and placenta after birth. *Lancet* 2, 871–873.

Zwicker, J. G., Miller, S. P., Grunau, R. E., Chau, V., Brant, R., Studholme, C., et al. (2016). Smaller cerebellar growth and poorer neurodevelopmental outcomes in very preterm infants exposed to neonatal morphine. *J. Pediatr.* 172, 81–87.e82. doi: 10.1016/j.jpeds.2015.12.024

7

The Role of Connexin and Pannexin Channels in Perinatal Brain Injury and Inflammation

*Kelly Q. Zhou[1], Colin R. Green[2], Laura Bennet[1], Alistair J. Gunn[1] and Joanne O. Davidson**

[1] *Department of Physiology, The University of Auckland, Auckland, New Zealand,*

[2] *Department of Ophthalmology, The University of Auckland, Auckland, New Zealand*

Correspondence:
Joanne O. Davidson
joanne.davidson@auckland.ac.nz

Perinatal brain injury remains a major cause of death and life-long disability. Perinatal brain injury is typically associated with hypoxia-ischemia and/or infection/inflammation. Both hypoxia-ischemia and infection trigger an inflammatory response in the brain. The inflammatory response can contribute to brain cell loss and chronic neuroinflammation leading to neurological impairments. It is now well-established that brain injury evolves over time, and shows a striking spread from injured to previously uninjured regions of the brain. There is increasing evidence that this spread is related to opening of connexin hemichannels and pannexin channels, both of which are large conductance membrane channels found in almost all cell types in the brain. Blocking connexin hemichannels within the first 3 h after hypoxia-ischemia has been shown to improve outcomes in term equivalent fetal sheep but it is important to also understand the downstream pathways linking membrane channel opening with the development of injury in order to identify new therapeutic targets. Open membrane channels release adenosine triphosphate (ATP), and other neuroactive molecules, into the extracellular space. ATP has an important physiological role, but has also been reported to act as a damage-associated molecular pattern (DAMP) signal mediated through specific purinergic receptors and so act as a primary signal 1 in the innate immune system inflammasome pathway. More crucially, extracellular ATP is a key inflammasome signal 2 activator, with purinergic receptor binding triggering the assembly of the multi-protein inflammasome complex. The inflammasome pathway and complex formation contribute to activation of inflammatory caspases, and the release of inflammatory cytokines, including interleukin (IL)-1β, tumor necrosis factor (TNF)-α, IL-18, and vascular endothelial growth factor (VEGF). We propose that the NOD-like receptor protein-3 (NLRP3) inflammasome, which has been linked to inflammatory responses in models of ischemic stroke and various inflammatory diseases, may be one mechanism by which connexin hemichannel opening especially mediates perinatal brain injury.

Keywords: connexin, pannexin, hemichannel, ischemia, inflammation, inflammasome, ATP

INTRODUCTION

Perinatal brain injury is associated with death or significant long-term neurodevelopmental impairment, affecting 1.15 million infants in the world in 2010 (Lee et al., 2013). It affects both term and preterm infants (born <37 weeks of completed gestation), with the greatest incidence in the most preterm infants (Larroque et al., 2008). In term born infants, perinatal brain injury is most often linked to hypoxia-ischemia (HI) (Vannucci, 2000; Shankaran et al., 2005), where the incidence of moderate to severe hypoxic-ischemic encephalopathy (HIE) is ~1–3 in 1,000 live births (Edwards et al., 2010). By contrast, in preterm infants, brain injury arises from the complex interaction of HI, infection/inflammation and preterm birth itself (Galinsky et al., 2018b). Strikingly, ~50% of extremely preterm infants (born <26 weeks of gestation) develop moderate to severe disability (Marlow et al., 2005).

Currently, there is only one established neuroprotective treatment for term babies born with HIE, which is therapeutic hypothermia. Clinically, this treatment is only partially effective, with a number needed to treat of ~8, meaning of 8 treated infants with HIE, one additional infant will survive without moderate to severe disability (Gunn et al., 2017; Natarajan et al., 2018). However, there are currently no proven treatments to reduce brain damage for preterm infants with HIE or perinatal infection/inflammation. Therefore, there is significant interest in developing complementary or novel treatments for perinatal brain injury after HI or infection/inflammation. For term infants, it is important to develop interventions with additive benefit to therapeutic hypothermia, as it is now standard therapy. Novel treatments are needed for term and preterm infection/inflammation.

After HI, there is a striking evolution of injury which progresses over time from injured to previously uninjured regions of the brain (Azzopardi et al., 1989; Thornton et al., 1998). The mechanisms behind this spread are not well-understood. Increasing evidence supports the opening of cell membrane channels after HI as one of the mediators of this propagation of injury, particularly connexin hemichannels, which are the unopposed half of a gap junction, forming large conductance channels in the cell membrane (Davidson et al., 2012, 2014; Wang et al., 2014; Li et al., 2015). Pannexin channels may also open under pathological conditions, although they appear to be tightly regulated (Qiu and Dahl, 2009) and their role in the developing brain remains unclear. In this review, we examine the hypothesis that prolonged opening of connexin hemichannels leads to a cascade of injurious mechanism, potentially through inflammation by activation, amplification and perpetuation of the inflammasome pathway.

An inflammatory response is seen in perinatal brain injury after HI as well as infection/inflammation, and if chronic inflammation is established can have deleterious effects (Hagberg et al., 2015; Bennet et al., 2018). Hemichannels release adenosine triphosphate (ATP) (Kang et al., 2008; Chekeni et al., 2010; Orellana et al., 2011; Bennett et al., 2012), which may act as a damage associated molecular pattern (DAMP), but is also a key inflammasome activator signal. The release of ATP through connexin hemichannels can perpetuate inflammation through purinergic signaling (Pedata et al., 2016). Purinergic signaling has been associated with the activation of microglia (Li et al., 2011; Kaiser et al., 2016) and the inflammasome complex—a multi-protein complex involved in initiating an innate immune system inflammatory response (Feng et al., 2015). This review will dissect the evidence for these pathways downstream of connexin hemichannel and pannexin channel opening and how they contribute to inflammation. One other membrane pore forming protein, Gasdermin D, has been implicated in the inflammasome pathway (Groslambert and Py, 2018; Kerur et al., 2018), but that channel is very small in comparison with the pannexin and connexin channels and appears to be primarily associated with apoptosis. As will become evident in this review, both *in vitro* and animal studies using connexin hemichannel or pannexin channel blockers, would suggest that other channels are likely to play minor roles in relation to ATP release, and inflammasome activation in particular.

EVOLUTION OF INJURY

Perinatal brain injury after HI is an evolving process that can be characterized into four phases (Bennet et al., 2010; Davidson et al., 2015b). The primary phase of injury occurs during the HI insult itself, when the failure of oxidative metabolism results in anoxic depolarization, edema and necrosis (Wassink et al., 2018). After restoration of blood flow and oxygen supply, there is a period of apparent transient recovery when oxidative metabolism is at least partially restored, known as the latent phase (Davidson et al., 2018a). However, the latent phase is the key time when the deleterious mechanisms leading to the spread of brain injury may be initiated; for example, the opening of connexin hemichannels, which will be discussed further below (Davidson et al., 2012).

Following the latent phase, there is a delayed ("secondary") deterioration of oxidative metabolism starting ~6–15 h after the insult (Azzopardi et al., 1989; Williams et al., 1991; Gunn et al., 1997). This phase is characterized by delayed cerebral energy failure followed by seizures and secondary cell swelling (Bennet et al., 2006; Davidson et al., 2015c). There is marked neuronal injury after HI at term, with the majority of neuronal loss occurring during the secondary phase, through a continuum of necrosis-apoptosis and autophagy (Northington et al., 2007, 2011).

The tertiary phase is a period of repair and reorganization, persisting for weeks to years after the initial insult (Fleiss and Gressens, 2012). During this period, surviving cells in the brain can rewire, but there may be a low level of ongoing cell death due to the loss of trophic support and problems with connectivity (Ness et al., 2001; Romanko et al., 2004). Long-term impairment in perinatal brain injury may also be associated with epigenetic changes (Fleiss and Gressens, 2012), but also persistent inflammation (Bennet et al., 2018) as reported for other types of brain injury and degenerative diseases (Patterson and Holahan, 2012; Freeman and Ting, 2016).

INFLAMMATION IN PERINATAL BRAIN INJURY

Perinatal brain injury associated with HI or infection/inflammation can trigger an inflammatory response. The innate immune response is the body's first line of defense against pathogens, reacting rapidly following exposure to invading organisms (Medzhitov, 2007). As part of the innate immune response, pattern recognition receptors

(PRRs) expressed on immune cells recognize both the conserved molecular structures found on the pathogen known as pathogen-associated molecular patterns (PAMPs), and the endogenous signals released by damaged tissues known as danger-associated molecular patterns (DAMPs) (Medzhitov, 2007; Takeuchi and Akira, 2010).

The activation of PRRs initiates the inflammatory response leading to release of inflammatory cytokines, such as interleukin (IL)-1β (Turner et al., 2014). This early phase of inflammation targets the invading pathogens and/or clears injured tissue, which is beneficial to the host. However, this inflammatory response also leads to the death of uninjured neural cells in a process known as "bystander cell loss" (Hagberg et al., 2015). It is believed that the initial pro-inflammatory response is followed by anti-inflammatory and reparative processes, and either eventual resolution of inflammation or chronic inflammation (Gilroy and De Maeyer, 2015; Hagberg et al., 2015).

Elevated levels of inflammatory markers after birth are associated with adverse neurodevelopmental outcomes. A prospective cohort study of 73 term infants exposed to perinatal asphyxia showed that those who died or were diagnosed with cerebral palsy at a 1 year follow up, were associated with higher levels of IL-1, IL-6 and tumor necrosis factor (TNF)-α in heel-stick blood samples collected on the first or second day of birth (Foster-Barber et al., 2001). In the same cohort, followed up at 30 months of age, those with higher serum cytokine levels of IL-1β, IL-6, and IL-8 at birth were associated with abnormal cognitive and motor outcomes (Bartha et al., 2004). The extremely low gestational age newborns (born before 28 weeks of gestation) (ELGANs) study is a large multi-center observational study. In this cohort, elevated blood concentrations of inflammatory proteins, measured in the first few weeks of life was associated with mental and motor impairments at 2 years old (O'Shea et al., 2012) and adverse cognitive outcome at 10 years of age (Kuban et al., 2017), as well as increased risk of behavioral problems, including autism (Korzeniewski et al., 2018). Cytokine levels were not measured at later time points to determine if inflammation was sustained. However, a study by Lin and colleagues has suggested that perinatal brain injury is associated with long-lasting alterations to the inflammatory response (Lin et al., 2010). Peripheral blood mononuclear cells from a small cohort of preterm born children with periventricular leukomalacia induced cerebral palsy, were shown to have higher mRNA levels of inflammatory molecules, both before and after lipopolysaccharide (LPS) stimulation (Lin et al., 2010). Non-resolving inflammation could be the result of a prolonged or excessive inflammatory response, which may lead to the disruption of pathways that normally induce inflammatory resolution (Nathan and Ding, 2010; Bennet et al., 2018).

CONNEXIN HEMICHANNELS

Connexin gap junctions connect the intracellular space of two adjacent cells allowing for the exchange of ions and molecules (Kumar and Gilula, 1996; Alexander and Goldberg, 2003; Davidson et al., 2013a). A connexin hemichannel is comprised of six connexin subunits. Connexin hemichannels from adjacent cells dock together to form a gap junction (Unger et al., 1999; Davidson et al., 2013a; Leybaert et al., 2017) (**Figure 1**). Humans have 21 connexin genes, and 11 of these are expressed in the brain (Theis et al., 2005). Connexin 43 (Cx43) has been of particular interest in the brain as it is abundantly expressed, especially in astrocytes, microglia and microvascular endothelium (Dermietzel et al., 2000; Nagy et al., 2003; Davidson et al., 2013a). Under physiological conditions, prior to forming a gap junction, hemichannels at the cell surface have a low probability of opening, shown by low membrane permeability during resting conditions in cultured cells (Decrock et al., 2009). It is not known whether this is the case *in vivo*, as cells may be exposed to a wide range of stimuli influencing hemichannel opening (Sáez et al., 2005). When hemichannels do open though, they form a large non-selective membrane channel capable of passing molecules up to about 1 kDa in size (Evans et al., 2006). There is increasing evidence that dysregulated hemichannel opening can be detrimental and they are often referred to as "pathological pores" (Paul et al., 1991; Decrock et al., 2015; Willebrords et al., 2016).

Connexin hemichannels are involved in the spread of brain injury after HI or infection in the adult and immature brain (Davidson et al., 2012, 2013a) (studies are summarized in **Table 1**). They open in response to stimuli mimicking exposure to ischemia and inflammation *in vitro*. For example, in cultured cells, oxygen-glucose deprivation (OGD), metabolic inhibition, low extracellular Ca^{2+}, and strong depolarization have all been proven to stimulate hemichannel opening (Contreras et al., 2002; Decrock et al., 2009; Orellana et al., 2010). Conditioned medium from LPS-activated microglia or TNF-α and IL-1β increased hemichannel activity in cultured astrocytes (Retamal et al., 2007). In addition, neuroinflammation induced by S. aureus intracerebral inoculation increased Cx43 hemichannel activity in astrocytes surrounding the abscess (Karpuk et al., 2011). The opening of connexin hemichannels allows for the influx of Na^+, Cl^-, and Ca^{2+} and the efflux of K^+ ions. This increases cell permeability, leading to the depolarization of the cell, and cell lysis (Paul et al., 1991; Gómez-Hernández et al., 2003). Molecules, such as ATP, glutamate and aspartate can be released; all of these molecules are associated with injury (Ye et al., 2003; Gomes et al., 2005; Zhao et al., 2005; Kang et al., 2008). Additionally, Cx43 hemichannels are likely involved in the propagation of seizures following severe HI in near-term fetal sheep (Davidson et al., 2012).

An upregulation of Cx43 has been shown to occur in adult and perinatal animals after HI and in adult human post-mortem studies of cerebral ischemia (Nakase et al., 2006, 2009; Davidson et al., 2012; Wang et al., 2014; Li et al., 2015). The timing of this Cx43 increase varies between studies, with Cx43 mRNA levels significantly increased at 6 h after carotid artery occlusion in near-term fetal sheep (Davidson et al., 2012). Protein levels progressively increased in the ischemic region from 8 h to 7 days after common carotid artery ligation and hypoxia (commonly referred to as Rice-Vannucci model of HI) in post-natal day (P)7 rats (equivalent to 33–34 weeks of human brain maturation) (Li et al., 2015). In the subventricular zone, however,

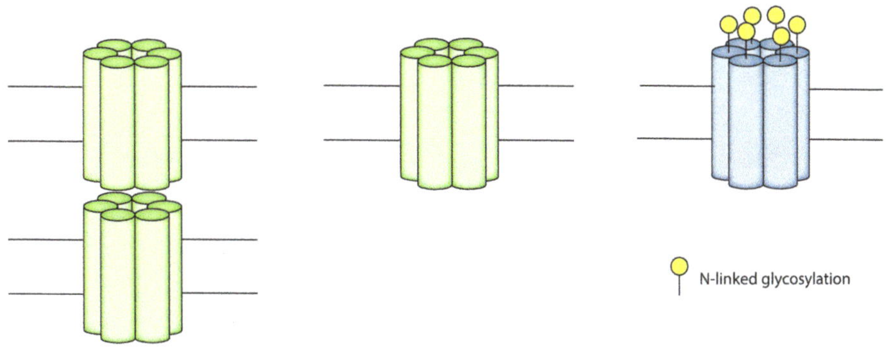

FIGURE 1 | Schematic depicting the Connexin 43 (Cx43) gap junction and hemichannel and pannexin 1 (Px1) channel. A connexon consists of six connexin subunits. A Cx43 gap junction is made up of two opposing connexons, each contributed from two adjacent cells. A Cx43 hemichannel is an unopposed connexon. A Px1 channel is formed by six pannexin subunits. Px1 does not form gap junctions due to N-linked glycosylation on the extracellular loop.

Wang and colleagues reported Cx43 protein expression was only significantly increased from 24 h after the same insult in P7 rats (Wang et al., 2014). However, there was no change in hippocampal Cx43 protein expression at all time-points between 10 min and 35 days after acute hypoxia in P10 rats (equivalent to human term brain maturation) (Zeinieh et al., 2010). Thus, the changes in Cx43 expression may be dependent on species, brain region, type and/or severity of insult. It should be noted that, the Rice-Vannucci model of HI in rodents produces a unilateral infarction in the brain but only moderate systemic hypoxia (Rice et al., 1981), whereas bilateral carotid artery occlusion in near-term fetal sheep produces a global cerebral insult resulting in a watershed pattern of brain injury, without systemic hypoxia (Williams et al., 1992). The reader should note that protein assays and immunohistochemical labeling do not allow ready discrimination between gap junctions and hemichannels, or channel function.

The blockade of Cx43 hemichannels, however, has been neuroprotective in a variety of different animal models of perinatal HI (Davidson et al., 2012, 2014; Li et al., 2015). Intracerebroventricular (i.c.v.) infusion (50 μmol/kg over 1 h, then 50 μmol/kg over 24 h) of the Cx43 mimetic peptide—Peptide5, started at 90 min after the end of carotid artery occlusion in near-term fetal sheep, was associated with improved neuronal and oligodendrocyte survival and, electroencephalogram (EEG) recovery and reduced seizure burden (Davidson et al., 2012). Similarly, Peptide5 infusion following the same protocol as above in preterm fetal sheep after umbilical cord occlusion improved EEG recovery and reduced neuronal and oligodendrocyte loss (Davidson et al., 2014). Reduced infarct size and improved motor and memory scores were observed in Gap 26 treated P7 rats [a connexin mimetic peptide which blocks hemichannels and gap junctions (Wang et al., 2013)], given i.p., 50 μg/kg, 1 h before HI (Li et al., 2015).

Cx43 hemichannel opening *in vivo* has been shown to occur after ischemia (in the latent phase), but not during ischemia. Pre-administration of Peptide5 was not neuroprotective when given 1 h before and during ischemia, but was neuroprotective when given after ischemia (Davidson et al., 2012, 2013b). Supporting this, hemichannels in astrocyte cultures subjected to OGD have been shown to open 1 h after OGD (Orellana et al., 2010). In addition, carbenoxolone (100 μmol/L) inhibition of connexin hemichannels did not attenuate ATP release during OGD in hippocampal slices (Frenguelli et al., 2007). Both Cx43 hemichannel and pannexin channel opening was reported to occur during hypoxia in endothelial cells with two thirds of ATP release connexin hemichannel mediated, but upon reperfusion, only Cx43 hemichannel opening occurred (Kim and Green, 2016). These studies indicate that Cx43 hemichannels likely do open after ischemia and may have an ongoing role in the evolution of injury after the insult. This is supported by the demonstration that prolonged infusion of Peptide5 (i.c.v., starting at 90 min) at a dose of 50 μmol/kg over 1 h, then 50 μmol/kg over 24 h of Peptide5 provided greater neuroprotection compared to a 1 h infusion only (50 μmol/kg) (Davidson et al., 2012). Furthermore, delayed administration of another known hemichannel blocker, Gap 26 (i.p., 50 μmol/kg) at 24 h after HI still had neuroprotective effects (Li et al., 2015). Interestingly, when Peptide5 administration (i.c.v., 50 μmol/kg for 1 h followed by 50 μmol/kg for 24 h) was delayed until 3 h after the end of ischemia in near-term fetal sheep, the neuroprotective effects were reduced when compared to earlier administration (Davidson et al., 2012, 2015a). The delayed administration reduced the seizure burden, but there was no clear effect on cell survival or EEG recovery (Davidson et al., 2012, 2015a).

The mechanisms behind how Cx43 hemichannels lead to neuronal and oligodendrocyte loss in HI is not well-understood. During and/or after HI there is impaired intracellular Ca^{2+} handling. This has been shown to contribute to mitochondrial dysfunction and necrotic and apoptotic cell death (Puka-Sundvall et al., 2000; Mallard et al., 2014). Potentially, the opening of hemichannels could lead to an influx of excessive intracellular Ca^{2+} accumulation leading directly to the neuronal and/or oligodendrocyte death (Galinsky et al.,

TABLE 1 | Summary of studies of Cx43 hemichannels and Px1 channels and purinergic receptors P2X4 and P2X7.

	Species	Age	Paradigm	Hemichannel activity/expression	Drug/knockout	Drug/knockout effect	References
Connexin 43 (Cx43)	Rat primary astrocyte culture	Embryonic day (E) 9	Metabolic inhibition	↑ Cx43 hemichannel opening during metabolic inhibition			Contreras et al., 2002
	Rat primary astrocyte culture	P1/2	Conditioned medium from LPS-activated microglia or TNF-α and IL-1β	↑ Cx43 hemichannel activity 24 h after treatment			Retamal et al., 2007
	Rat primary astrocyte culture	P1/2	Hypoxia and artificial cerebrospinal fluid medium mimicking ischemic conditions	↑ Cx43 hemichannel opening 1 h after reoxygenation			Orellana et al., 2010*
	Human microvascular endothelial cells		Hypoxic acidic ion-shifted ringer solution	↑ ATP release from Cx43 hemichannels during treatment and after reperfusion			Kim and Green, 2016*
	C6 glioma cells transfected with Cx43		Voltage activation of Cx43 hemichannels	↑ ATP release from Cx43 hemichannels			Kang et al., 2008
	Human adult retinal pigment epithelial cells		High glucose, TNF-α and IL-1β	↑ ATP release from Cx43 hemichannels	Peptide 5 (5–50 μM), administered at the same time as high glucose and cytokine treatment	↓ NLRP3 oligomerization ↓ Cytokine release	Mugisho et al., 2018
	Mouse acute brain slice	8–12 weeks	*S. aureus in vivo* intracerebral inoculation	↑ Cx43 hemichannel activity			Karpuk et al., 2011*
	Sheep	Near-term	Carotid artery occlusion	↑ mRNA expression (6 h after end of occlusion)	Peptide5 i.c.v. (50 μmol/kg over 1 h, then 50 μmol/kg over 24 h) started 90 min after end of occlusion	↑ Neuronal and oligodendrocyte survival Improved electroencephalogram recovery ↓ Seizure burden	Davidson et al., 2012; Galinsky et al., 2017
	Sheep	Near-term	Carotid artery occlusion		Peptide5 i.c.v. (50 μmol/kg over 1 h, then 50 μmol/kg over 24 h) started 3 h after end of occlusion	↓ Seizure burden	Davidson et al., 2015a
	Sheep	Near-term	Carotid artery occlusion		Peptide5 i.c.v. (50 μmol/kg/h) given 1 h before, and during occlusion only	No neuroprotection	Davidson et al., 2013b
	Sheep	Preterm	Umbilical cord occlusion		Peptide5 i.c.v. (50 μmol/kg over 1 h, then 50 μmol/kg over 24 h) started 90 min after end of occlusion	↑ Neuronal and oligodendrocyte Improved electroencephalogram recovery	Davidson et al., 2013a
	Rat	P7	Common carotid artery ligation and hypoxia	↑ Protein expression (24–48 h after HI)			Wang et al., 2014
	Rat	P7	Common carotid artery ligation and hypoxia	↑ Protein expression (8 h to 7 d after HI)	Gap 26 i.p. (50 μg/kg, 1 h) before HI	↓ Infarct size ↑ Motor and memory scores	Li et al., 2015

(Continued)

TABLE 1 | Continued

	Species	Age	Paradigm	Hemichannel activity/expression	Drug/knockout	Drug/knockout effect	References
	Rat	P10	Acute hypoxia	No change (10 min to 35 d after HI)			Zeinieh et al., 2010
Pannexin 1 (Px1)	Rat primary neurons	P20-25	N-methyl-D-aspartate receptor (NMDAR) activation	↑ Px1 channel opening			Thompson et al., 2008
	Rat primary neurons	P15-20	OGD	↑ Px1 channel opening during OGD			Thompson et al., 2006
	Mouse hippocampal slice	P13-14	High K^+ medium	↑ Px1 channel opening			Santiago et al., 2011
	Mouse primary astrocytes		OGD		Probenecid (10 μM)	↓ IL-1β release ↓ NLRP3 protein expression	Jian et al., 2016
	Mouse acute brain slice	8–12 weeks	*S. aureus in vivo* intracerebral inoculation	↑ Px1 channel activity			Karpuk et al., 2011*
	Xenopus oocytes expressing Px1		High K^+ medium	↑ ATP release during treatment from Px1 channels			Bao et al., 2004
	Rat primary astrocyte culture	P1/2	Hypoxia and artificial cerebrospinal fluid medium mimicking ischemic conditions	No Px1 channel opening at 1 h after reoxygenation			Orellana et al., 2010*
	Human microvascular endothelial cells		Hypoxic acidic ion-shifted ringer solution	↑ ATP release from Px1 channels during treatment but not after reperfusion			Kim and Green, 2016*
	Mice	Adult	MCAO		Mefloquine i.p. (1 mg/kg/d) given during the start of MCAO	↓ Infarction size ↑ Motor scores * No additive effect with P2X7R blockade	Cisneros-Mejorado et al., 2015a*
	Rat	Adult	MCAO		Probencid (i.v., 2 mg/kg) given before reperfusion	↑ Neuronal survival	Wei et al., 2015
	Mice	Adult	MCAO	↑ Px1 protein expression in females vs. male on ischemic and non-ischemic hemispheres	Probenicid i.p. (250 mg/kg) at 1.5 and 5 h	↓ Infarct volume (female only)	Freitas-Andrade et al., 2017
Purinergic receptor (P2X4R)	Rat hippocampal slice	P8-10	OGD	↑ Protein expression at 24 h			Cavaliere et al., 2003
	Mice	Adult	MCAO	↑ Protein expression at 6, 24, and 72 h	Global P2X4R knockout Myeloid cell P2X4R knockout	↓ Infarct volume ↓ IL-1β and TNF-α release ↓ Infarct volume (females only)	Verma et al., 2017

(Continued)

TABLE 1 | Continued

	Species	Age	Paradigm	Hemichannel activity/expression	Drug/knockout	Drug/knockout effect	References
	Rat primary microglia	P2-3			TNP-ATP (20 μM)	↓ Change of microglia to rounded morphology ↓ IL-1β and TNF-α protein expression	Li et al., 2011
	Rat	P0	Hypoxia	↑ Protein expression from 4 h to 14 d			Li et al., 2011
	Rat	P3	Common carotid artery occlusion and hypoxia	↑ Protein expression 5 and 7 d after HI			Wixey et al., 2009
Puringeric receptor (P2X7R)	Neuronal culture		OGD		Brilliant Blue G (50 nM or 5 μM) during OGD	↓ Cell death	Arbeloa et al., 2012
	Rat	Adult	MCAO		Brilliant Blue G i.p. (30 mg/kg) during MCAO	↓ Neuronal loss ↓ Infarct volume	Arbeloa et al., 2012
	Rat	P0	Intrauterine asphyxia	↑ Protein expression immediately after asphyxia			Frizzo et al., 2010
	Rat	Adult	MCAO	↑ Protein expression 4 d after MCAO			Franke et al., 2004
	Rat	Adult	Common carotid and vertebral arteries occlusion	↑ Protein expression from 6 h to 7 d after insult	Brilliant Blue G treatment i.v. (50 mg/kg) administered daily, for 3 d immediately after occlusion	↓ Neuronal loss	Yu et al., 2013
	Rat	Adult	MCAO		A-438079 (3 μg, i.c.v.) or Brilliant Blue G (10 μg, i.c.v.), or Oxidized ATP (1 μg, i.c.v.), prior to HI	↓ Neuronal loss ↑ Motor performance	Chu et al., 2012
	Rat	Adult	MCAO	*De novo* expression of P2X7R on microglia			Melani et al., 2006
	Rat	Adult	Intracerebral hemorrhage		P2X7R siRNA i.c.v. (1,000 pmol)	↓ NLRP3 inflammasome activation ↓ IL-1β and IL-18 release	Feng et al., 2015
	Neuronal culture		OGD	↑ Protein expression after 3, 6, and 12 h of OGD			Ye et al., 2017
	Mice	Adult	Photothrombotic cerebral ischemia	↑ Protein expression from 1 to 5 d after insult	Brilliant Blue G (45.5 mg/kg, i.p.) given at 1, 3, and 5 d	↓ Infarct volume ↓ Protein expression of NLRP3, ASC, and caspase 1 p20	Ye et al., 2017
	Mice	Adult	MCAO		Brilliant Blue G (30 mg/kg twice per day, i.p.) during MCAO	↓ Infarction size ↑ Motor scores * No additive effect with Px1 blockade	Cisneros-Mejorado et al., 2015a*
	Mice	Adult	MCAO		P2X7R knockout	↓ Microglia activation	Kaiser et al., 2016

Studies that report interactions between connexin hemichannels, pannexin channels, and/or purinergic receptors.

2018a). In support, GABAergic striatal neurons expressing intracellular calcium binding proteins are shown to be highly susceptible to HI injury in near-term fetal sheep (Galinsky et al., 2017).

ATP has been widely associated with both inflammasome signal 1 priming which results in transcriptional upregulation of pro-IL-1β and pro-IL-18 and molecules in the inflammasome pathway itself, and inflammasome signal 2 activation that results in assembly of the NLRP3-ASC-pro-caspasel inflammasome complex within the cell cytoplasm, and activation of caspase 1. Cx43 hemichannel mediated ATP release in particular has been associated with NOD-like receptor protein-3 (NLRP3) inflammasome complex assembly as shown in retinal pigment epithelial cells (Mugisho et al., 2018), and with inflammasome activation *in vivo* in a model of chronic pain (Tonkin et al., 2018). Neuron and oligodendrocyte damage after perinatal brain injury may also be due to this innate immune system inflammatory response, and is discussed further in section Activation of the Inflammasome below.

PANNEXIN CHANNELS

Pannexin channels may have similar functions to connexin hemichannels, but their role in perinatal brain injury is not well-understood. Pannexins share homology with the gap junction proteins in invertebrates called innexins (Panchin, 2005), and have a similar topological structure to connexins, despite not sharing sequence homology (Panchin, 2005) (**Figure 1**). Unlike connexins, pannexins have N-glycosylation on the extracellular loop, which appears to prevent the formation of cell-cell junctions (Boassa et al., 2007) although there is some evidence for pannexin junction formation in C2C12 cells in culture (Ishikawa et al., 2011). There are three subtypes of pannexin, of which pannexin 1 (Px1) and pannexin 2 (Px2) are found to be expressed in the adult and developing brain (Bruzzone et al., 2003; Vogt et al., 2005). Px1 is predominantly expressed in the plasma membrane, whereas Px2 is mainly expressed in intracellular membranes (Boassa et al., 2007).

Opening of pannexin channels can be induced by a range of stimuli *in vitro*—including OGD, high extracellular K^+ concentration, hypoglycemia, cell swelling and the stimulation of NMDA receptors (Thompson et al., 2006, 2008; Kawamura et al., 2010; Santiago et al., 2011). Px1 channels are permeable to ions, and molecules, such as ATP and glucose (Bruzzone et al., 2003; Bao et al., 2004; Riquelme et al., 2013) and the opening of Px1 channels contributes to anoxic depolarization, which can lead to cell death (Thompson et al., 2008; Weilinger et al., 2012). In astrocytes on the border of abscess regions caused by S. aureus intracerebral inoculation in mice, there is increased Cx43 hemichannel and Px1 channel activity (Karpuk et al., 2011). Increased Px1 channel activity in apoptotic lymphocytes *in vitro* has been associated with providing "find me" signals through ATP release to attract macrophages (Chekeni et al., 2010). In addition, Px1 channel opening has been linked to the activation of the NLRP3 inflammasome and IL-1β release in astrocytes subjected to OGD (Jian et al., 2016).

In adult rodent models of stroke, blocking Px1 has neuroprotective effects (Cisneros-Mejorado et al., 2015a; Wei et al., 2015; Freitas-Andrade et al., 2017). However, to the best of our knowledge, the effect of Px1 blockade after HI has not been examined in the developing brain. Mefloquine (Px1 blocker) injections given during the start of middle cerebral artery occlusion (MCAO) (i.p., 1 mg/kg/day) in adult mice reduced infarction size and improved motor scores (Cisneros-Mejorado et al., 2015a). It should be noted, however, that mefloquine may also inhibit connexin hemichannel opening (Cruikshank et al., 2004). The effectiveness of Px1 blockade is time dependent, as the administration of probenecid, another non-specific Px1 blocker, was most protective against the death of hippocampal CA1 neurons when given before reperfusion (i.v., 2 mg/kg) in adult rats subjected to MCAO (Wei et al., 2015). There was partial protection when administered at 2 h, but no effect when delayed until 6 h after the insult (Wei et al., 2015). Probenecid administration for 7 days starting at 6 h, however, was more protective than a single dose at 6 h. There was also reduced inflammation, shown by reduced astrocytic and microglial immunoreactivity (Wei et al., 2015). The role of Px1 may also be sex dependent, as Px1 protein levels were higher in female than male mice before and after MCAO (Freitas-Andrade et al., 2017). Both Px1 knockout mice and probenecid treated mice (at 1.5 and 5 h, 250 mg/kg, i.p.), had reduced infarct volumes after MCAO compared to control, but the effect was not seen in males (Freitas-Andrade et al., 2017). It is unclear what mechanisms are involved in producing this sex difference, but it may be related to differences in caspase-dependent cell death pathways and estrogen receptor β signaling in females (Freitas-Andrade et al., 2017).

The interaction of connexin hemichannels and pannexin cell channels has been examined in astrocyte cultures exposed to hypoxia and artificial cerebral spinal fluid medium that mimics ischemic conditions in the brain (Orellana et al., 2010). After reoxygenation, there was increased hemichannel activity, indicated by increased uptake of ethidium bromide, which peaked at 1 h after rexoygenation. This hemichannel activity was mediated by Cx43 hemichannels and not pannexin channels, as dye uptake was reduced by Cx43 hemichannel blockade or Cx43 knockout, but not pannexin blockade (Orellana et al., 2010). This is consistent with the endothelial cell hypoxia-reperfusion study referred to above, where pannexin channel opening was reported during hypoxia, but not reperfusion (Kim and Green, 2016). Furthermore, connexin hemichannels, but not pannexin channels, have been implicated in the inflammasome pathway in muscular dystrophy (Cea et al., 2016), and inflammatory cytokine release normally associated with the inflammasome pathway in rodent models of Parkinson's disease (Maatouk et al., 2018) and Alzheimer's disease (Yi et al., 2016). Finally, pannexin channels are self-regulated, and whilst they may release ATP, they are also closed by the presence of ATP in the extracellular milieu (Qiu and Dahl, 2009). Taken overall, it is possible that pannexin channel opening may play a role in inflammasome pathway initiation, but amplification and perpetuation in chronic disease conditions may be primarily connexin hemichannel mediated. This is likely to apply to perinatal brain injury and inflammation too, but remains to be proven.

ASTROCYTES AND INFLAMMATION

Astrocytes play an important physiological role in maintaining the homeostasis of the microenvironment in the brain. Astrocytes are the most abundant cell type and account for half of the cells in the central nervous system (Markiewicz and Lukomska, 2006). They are electrically non-excitable cells, but have a role in propagating Ca^{2+} waves through gap junctions between astrocytes-astrocytes and astrocytes-neurons (Nedergaard, 1994), and extracellularly between isolated cells (Hassinger et al., 1996). Astrocytes maintain K^{+} ionic balance (Wallraff et al., 2006), and have an important role in the reuptake and recycling of glutamate (Rothstein et al., 1994). Additionally, astrocytes provide metabolic support for neurons by producing lactate, which is taken up by neurons to produce ATP (Mächler et al., 2016).

Astrocytes can also contribute to the inflammatory response after perinatal brain injury. Reactive astrogliosis can occur where astrocytes undergo hypertrophy, increase expression of glial fibrillary protein and form a glial scar around a focal injury (Romero et al., 2014). However, astrogliosis responses have varied between different experimental paradigms. GFAP expression was increased but numbers of GFAP positive cells did not change in P7 rats at 24 h after HI (Odorcyk et al., 2017). There were increased GFAP positive cells and area fraction in preterm fetal sheep at 3 days after umbilical cord occlusion (Wassink et al., 2017). In contrast, there were no changes in the number and area fraction of GFAP positive cells in near-term fetal sheep at 7 days after carotid artery occlusion (Davidson et al., 2016). Moreover, there was a reduction in area fraction and the size of astrocytes in neonatal pigs at 3 days after hypoxia (Sullivan et al., 2010).

Astrocytes predominantly express Cx43, with some expression of Cx26, Cx30, Cx40, and Cx45 (Nagy et al., 1997, 2003; Dermietzel et al., 2000). The opening of astrocytic Cx43 hemichannels after HI may compromise the ability of astrocytes to maintain homeostasis and neuronal support. This in turn, can have detrimental effects on neuronal and oligodendrocyte survival, the propagation of seizures and secondary energy failure (Davidson et al., 2013a). Additionally, astrocytes cultures subjected to OGD/reperfusion increased ATP release through Cx43 hemichannels. Further, treating OGD/reperfusion microglial cultures with ATP or medium from astrocytes subjected to OGD/reperfusion induced microglial activation (Yin et al., 2018b). The potential mechanisms of microglial activation through ATP signaling is discussed further below.

MICROGLIA AND INFLAMMATION

Microglia are the innate immune cells of the brain; having an important role in immune surveillance under normal conditions (Nimmerjahn et al., 2005). Aside from their immune function, they are important for apoptosis and pruning of excessive neurons and synapses, and the phagocytosis of debris during brain development (Baburamani et al., 2014). After brain injury, however, microglia undergo proliferation and activation during the inflammatory response (Baburamani et al., 2014). Resting microglia commonly have ramified morphology and become amoeboid when activated. However, during development, microglia migrate in the brain in amoeboid form and change into a ramified morphology (Pierre et al., 2017).

Activated microglia have various roles, where the classically activated, or M1-like polarization facilitates the progression of inflammation and the alternatively activated, or M2-like polarization is involved in the resolution of inflammation (Bonestroo et al., 2013; Jaworska et al., 2017). The M1-like microglia express cluster of differentiation (CD)86, CD16, CD32, produce reactive oxygen species and nitric oxide synthase, proteases, a range of interleukins and inflammatory cytokines, such as IL-1β, IL-6, and TNF-α (Czeh et al., 2011; Barakat and Redzic, 2015; Fumagalli et al., 2015). The M2-like polarization express CD206 and arginase 1 and produce anti-inflammatory IL-10 and growth factors, favoring repair (Czeh et al., 2011; Barakat and Redzic, 2015; Fumagalli et al., 2015). However, the view that there is a clear polarization of the microglia phenotypes has been challenged in recent years, and currently it is hypothesized that microglial polarization is a continuum with M1 on one end, and M2 on the other (Cherry et al., 2014; Hellström et al., 2016).

In P7 rats, there was a marked increase in CD45/CD11b positive cells in injured areas at 24 h after transient MCAO. These cells were predominantly microglia and not infiltrated blood monocytes (Denker et al., 2007). Supporting this, microglia/macrophage counts were significantly elevated in the hippocampus from 1 day after common carotid artery ligation and hypoxia in P9 mice (human term brain maturation equivalent) (Ferrazzano et al., 2013). There may be a biphasic response of microglial upregulation, with an initial increase in microglial number in the hippocampus at 2 days, followed by a delayed increased in the striatum and cortex at 9 days, after common carotid artery ligation and hypoxia in P9 mice (Cikla et al., 2016). Similarly, classically activated CD11b/CD86 positive microglia from whole brain homogenates were upregulated at 24 h, followed by a secondary peak at 1 week, which was resolved to control levels by 2 weeks after HI (Rice-Vannucci model) in P10 mice (Winerdal et al., 2012). However, the alternative microglial activation markers were not assessed in that study. Significantly elevated counts of ionized calcium-binding adapter molecule 1 (Iba1) positive microglia in the intragyral white matter of the first and second parasagittal gyrus, and the periventricular white matter were present after 1 week of recovery from global cerebral ischemia in near-term fetal sheep (Davidson et al., 2015c, 2016). Moreover, Iba1 positive microglial number was still elevated in the same white matter regions as above at 21 days after severe HI induced by acute umbilical cord occlusion in preterm fetal sheep (van den Heuij et al., 2019). This longer term recovery highlights the chronic nature of inflammation after perinatal HI insults.

The functions of activated microglia appear to change over time after HI. The activation characterization of microglia and infiltrated macrophages has been assessed in P9 mice after common carotid artery occlusion followed by hypoxia (Hellström et al., 2016). There was an increase in mRNA levels of both pro and anti-inflammatory genes at 24 h after the insult. Furthermore, there was a significant increase in classically activated CD86 positive microglia. In contrast, although absolute numbers of alternatively activated CD206 positive microglia increased, their relative proportion was reduced. Surprisingly, there was a population of microglia which did not express CD86 or CD206, highlighting the complexity of microglia activation polarization (Hellström et al., 2016). The early rise of pro-inflammatory markers is supported by an increase of IL-1β and TNF-α mRNA expression between 1 and 24 h after HI in P7 rats (Rice-Vannucci model) (Bona et al., 1999). In another study, using the same paradigm to induce HI in P7 rats, both pro-inflammatory (IL-1β, TNF-α) and anti-inflammatory (IL-10) mRNA expression increased at 3 h after the insult. At 24 h, TNF-α expression was still elevated, but was lower than at 3 h. In addition, anti-inflammatory cytokine TGF-β expression also increased at 24 h along with an increase of CD206 and Iba1 positive microglia (Bonestroo et al., 2013). However, in P7 rats, the majority of CD86 positive microglia were co-localized with IL-1β and only a small number were co-localized with arginase-1, at 6 days after carotid artery ligation and hypoxia (Jaworska et al., 2017). Although some studies indicate a trend toward resolution of inflammation over time, microglia remain upregulated even 3 weeks after HI in preterm fetal sheep (van den Heuij et al., 2019), and so further experimental studies are needed to determine the function of microglia at these later time points.

The increase in inflammatory cytokine release highlighted in the studies above is consistent with NLRP3 inflammasome activation (Shao et al., 2018). Both astrocytes and microglia are known to play key roles in the inflammasome pathway (for review see Song et al., 2017).

ATP RELEASE FROM MEMBRANE CHANNELS

Both connexin hemichannels and pannexin channels can contribute to ATP release into the extracellular space (Kang et al., 2008; Chekeni et al., 2010; Orellana et al., 2011; Bennett et al., 2012), although, as discussed above, pannexin channels may also be regulated (closed) by extracellular ATP (Qiu and Dahl, 2009). ATP is a high energy molecule, essential for driving many cellular processes in the body. It also has a crucial neurotransmitter and neuromodulatory role in the brain (Melani et al., 2005; Pedata et al., 2016). ATP can be co-released with other neurotransmitters or function as an extracellular signaling molecule on its own (Burnstock, 2009; Suurväli et al., 2017). However, under pathological conditions, it may have injurious effects acting as a DAMP (Melani et al., 2005; Pedata et al., 2016) but more crucially as an inflammasome signal 2 activator. Extracellular ATP can activate purinergic receptors, which can perpetuate inflammasome activity in a number of brain cell types, including microglia (Bours et al., 2011) (**Figure 2**).

The bulk of ATP production occurs in mitochondria through oxidative metabolism, but a small amount is produced through anaerobic glycolysis. The disruption of oxygen and glucose delivery during HI affects oxidative metabolism, attenuating the production of ATP (Bainbridge et al., 2014; Wassink et al., 2014). ATP is critical for the function of Na^+/K^+-ATPase, which maintain ionic gradients. When ATP is depleted, the failure to maintain cellular ionic homeostasis causes cytotoxic edema, which is indicated by a rise in cortical impedance starting soon after the onset of ischemia in near-term fetal sheep (Williams et al., 1993; Davidson et al., 2018b). We have previously shown that during profound asphyxia in near-term fetal sheep, there was a rapid increase in oxidized cytochrome oxidase at 2–6 min from the start of asphyxia (Drury et al., 2012). The increase in oxidized cytochrome oxidase indicate that there was a decreased availability of reducing equivalents in the mitochondrial electron transport chain, impairing ATP production. Additionally, a phosphorus magnetic resonance spectroscopy study showed that cerebral phosphocreatine and total nucleotide triphosphate decreased, whereas inorganic phosphate increased during HI in neonatal piglets (Bainbridge et al., 2014). During secondary energy failure at 24 and 48 h after HI in neonatal piglets, the cerebral phosphocreatine/inorganic phosphate and nucleotide triphosphate/exchangeable phosphate pool also decreased (Lorek et al., 1994).

Paradoxically, at a time when ATP production is impaired, there is augmented ATP release into the extracellular space after permanent MCAO in the adult rat brain (Melani et al., 2005, 2012). Microdialysis samples collected from the striatum showed that ATP concentrations were an average of 30 nmol/L before ischemia, which increased to an average of 50 nmol/L after permanent MCAO (Melani et al., 2012). When an ecto-ATPase inhibitor—hexapotassium dihydrogen monotitanoundecatungstocobaltate (II) tridecahydrate (PV4, 100 μmol/L) was used, the extracellular ATP concentrations were between 320 and 450 nmol/L (Melani et al., 2012). This is within the range of what was detected in hippocampal slices during reoxygenation after OGD (700 nmol/L), using a biosensor measured in real time (Frenguelli et al., 2007). However, extracellular ATP release has not been examined after HI in the developing brain.

The increase in extracellular ATP can lead to a subsequent increase in adenosine, as ATP is catabolized into adenosine, through the ATP → ADP → AMP → adenosine pathway, mediated by ecto-nucleotidase enzymes (Pedata et al., 2016). Adenosine concentrations increased by 90% during a 1 h period of fetal hypoxia induced by reduction of maternal fraction of inspired oxygen, compared to levels during normoxia in 0.8 gestation fetal sheep (Koos et al., 1997). The rise in adenosine concentrations was attributed to the degradation of AMP, as blocking the degradation of AMP to adenosine with adenosine 5′-(α,β-methylene) diphosphate (AOPCP), an ecto-5′-nucleotidase inhibitor, attenuated the hypoxia-induced rise in adenosine (Koos et al., 1997). In support, in the first hour after permanent MCAO in the adult rat brain, extracellular adenosine was mainly derived from ATP hydrolysis (Melani et al., 2012). This is in contrast to physiological conditions, when adenosine can be directly released from intracellular stores (Melani et al., 2012). Adenosine is very important to the initial metabolic suppression

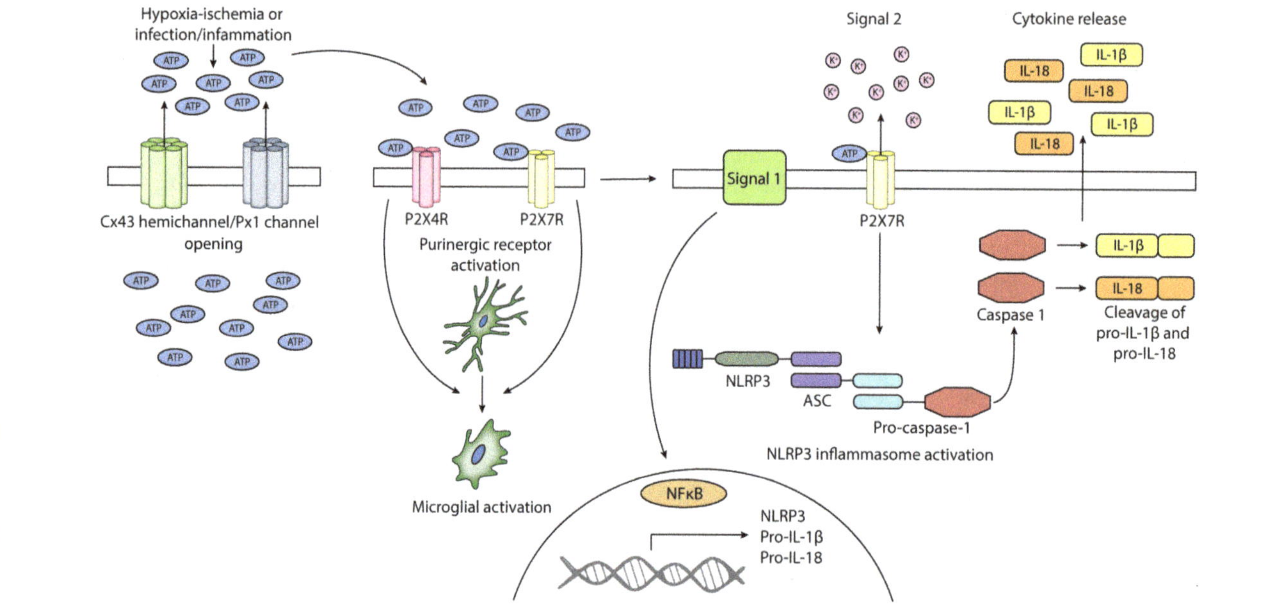

FIGURE 2 | Schematic diagram of the potential involvement of connexin 43 hemichannels and pannexin 1 channels and purinergic receptors P2X4 and P2X7 in the activation of microglia and NLRP3 inflammasome. Cx43 hemichannels and Px1 channels may open after exposure to HI or infection/inflammation. The opening of these channels leads to the release of ATP into the extracellular space. Extracellular ATP can activate purinergic receptors P2X4R and P2X7R. The activation of P2X4R and P2X7R can lead to the activation of microglia. Signal 1 of NLRP3 inflammasome activation is provided by PAMPs or DAMPs, which leads to the upregulation of NLRP3, pro-IL-1β, and pro-IL-18. Signal 2 is mediated by ATP activation of P2X7R and can lead to the assembly of NLRP3, ASC, and pro-caspase 1, forming the NLRP3 inflammasome. Pro-caspase 1 is activated into caspase 1, which cleaves pro-IL-1β and pro-IL-18 into their mature forms. Mature IL-1β and IL-18 is secreted.

that occurs at the beginning of an HI insult (Hunter et al., 2003). Blocking this response with the adenosine A1 receptor antagonist 8-cyclopentyl-1,3-dipropylxanthine (DPCPX) (2.5 mg/mL) in near-term fetal sheep before and during profound asphyxia, was associated with increased neuronal loss compared to the vehicle group (Hunter et al., 2003). Further studies are needed to examine the interaction of ATP and adenosine *in vivo*, in the developing brain after HI, and to investigate inflammasome complex assembly under those conditions. In parallel, it is necessary to consider the purinergic receptors themselves (see section Purinergic Receptors).

PURINERGIC RECEPTORS

Purinergic P1 and P2 receptors are activated by adenosine and ATP, respectively. Within the group of P2 receptors, there are P2X receptors, which are ionotropic and P2Y, which are metabotropic (Pedata et al., 2016). In this review, we will focus on the P2X receptors, which form trimeric cationic channels in the cell membrane (Habermacher et al., 2016). Of the seven P2X subtypes (P2X1-7), P2X4 receptor (P2X4R), and P2X7 receptor (P2X7R) have been more widely studied in the brain (Pedata et al., 2016). These channels open in response to ATP binding and are permeable to Na^+, K^+, and especially Ca^{2+} (Hattori and Gouaux, 2012). The activation of purinergic receptors can lead to the opening of more connexin hemichannels (and at least potentially pannexin channels), triggering further release of ATP in a process known as "ATP-induced ATP release" in a positive feedback loop (Stout et al., 2002; Baroja-Mazo et al., 2013).

P2X4 Receptor

P2X4R is one of the most sensitive P2X receptors, as it binds ATP in the nanomolar range, whereas P2X7R binds at a micromolar range (Suurväli et al., 2017). It also has the highest permeability to Ca^{2+}, and is the most abundantly expressed P2X subtype in the brain (Egan and Khakh, 2004; Cheng et al., 2014), found on neurons and glial cells, in various brain regions (Bo et al., 2003; Stokes et al., 2017; Suurväli et al., 2017). Under physiological conditions, P2X4R may have an important role in neurotransmission pathways (Suurväli et al., 2017). P2X4 knockout mice show deficits in sensorimotor tasks and social interactions, which was associated with altered subunit expression of glutamate and gamma-aminobutyric acid (GABA) receptors (Wyatt et al., 2013). As P2X4R is expressed abundantly in cells of myeloid origin, such as microglia and monocytes, they may play important roles in pro-inflammatory cytokine release following injury (Cavaliere et al., 2003).

P2X4R has been targeted for neuroprotection after HI. Global P2X4R knockout mice have a reduction in infarct volume and IL-1β and TNF-α release after MCAO compared to wild type mice (Verma et al., 2017). However, when P2X4R was knocked out in myeloid cells only, the neuroprotective effect was only seen in females. The role of P2X4R is complex, as the P2X4R knockout was associated with increased depressive-like behavior compared to wild type mice measured at 30 days after MCAO (Verma et al., 2017). In addition, P2X4R on vascular endothelial cells was involved in neuroprotection via ischemic preconditioning after MCAO in adult mice, as the inhibition of P2X4R abolished this effect (Ozaki et al., 2016).

P2X4 Receptor and Activation of Microglia

Microglia and peripheral monocytes have been shown to express P2X4R, and electrical currents can be induced by ATP activation of P2X4R (Wang et al., 2004; Cheng et al., 2014). The expression of P2X4R is upregulated in organotypic hippocampal culture at 24 h after OGD (Cavaliere et al., 2003) In P0 rats, P2X4R protein expression increased from 4 h after hypoxia until 14 days (Li et al., 2011). However, in P3 rats, there was a significant increase in P2X4R protein expression only at 5 days after common carotid artery occlusion and hypoxia (Wixey et al., 2009). In both neonatal rat studies, P2X4R expression was predominantly colocalized with microglia (Wixey et al., 2009; Li et al., 2011). Although the increase in P2X4R at 5 days was not temporally correlated with the early increase in Iba1 protein expression seen at 2 days after HI, it correlated with the delayed increase in Iba1 protein expression from 6 days after HI. It was postulated that these P2X4R positive microglia may be a distinct population of microglia involved in neuroinflammation (Wixey et al., 2009). Furthermore, P2X4R blockade with trinitrophenyl (TNP)-ATP (20 μM) prevented the change of primary microglial cells to a more rounded morphology after hypoxia, and attenuated the increased IL-1β and TNF-α protein expression (Li et al., 2011).

P2X7 Receptor

Although, P2X7R has a lower affinity of 0.1–1 mM for ATP, when compared to P2X4R, the increased extracellular ATP levels after ischemia may be sufficient to activate it (Surprenant and North, 2009; Melani et al., 2012). The deleterious roles of the P2X7R include increasing intracellular Ca^{2+} concentrations, glutamate release and inflammasome activation (Di Virgilio, 2007; Matute et al., 2007; Rossi and Volterra, 2009; Ye et al., 2017). Additionally, prolonged ATP activation of P2X7R can transform the cationic channel into a large membrane pore, permeable to molecules 900 Da in size (Yan et al., 2010).

Animal studies have shown that P2X7R is upregulated after ischemia in the immature and adult brain. In a fetal rat model of intrauterine asphyxia, P2X7R expression in the hippocampus was upregulated 3-fold immediately after asphyxia, but returned to control levels at 60 min (Frizzo et al., 2010). In adult rats, however, cortical P2X7R expression was increased 5-fold compared to controls at 4 days after permanent MCAO (Franke et al., 2004). Whereas, in adult mice subjected to photothrombotic cerebral ischemia, cortical P2X7R expression was upregulated from 1 day post-ischemia until 5 days (Ye et al., 2017). In cortical neuronal culture, there was a significant upregulation of P2X7R after exposure to OGD (Ye et al., 2017). P2X7R expression was increased in the CA1 region of the hippocampus from 6 h and maintained until 7 days after global cerebral ischemia in adult rats (Yu et al., 2013). The differences in the timing of P2X7R upregulation could be due age, species, brain region and type of insult.

Blocking P2X7R has been shown to be beneficial for ischemic brain injury *in vitro* and in adult animals. In neuronal culture, Brilliant Blue G—a P2X7R blocker (50 nM or 5 μM), applied during OGD, reduced cell death measured at 24 h after OGD (Arbeloa et al., 2012). This was replicated *in vivo*; Brilliant Blue G (30 mg/kg, i.p.) administered at 30 min during a 90 min MCAO and continued daily in adult rats reduced infarct volume and neuronal loss when measured at 3 days after the insult (Arbeloa et al., 2012). In support, Brilliant Blue G treatment (50 mg/kg, i.v.) administered daily, for 3 days, starting immediately after occluding bilateral common carotid and vertebral arteries in adult rats, partially attenuated CA1 neuronal loss in the hippocampus at 7 days after injury (Yu et al., 2013). Although Brilliant Blue G has higher affinity for P2X7R, it can also bind to other P2X receptors at higher concentrations (Chu et al., 2012). However, the administration of a more selective P2X7R antagonist—A-438079 (3 μg, i.c.v.), prior to transient common carotid artery occlusion in adult rats, had similar neuroprotective effects to Brilliant Blue G (10 μg, i.c.v.) and Oxidized ATP (1 μg, i.c.v.), in terms of neuronal survival and motor performance (Chu et al., 2012). Additionally, in an adult rat model of intracerebral hemorrhage, silencing the P2X7R gene reduced NLRP3 inflammasome activation and release of IL-1β and IL-18 at 24 h after the insult (Feng et al., 2015). It is difficult to disentangle the timing of when P2X7R is involved in injury, as most of these studies above started blocking P2X7R either during or immediately after ischemia.

Several studies have shown that connexin hemichannels and pannexin channels are involved in purinergic signaling. For example, IL-1β release induced by P2X7R activation was associated with Px1 channels in macrophages (Pelegrin and Surprenant, 2006). When a Px1 blocker—mefloquine (1 mg/kg, i.p.) was co-administered with Brilliant Blue G (30 mg/kg twice per day, i.p.) to block P2X7R, starting at 30 min during 60 min of MCAO, there was no additive benefit when compared to administering either drug alone in adult mice after MCAO (Cisneros-Mejorado et al., 2015a). However, as stated earlier, mefloquine can also target connexin hemichannels (Cruikshank et al., 2004). A potential mechanism of injury may be ATP release, as both the prevention of ATP release, or inhibition of P2X7R may have beneficial effects (Cisneros-Mejorado et al., 2015b). For example, targeting Cx43 using Peptide5 at 0 h (10 mg/kg), 2 h (5 mg/kg), and 4 h (2.5 mg/kg, i.p.), after spinal cord injury in rats was associated with a reduction is tissue damage and improved functional recovery (Mao et al., 2017). Similarly, the administration of Brilliant Blue G to inhibit P2X7R (10 or 50 mg/kg daily for 3 days) starting 10–15 min after spinal cord injury in rats, reduced tissue damage and improved motor performance (Peng et al., 2009).

P2X7 Receptor and Activation of Microglia

In adult rats after MCAO, the expression of P2X7R was colocalized with microglia at 1 and 4 days, neurons at 4 and 7 days, and astrocytes at 4 days after the insult (Franke et al., 2004). *De novo* expression of P2X7R was observed on activated microglia at 24 h after MCAO in adult rats, with no expression seen in control animals (Melani et al., 2006). It has been debated as to whether the overexpression of P2X7R drives the activation of microglia, or whether the overexpression of P2X7R is a result of microglial activation (Bai and Li, 2013). In support of the role of P2X7R in microglia activation, the overexpression of P2X7R by transfection of microglia in culture resulted in activation and proliferation of microglia (Monif et al., 2009). Additionally, P2X7R knockout mice showed significantly attenuated microglial activation at 72 h following MCAO compared to wild type mice (Kaiser et al., 2016). In the developing brain, both P2X7R and P2X4R were constitutively expressed in microglia in P3 rats, but P2X4R immunofluorescence was more intense than P2X7R. However, only the changes in P2X4R expression was examined after exposure to hypoxia in P0 rats (Li et al., 2011).

ACTIVATION OF THE INFLAMMASOME

The family of PRRs include Toll-like receptors (TRLs), NOD-like receptors (NLRs), and retinoic acid-inducible gene-I-like receptors (RLRs) which recognize PAMPs or DAMPs (Hagberg et al., 2015; Mallard et al., 2018). There is growing interest in the role of NLRs in inflammatory diseases, but relatively little is known about their role in perinatal brain injury. Inflammasomes are a multimeric complex of proteins which oligomerize after sensing PAMP or DAMP signals (Jo et al., 2016). Typically, NLR inflammsomes are formed by the assembly of the NLR family protein, apoptosis-associated speck-like protein containing a caspase recruitment domain (ASC) and pro-caspase 1. The 22 members of the NLR family are distinguished by their N-terminal effector domains, and grouped into NLRA, NLRB, NLRC and NLRP (Ting et al., 2008). One of the better characterized inflammasomes in the NLR family is the NOD-like receptor protein-3 (NLRP3) inflammasome. The activation of the NLRP3 inflammasome leads to the activation of caspase 1, the cleavage and release of mature IL-1β and IL-18 and subsequent release of other cytokines (Jo et al., 2016; Mugisho et al., 2018).

There are two steps to NLRP3 inflammasome activation. Signal 1 is a priming step, induced by PAMPS, such as microbial toxins and surface proteins, TLR ligands and viral RNA (Martinon et al., 2009; Jun et al., 2012; Chakrabarti et al., 2015) or DAMPs, such as amyloid-β, hyaluronan, monosodium urate, calcium pyrophosphate dehydrate and extracellular ATP (Martinon et al., 2009; Gong et al., 2018). Endogenous inflammatory cytokines including TNF-α and IL-1β can also act as priming signals (Franchi et al., 2009; He et al., 2016; Gong et al., 2018). The priming signal leads to the upregulation of NLRP3 and pro-IL-1β and pro-IL-18 expression through the nuclear factor kappa-light-chain-(NF-κB) translocation to the nucleus to trigger their transcription (He et al., 2016). Signal 2 of the NLRP3 inflammasome is the activation signal. This leads to assembly of the inflammasome complex. A clear model for activation remains unclear; much of the literature suggests that many of the same molecules involved in priming may have a secondary role in activation (Shao et al., 2018). That seems unlikely. Thus, is remains a significant question to define which molecular mechanism(s) trigger activation of the NLRP3 inflammasome (He et al., 2016; Jo et al., 2016). More recently, the list of potential activator signals has been narrowed down. Key players are now suggested to include: ATP, calcium signaling, and reactive oxygen species (He et al., 2016; Jo et al., 2016; Groslambert and Py, 2018). Mitochondrial dysfunction, lysosomal rupture and K^+ efflux are also reported to be activators (He et al., 2016; Gao et al., 2017), although it is unclear to what extent some of these may be effects of inflammation rather than initiators *per se*.

Potassium efflux can be mediated through the opening of endogenous ion channels or through bacterial pore forming toxins (Gao et al., 2017). Purinergic receptors have been associated with the efflux of K^+ (Yan et al., 2008) as have connexin hemichannels (Schalper et al., 2010; Leybaert et al., 2017). It is unclear how the reduction in intracellular K^+ leads to the activation of the inflammasome although studies have shown that it is a necessary step for the kinase Never In Mitosis A-Related Kinase 7 to bind to NLRP3, required for the assembly of the inflammasome (He et al., 2016; Shi et al., 2016). Additionally, K^+ efflux can lead to the disruption of mitochondrial function and production of mitochondrial reactive oxygen species (Tang et al., 2017). It is also of note that potassium efflux is induced by ATP suggesting that ATP release may therefore be the primary or upstream activator not only for potassium efflux, but also mitochondrial dysfunction and reactive oxygen species. Our work has shown that reducing ATP release on its own alone (by blocking connexin hemichannels alone) is sufficient to shut down inflammasome complex assembly, while the addition of exogenous ATP sufficient to reestablish assembly (Mugisho et al., 2018), consistent with the evidence that purinergic receptors play a key role, as outlined above and in **Table 1**.

Inflammasome Activation in Brain Injury

A large body of evidence in the adult brain shows that inflammation is a least in part mediated by the NLRP3 inflammasome in animal models of stroke, traumatic brain injury and subarachnoid hemorrhage with upregulation of mRNA or protein expression of NLRP3, ASC, caspase-1 and associated inflammatory cytokines, such as TNF-α, IL-18 and IL-6 (Gao et al., 2017; Ye et al., 2017; Ismael et al., 2018; Lee et al., 2018; Wang et al., 2018; Xu et al., 2018; Yin et al., 2018a). Additionally, clinical data show that children with severe traumatic brain injury (open/closed head injury not specified) had elevated levels of NLRP3 in cerebrospinal fluid collected between 0 to ~72 h after the injury (Wallisch et al., 2017). NLRP3 and IL-1β mRNA expression was increased in the hippocampus, striatum and the thalamus at 24 h after common carotid artery ligation followed by hypoxia in P9 neonatal mice (Ystgaard et al., 2015). Supporting this, NLRP3 immunofluorescence increased at 24 h after common carotid artery ligation and hypoxia in P7 rats, which was predominantly colocalized with microglia (Chen et al., 2018). Additionally, there was an increase in IL-1β, caspase 1 and NLRP3 protein expression (Chen et al., 2018).

Targeting the NLRP3 inflammasome has neuroprotective effects in ischemic brain injury either through selective inhibition of NLRP3, or through anti-inflammatory drugs which affect the NLRP3 pathway (Ye et al., 2017; Chen et al., 2018; Ismael et al., 2018). The selective inhibition of NLRP3 using MCC950 (50 mg/kg, i.p. *in vivo* and 1 μM *in vitro*) reduced neuronal apoptosis when delivered after photothrombotic cerebral ischemia in adult mice, and before OGD in neuronal cultures (Ye et al., 2017). In support, MCC950 (50 mg/kg, i.p.) administration at 1 and 3 h was associated with a reduction in infarction size and cerebral edema, and improved neurological deficit scores, after MCAO in adult mice. These findings were in turn associated with a decrease in protein levels of NLRP3, caspase 1 and ASC at 24 h after the insult (Ismael et al., 2018). Ginkgolide B—a component of Ginkgo biloba extracts (5–10 mg/kg, i.p.), which has anti-inflammatory effects, was administered to P7 rats 30 min prior to common carotid artery ligation and hypoxia and was associated with the attenuation of the increased expression of NLRP3, caspase 1 and IL-1β at 24 h after injury. These changes were accompanied by reduced infarct size and cerebral edema measured at 72 h (Chen et al., 2018). In contrast, NLRP3 knockout was not associated with neuroprotection in P9 mice, as infarction volume was not significantly different compared to wild type mice at 24 h after common carotid artery ligation and hypoxia (Ystgaard et al., 2015) and in some cases other NLRs or other pathways may be implicated.

Inflammasome Activation in Perinatal Infection/Inflammation

The studies discussed in this review predominantly focused on the role of connexin hemichannels and pannexin channels and purinergic receptors in experimental models of HI. Given that HI and infection/inflammation both lead to neuroinflammation, it is possible that both may be perpetuated through inflammasome pathway activation. In this section, we discuss the evidence for inflammasome activation in infection/inflammation in clinical and experimental studies.

Inflammasome activation, at least in adults, is an important inflammatory response to combat infection. For example, adult mice deficient in NLRP3, ASC, or caspase 1 have reduced survival rates compared to wild type mice after Group B Streptococcus infection (Costa et al., 2012). Group B Streptococcus is a Gram-positive bacterium that is common cause of life-threatening sepsis and meningitis in neonates and pregnant women (Henneke and Berner, 2006). Preterm and very-low-birthweight neonates are susceptible to neonatal sepsis likely due to increased risk of exposure to microbes (for example via mechanical ventilation, intravenous catheters and parenteral feeding). Secondly, they may have deficits in their innate and adaptive immune responses leading to insufficient inflammatory mediators (Wynn and Wong, 2010; Strunk et al., 2011). In view of the latter, a study of 21 preterm infants born 24–32 weeks showed that preterm umbilical cord blood monocytes, had a reduction in IL-1β secretion and an induction of NLRP3 expression, compared to term infants and adult peripheral monocytes after ATP/LPS stimulation (Sharma et al., 2015). However, IL-1β secretion from preterm peripheral blood monocytes (24–29 weeks of gestation) collected at an average of 15 post-natal days was comparable to adult monocytes, suggesting that the impairment in IL-1β secretion is restored shortly after birth (Sharma et al., 2015). A study of 72 neonates showed that IL-1β secretion from peripheral blood mononuclear cells did not differ between extremely preterm (born <28 weeks) and very preterm infants (28–32 weeks) on the fifth day of life. However, the peripheral blood mononuclear cells (collected within 24 h of late onset sepsis) from the extremely preterm group secreted higher levels of IL-1β, than the very preterm neonates (Zasada et al., 2018). It is unclear whether this gestational age dependent response is related to the higher counts of circulating mononuclear cells found in the extremely preterm group.

Conversely, the excessive activation of the inflammasome and release of pro-inflammatory cytokines in neonatal sepsis, can lead to multi-organ failure and death (Gentile et al., 2015). Caspase-1/11 knockout mice (P5-7) exposed to cecal slurry to induce polymicrobial intra-abdominal neonatal sepsis had greater survival rates compared to wild type mice (Gentile et al., 2015). Additionally, there was reduced IL-1β and IL-18 release at 2, 6, 18, and 24 h after the induction of sepsis. Surprisingly, genetic ablation of ASC or NLRP3 was not associated with a protective effect (Gentile et al., 2015). The knockout of ASC or NLRP3 may be insufficient for the complete elimination of caspase 1 activity as it is not solely activated by the NLRP3 inflammasome (Gentile et al., 2015). Further adverse effects are evidenced from infants who have rare genetic mutations leading to over activation of the NLRP3 inflammasome which manifests as neonatal-onset multi-system inflammatory disease (Aróstegui et al., 2010).

Recent evidence has demonstrated that increased inflammasome activity is associated with chorioamnionitis (Gomez-Lopez et al., 2017). A study of 70 pregnant women who had undergone preterm labor showed that the chorioamniotic membranes from those with acute histological chorioamnionitis compared to those without, had greater mRNA levels of inflammasome components, including NLRP3, and other NLR proteins, caspase 1, IL-1β, IL-18, and increased ASC and caspase 1 complex formation (Gomez-Lopez et al., 2017). Additionally, a study of amniotic fluid from 143 women showed that those who had undergone spontaneous preterm labor, with intra-amniotic infection/inflammation (positive culture for microorganisms in the amniotic fluid, or a white blood cell count of >100 cells/mm^3) had significantly higher caspase 1 levels compared to those without intra-amniotic infection/inflammation, delivering at term or preterm (Gotsch et al., 2008). Furthermore, umbilical cord blood monocytes from preterm infants with histological chorioamnionitis showed reduced caspase 1 activity compared to those without histological chorioamnionitis (Sharma et al., 2015).

Although NLRP3 mediated inflammation may be implicated in many diseases, further study of its involvement in perinatal brain injury after HI and infection/inflammation is necessary. Disentangling the temporal effects of inflammation is particularly important, as discussed earlier the role of inflammation can be both beneficial and deleterious.

CONCLUSION

Connexin and pannexin membrane channels can contribute to the evolution of perinatal brain injury. Connexin hemichannel, and to a lesser extent pannexin channel, blockade, has been associated with neuroprotection in a number of models of brain injury. A potential mechanism of injury perpetuated by connexin hemichannels could be release of what may be a key inflammasome signal 2 activator, ATP. Extracellular ATP activates purinergic receptors, which in turn have been shown to be involved with the activation of microglia and the inflammasome complex. Blockade of purinergic receptors P2X4 and P2X7 has been protective in adult animal models of stroke but further studies are required to investigate the involvement of purinergic receptors in the propagation of perinatal brain injury, and in particular the timing of their contribution to spreading injury. However, although P2X4R and P2X7R have been implicated in microglial activation following HI insults, and could be targets for modulating microglial responses after perinatal brain injury, connexin hemichannel perpetuation of the inflammasome would be upstream of both. Increasing evidence suggests that modulating the cascade upstream of inflammasome activation may attenuate brain injury mediated through inflammation. Inflammasome activation should be investigated further in perinatal brain injury, as it may be an important mediator of deleterious inflammatory responses.

AUTHOR CONTRIBUTIONS

JD and KZ conceptualized this topical review. KZ, JD, AG, LB, and CG undertook manuscript writing and preparation of figures. All authors reviewed and edited this manuscript.

FUNDING

The authors' studies discussed in this review was funded by The Health Research Council of New Zealand, grant numbers: 16/003, 12/613, 14/216, 17/601 and the Marsden Fund, grant number 17-UOA232. JD holds a Sir Charles Hercus Fellowship from the Health Research Council of New Zealand (16/003). CG acknowledges support from Wendy and Bruce Hadden. KZ was supported by a University of Auckland Doctoral Scholarship.

REFERENCES

Alexander, D. B., and Goldberg, G. S. (2003). Transfer of biologically important molecules between cells through gap junction channels. *Curr. Med. Chem.* 10, 2045–2058. doi: 10.2174/0929867033456927

Arbeloa, J., Pérez-Samartín, A., Gottlieb, M., and Matute, C. (2012). P2X7 receptor blockade prevents ATP excitotoxicity in neurons and reduces brain damage after ischemia. *Neurobiol. Dis.* 45, 954–961. doi: 10.1016/j.nbd.2011.12.014

Aróstegui, J. I., Lopez Saldana, M. D., Pascal, M., Clemente, D., Aymerich, M., Balaguer, F., et al. (2010). A somatic NLRP3 mutation as a cause of a sporadic case of chronic infantile neurologic, cutaneous, articular syndrome/neonatal-onset multisystem inflammatory disease: novel evidence of the role of low-level mosaicism as the pathophysiologic mechanism underlying mendelian inherited diseases. *Arthritis Rheum.* 62, 1158–1166. doi: 10.1002/art.27342

Azzopardi, D., Wyatt, J. S., Cady, E. B., Delpy, D. T., Baudin, J., Stewart, A. L., et al. (1989). Prognosis of newborn infants with hypoxic-ischemic brain injury assessed by phosphorus magnetic resonance spectroscopy. *Pediatr. Res.* 25, 445–451. doi: 10.1203/00006450-198905000-00004

Baburamani, A. A., Supramaniam, V. G., Hagberg, H., and Mallard, C. (2014). Microglia toxicity in preterm brain injury. *Reprod. Toxicol.* 48, 106–112. doi: 10.1016/j.reprotox.2014.04.002

Bai, H. Y., and Li, A. P. (2013). P2X(7) receptors in cerebral ischemia. *Neurosci. Bull.* 29, 390–398. doi: 10.1007/s12264-013-1338-7

Bainbridge, A., Tachtsidis, I., Faulkner, S. D., Price, D., Zhu, T., Baer, E., et al. (2014). Brain mitochondrial oxidative metabolism during and after cerebral hypoxia-ischemia studied by simultaneous phosphorus magnetic-resonance and broadband near-infrared spectroscopy. *Neuroimage* 102, 173–183. doi: 10.1016/j.neuroimage.2013.08.016

Bao, L., Locovei, S., and Dahl, G. (2004). Pannexin membrane channels are mechanosensitive conduits for ATP. *FEBS Lett.* 572, 65–68. doi: 10.1016/j.febslet.2004.07.009

Barakat, R., and Redzic, Z. (2015). Differential cytokine expression by brain microglia/macrophages in primary culture after oxygen glucose deprivation and their protective effects on astrocytes during anoxia. *Fluids Barriers CNS* 12:6. doi: 10.1186/s12987-015-0002-1

Baroja-Mazo, A., Barberà-Cremades, M., and Pelegrin, P. (2013). The participation of plasma membrane hemichannels to purinergic signaling. *Biochim. Biophys. Acta* 1828, 79–93. doi: 10.1016/j.bbamem.2012.01.002

Bartha, A. I., Foster-Barber, A., Miller, S. P., Vigneron, D. B., Glidden, D. V., Barkovich, A. J., et al. (2004). Neonatal encephalopathy: association of cytokines with MR spectroscopy and outcome. *Pediatr. Res.* 56, 960–966. doi: 10.1203/01.PDR.0000144819.45689.BB

Bennet, L., Booth, L., and Gunn, A. J. (2010). Potential biomarkers for hypoxic-ischemic encephalopathy. *Semin. Fetal Neonatal Med.* 15, 253–260. doi: 10.1016/j.siny.2010.05.007

Bennet, L., Dhillon, S., Lear, C. A., Van Den Heuij, L., King, V., Dean, J. M., et al. (2018). Chronic inflammation and impaired development of the preterm brain. *J. Reprod. Immunol.* 125, 45–55. doi: 10.1016/j.jri.2017.11.003

Bennet, L., Roelfsema, V., Pathipati, P., Quaedackers, J., and Gunn, A. J. (2006). Relationship between evolving epileptiform activity and delayed loss of mitochondrial activity after asphyxia measured by near-infrared spectroscopy in preterm fetal sheep. *J. Physiol.* 572, 141–154. doi: 10.1113/jphysiol.2006.105197

Bennett, M. V., Garré, J. M., Orellana, J. A., Bukauskas, F. F., Nedergaard, M., and Saez, J. C. (2012). Connexin and pannexin hemichannels in inflammatory responses of glia and neurons. *Brain Res.* 1487, 3–15. doi: 10.1016/j.brainres.2012.08.042

Bo, X., Kim, M., Nori, S. L., Schoepfer, R., Burnstock, G., and North, R. A. (2003). Tissue distribution of P2X4 receptors studied with an ectodomain antibody. *Cell Tissue Res.* 313, 159–165. doi: 10.1007/s00441-003-0758-5

Boassa, D., Ambrosi, C., Qiu, F., Dahl, G., Gaietta, G., and Sosinsky, G. (2007). Pannexinl channels contain a glycosylation site that targets the hexamer to the plasma membrane. *J. Biol. Chem.* 282, 31733–31743. doi: 10.1074/jbc.M702422200

Bona, E., Andersson, A. L., Blomgren, K., Gilland, E., Puka-Sundvall, M., Gustafson, K., et al. (1999). Chemokine and inflammatory cell response to hypoxia-ischemia in immature rats. *Pediatr. Res.* 45, 500–509. doi: 10.1203/00006450-199904010-00008

Bonestroo, H. J., Nijboer, C. H., van Velthoven, C. T., Kavelaars, A., Hack, C. E., Van Bel, F., et al. (2013). Cerebral and hepatic inflammatory response after neonatal hypoxia-ischemia in newborn rats. *Dev. Neurosci.* 35, 197–211. doi: 10.1159/000346685

Bours, M. J., Dagnelie, P. C., Giuliani, A. L., Wesselius, A., and Di Virgilio, F. (2011). P2 receptors and extracellular ATP: a novel homeostatic pathway in inflammation. *Front. Biosci. (Schol. Ed.)* 3, 1443–1456. doi: 10.2741/s235.

Bruzzone, R., Hormuzdi, S. G., Barbe, M. T., Herb, A., and Monyer, H. (2003). Pannexins, a family of gap junction proteins expressed in brain. *Proc. Natl. Acad. Sci. U.S.A.* 100, 13644–13649. doi: 10.1073/pnas.2233464100

Burnstock, G. (2009). Purinergic cotransmission. *F1000 Biol. Rep.* 1:46. doi: 10.3410/B1-46

Cavaliere, F., Florenzano, F., Amadio, S., Fusco, F. R., Viscomi, M. T., D'ambrosi, N., et al. (2003). Up-regulation of P2X2, P2X4 receptor and ischemic cell death: prevention by P2 antagonists. *Neuroscience* 120, 85–98. doi: 10.1016/S0306-4522(03)00228-8

Cea, L. A., Balboa, E., Puebla, C., Vargas, A. A., Cisterna, B. A., Escamilla, R., et al. (2016). Dexamethasone-induced muscular atrophy is mediated by functional expression of connexin-based hemichannels. *Biochim. Biophys. Acta* 1862, 1891–1899. doi: 10.1016/j.bbadis.2016.07.003

Chakrabarti, A., Banerjee, S., Franchi, L., Loo, Y. M., Gale, M. Jr., Nunez, G., et al. (2015). RNase L activates the NLRP3 inflammasome during viral infections. *Cell Host Microbe* 17, 466–477. doi: 10.1016/j.chom.2015.02.010

Chekeni, F. B., Elliott, M. R., Sandilos, J. K., Walk, S. F., Kinchen, J. M., Lazarowski, E. R., et al. (2010). Pannexin 1 channels mediate 'find-me' signal release and membrane permeability during apoptosis. *Nature* 467, 863–867. doi: 10.1038/nature09413

Chen, A., Xu, Y., and Yuan, J. (2018). Ginkgolide B ameliorates NLRP3 inflammasome activation after hypoxic-ischemic brain injury in the neonatal male rat. *Int. J. Dev. Neurosci.* 69, 106–111. doi: 10.1016/j.ijdevneu.2018.07.004

Cheng, R. D., Ren, J. J., Zhang, Y. Y., and Ye, X. M. (2014). P2X4 receptors expressed on microglial cells in post-ischemic inflammation of brain ischemic injury. *Neurochem. Int.* 67, 9–13. doi: 10.1016/j.neuint.2014.01.011

Cherry, J. D., Olschowka, J. A., and O'banion, M. K. (2014). Neuroinflammation and M2 microglia: the good, the bad, and the inflamed. *J. Neuroinflammation* 11:98. doi: 10.1186/1742-2094-11-98

Chu, K., Yin, B., Wang, J., Peng, G., Liang, H., Xu, Z., et al. (2012). Inhibition of P2X7 receptor ameliorates transient global cerebral ischemia/reperfusion injury via modulating inflammatory responses in the rat hippocampus. *J. Neuroinflammation* 9:69. doi: 10.1186/1742-2094-9-69

Cikla, U., Chanana, V., Kintner, D. B., Covert, L., Dewall, T., Waldman, A., et al. (2016). Suppression of microglia activation after hypoxia-ischemia results in age-dependent improvements in neurologic injury. *J. Neuroimmunol.* 291, 18–27. doi: 10.1016/j.jneuroim.2015.12.004

Cisneros-Mejorado, A., Gottlieb, M., Cavaliere, F., Magnus, T., Koch-Nolte, F., Scemes, E., et al. (2015a). Blockade of P2X7 receptors or pannexin-1 channels similarly attenuates postischemic damage. *J. Cereb. Blood Flow Metab.* 35, 843–850. doi: 10.1038/jcbfm.2014.262

Cisneros-Mejorado, A., Pérez-Samartín, A., Gottlieb, M., and Matute, C. (2015b). ATP signaling in brain: release, excitotoxicity and potential therapeutic targets. *Cell. Mol. Neurobiol.* 35, 1–6. doi: 10.1007/s10571-014-0092-3

Contreras, J. E., Sánchez, H. A., Eugenin, E. A., Speidel, D., Theis, M., Willecke, K., et al. (2002). Metabolic inhibition induces opening of unapposed connexin 43 gap junction hemichannels and reduces gap junctional communication in cortical astrocytes in culture. *Proc. Natl. Acad. Sci. U.S.A.* 99, 495–500. doi: 10.1073/pnas.012589799

Costa, A., Gupta, R., Signorino, G., Malara, A., Cardile, F., Biondo, C., et al. (2012). Activation of the NLRP3 inflammasome by group B streptococci. *J. Immunol.* 188, 1953–1960. doi: 10.4049/jimmunol.1102543

Cruikshank, S. J., Hopperstad, M., Younger, M., Connors, B. W., Spray, D. C., and Srinivas, M. (2004). Potent block of Cx36 and Cx50 gap junction channels by mefloquine. *Proc. Natl. Acad. Sci. U.S.A.* 101, 12364–12369. doi: 10.1073/pnas.0402044101

Czeh, M., Gressens, P., and Kaindl, A. M. (2011). The yin and yang of microglia. *Dev. Neurosci.* 33, 199–209. doi: 10.1159/000328989

Davidson, J. O., Dean, J. M., Fraser, M., Wassink, G., Andelius, T. C., Dhillon, S. K., et al. (2018a). Perinatal brain injury: mechanisms and therapeutic approaches. *Front. Biosci. (Landmark Ed.)* 23, 2204–2226. doi: 10.2741/4700

Davidson, J. O., Draghi, V., Whitham, S., Dhillon, S. K., Wassink, G., Bennet, L., et al. (2018b). How long is sufficient for optimal neuroprotection with cerebral cooling after ischemia in fetal sheep? *J. Cereb. Blood Flow Metab.* 38, 1047–1059. doi: 10.1177/0271678X17707671

Davidson, J. O., Drury, P. P., Green, C. R., Nicholson, L. F., Bennet, L., and Gunn, A. J. (2014). Connexin hemichannel blockade is neuroprotective after asphyxia in preterm fetal sheep. *PLoS ONE* 9:e96558. doi: 10.1371/journal.pone.0096558

Davidson, J. O., Green, C. R., Bennet, L., Nicholson, L. F., Danesh-Meyer, H., Carroll, S. J., et al. (2013a). A key role for connexin hemichannels in spreading ischemic brain injury. *Curr. Drug Targets* 14, 36–46. doi: 10.2174/138945013804806479

Davidson, J. O., Green, C. R., Nicholson, L. F., Bennet, L., and Gunn, A. J. (2013b). Connexin hemichannel blockade is neuroprotective after, but not during, global cerebral ischemia in near-term fetal sheep. *Exp. Neurol.* 248, 301–308. doi: 10.1016/j.expneurol.2013.06.026

Davidson, J. O., Green, C. R., Nicholson, L. F., O'carroll, S. J., Fraser, M., Bennet, L., et al. (2012). Connexin hemichannel blockade improves outcomes in a model of fetal ischemia. *Ann. Neurol.* 71, 121–132. doi: 10.1002/ana.22654

Davidson, J. O., Rout, A. L., Wassink, G., Yuill, C. A., Zhang, F. G., Green, C. R., et al. (2015a). Non-additive effects of delayed connexin hemichannel blockade and hypothermia after cerebral ischemia in near-term fetal sheep. *J. Cereb. Blood Flow Metab.* 35, 2052–2061. doi: 10.1038/jcbfm.2015.171

Davidson, J. O., Wassink, G., Van Den Heuij, L. G., Bennet, L., and Gunn, A. J. (2015b). Therapeutic hypothermia for neonatal hypoxic-ischemic encephalopathy-where to from here? *Front. Neurol.* 6:198. doi: 10.3389/fneur.2015.00198

Davidson, J. O., Wassink, G., Yuill, C. A., Zhang, F. G., Bennet, L., and Gunn, A. J. (2015c). How long is too long for cerebral cooling after ischemia in fetal sheep? *J. Cereb. Blood Flow Metab.* 35, 751–758. doi: 10.1038/jcbfm.2014.259

Davidson, J. O., Yuill, C. A., Zhang, F. G., Wassink, G., Bennet, L., and Gunn, A. J. (2016). Extending the duration of hypothermia does not further improve white matter protection after ischemia in term-equivalent fetal sheep. *Sci. Rep.* 6:25178. doi: 10.1038/srep25178

Decrock, E., De Bock, M., Wang, N., Bultynck, G., Giaume, C., Naus, C. C., et al. (2015). Connexin and pannexin signaling pathways, an architectural blueprint for CNS physiology and pathology? *Cell. Mol. Life Sci.* 72, 2823–2851. doi: 10.1007/s00018-015-1962-7

Decrock, E., De Vuyst, E., Vinken, M., Van Moorhem, M., Vranckx, K., Wang, N., et al. (2009). Connexin 43 hemichannels contribute to the propagation of apoptotic cell death in a rat C6 glioma cell model. *Cell Death Differ.* 16, 151–163. doi: 10.1038/cdd.2008.138

Denker, S. P., Ji, S., Dingman, A., Lee, S. Y., Derugin, N., Wendland, M. F., et al. (2007). Macrophages are comprised of resident brain microglia not infiltrating peripheral monocytes acutely after neonatal stroke. *J. Neurochem.* 100, 893–904. doi: 10.1111/j.1471-4159.2006.04162.x

Dermietzel, R., Gao, Y., Scemes, E., Vieira, D., Urban, M., Kremer, M., et al. (2000). Connexin43 null mice reveal that astrocytes express multiple connexins. *Brain Res. Brain Res. Rev.* 32, 45–56. doi: 10.1016/S0165-0173(99)00067-3

Di Virgilio, F. (2007). Liaisons dangereuses: P2X(7) and the inflammasome. *Trends Pharmacol. Sci.* 28, 465–472. doi: 10.1016/j.tips.2007.07.002

Drury, P. P., Bennet, L., Booth, L. C., Davidson, J. O., Wassink, G., and Gunn, A. J. (2012). Maturation of the mitochondrial redox response to profound asphyxia in fetal sheep. *PLOS ONE* 7:e39273. doi: 10.1371/journal.pone.0039273

Edwards, A. D., Brocklehurst, P., Gunn, A. J., Halliday, H., Juszczak, E., Levene, M., et al. (2010). Neurological outcomes at 18 months of age after moderate hypothermia for perinatal hypoxic ischaemic encephalopathy: synthesis and meta-analysis of trial data. *BMJ* 340:c363. doi: 10.1136/bmj.c363

Egan, T. M., and Khakh, B. S. (2004). Contribution of calcium ions to P2X channel responses. *J. Neurosci.* 24, 3413–3420. doi: 10.1523/JNEUROSCI.5429-03.2004

Evans, W. H., De Vuyst, E., and Leybaert, L. (2006). The gap junction cellular internet: connexin hemichannels enter the signalling limelight. *Biochem. J.* 397, 1–14. doi: 10.1042/BJ20060175

Feng, L., Chen, Y., Ding, R., Fu, Z., Yang, S., Deng, X., et al. (2015). P2X7R blockade prevents NLRP3 inflammasome activation and brain injury in a rat model of intracerebral hemorrhage: involvement of peroxynitrite. *J. Neuroinflammation* 12:190. doi: 10.1186/s12974-015-0409-2

Ferrazzano, P., Chanana, V., Uluc, K., Fidan, E., Akture, E., Kintner, D. B., et al. (2013). Age-dependent microglial activation in immature brains after hypoxia- ischemia. *CNS Neurol. Disord. Drug Targets* 12, 338–349. doi: 10.2174/1871527311312030007

Fleiss, B., and Gressens, P. (2012). Tertiary mechanisms of brain damage: a new hope for treatment of cerebral palsy? *Lancet Neurol.* 11, 556–566. doi: 10.1016/S1474-4422(12)70058-3

Foster-Barber, A., Dickens, B., and Ferriero, D. M. (2001). Human perinatal asphyxia: correlation of neonatal cytokines with MRI and outcome. *Dev. Neurosci.* 23, 213–218. doi: 10.1159/000046146

Franchi, L., Eigenbrod, T., and Núñez, G. (2009). Cutting edge: TNF-alpha mediates sensitization to ATP and silica via the NLRP3 inflammasome in the absence of microbial stimulation. *J. Immunol.* 183, 792–796. doi: 10.4049/jimmunol.0900173

Franke, H., Günther, A., Grosche, J., Schmidt, R., Rossner, S., Reinhardt, R., et al. (2004). P2X7 receptor expression after ischemia in the cerebral cortex of rats. *J. Neuropathol. Exp. Neurol.* 63, 686–699. doi: 10.1093/jnen/63.7.686

Freeman, L. C., and Ting, J. P. (2016). The pathogenic role of the inflammasome in neurodegenerative diseases. *J. Neurochem.* 136, 29–38. doi: 10.1111/jnc.13217

Freitas-Andrade, M., Bechberger, J. F., Macvicar, B. A., Viau, V., and Naus, C. C. (2017). Pannexin1 knockout and blockade reduces ischemic stroke injury in female, but not in male mice. *Oncotarget* 8, 36973–36983. doi: 10.18632/oncotarget.16937

Frenguelli, B. G., Wigmore, G., Llaudet, E., and Dale, N. (2007). Temporal and mechanistic dissociation of ATP and adenosine release during ischaemia in the mammalian hippocampus. *J. Neurochem.* 101, 1400–1413. doi: 10.1111/j.1471-4159.2006.04425.x

Frizzo, J. K., Cardoso, M. P., De Assis, A. M., Perry, M. L., Volonté, C., and Frizzo, M. E. (2010). Effects of acute perinatal asphyxia in the rat hippocampus. *Cell. Mol. Neurobiol.* 30, 683–692. doi: 10.1007/s10571-009-9492-1

Fumagalli, S., Perego, C., Pischiutta, F., Zanier, E. R., and De Simoni, M. G. (2015). The ischemic environment drives microglia and macrophage function. *Front. Neurol.* 6:81. doi: 10.3389/fneur.2015.00081

Galinsky, R., Davidson, J. O., Dean, J. M., Green, C. R., Bennet, L., and Gunn, A. J. (2018a). Glia and hemichannels: key mediators of perinatal encephalopathy. *Neural Regen. Res.* 13, 181–189. doi: 10.4103/1673-5374.226378

Galinsky, R., Davidson, J. O., Lear, C. A., Bennet, L., Green, C. R., and Gunn, A. J. (2017). Connexin hemichannel blockade improves survival of striatal GABA-ergic neurons after global cerebral ischaemia in term-equivalent fetal sheep. *Sci. Rep.* 7:6304. doi: 10.1038/s41598-017-06683-1

Galinsky, R., Lear, C. A., Dean, J. M., Wassink, G., Dhillon, S. K., Fraser, M., et al. (2018b). Complex interactions between hypoxia-ischemia and inflammation in preterm brain injury. *Dev. Med. Child Neurol.* 60, 126–133. doi: 10.1111/dmcn.13629

Gao, L., Dong, Q., Song, Z., Shen, F., Shi, J., and Li, Y. (2017). NLRP3 inflammasome: a promising target in ischemic stroke. *Inflamm. Res.* 66, 17–24. doi: 10.1007/s00011-016-0981-7

Gentile, L. F., Cuenca, A. L., Cuenca, A. G., Nacionales, D. C., Ungaro, R., Efron, P. A., et al. (2015). Improved emergency myelopoiesis and survival in neonatal sepsis by caspase-1/11 ablation. *Immunology* 145, 300–311. doi: 10.1111/imm.12450

Gilroy, D., and De Maeyer, R. (2015). New insights into the resolution of inflammation. *Semin. Immunol.* 27, 161–168. doi: 10.1016/j.smim.2015.05.003

Gomes, P., Srinivas, S. P., Van Driessche, W., Vereecke, J., and Himpens, B. (2005). ATP release through connexin hemichannels in corneal endothelial cells. *Invest. Ophthalmol. Vis. Sci.* 46, 1208–1218. doi: 10.1167/iovs.04-1181

Gómez-Hernández, J. M., De Miguel, M., Larrosa, B., Gonzalez, D., and Barrio, L. C. (2003). Molecular basis of calcium regulation in connexin-32 hemichannels. *Proc. Natl. Acad. Sci. U.S.A.* 100, 16030–16035. doi: 10.1073/pnas.2530348100

Gomez-Lopez, N., Romero, R., Xu, Y., Garcia-Flores, V., Leng, Y., Panaitescu, B., et al. (2017). Inflammasome assembly in the chorioamniotic membranes during spontaneous labor at term. *Am. J. Reprod. Immunol.* 77:e12648. doi: 10.1111/aji.12648

Gong, T., Yang, Y., Jin, T., Jiang, W., and Zhou, R. (2018). Orchestration of NLRP3 inflammasome activation by ion fluxes. *Trends Immunol.* 39, 393–406. doi: 10.1016/j.it.2018.01.009

Gotsch, F., Romero, R., Chaiworapongsa, T., Erez, O., Vaisbuch, E., Espinoza, J., et al. (2008). Evidence of the involvement of caspase-1 under physiologic and pathologic cellular stress during human pregnancy: a link between the inflammasome and parturition. *J. Matern. Fetal Neonatal Med.* 21, 605–616. doi: 10.1080/14767050802212109

Groslambert, M., and Py, B. F. (2018). Spotlight on the NLRP3 inflammasome pathway. *J. Inflamm. Res.* 11, 359–374. doi: 10.2147/JIR.S141220

Gunn, A. J., Gunn, T. R., De Haan, H. H., Williams, C. E., and Gluckman, P. D. (1997). Dramatic neuronal rescue with prolonged selective head cooling after ischemia in fetal lambs. *J. Clin. Invest.* 99, 248–256. doi: 10.1172/JCI119153

Gunn, A. J., Laptook, A. R., Robertson, N. J., Barks, J. D., Thoresen, M., Wassink, G., et al. (2017). Therapeutic hypothermia translates from ancient history in to practice. *Pediatr. Res.* 81, 202–209. doi: 10.1038/pr.2016.198

Habermacher, C., Dunning, K., Chataigneau, T., and Grutter, T. (2016). Molecular structure and function of P2X receptors. *Neuropharmacology* 104, 18–30. doi: 10.1016/j.neuropharm.2015.07.032

Hagberg, H., Mallard, C., Ferriero, D. M., Vannucci, S. J., Levison, S. W., Vexler, Z. S., et al. (2015). The role of inflammation in perinatal brain injury. *Nat. Rev. Neurol.* 11, 192–208. doi: 10.1038/nrneurol.2015.13

Hassinger, T. D., Guthrie, P. B., Atkinson, P. B., Bennett, M. V., and Kater, S. B. (1996). An extracellular signaling component in propagation of astrocytic calcium waves. *Proc. Natl. Acad. Sci. U.S.A.* 93, 13268–13273. doi: 10.1073/pnas.93.23.13268

Hattori, M., and Gouaux, E. (2012). Molecular mechanism of ATP binding and ion channel activation in P2X receptors. *Nature* 485, 207–212. doi: 10.1038/nature11010

He, Y., Hara, H., and Núñez, G. (2016). Mechanism and regulation of NLRP3 inflammasome activation. *Trends Biochem. Sci.* 41, 1012–1021. doi: 10.1016/j.tibs.2016.09.002

Hellström, E. N., Smith, P. L., Fleiss, B., Nair, S., Svedin, P., Wang, W., et al. (2016). Temporal characterization of microglia/macrophage phenotypes in a mouse model of neonatal hypoxic-ischemic brain injury. *Front. Cell. Neurosci.* 10:286. doi: 10.3389/fncel.2016.00286

Henneke, P., and Berner, R. (2006). Interaction of neonatal phagocytes with group B streptococcus: recognition and response. *Infect. Immun.* 74, 3085–3095. doi: 10.1128/IAI.01551-05

Hunter, C. J., Bennet, L., Power, G. G., Roelfsema, V., Blood, A. B., Quaedackers, J. S., et al. (2003). Key neuroprotective role for endogenous adenosine A1 receptor activation during asphyxia in the fetal sheep. *Stroke* 34, 2240–2245. doi: 10.1161/01.STR.0000083623.77327.CE

Ishikawa, M., Iwamoto, T., Nakamura, T., Doyle, A., Fukumoto, S., and Yamada, Y. (2011). Pannexin 3 functions as an ER Ca(2+) channel, hemichannel, and gap junction to promote osteoblast differentiation. *J. Cell Biol.* 193, 1257–1274. doi: 10.1083/jcb.201101050

Ismael, S., Zhao, L., Nasoohi, S., and Ishrat, T. (2018). Inhibition of the NLRP3-inflammasome as a potential approach for neuroprotection after stroke. *Sci. Rep.* 8:5971. doi: 10.1038/s41598-018-24350-x

Jaworska, J., Ziemka-Nalecz, M., Sypecka, J., and Zalewska, T. (2017). The potential neuroprotective role of a histone deacetylase inhibitor, sodium butyrate, after neonatal hypoxia-ischemia. *J. Neuroinflammation* 14:34. doi: 10.1186/s12974-017-0807-8

Jian, Z., Ding, S., Deng, H., Wang, J., Yi, W., Wang, L., et al. (2016). Probenecid protects against oxygen-glucose deprivation injury in primary astrocytes by regulating inflammasome activity. *Brain Res.* 1643, 123–129. doi: 10.1016/j.brainres.2016.05.002

Jo, E. K., Kim, J. K., Shin, D. M., and Sasakawa, C. (2016). Molecular mechanisms regulating NLRP3 inflammasome activation. *Cell Mol. Immunol.* 13, 148–159. doi: 10.1038/cmi.2015.95

Jun, H. K., Lee, S. H., Lee, H. R., and Choi, B. K. (2012). Integrin alpha5beta1 activates the NLRP3 inflammasome by direct interaction with a bacterial surface protein. *Immunity* 36, 755–768. doi: 10.1016/j.immuni.2012.05.002

Kaiser, M., Penk, A., Franke, H., Krugel, U., Norenberg, W., Huster, D., et al. (2016). Lack of functional P2X7 receptor aggravates brain edema development after middle cerebral artery occlusion. *Purinergic Signal.* 12, 453–463. doi: 10.1007/s11302-016-9511-x

Kang, J., Kang, N., Lovatt, D., Torres, A., Zhao, Z., Lin, J., et al. (2008). Connexin 43 hemichannels are permeable to ATP. *J. Neurosci.* 28, 4702–4711. doi: 10.1523/JNEUROSCI.5048-07.2008

Karpuk, N., Burkovetskaya, M., Fritz, T., Angle, A., and Kielian, T. (2011). Neuroinflammation leads to region-dependent alterations in astrocyte gap junction communication and hemichannel activity. *J. Neurosci.* 31, 414–425. doi: 10.1523/JNEUROSCI.5247-10.2011

Kawamura, M. Jr., Ruskin, D. N., and Masino, S. A. (2010). Metabolic autocrine regulation of neurons involves cooperation among pannexin hemichannels, adenosine receptors, and KATP channels. *J. Neurosci.* 30, 3886–3895. doi: 10.1523/JNEUROSCI.0055-10.2010

Kerur, N., Fukuda, S., Banerjee, D., Kim, Y., Fu, D., Apicella, I., et al. (2018). cGAS drives noncanonical-inflammasome activation in age-related macular degeneration. *Nat. Med.* 24, 50–61. doi: 10.1038/nm.4450

Kim, Y., and Green, C. R. (2016). "Assessing connexin hemichannel function during ischemic injury and reperfusion," in *Gap Junction Channels and Hemichannels*, eds D. Bai and J. C. Saez (Boca Raton, FL: CRC Press; Taylor & Francis Group), 169–188.

Koos, B. J., Kruger, L., and Murray, T. F. (1997). Source of extracellular brain adenosine during hypoxia in fetal sheep. *Brain Res.* 778, 439–442. doi: 10.1016/S0006-8993(97)01207-9

Korzeniewski, S. J., Allred, E. N., O'shea, T. M., Leviton, A., and Kuban, K. C. K. (2018). Elevated protein concentrations in newborn blood and the risks of autism spectrum disorder, and of social impairment, at age 10 years among infants born before the 28th week of gestation. *Transl. Psychiatry* 8:115. doi: 10.1038/s41398-018-0156-0

Kuban, K. C., Joseph, R. M., O'shea, T. M., Heeren, T., Fichorova, R. N., Douglass, L., et al. (2017). Circulating inflammatory-associated proteins in the first month of life and cognitive impairment at age 10 years in children born extremely preterm. *J. Pediatr.* 180, 116–123 e111. doi: 10.1016/j.jpeds.2016.09.054

Kumar, N. M., and Gilula, N. B. (1996). The gap junction communication channel. *Cell* 84, 381–388. doi: 10.1016/S0092-8674(00)81282-9

Larroque, B., Ancel, P. Y., Marret, S., Marchand, L., Andre, M., Arnaud, C., et al. (2008). Neurodevelopmental disabilities and special care of 5-year-old children born before 33 weeks of gestation (the EPIPAGE study): a longitudinal cohort study. *Lancet* 371, 813–820. doi: 10.1016/S0140-6736(08)60380-3

Lee, A. C., Kozuki, N., Blencowe, H., Vos, T., Bahalim, A., Darmstadt, G. L., et al. (2013). Intrapartum-related neonatal encephalopathy incidence and impairment at regional and global levels for 2010 with trends from 1990. *Pediatr. Res.* 74, 50–72. doi: 10.1038/pr.2013.206

Lee, S. W., Gajavelli, S., Spurlock, M. S., Andreoni, C., De Rivero Vaccari, J. P., Bullock, M. R., et al. (2018). Microglial inflammasome activation in penetrating ballistic-like brain injury. *J. Neurotrauma* 35, 1681–1693. doi: 10.1089/neu.2017.5530

Leybaert, L., Lampe, P. D., Dhein, S., Kwak, B. R., Ferdinandy, P., Beyer, E. C., et al. (2017). Connexins in cardiovascular and neurovascular health and disease: pharmacological implications. *Pharmacol. Rev.* 69, 396–478. doi: 10.1124/pr.115.012062

Li, F., Wang, L., Li, J. W., Gong, M., He, L., Feng, R., et al. (2011). Hypoxia induced amoeboid microglial cell activation in postnatal rat brain is mediated by ATP receptor P2X4. *BMC Neurosci.* 12:111. doi: 10.1186/1471-2202-12-111

Li, X., Zhao, H., Tan, X., Kostrzewa, R. M., Du, G., Chen, Y., et al. (2015). Inhibition of connexin43 improves functional recovery after ischemic brain injury in neonatal rats. *Glia* 63, 1553–1567. doi: 10.1002/glia.22826

Lin, C. Y., Chang, Y. C., Wang, S. T., Lee, T. Y., Lin, C. F., and Huang, C. C. (2010). Altered inflammatory responses in preterm children with cerebral palsy. *Ann. Neurol.* 68, 204–212. doi: 10.1002/ana.22049

Lorek, A., Takei, Y., Cady, E. B., Wyatt, J. S., Penrice, J., Edwards, A. D., et al. (1994). Delayed ("secondary") cerebral energy failure after acute hypoxia-ischemia in the newborn piglet: continuous 48-hour studies by phosphorus magnetic resonance spectroscopy. *Pediatr. Res.* 36, 699–706. doi: 10.1203/00006450-199412000-00003

Maatouk, L., Yi, C., Carrillo-De Sauvage, M. A., Compagnion, A. C., Hunot, S., Ezan, P., et al. (2018). Glucocorticoid receptor in astrocytes regulates midbrain dopamine neurodegeneration through connexin hemichannel activity. *Cell Death Differ.* 26, 580–596. doi: 10.1038/s41418-018-0150-3

Mächler, P., Wyss, M. T., Elsayed, M., Stobart, J., Gutierrez, R., Von Faber-Castell, A., et al. (2016). *In vivo* evidence for a lactate gradient from astrocytes to neurons. *Cell Metab.* 23, 94–102. doi: 10.1016/j.cmet.2015.10.010

Mallard, C., Davidson, J. O., Tan, S., Green, C. R., Bennet, L., Robertson, N. J., et al. (2014). Astrocytes and microglia in acute cerebral injury underlying cerebral palsy associated with preterm birth. *Pediatr. Res.* 75, 234–240. doi: 10.1038/pr.2013.188

Mallard, C., Tremblay, M. E., and Vexler, Z. S. (2018). Microglia and neonatal brain injury. *Neuroscience.* doi: 10.1016/j.neuroscience.2018.01.023. [Epub ahead of print].

Mao, Y., Nguyen, T., Tonkin, R. S., Lees, J. G., Warren, C., O'carroll, S. J., et al. (2017). Characterisation of Peptide5 systemic administration for treating traumatic spinal cord injured rats. *Exp. Brain Res.* 235, 3033–3048. doi: 10.1007/s00221-017-5023-3

Markiewicz, I., and Lukomska, B. (2006). The role of astrocytes in the physiology and pathology of the central nervous system. *Acta Neurobiol. Exp. (Warsz).* 66, 343–358.

Marlow, N., Wolke, D., Bracewell, M. A., and Samara, M. (2005). Neurologic and developmental disability at six years of age after extremely preterm birth. *N. Engl. J. Med.* 352, 9–19. doi: 10.1056/NEJMoa041367

Martinon, F., Mayor, A., and Tschopp, J. (2009). The inflammasomes: guardians of the body. *Annu. Rev. Immunol.* 27, 229–265. doi: 10.1146/annurev.immunol.021908.132715

Matute, C., Torre, I., Perez-Cerda, F., Pérez-Samartín, A., Alberdi, E., Etxebarria, E., et al. (2007). P2X(7) receptor blockade prevents ATP excitotoxicity in oligodendrocytes and ameliorates experimental autoimmune encephalomyelitis. *J. Neurosci.* 27, 9525–9533. doi: 10.1523/JNEUROSCI.0579-07.2007

Medzhitov, R. (2007). Recognition of microorganisms and activation of the immune response. *Nature* 449, 819–826. doi: 10.1038/nature06246

Melani, A., Amadio, S., Gianfriddo, M., Vannucchi, M. G., Volontè, C., Bernardi, G., et al. (2006). P2X7 receptor modulation on microglial cells and reduction of brain infarct caused by middle cerebral artery occlusion in rat. *J. Cereb. Blood Flow Metab.* 26, 974–982. doi: 10.1038/sj.jcbfm.9600250

Melani, A., Corti, F., Stephan, H., Müller, C. E., Donati, C., Bruni, P., et al. (2012). Ecto-ATPase inhibition: ATP and adenosine release under physiological and ischemic *in vivo* conditions in the rat striatum. *Exp. Neurol.* 233, 193–204. doi: 10.1016/j.expneurol.2011.09.036

Melani, A., Turchi, D., Vannucchi, M. G., Cipriani, S., Gianfriddo, M., and Pedata, F. (2005). ATP extracellular concentrations are increased in the rat striatum during *in vivo* ischemia. *Neurochem. Int.* 47, 442–448. doi: 10.1016/j.neuint.2005.05.014

Monif, M., Reid, C. A., Powell, K. L., Smart, M. L., and Williams, D. A. (2009). The P2X7 receptor drives microglial activation and proliferation: a trophic role for P2X7R pore. *J. Neurosci.* 29, 3781–3791. doi: 10.1523/JNEUROSCI.5512-08.2009

Mugisho, O. O., Green, C. R., Kho, D. T., Zhang, J., Graham, E. S., Acosta, M. L., et al. (2018). The inflammasome pathway is amplified and perpetuated in an autocrine manner through connexin43 hemichannel mediated ATP release. *Biochim. Biophys. Acta* 1862, 385–393. doi: 10.1016/j.bbagen.2017.11.015

Nagy, J. I., Ionescu, A. V., Lynn, B. D., and Rash, J. E. (2003). Coupling of astrocyte connexins Cx26, Cx30, Cx43 to oligodendrocyte Cx29, Cx32, Cx47: implications from normal and connexin32 knockout mice. *Glia* 44, 205–218. doi: 10.1002/glia.10278

Nagy, J. I., Ochalski, P. A., Li, J., and Hertzberg, E. L. (1997). Evidence for the co-localization of another connexin with connexin-43 at astrocytic gap junctions in rat brain. *Neuroscience* 78, 533–548. doi: 10.1016/S0306-4522(96)00584-2

Nakase, T., Maeda, T., Yoshida, Y., and Nagata, K. (2009). Ischemia alters the expression of connexins in the aged human brain. *J. Biomed. Biotechnol.* 2009:147946. doi: 10.1155/2009/147946

Nakase, T., Yoshida, Y., and Nagata, K. (2006). Enhanced connexin 43 immunoreactivity in penumbral areas in the human brain following ischemia. *Glia* 54, 369–375. doi: 10.1002/glia.20399

Natarajan, G., Laptook, A., and Shankaran, S. (2018). Therapeutic hypothermia: how can we optimize this therapy to further improve outcomes? *Clin. Perinatol.* 45, 241–255. doi: 10.1016/j.clp.2018.01.010

Nathan, C., and Ding, A. (2010). Nonresolving inflammation. *Cell* 140, 871–882. doi: 10.1016/j.cell.2010.02.029

Nedergaard, M. (1994). Direct signaling from astrocytes to neurons in cultures of mammalian brain cells. *Science* 263, 1768–1771. doi: 10.1126/science.8134839

Ness, J. K., Romanko, M. J., Rothstein, R. P., Wood, T. L., and Levison, S. W. (2001). Perinatal hypoxia-ischemia induces apoptotic and excitotoxic death of periventricular white matter oligodendrocyte progenitors. *Dev. Neurosci.* 23, 203–208. doi: 10.1159/000046144

Nimmerjahn, A., Kirchhoff, F., and Helmchen, F. (2005). Resting microglial cells are highly dynamic surveillants of brain parenchyma *in vivo*. *Science* 308, 1314–1318. doi: 10.1126/science.1110647

Northington, F. J., Chavez-Valdez, R., and Martin, L. J. (2011). Neuronal cell death in neonatal hypoxia-ischemia. *Ann. Neurol.* 69, 743–758. doi: 10.1002/ana.22419

Northington, F. J., Zelaya, M. E., O'riordan, D. P., Blomgren, K., Flock, D. L., Hagberg, H., et al. (2007). Failure to complete apoptosis following neonatal hypoxia-ischemia manifests as "continuum" phenotype of cell death and occurs with multiple manifestations of mitochondrial dysfunction in rodent forebrain. *Neuroscience* 149, 822–833. doi: 10.1016/j.neuroscience.2007.06.060

Odorcyk, F. K., Nicola, F., Duran-Carabali, L. E., Figueiro, F., Kolling, J., Vizuete, A., et al. (2017). Galantamine administration reduces reactive astrogliosis and upregulates the anti-oxidant enzyme catalase in rats submitted to neonatal hypoxia ischemia. *Int. J. Dev. Neurosci.* 62, 15–24. doi: 10.1016/j.ijdevneu.2017.07.006

Orellana, J. A., Froger, N., Ezan, P., Jiang, J. X., Bennett, M. V., Naus, C. C., et al. (2011). ATP and glutamate released via astroglial connexin 43 hemichannels mediate neuronal death through activation of pannexin 1 hemichannels. *J. Neurochem.* 118, 826–840. doi: 10.1111/j.1471-4159.2011.07210.x

Orellana, J. A., Hernandez, D. E., Ezan, P., Velarde, V., Bennett, M. V., Giaume, C., et al. (2010). Hypoxia in high glucose followed by reoxygenation in normal glucose reduces the viability of cortical astrocytes through increased permeability of connexin 43 hemichannels. *Glia* 58, 329–343. doi: 10.1002/glia.20926

O'Shea, T. M., Allred, E. N., Kuban, K. C., Dammann, O., Paneth, N., Fichorova, R., et al. (2012). Elevated concentrations of inflammation-related proteins in postnatal blood predict severe developmental delay at 2 years of age in extremely preterm infants. *J. Pediatr.* 160, 395–401 e394. doi: 10.1016/j.jpeds.2011.08.069

Ozaki, T., Muramatsu, R., Sasai, M., Yamamoto, M., Kubota, Y., Fujinaka, T., et al. (2016). The P2X4 receptor is required for neuroprotection via ischemic preconditioning. *Sci. Rep.* 6:25893. doi: 10.1038/srep25893

Panchin, Y. V. (2005). Evolution of gap junction proteins–the pannexin alternative. *J. Exp. Biol.* 208, 1415–1419. doi: 10.1242/jeb.01547

Patterson, Z. R., and Holahan, M. R. (2012). Understanding the neuroinflammatory response following concussion to develop treatment strategies. *Front. Cell. Neurosci.* 6:58. doi: 10.3389/fncel.2012.00058

Paul, D. L., Ebihara, L., Takemoto, L. J., Swenson, K. I., and Goodenough, D. A. (1991). Connexin46, a novel lens gap junction protein, induces voltage-gated currents in nonjunctional plasma membrane of Xenopus oocytes. *J. Cell Biol.* 115, 1077–1089. doi: 10.1083/jcb.115.4.1077

Pedata, F., Dettori, I., Coppi, E., Melani, A., Fusco, I., Corradetti, R., et al. (2016). Purinergic signalling in brain ischemia. *Neuropharmacology* 104, 105–130. doi: 10.1016/j.neuropharm.2015.11.007

Pelegrin, P., and Surprenant, A. (2006). Pannexin-1 mediates large pore formation and interleukin-1beta release by the ATP-gated P2X7 receptor. *EMBO J.* 25, 5071–5082. doi: 10.1038/sj.emboj.7601378

Peng, W., Cotrina, M. L., Han, X., Yu, H., Bekar, L., Blum, L., et al. (2009). Systemic administration of an antagonist of the ATP-sensitive receptor P2X7 improves recovery after spinal cord injury. *Proc. Natl. Acad. Sci. U.S.A.* 106, 12489–12493. doi: 10.1073/pnas.0902531106

Pierre, W. C., Smith, P. L., Londono, I., Chemtob, S., Mallard, C., and Lodygensky, G. A. (2017). Neonatal microglia: the cornerstone of brain fate. *Brain. Behav. Immun.* 59, 333–345. doi: 10.1016/j.bbi.2016.08.018

Puka-Sundvall, M., Gajkowska, B., Cholewinski, M., Blomgren, K., Lazarewicz, J. W., and Hagberg, H. (2000). Subcellular distribution of calcium and ultrastructural changes after cerebral hypoxia-ischemia in immature rats. *Brain Res. Dev. Brain Res.* 125, 31–41. doi: 10.1016/S0165-3806(00)00110-3

Qiu, F., and Dahl, G. (2009). A permeant regulating its permeation pore: inhibition of pannexin 1 channels by ATP. *Am. J. Physiol. Cell Physiol.* 296, C250–C255. doi: 10.1152/ajpcell.00433.2008

Retamal, M. A., Froger, N., Palacios-Prado, N., Ezan, P., Sáez, P. J., Sáez, J. C., et al. (2007). Cx43 hemichannels and gap junction channels in astrocytes are regulated oppositely by proinflammatory cytokines released from activated microglia. *J. Neurosci.* 27, 13781–13792. doi: 10.1523/JNEUROSCI.2042-07.2007

Rice, J. E., Vannucci, R. C., and Brierley, J. B. (1981). The influence of immaturity on hypoxic-ischemic brain damage in the rat. *Ann. Neurol.* 9, 131–141. doi: 10.1002/ana.410090206

Riquelme, M. A., Cea, L. A., Vega, J. L., Boric, M. P., Monyer, H., Bennett, M. V., et al. (2013). The ATP required for potentiation of skeletal muscle contraction is released via pannexin hemichannels. *Neuropharmacology* 75, 594–603. doi: 10.1016/j.neuropharm.2013.03.022

Romanko, M. J., Rothstein, R. P., and Levison, S. W. (2004). Neural stem cells in the subventricular zone are resilient to hypoxia/ischemia whereas progenitors are vulnerable. *J. Cereb. Blood Flow Metab.* 24, 814–825. doi: 10.1097/01.WCB.0000123906.17746.00

Romero, J., Muñiz, J., Logica Tornatore, T., Holubiec, M., Gonzalez, J., Barreto, G. E., et al. (2014). Dual role of astrocytes in perinatal asphyxia injury and neuroprotection. *Neurosci. Lett.* 565, 42–46. doi: 10.1016/j.neulet.2013.10.046

Rossi, D., and Volterra, A. (2009). Astrocytic dysfunction: insights on the role in neurodegeneration. *Brain Res. Bull.* 80, 224–232. doi: 10.1016/j.brainresbull.2009.07.012

Rothstein, J. D., Martin, L., Levey, A. I., Dykes-Hoberg, M., Jin, L., Wu, D., et al. (1994). Localization of neuronal and glial glutamate transporters. *Neuron* 13, 713–725. doi: 10.1016/0896-6273(94)90038-8

Sáez, J. C., Retamal, M. A., Basilio, D., Bukauskas, F. F., and Bennett, M. V. (2005). Connexin-based gap junction hemichannels: gating mechanisms. *Biochim. Biophys. Acta* 1711, 215–224. doi: 10.1016/j.bbamem.2005.01.014

Santiago, M. F., Veliskova, J., Patel, N. K., Lutz, S. E., Caille, D., Charollais, A., et al. (2011). Targeting pannexin1 improves seizure outcome. *PLoS ONE* 6:e25178. doi: 10.1371/journal.pone.0025178

Schalper, K. A., Sanchez, H. A., Lee, S. C., Altenberg, G. A., Nathanson, M. H., and Saez, J. C. (2010). Connexin 43 hemichannels mediate the Ca^{2+} influx induced by extracellular alkalinization. *Am. J. Physiol. Cell Physiol.* 299, C1504–C1515. doi: 10.1152/ajpcell.00015.2010

Shankaran, S., Laptook, A. R., Ehrenkranz, R. A., Tyson, J. E., Mcdonald, S. A., Donovan, E. F., et al. (2005). Whole-body hypothermia for neonates with hypoxic-ischemic encephalopathy. *N. Engl. J. Med.* 353, 1574–1584. doi: 10.1056/NEJMcps050929

Shao, B. Z., Cao, Q., and Liu, C. (2018). Targeting NLRP3 inflammasome in the treatment of CNS diseases. *Front. Mol. Neurosci.* 11:320. doi: 10.3389/fnmol.2018.00320

Sharma, A. A., Jen, R., Kan, B., Sharma, A., Marchant, E., Tang, A., et al. (2015). Impaired NLRP3 inflammasome activity during fetal development regulates IL-1beta production in human monocytes. *Eur. J. Immunol.* 45, 238–249. doi: 10.1002/eji.201444707

Shi, H., Wang, Y., Li, X., Zhan, X., Tang, M., Fina, M., et al. (2016). NLRP3 activation and mitosis are mutually exclusive events coordinated by NEK7, a new inflammasome component. *Nat. Immunol.* 17, 250–258. doi: 10.1038/ni.3333

Song, L., Pei, L., Yao, S., Wu, Y., and Shang, Y. (2017). NLRP3 inflammasome in neurological diseases, from functions to therapies. *Front. Cell. Neurosci.* 11:63. doi: 10.3389/fncel.2017.00063

Stokes, L., Layhadi, J. A., Bibic, L., Dhuna, K., and Fountain, S. J. (2017). P2X4 receptor function in the nervous system and current breakthroughs in pharmacology. *Front. Pharmacol* 8:291. doi: 10.3389/fphar.2017.00291

Stout, C. E., Costantin, J. L., Naus, C. C., and Charles, A. C. (2002). Intercellular calcium signaling in astrocytes via ATP release through connexin hemichannels. *J. Biol. Chem.* 277, 10482–10488. doi: 10.1074/jbc.M109902200

Strunk, T., Currie, A., Richmond, P., Simmer, K., and Burgner, D. (2011). Innate immunity in human newborn infants: prematurity means more than immaturity. *J. Matern. Fetal Neonatal Med.* 24, 25–31. doi: 10.3109/14767058.2010.482605

Sullivan, S. M., Björkman, S. T., Miller, S. M., Colditz, P. B., and Pow, D. V. (2010). Morphological changes in white matter astrocytes in response to hypoxia/ischemia in the neonatal pig. *Brain Res.* 1319, 164–174. doi: 10.1016/j.brainres.2010.01.010

Surprenant, A., and North, R. A. (2009). Signaling at purinergic P2X receptors. *Annu. Rev. Physiol.* 71, 333–359. doi: 10.1146/annurev.physiol.70.113006.100630

Suurväli, J., Boudinot, P., Kanellopoulos, J., and Ruutel Boudinot, S. (2017). P2X4: A fast and sensitive purinergic receptor. *Biomed. J.* 40, 245–256. doi: 10.1016/j.bj.2017.06.010

Takeuchi, O., and Akira, S. (2010). Pattern recognition receptors and inflammation. *Cell* 140, 805–820. doi: 10.1016/j.cell.2010.01.022

Tang, T., Lang, X., Xu, C., Wang, X., Gong, T., Yang, Y., et al. (2017). CLICs-dependent chloride efflux is an essential and proximal upstream event for NLRP3 inflammasome activation. *Nat. Commun.* 8:202. doi: 10.1038/s41467-017-00227-x

Theis, M., Sohl, G., Eiberger, J., and Willecke, K. (2005). Emerging complexities in identity and function of glial connexins. *Trends Neurosci.* 28, 188–195. doi: 10.1016/j.tins.2005.02.006

Thompson, R. J., Jackson, M. F., Olah, M. E., Rungta, R. L., Hines, D. J., Beazely, M. A., et al. (2008). Activation of pannexin-1 hemichannels augments aberrant bursting in the hippocampus. *Science* 322, 1555–1559. doi: 10.1126/science.1165209

Thompson, R. J., Zhou, N., and Macvicar, B. A. (2006). Ischemia opens neuronal gap junction hemichannels. *Science* 312, 924–927. doi: 10.1126/science.1126241

Thornton, J. S., Ordidge, R. J., Penrice, J., Cady, E. B., Amess, P. N., Punwani, S., et al. (1998). Temporal and anatomical variations of brain water apparent diffusion coefficient in perinatal cerebral hypoxic-ischemic injury: relationships to cerebral energy metabolism. *Magn. Reson. Med.* 39, 920–927. doi: 10.1002/mrm.1910390609

Ting, J. P., Lovering, R. C., Alnemri, E. S., Bertin, J., Boss, J. M., Davis, B. K., et al. (2008). The NLR gene family: a standard nomenclature. *Immunity* 28, 285–287. doi: 10.1016/j.immuni.2008.02.005

Tonkin, R. S., Bowles, C., Perera, C. J., Keating, B. A., Makker, P. G. S., Duffy, S. S., et al. (2018). Attenuation of mechanical pain hypersensitivity by treatment with Peptide5, a connexin-43 mimetic peptide, involves inhibition of NLRP3 inflammasome in nerve-injured mice. *Exp. Neurol.* 300, 1–12. doi: 10.1016/j.expneurol.2017.10.016

Turner, M. D., Nedjai, B., Hurst, T., and Pennington, D. J. (2014). Cytokines and chemokines: at the crossroads of cell signalling and inflammatory disease. *Biochim. Biophys. Acta* 1843, 2563–2582. doi: 10.1016/j.bbamcr.2014.05.014

Unger, V. M., Kumar, N. M., Gilula, N. B., and Yeager, M. (1999). Three-dimensional structure of a recombinant gap junction membrane channel. *Science* 283, 1176–1180. doi: 10.1126/science.283.5405.1176

van den Heuij, L. G., Fraser, M., Miller, S. L., Jenkin, G., Wallace, E. M., Davidson, J. O., et al. (2019). Delayed intranasal infusion of human amnion epithelial cells improves white matter maturation after asphyxia in preterm fetal sheep. *J. Cereb. Blood Flow Metab.* 39, 223–239. doi: 10.1177/0271678X17729954

Vannucci, R. C. (2000). Hypoxic-ischemic encephalopathy. *Am. J. Perinatol.* 17, 113–120. doi: 10.1055/s-2000-9293

Verma, R., Cronin, C. G., Hudobenko, J., Venna, V. R., Mccullough, L. D., and Liang, B. T. (2017). Deletion of the P2X4 receptor is neuroprotective acutely, but induces a depressive phenotype during recovery from ischemic stroke. *Brain. Behav. Immun.* 66, 302–312. doi: 10.1016/j.bbi.2017.07.155

Vogt, A., Hormuzdi, S. G., and Monyer, H. (2005). Pannexin1 and Pannexin2 expression in the developing and mature rat brain. *Brain Res. Mol. Brain Res.* 141, 113–120. doi: 10.1016/j.molbrainres.2005.08.002

Wallisch, J. S., Simon, D. W., Bayir, H., Bell, M. J., Kochanek, P. M., and Clark, R. S. B. (2017). Cerebrospinal fluid NLRP3 is increased after severe traumatic brain injury in infants and children. *Neurocrit. Care* 27, 44–50. doi: 10.1007/s12028-017-0378-7

Wallraff, A., Kohling, R., Heinemann, U., Theis, M., Willecke, K., and Steinhauser, C. (2006). The impact of astrocytic gap junctional coupling on potassium buffering in the hippocampus. *J. Neurosci.* 26, 5438–5447. doi: 10.1523/JNEUROSCI.0037-06.2006

Wang, D., Xu, X., Wu, Y. G., Lyu, L., Zhou, Z. W., and Zhang, J. N. (2018). Dexmedetomidine attenuates traumatic brain injury: action pathway and mechanisms. *Neural Regen. Res.* 13, 819–826. doi: 10.4103/1673-5374.232529

Wang, J., Ma, A., Xi, J., Wang, Y., and Zhao, B. (2014). Connexin 43 and its hemichannels mediate hypoxia-ischemia-induced cell death in neonatal rats. *Child Neurol. Open* 1:2329048X14544955. doi: 10.1177/2329048X14544955

Wang, L., Jacobsen, S. E., Bengtsson, A., and Erlinge, D. (2004). P2 receptor mRNA expression profiles in human lymphocytes, monocytes and $CD34^+$ stem and progenitor cells. *BMC Immunol.* 5:16. doi: 10.1186/1471-2172-5-16

Wang, N., De Bock, M., Decrock, E., Bol, M., Gadicherla, A., Bultynck, G., et al. (2013). Connexin targeting peptides as inhibitors of voltage- and intracellular Ca^{2+}-triggered Cx43 hemichannel opening. *Neuropharmacology* 75, 506–516. doi: 10.1016/j.neuropharm.2013.08.021

Wassink, G., Davidson, J. O., Dhillon, S. K., Fraser, M., Galinsky, R., Bennet, L., et al. (2017). Partial white and grey matter protection with prolonged infusion of recombinant human erythropoietin after asphyxia in preterm fetal sheep. *J. Cereb. Blood Flow Metab.* 37, 1080–1094. doi: 10.1177/0271678X16650455

Wassink, G., Davidson, J. O., Lear, C. A., Juul, S. E., Northington, F., Bennet, L., et al. (2018). A working model for hypothermic neuroprotection. *J. Physiol.* 596, 5641–5654 doi: 10.1113/JP274928

Wassink, G., Gunn, E. R., Drury, P. P., Bennet, L., and Gunn, A. J. (2014). The mechanisms and treatment of asphyxial encephalopathy. *Front. Neurosci.* 8:40. doi: 10.3389/fnins.2014.00040

Wei, R., Wang, J., Xu, Y., Yin, B., He, F., Du, Y., et al. (2015). Probenecid protects against cerebral ischemia/reperfusion injury by inhibiting lysosomal and inflammatory damage in rats. *Neuroscience* 301, 168–177. doi: 10.1016/j.neuroscience.2015.05.070

Weilinger, N. L., Tang, P. L., and Thompson, R. J. (2012). Anoxia-induced NMDA receptor activation opens pannexin channels via Src family kinases. *J. Neurosci.* 32, 12579–12588. doi: 10.1523/JNEUROSCI.1267-12.2012

Willebrords, J., Crespo Yanguas, S., Maes, M., Decrock, E., Wang, N., Leybaert, L., et al. (2016). Connexins and their channels in inflammation. *Crit. Rev. Biochem. Mol. Biol.* 51, 413–439. doi: 10.1080/10409238.2016.1204980

Williams, C. E., Gunn, A., and Gluckman, P. D. (1991). Time course of intracellular edema and epileptiform activity following prenatal cerebral ischemia in sheep. *Stroke* 22, 516–521. doi: 10.1161/01.STR.22.4.516

Williams, C. E., Gunn, A. J., Mallard, C., and Gluckman, P. D. (1992). Outcome after ischemia in the developing sheep brain: an electroencephalographic and histological study. *Ann. Neurol.* 31, 14–21. doi: 10.1002/ana.410310104

Williams, C. E., Mallard, C., Tan, W., and Gluckman, P. D. (1993). Pathophysiology of perinatal asphyxia. *Clin. Perinatol.* 20, 305–325. doi: 10.1016/S0095-5108(18)30395-6

Winerdal, M., Winerdal, M. E., Kinn, J., Urmaliya, V., Winqvist, O., and Aden, U. (2012). Long lasting local and systemic inflammation after cerebral hypoxic ischemia in newborn mice. *PLoS ONE* 7:e36422. doi: 10.1371/journal.pone.0036422

Wixey, J. A., Reinebrant, H. E., Carty, M. L., and Buller, K. M. (2009). Delayed P2X4R expression after hypoxia-ischemia is associated with microglia in the immature rat brain. *J. Neuroimmunol.* 212, 35–43. doi: 10.1016/j.jneuroim.2009.04.016

Wyatt, L. R., Godar, S. C., Khoja, S., Jakowec, M. W., Alkana, R. L., Bortolato, M., et al. (2013). Sociocommunicative and sensorimotor impairments in male P2X4-deficient mice. *Neuropsychopharmacology* 38, 1993–2002. doi: 10.1038/npp.2013.98

Wynn, J. L., and Wong, H. R. (2010). Pathophysiology and treatment of septic shock in neonates. *Clin. Perinatol.* 37, 439–479. doi: 10.1016/j.clp.2010.04.002

Xu, X., Yin, D., Ren, H., Gao, W., Li, F., Sun, D., et al. (2018). Selective NLRP3 inflammasome inhibitor reduces neuroinflammation and improves long-term neurological outcomes in a murine model of traumatic brain injury. *Neurobiol. Dis.* 117, 15–27. doi: 10.1016/j.nbd.2018.05.016

Yan, Z., Khadra, A., Li, S., Tomic, M., Sherman, A., and Stojilkovic, S. S. (2010). Experimental characterization and mathematical modeling of P2X7 receptor channel gating. *J. Neurosci.* 30, 14213–14224. doi: 10.1523/JNEUROSCI.2390-10.2010

Yan, Z., Li, S., Liang, Z., Tomic, M., and Stojilkovic, S. S. (2008). The P2X7 receptor channel pore dilates under physiological ion conditions. *J. Gen. Physiol.* 132, 563–573. doi: 10.1085/jgp.200810059

Ye, X., Shen, T., Hu, J., Zhang, L., Zhang, Y., Bao, L., et al. (2017). Purinergic 2X7 receptor/NLRP3 pathway triggers neuronal apoptosis after ischemic stroke in the mouse. *Exp. Neurol.* 292, 46–55. doi: 10.1016/j.expneurol.2017.03.002

Ye, Z. C., Wyeth, M. S., Baltan-Tekkok, S., and Ransom, B. R. (2003). Functional hemichannels in astrocytes: a novel mechanism of glutamate release. *J. Neurosci.* 23, 3588–3596. doi: 10.1523/JNEUROSCI.23-09-03588.2003

Yi, C., Mei, X., Ezan, P., Mato, S., Matias, I., Giaume, C., et al. (2016). Astroglial connexin43 contributes to neuronal suffering in a mouse model of Alzheimer's disease. *Cell Death Differ.* 23, 1691–1701. doi: 10.1038/cdd.2016.63

Yin, D., Zhou, S., Xu, X., Gao, W., Li, F., Ma, Y., et al. (2018a). Dexmedetomidine attenuated early brain injury in rats with subarachnoid haemorrhage by suppressing the inflammatory response: the TLR4/NF-kappaB pathway and the NLRP3 inflammasome may be involved in the mechanism. *Brain Res.* 1698, 1–10. doi: 10.1016/j.brainres.2018.05.040

Yin, X., Feng, L., Ma, D., Yin, P., Wang, X., Hou, S., et al. (2018b). Roles of astrocytic connexin-43, hemichannels, and gap junctions in oxygen-glucose deprivation/reperfusion injury induced neuroinflammation and the possible regulatory mechanisms of salvianolic acid B and carbenoxolone. *J. Neuroinflammation* 15:97. doi: 10.1186/s12974-018-1127-3

Ystgaard, M. B., Sejersted, Y., Loberg, E. M., Lien, E., Yndestad, A., and Saugstad, O. D. (2015). Early upregulation of NLRP3 in the brain of neonatal mice exposed to hypoxia-ischemia: no early neuroprotective effects of NLRP3 deficiency. *Neonatology* 108, 211–219. doi: 10.1159/000437247

Yu, Q., Guo, Z., Liu, X., Ouyang, Q., He, C., Burnstock, G., et al. (2013). Block of P2X7 receptors could partly reverse the delayed neuronal death in area CA1 of the hippocampus after transient global cerebral ischemia. *Purinergic Signal.* 9, 663–675. doi: 10.1007/s11302-013-9379-y

Zasada, M., Lenart, M., Rutkowska-Zapala, M., Stec, M., Mol, N., Czyz, O., et al. (2018). Analysis of selected aspects of inflammasome function in the monocytes from neonates born extremely and very prematurely. *Immunobiology* 223, 18–24. doi: 10.1016/j.imbio.2017.10.019

Zeinieh, M. P., Talhouk, R. S., El-Sabban, M. E., and Mikati, M. A. (2010). Differential expression of hippocampal connexins after acute hypoxia in the developing brain. *Brain Dev.* 32, 810–817. doi: 10.1016/j.braindev.2009.11.003

Zhao, H. B., Yu, N., and Fleming, C. R. (2005). Gap junctional hemichannel-mediated ATP release and hearing controls in the inner ear. *Proc. Natl. Acad. Sci. U.S.A.* 102, 18724–18729. doi: 10.1073/pnas.0506481102

8

Bestrophin-3 Expression in a Subpopulation of Astrocytes in the Neonatal Brain After Hypoxic-Ischemic Injury

Veronika Golubinskaya[1], Regina Vontell[2], Veena Supramaniam[2], Josephine Wyatt-Ashmead[3], Helena Gustafsson[1], Carina Mallard[1] and Holger Nilsson[1]*

[1] *Department of Physiology, Institute of Neuroscience and Physiology, The Sahlgrenska Academy, University of Gothenburg, Gothenburg, Sweden,* [2] *Division of Imaging Sciences & Biomedical Engineering, Centre for the Developing Brain, King's College London, King's Health Partners, St Thomas' Hospital, London, United Kingdom,* [3] *Wigglesworth Perinatal-Padiatric Pathology Service, Imperial College Healthcare NHS Trust, London, United Kingdom*

***Correspondence:**
Veronika Golubinskaya
veronika.golubinskaya@gu.se

Bestrophin-3, a potential candidate for a calcium-activated chloride channel, recently was suggested to have cell-protective functions. We studied the expression and alternative splicing of bestrophin-3 in neonatal mouse brain and after hypoxic-ischemic (HI) injury and in human neonatal brain samples. HI brain injury was induced in 9-day old mice by unilateral permanent common carotid artery occlusion in combination with exposure to 10% oxygen for 50 min. Endoplasmic reticulum stress was induced by thapsigargin treatment in primary culture of mouse brain astrocytes. We also investigated expression of bestrophin-3 protein in a sample of human neonatal brain tissue. Bestrophin-3 protein expression was detected with immunohistochemical methods and western blot; mRNA expression and splicing were analyzed by RT-PCR. HI induced a brain tissue infarct and a pronounced increase in the endoplasmic reticulum-associated marker CHOP. Three days after HI a population of astrocytes co-expressed bestrophin-3 and nestin in a penumbra-like area of the injured hemisphere. However, total levels of Bestrophin-3 protein in mouse cortex were reduced after injury. Mouse astrocytes in primary culture also expressed bestrophin-3 protein, the amount of which was reduced by endoplasmic reticulum stress. Bestrophin-3 protein was detected in astrocytes in the hippocampal region of the human neonatal brain which had patchy white matter gliosis and neuronal loss in the Sommer's sector of the Ammon's horn (CA1). Analysis of bestrophin-3 mRNA in mouse brain with and without injury showed the presence of two truncated spliced variants, but no full-length mRNA. Total amount of bestrophin-3 mRNA increased after HI, but showed only minor injury-related change. However, the splice variants of bestrophin-3 mRNA were differentially regulated after HI depending on the presence of tissue injury. Our results show that bestrophin-3 is expressed in neonatal mouse brain after injury and in the human neonatal brain with pathology. In mouse brain bestrophin-3 protein is upregulated in a specific astrocyte population after injury and is co-expressed with nestin. Splice variants of bestrophin-3 mRNA respond differently to HI, which might indicate their different roles in tissue injury.

Keywords: bestrophin-3 (Best3), alternative splicing, astroglia, endoplasmic reticulum (ER) stress, hypoxia-ischemia

INTRODUCTION

Bestrophins are anion channels that generally serve as chloride channels involved in regulation of cell excitability or cell volume regulation (Duran et al., 2010). Mainly three isoforms have been identified, and on the mRNA level all have been shown to be expressed in the brain (Krämer et al., 2004). Best1 is the most studied, and can function not only as a chloride channel, but also as a release mechanism for glutamate (Oh et al., 2012; Han et al., 2013) and GABA (Park et al., 2009; Lee et al., 2010) in brain astrocytes. It seems to be of special importance in reactive astrocytes, where redistribution of Best1 parallels enhanced GABA production (Oh and Lee, 2017). Data on Best2 and Best3 in brain are scarce.

Best3 mRNA is subject to alternative splicing in mouse and human, resulting in a number of splice variants of unclear function. Some splice variants of Best3 have the channel pore region spliced out, likely causing them to lose ability to act as ion channels (Srivastava et al., 2008). A specific splice variant has been suggested to control intracellular calcium release in myoblasts, possibly preventing calcium overload (Wu et al., 2016). Best3 has recently also been implicated in various cell-protective mechanisms outside the brain. This mainly stems from three studies: (a) Best3 has anti-apoptotic function in basilar artery smooth muscle cells stressed by hydrogen peroxide (Jiang et al., 2013), (b) Best3 ameliorates TNFα-induced inflammation in endothelial cells (Song et al., 2014), and (c) Best3 decides cell fate in an endoplasmic reticulum (ER) stress model in renal proximal tubule cells (Lee et al., 2012).

One of the consequences of cerebral ischemia is ER stress and the unfolded protein response (UPR) in brain cells. These processes have a complex role in cell injury, promoting either survival or death of the cells in the brain, depending on injury conditions (DeGracia and Montie, 2004). ER stress has been demonstrated also in astrocytes, resulting in increased production of cytokines and less neurotropic factors (Singh et al., 2018), potentially enhancing tissue injury. At the same time ER stress can have a protective preconditioning effect in cell injury (Lehotský et al., 2009; Leonard et al., 2014). Both ER stress (Chavez-Valdez et al., 2016) and apoptosis (Zhu et al., 2005) are important mechanisms following injury in the developing brain.

The role of Best3 in brain injury is unknown. Since Best3 has been implicated in cell protection after ER stress, we hypothesized that it could serve as a marker for cells involved in the response to brain injury. We used a well-established model of neonatal hypoxia-ischemia in mice. Unilateral brain injury was induced by a combination of hypoxia and ischemia (HI) (Rice et al., 1981; Sheldon et al., 1998; Hedtjärn et al., 2002). The resultant brain injury is characterized by increased gliosis and apoptosis-dependent brain injury (Blomgren et al., 2001).

Our work shows for the first time the expression of Best3 in neonatal brain in mice and humans, and describes changes in Best3 expression and alternative splicing following brain injury.

MATERIALS AND METHODS

Animals

C57Bl6J mice were obtained from the Jackson Laboratory, United States, and bred in-house at the laboratory of Experimental Biomedicine (EBM) at Sahlgrenska Academy, University of Gothenburg, Sweden.

In total 76 mouse pups of either sex were used in the experiments. Animals were randomly allocated into groups, and different animals were used for mRNA and protein expression analysis. For the mRNA expression analysis, a total of 41 pups (21 male, 20 females) were used, among those 26 pups in the HI group (12 males, 14 females) and 15 pups in the sham-operated group (9 males, 6 females). These were divided into separate groups for the various time points. The 6 h time point: 5 pups in the HI group (3 males, 2 females) and 3 pups in the sham group (2 males, 1 female); 12 h time point: HI 6 pups (3 males, 3 females), sham 4 pups (2 males, 2 females); 24 h time point: HI 6 pups (3 males, 3 females), sham 3 pups (2 males, 1 female); 72 h time point: HI 5 pups (2 males, 3 females), sham 3 pups (1 male, 2 females); 7 days time point: HI 4 pups (1 male, 3 females), sham 2 pups (2 males). For protein expression analysis by western blot a total of 18 pups were used, HI 14 pups (8 males, 6 females), sham 4 pups (2 males and 2 females). In experiments with immunostaining 9 pups of either sex were used. In experiments with astrocyte primary culture 8 pups of either sex were used.

Animals were euthanised either by an overdose of barbiturates or by direct decapitation (in experiments with primary cell culture of brain cells). All animal experiments and methods for animal euthanasia were approved by the Animal Ethics Committee in Gothenburg.

Model of Neonatal Hypoxia-Ischemia (HI) Injury

Nine-day old mice of either sex were exposed to HI treatment according to the Rice-Vanucci model (Rice et al., 1981; Sheldon et al., 1998). Under isoflurane anesthesia (1.5% in a 1:1 mixture of N_2 and O_2) the left common carotid artery was permanently ligated with proline 6.0 suture, then the incision was closed and treated with local anesthetic. The pups were returned to their mothers for 1 h recovery. After that pups were placed for 50 min in a 36° C -heated incubator containing a humidified gas mixture of O_2 (10%) in N_2. Subsequently pups stayed with their mothers until removed for tissue sampling. No mortality was observed after HI under the conditions used. Control sham-operated animals underwent the same surgical procedure except for the ligation of the carotid artery, and later they were kept under warm conditions in normal air at the same time as HI treatment was performed. Animals were euthanised at the time points of 6, 12, 24 and 72 h after HI.

In this model, the left hemisphere, ipsilateral to the artery ligation, receives a reduced blood flow, which in combination with hypoxia results in unilateral injury to this hemisphere. The contralateral (right) hemisphere does not experience a fall in cerebral blood flow (Ek et al., 2015), and no gross morphological injury is observed in this hemisphere

(Vannucci and Hagberg, 2004). Left and right hemispheres from sham-operated mice were used as non-treated controls.

Primary Culture of Mouse Brain Astrocytes

Experiments were based on previously described procedures for primary culture of murine brain cells (Lund et al., 2006; de Vellis et al., 2010). 1–2 days old mouse pups were decapitated, the brain was quickly removed and washed in cold Hanks' balanced salt solution (HBSS, Sigma-Aldrich) containing 1% antibiotics (penicillin-streptomycin, Sigma-Aldrich). Then the cerebellum was removed, and the rest of the brain tissue was mechanically homogenized by pipetting in warm Dulbecco's modified Eagle's medium (DMEM, Sigma-Aldrich, D5796) containing 1% antibiotics and 20% fetal bovine serum (FBS, Gibco, Life Technologies). Further culture medium always contained 1% of antibiotics. A homogenate of 1–2 brains was filtered through a 70 μm-diameter filter and diluted up to the final volume of 24 ml in DMEM with 20% FBS, and finally transferred to 75 cm^2 flask (Sarstedt AB, Helsingborg, Sweden). Cells were left growing in 5% CO_2/95% air at 37°C for 7 days, then medium was changed to DMEM with 10% FBS, and cells were allowed to grow for an additional week. After that flasks were shaken for 24 h at 250 rpm in 5% CO_2/95% air at 37°C. The medium was removed, cells were washed 2–3 times with warm HBSS and incubated in 0.05% Trypsin+EDTA (in HBSS) for 20-30 min in 5% CO_2/95% air at 37°C with gentle shaking, until the cells fully detached from the flask bottom. Then trypsin activity was blocked by adding an equivalent volume of DMEM with 10% FBS. After that cell suspension was transferred to 50 ml tubes and centrifuged at 250 g for 5 min. The supernatant was discarded, the cell pellet was resuspended in DMEM with 10% FBS, and the number of cells per 1 ml was measured (Scepter TM Automated Cell Counter, Merck Millipore). Cells were plated either 50,000 cells per well in 12-well plate (Corning Inc., United States) for further studying the mRNA or protein expression, or 10,000 cells per well in 8-well glass slide chamber (BD Falcon TM culture slides, BD Biosciences, United States) for further immunostaining. Cells were left to attach and grow for 3 days, and then the treatments were performed. The resulting cell culture contained about 95% of GFAP-positive astrocytes, among the remaining cells microglia could be detected (de Vellis et al., 2010).

The ER stress was induced in the cells by treatment with thapsigargin (TG, 200 nM, Sigma-Aldrich) in serum-free DMEM; control cells received the same medium. In this concentration TG induces ER stress in cultured astrocytes and increases ER-stress markers (Johnson et al., 2014). Forty-eight hours after the treatment cells were harvested for mRNA and western blot analysis.

Preparation of the Samples for Immunostaining in Mouse Brain Tissue

For brain tissue samples the animals were euthanised by an overdose of barbiturates i.p. and immediately transcardially perfused first with saline, then with PFA (Sigma-Aldrich) 4% in PBS. Brains were then removed and kept in 4% PFA for 1 day at 4°C. Then tissues were dehydrated in graded ethanol and xylene substitute Tissue-Clear® (Tissue-Tek® Sacura) and embedded in paraffin. Coronal sections (5 μm) of the brain were prepared and mounted on glass slides.

For immunochemistry in primary astrocyte culture the cell medium was replaced with 4% PFA, and the cells were fixed for 15 min at room temperature and stored in PBS at 4°C for 1–2 weeks until the staining was performed.

Immunostaining

Immunostaining in mouse brain sections was performed as described in Golubinskaya et al. (2015). In short, PFA-fixed tissue and cell preparations were deparaffinised and received standard antigen retrieval treatment: the preparations on the glass slides were placed in 50 mM citrate buffer (pH 6.0) and heated to 98–99°C for 30 min. Then the preparations were permeabilized and incubated with primary antibody for 24–36 h at 4°C. One of the specimens in each experiment was processed the same way, but without primary antibodies in the incubation buffer, to control for possible non-specific binding of the secondary antibody.

The primary anti-mouse antibodies used were obtained from commercial sources: Best3 (Rabbit polyclonal, IgG, Bst-301AP, lot# A532.Fb.AP, FabGennix International Inc., United States), Nestin (Goat polyclonal, IgG, G-20: sc-21248, Santa Cruz Biotechnology Inc., United States), GFAP (Mouse monoclonal IgG, G3893, Sigma-Aldrich), Iba-1 (Goat polyclonal IgG, orb19198, Biorbyt), NeuN (Mouse monoclonal IgG, MAB377, Millipore). The anti-Best3 antibody does not distinguish between Best3 splice isoforms studied in this paper, as the antigen is localized at the very end of the C-terminal region. An antibody directed to the same region in human Best3 (BEST-312AP, FabGennix), which differs in amino acid sequence, was used as a non-specific IgG control. We have previously shown the specificity of staining with BEST-301AP as it was inhibited by blocking peptide (Golubinskaya et al., 2015).

Secondary antibodies (488 or 594 DyLight-labeled secondary antibody made in donkey, Jackson Immunoresearch, United Kingdom) were incubated with specimens for 60 min at room temperature. Nuclei were detected by DAPI (Invitrogen) in dilution 1:75000. ProLongTM Gold antifade reagent (Invitrogen, Molecular Probes) was used for mounting the slides.

Conventional images were obtained by Olympus BX60 conventional fluorescence microscope (camera Olympus DP50) and Zeiss Imager.Z2 conventional fluorescence microscope (camera AxioCam MRM, Zeiss). Confocal images were obtained with a Zeiss LSM 800 microscope.

mRNA Expression Analysis

The animals were transcardially perfused with saline. Brains were quickly removed and dissected: cerebellum and the frontal part with olfactory bulbs were removed, then on the coronal projection of the brain the sector containing the cortex and hippocampus injury was dissected out. Tissue was immediately frozen in dry ice and stored for further investigation. Primary astrocyte cells were briefly washed three times with cold PBS and then lysed directly in the wells by RLT buffer (Qiagen GmbH,

Germany) containing 1% of beta-mercaptoethanol (Sigma-Aldrich) and then frozen for storage.

For total RNA extraction brain samples were briefly homogenized mechanically on ice in RNAase-free PBS, then a third of the sample was transferred to QIAzol Lysis Reagent (Qiagen GmbH, Germany) and homogenized additionally. Cultured astrocytes were homogenized in beta-mercaptoethanol-containing RLT buffer by intense vortexing. The samples were further processed according to RNeasy Lipid tissue Mini Kit (brain samples) or RNeasy Mini Kit protocol (cultured cells), both with DNAse digestion (QIAGEN GmbH, Germany). Concentration of the extracted total RNA was detected spectrophotometrically as the absorbance at 260 and 280 nm (NanoDrop 1000 spectrophotometer, Wilmington, Del., United States). For cDNA synthesis QuantiTect Rev.Transcription Kit (QIAGEN GmbH, Germany) was used, total amount of RNA used in RT reaction for each sample was 1 μg.

Primers and analysis of PCR products (**Figure 2A**) were made as described previously (Golubinskaya et al., 2015) in accordance with the predicted mRNA sequence for mouse bestrophin-3 (NM_001007583.1). Also PCR and qPCR analysis of alternative splicing of Best3 mRNA was performed as described by Golubinskaya et al. (2015). For qPCR analysis of Best3, expression primer pairs C (for detecting total mRNA of Best3), G (for variant with exon 6 is present, "+6" variant) and I (for variant missing exon 6, "−6" variant) were used. For quantification of nestin (Mm_Nes_2_SG), CHOP (Mm_Ddit3_2_SG) and a housekeeping gene GAPDH (Mm_Gapdh_3_SG) the commercial primers (QuantiTect Primer Assays from QIAGEN GmbH, Germany) were used.

For each sample the results were calculated as the difference in crossing-point (Cp) numbers between the housekeeping gene and the gene of interest (delta Cp). Then from each individual delta Cp the delta Cp value of the corresponding control samples was subtracted as shown below (delta delta Cp). The resulting values are equal to $\log_2$ of the concentration ratio of the gene of interest between treated and control groups and reflect the change in treated samples in relation to the corresponding control samples.

(1) Effect of HI:
Log_2(fold change) = delta Cp (left hemisphere of HI-treated or sham-operated mouse) − average delta Cp in the left hemisphere of time point-matched sham-operated mice;
(2) Effect of HI in the uninjured hemisphere:
Log_2(fold change) = delta Cp (right hemisphere of HI-treated mouse or right hemisphere of sham-operated mouse) − average delta Cp in the right hemisphere of time point-matched sham-operated mice;
(3) Effect of TG in the cell culture:
Log_2(fold change) = delta Cp (sample of treated or control cells) − average delta Cp in all control samples.

Protein Expression Analysis in Mouse Brain After HI by Western Blot

Brain tissue was obtained and dissected in the same way as in experiments with mRNA expression analysis. Then the tissue samples were either frozen for further analysis of total protein or were directly homogenized on ice for further subcellular fractionation of proteins. Samples from right (control) and left (injured) hemispheres were processed separately for each animal.

For subcellular fractionation of the proteins the simplified variant of protocol described by Cox and Emili (2006) was used. Briefly, tissue was homogenized in 250-STMDPS buffer (250 mM sucrose, 50 mM TrisBase, 5 mM $MgCl_2$, DTT 1 mM, spermine 50 μg/μl, spermidine 50 μg/μl, PMSF 0,1 mM, pH 7.4) in glass Dounce homogenizer tube. The aliquot of homogenate was saved frozen for later total protein analysis. The rest of homogenate was centrifuged at 800 × *g*, 15 min at 4°C, twice after which the supernatant representing the cytoplasmic fraction was saved frozen.

For extraction of total protein from brains after HI, frozen brain tissue and the total protein aliquot from subcellular fractionation were homogenized in the lysis buffer containing Tris-HCl 50 mM, NaCl 150 mM, Triton X-100 1%, Igepal 0,25%, phosphatase inhibitor and protease inhibitor cocktails (Roche, Germany), pH 7.5.

For extraction of total protein from primary astrocytes the cells were washed 2–3 times in PBS, then collected in PBS containing Triton X-100 0.5%, Igepal 0,12%, PMSF 0.1% and protease inhibitor cocktail 0.5% and then stored frozen.

Then all the samples (total protein from HI brains and from primary astrocytes, cytoplasmic and total protein fractions) were additionally mechanically homogenized by vortexing and by passing through 27–29G syringe needle. After that protein concentration in the samples was measured by BCA method. Then samples were prepared in Laemmli sample buffer 4× (Bio-Rad Laboratories, United States) with 10% DTT, heated for 5 min at 95°C and run through the 4–20% Criterion TGS Stain-free gel in amounts of 10 μg/well for total protein and cytoplasmic fractions and 1 μg/well for total protein samples from primary astrocytes. Protein was transferred to 0.2 μm PVDF membrane (Bio-Rad) by Trans-Blot Turbo Transfer System (Bio-Rad). Then membrane was washed in TBS-T buffer, blocked by 5% milk solution and stained with primary antibody against Best3 (5000 dilution in PBS with 3% BSA and 0.1% sodium azide). Bst-301AP (FabGennix International Inc., United States) was used for detection of Best3 in primary astrocyte samples, and ARP50108_P050 (Aviva Systems Biology, United States) was used for analysis of Best3 in HI brain tissue samples. We have previously shown specificity of Western blot detection with Bst-301AP by inhibition with blocking peptide (Matchkov et al., 2008); **Supplementary Image S2** here shows the same for ARP50108_P050. For visualization of Best3 peroxidase-labeled secondary antibody (Vector Laboratories, United States) and SuperSignalR West Dura Extended Duration Substrate (Thermo Scientific, United States) were used. The images were captured by ChemiDoc^{TM} Imaging System, Bio-Rad. Precision Plus Unstained and Precision Plus All blue Protein Ladders from Bio-Rad were used to estimate the molecular weight of visualized proteins. Bands were identified and their area-intensity product normalized to total protein using ImageLab software (Bio-Rad).

Statistical Analysis

In the experiments n equals number of animals (brain tissue samples) or wells (cell culture studies). Data of qPCR experiments (delta Cp values) was analyzed by three-way mixed ANOVA (analyzing brain hemispheres (within subjects), treatment and time (between subjects) using GLM for repeated measurements using IBM SPS Statistics 25; simple effects were analyzed from estimated marginal means with Bonferroni adjustment. Data from western blot were analyzed by two-way mixed ANOVA. Analyses of two groups were by means of Student's t-test. Data is presented on the graphs as individual values with group means ± SEM. A P-value of less than 0.05 was regarded as significant. In **Figure 3** values for treated animals are plotted as differences from the corresponding means of sham animals; the detailed statistical results for **Figure 3** are given in the **Supplementary Table S1**.

Immunostaining in Human Neonatal Post-mortem Brain Tissue With Pathology

Informed parental consent was acquired in accordance with the National Health Services United Kingdom guidelines and research study ethics was obtained from the National Research Ethics Services (West London), United Kingdom (ethics number 07/H0707/139; Postmortem Magnetic Imaging Study of the Developing Brain). The postmortem case assessed in this study was a term stillbirth/intrauterine death (at 41.7 weeks

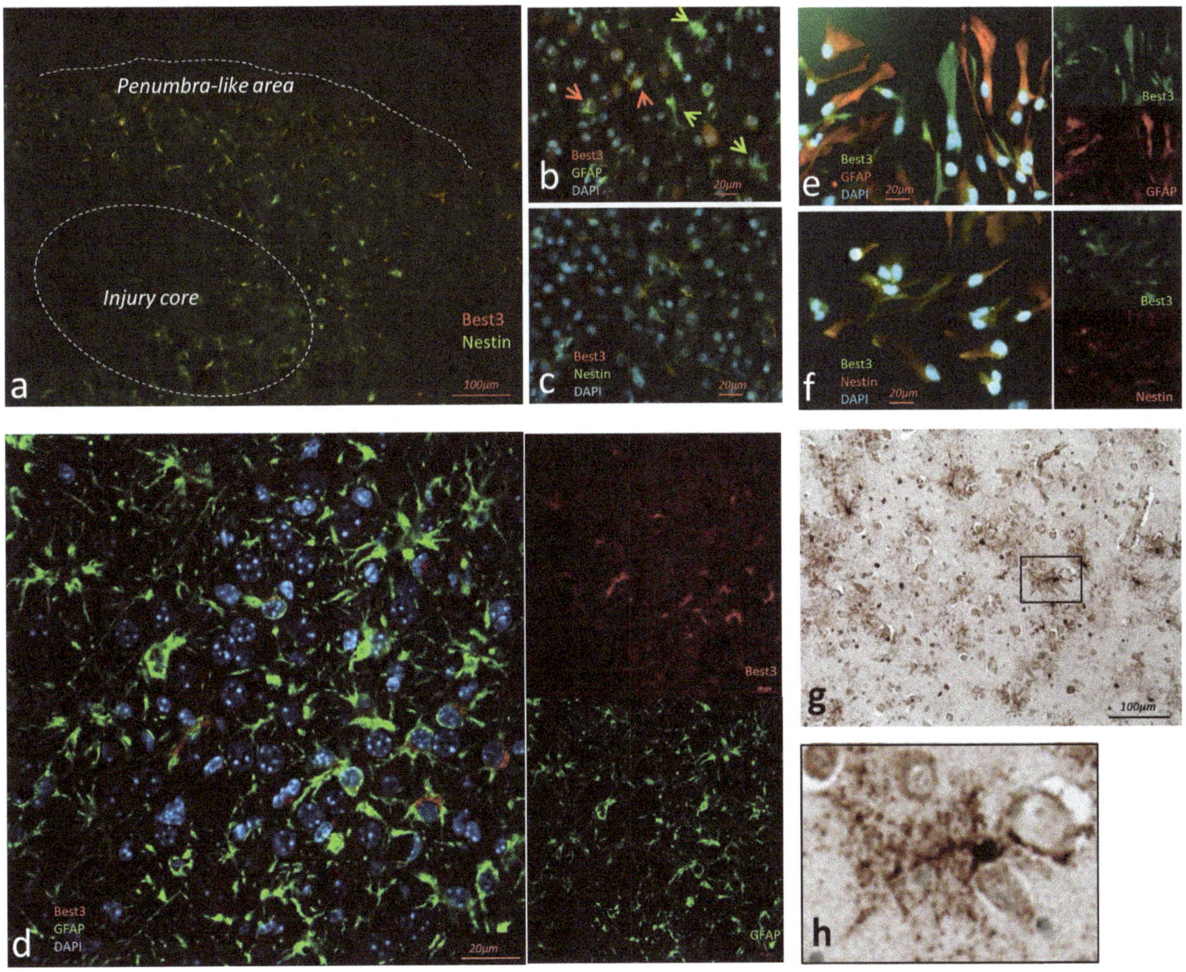

FIGURE 1 | Immunohistochemical evidence for Best3 expression in newborn mouse and human brain after injury. Best3 is expressed in mouse brain cortex after HI **(a–d)**, in mouse primary astrocyte culture **(e,f)** and in brain of newborn child with birth pathology **(g,h)**. Best3 was expressed in the injured mouse brain 3 days after HI **(a)** in a subpopulation of GFAP-positive cells **(b,d)**. Some cells expressed both Best3 and GFAP (**b**, red arrows), while other GFAP-positive cells did not express Best3 (**b**, green arrows). Best3-positive cells also expressed the intermediate filament nestin and were localized mostly in cortex and hippocampus in a penumbra-like area of the injury **(a,c)**. Confocal image of the penumbra-like area **(d)** shows Best3 intracellularly in the perinuclear area. Similar to the brain tissue astrocytes, some, but not all GFAP-positive astrocytes in a primary culture were expressing Best3 **(e)**. These cells also expressed the intermediate filament nestin **(f)**. Best3 is stained red, nestin and GFAP green **(a–d)**, Best3 is stained green, nestin and GFAP red **(e,f)**, nuclear staining with DAPI blue, magnification 10× **(a)**, 40× **(b,c)**, 60× **(d)**. Best3 was also expressed in astrocyte-like cells in cortical areas of the brain of a term infant with white matter gliosis (**g**, enlarged Best3-positive structure in **h**). Peroxidase-based immunostaining captured at magnification 20×.

gestational age; male) associated with amniotic fluid infection. The pregnancy was otherwise uncomplicated and there were no major congenital anomalies, chromosomal defects or overt culture-positive sepsis evident in the infant. The clinical pathologist noted that there was slight congestion and oedema seen throughout the brain and there was evidence of patchy white matter gliosis. However, except for the hippocampal region which had overt neuronal loss in the Sommer's sector of the Ammon's Horn, the rest of the brain was unremarkable (i.e., no hypoxic-ischemic neurons or apoptotic neurons were seen). Samples containing the Ammon's Horn, thalamus and lentiform nucleus were used in this study. Postmortem tissue preparation has previously been described (Vontell et al., 2015) and the standard immunohistochemistry procedure for neonatal brain tissue has been described elsewhere (Supramaniam et al., 2013; Vontell et al., 2013). The tissue slides were incubated with the human-specific antiBest3 primary antibody (1:200 rabbit polyclonal, ab101828 from Abcam, Cambridge, United Kingdom) overnight, followed by incubation with secondary biotinylated antibody (1:1000 goat-anti-rabbit, BA-1000, Vector Laboratories, Burlingame, CA, United States) for 1 h, and then processed as described in Vontell et al. (2015).

RESULTS

Expression of Best3 Is Seen in the Ventricles of Non-injured Mouse Brain

In non-injured mouse brains (in sham-operated animals and in the right, contralateral hemisphere of the brain of HI mice) immunohistochemical analysis revealed presence of Best3 protein in ependymal cells and occasionally in radial-glia on the surface of the brain ventricles (**Supplementary Image S1**), but no obvious staining in other brain cells was detected. A similar

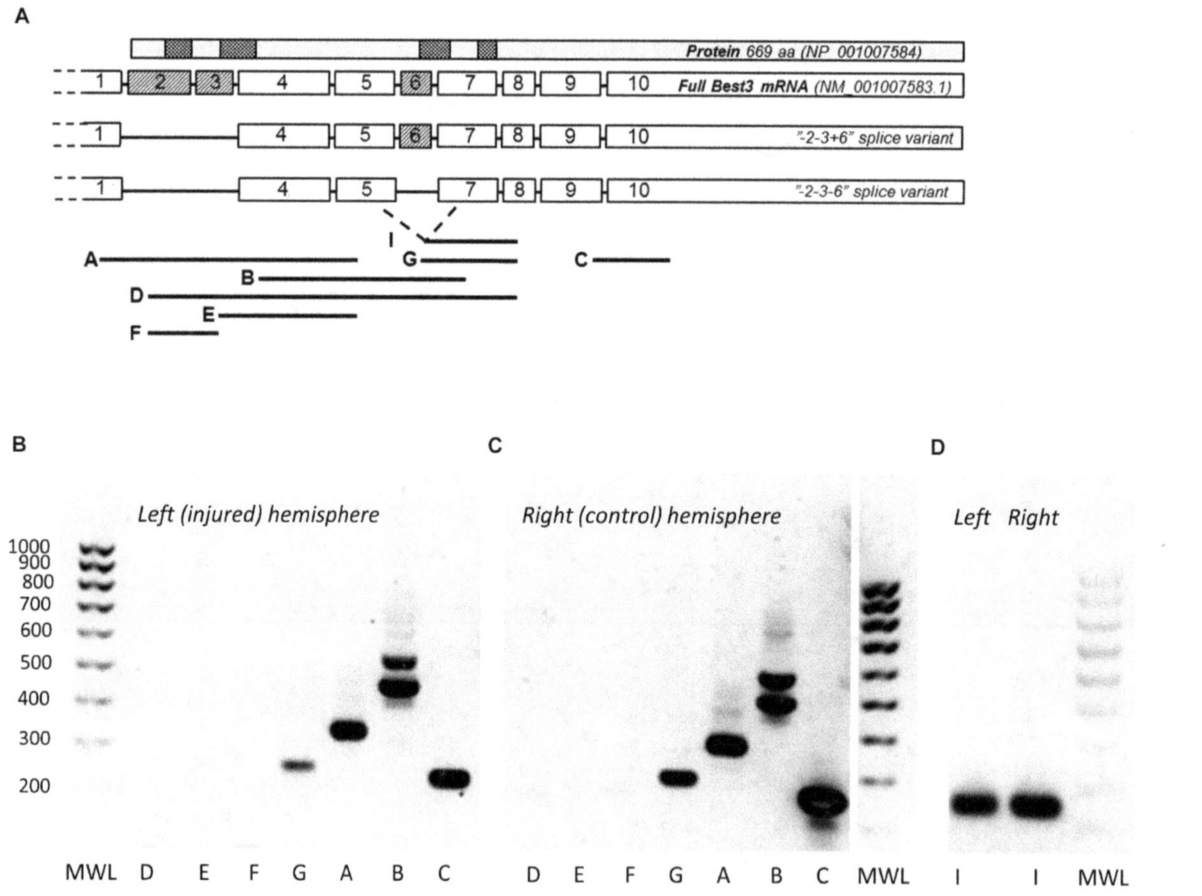

FIGURE 2 | PCR analysis of Best3 mRNA alternative splicing in mouse brain with and without HI injury. Alternative splicing of Best3 mRNA was studied by a set of primers **(A)** spanning the areas of expected splicing of exons 2, 3, and 6 in different combinations as described in detail previously (Golubinskaya et al., 2015). The results of these PCR experiments are presented in **(B–D)**. Total Best3 mRNA can be detected by primer pair C localized in exons 9 and 10 in both healthy **(C)** and injured brain **(B)**. Splice variants of Best3 with exons 2 and 3 present were not detected, neither in healthy brain nor in injury (pairs of primers: A, localized in exons 1 and 5; D in exons 2 and 7; E in exons 3 and 5; F in exons 2 and 3). Exon 6 can be either present or spliced out in Best3 mRNA. Primer pair B spanning exons 4–7 gives two bands, the heavier band corresponds to "+6" and the lighter one to "–6" splice variants. The pair of primers G localized in exons 6 and 8 shows a band corresponding to "+6" splice variant. Primer pair I detects the "–6" variant **(D)**. Primer pairs G and I can potentially detect more than one transcript corresponding to "+6" and "–6" variants depending on possible splicing of exon 10. Positive controls for these primers have been published previously by our group (Golubinskaya et al., 2015). MWL, molecular weight ladder.

pattern was seen in HI-injured mouse brain (left, ipsilateral hemisphere). We also have a preliminary observation of similar staining for Best3 in brain ependymal cells in the brains of adult naive mice.

Immunofluorescent Analysis Shows Best3 Protein Expression in Mouse Brain Astrocytes After Injury

After HI Best3-positive cells were detected in the injured hemisphere, primarily in the cortex and hippocampus in the penumbra-like area of injury (**Figure 1a**) and this expression pattern was similar in male and female pups. Best3-positive cells were first seen at 24 h after injury, but the staining was most pronounced 72 h after the HI event. Seven days after injury almost no injury-associated Best3-positive cells were evident. Best3 immunoreactivity was not detected in the contralateral non-injured hemisphere in cortical and hippocampal regions.

Best3-positive cells also expressed the intermediate filament nestin (**Figures 1a,c**). Best3 expression in astrocytes was supported by the observation that Best3 staining did not overlap with neuronal markers NeuN or calretinin, nor with Iba-1, a marker for microglia. With regard to the astrocyte marker GFAP, it was clear that Best3 was expressed in some but not in all GFAP-positive cells (**Figures 1b,d**). This suggests that after injury Best3 is expressed in a subpopulation of astrocytes that express nestin. The possibility that some of these cells could be of other type (neural progenitors etc.) cannot be neglected, but the combination of astrocyte markers and cell size and morphology suggests that the majority of Best3-positive cells were astrocytes.

Immunofluorescent Analysis Shows Best3 Protein Expression in Mouse Astrocytes in Primary Culture

Best3 expression in brain astrocytes was further confirmed by Best3-positive staining in a primary culture of mouse astrocytes (**Figures 1e,f**). As in the brain tissue, Best3 in cultured astrocytes was co-expressed with nestin (**Figure 1h**), while overlap with GFAP was not complete (**Figure 1e**).

Expression of Best3 Is Seen in the Human Brain

Immunohistochemical analysis showed expression of Best3 protein in astrocytes (**Figures 1g,h**) in the thalamic and hippocampal region of the post-mortem neonatal human brain. Best3 was highly expressed in hypertrophic astrocytes, where it was observed in the cell bodies and extended into the filamentous processes.

Expression and Alternative Splicing of Best3 mRNA in the Mouse Brain Tissue Is Changed After HI in the Injured and Non-injured Hemispheres

Alternative Splicing of Best3 mRNA

The PCR analysis of Best3 mRNA was made by using specifically made primer pairs published previously (Golubinskaya et al., 2015) spanning the expected areas of splicing of exons 2, 3, and 6 (**Figure 2A**) based on earlier published data on alternative splicing in Best3 mRNA in mouse tissues (Krämer et al., 2004; Srivastava et al., 2008). We did not investigate the possible splicing of exon 10 that recently has been described by Wu et al. (2016), so in our PCR experiments the "−2−3+6" and "−2−3−6" splice variants of mRNA could represent corresponding groups of splice variants where also exon 10 is alternatively spliced. Analysis of the ipsilateral, injured hemisphere and the contralateral non-injured hemisphere (**Figures 2B–D**) showed the presence of two splice variants of Best3 in both hemispheres: one longer variant where exon 6 was present ("+6" variant) and another shorter one, "−6" variant, where exon 6 was spliced out. This conclusion was made from the observation that primer pair B, covering exons 4–7, gave two bands of corresponding weights. The presence of the "+6" splice isoform was confirmed by the band corresponding to the primer pair G with forward primer placed in exon 6, and the presence of the "−6" isoform by the band corresponding to primer pair I targeting the junction of exons 5 and 7. The "+6" variant was dominating in brain tissue.

At the same time no full-length mRNA for Best3 could be detected in either hemisphere, as exons 2 and 3 were absent in both "−6" and "+6" splice variants. Primer pair A, spanning exons 1 and 5, gave only one band with a weight corresponding to the splice variant with both exons 2 and 3 absent. Neither primer pairs D and E, where one of the primers in each pair was complementary to the sequence in exon 2 or 3, nor primer pair F spanning exons 2 and 3, revealed any band by PCR analysis.

Time Course of Changes in Best3 mRNA Expression in the Non-injured Brain Hemisphere After HI

By comparing the right contralateral hemispheres of HI-treated mice to the right hemispheres of sham-operated mice, one can estimate the effect of HI on the uninjured hemisphere (**Figure 3**, blue marking compared to the zero level). In our experiments HI induced early changes in Best3 mRNA expression in the contralateral (right) hemisphere. Total Best3 (**Figure 3A**) showed a biphasic response with an early increase at 6 and 12 h and down-regulation at 72 h. The two splice variants followed similar initial time courses, increasing at 6 and 12 h after HI, but after 24 h the values were back to control level and no further changes occurred during the later time points (**Figures 3B,C**).

Nestin expression was transiently downregulated at 6, 12, and 24 h, returning to its control values at 72 h after HI (**Figure 3D**). There were no signs of pronounced ER stress in the non-injured brain hemisphere after HI, as expression of the ER-stress marker CHOP did not increase, but rather slightly decreased at the early time points after HI (**Figure 3E**).

Time Course of Changes in Best3 mRNA Expression in Brain Injured After HI

The total effect of HI can be studied by comparing the left ipsilateral (injured) hemisphere of HI-exposed mice with the left hemisphere of sham-operated animals (**Figure 3**, red marking compared to the zero level). Total mRNA for Best3 increased transiently at 6 h after HI, and then remained at control level

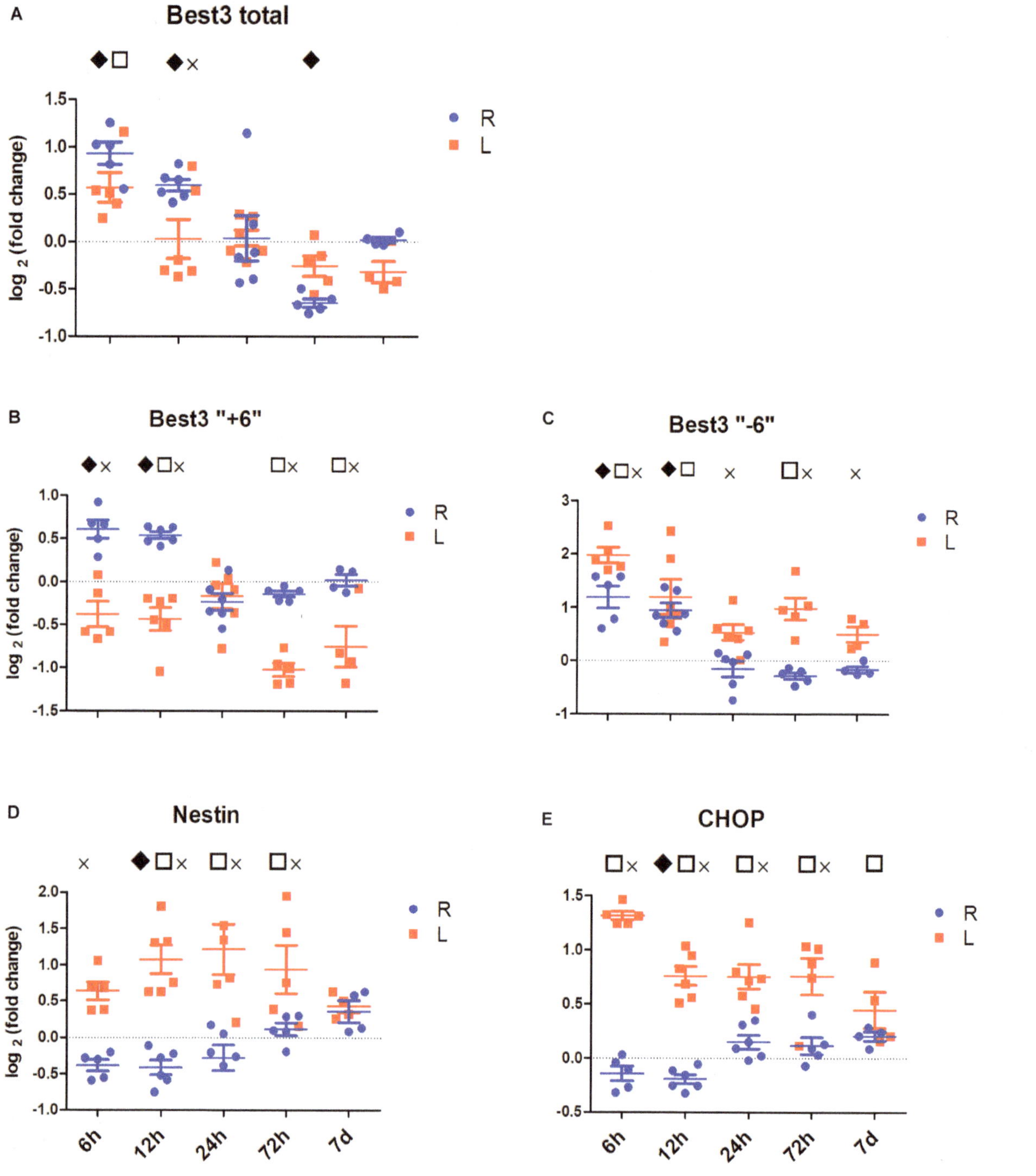

FIGURE 3 | The expression of Best3 mRNA in mouse brain tissue at different time points after HI. Figures show relative expression of the studied mRNAs in uninjured (R, blue) and injured (L, red) hemispheres in relation to the average expression in corresponding hemispheres of sham animals at the respective time points (sham group mean set to zero in the figure). Statistical analysis was performed by mixed-model three-way ANOVA on *Cp* values; main effects were based on subsequently estimated marginal means. Symbols above graphs indicate significant difference between uninjured and sham (R vs. sham group at zero, ♦), between injured and sham (L vs. sham group at zero, □), and between uninjured and injured (R vs. L, ×), all symbols indicate $P < 0.05$. The total mRNA for Best3 increased in both hemispheres at early time points after HI, but returned to control values already 24 h after HI, and even showed a transient decrease at 72 h **(A)**. The long "+6" splice variant increased only in the uninjured hemisphere, while in the injured hemisphere it decreased and stayed decreased through all time point except 24 h **(B)**. The short "–6" splice variant transiently increased at 6 and 12 h, and in the injured hemisphere also again at 72 h **(C)**. Expression of mRNA for nestin **(D)** decreased at early time points in non-injured hemisphere, but returned to control values at 72 h after HI, while it increased in the injured hemisphere during this period to return to control values at 7 days after injury. The ER-stress marker CHOP slightly decreased during the early period after HI in the non-injured hemisphere, but was elevated throughout the studied period in the injured hemisphere **(E)**. A total of 41 pups (26 HI, 15 sham) were used; for details see section "Materials and Methods." Detailed statistical results are given in the (**Supplementary Table S1**).

(**Figure 3A**). The long and the short splice variants of Best3 showed opposite changes: the "+6" variant was downregulated (**Figure 3B**), and "−6" was markedly upregulated (**Figure 3C**). At 24 h after injury the expression of both splice variants was close to the control values (**Figures 3B,C**).

Both nestin (**Figure 3D**) and ER-stress marker CHOP (**Figure 3E**) were upregulated already at 6 h and stayed upregulated through most of the investigated period. Nestin developed its maximal expression between 12 and 72 h, while CHOP showed maximum expression at 6 h after HI, after which its expression decreased over time toward baseline.

Time Course of Injury-Related Changes in Best3 mRNA Expression in the Brain After HI

By comparing the left ipsilateral (injured; **Figure 3**, red marking) with the right contralateral (non-injured; **Figure 3**, blue marking) hemisphere in the same animal the changes produced by the development of tissue injury can be estimated. **Figure 3** shows that injury reduced the expression of total Best3 mRNA at 12 h only (**Figure 3A**). Best3 splice variants changed in opposite directions: the long "+6" splice variant was downregulated in a biphasic manner with a transient return to control values at 24 h after HI (**Figure 3B**), while the expression of the short "−6" splice variant, on the other hand, slightly increased at 6 h and from 24 h onwards compared to the non-injured hemisphere (**Figure 3C**).

Nestin gradually increased in response to injury, reaching maximal expression between 12 and 24 h, and returning to its control values by 7 days after HI (**Figure 3D**). Injury was associated with ER stress as indicated by CHOP expression, which was maximally increased at 6 h, and then gradually decreased, returning to its control values at 7 days after HI (**Figure 3E**). Details of the statistical analysis are given in the **Supplementary Table S1**.

ER Stress Alters Expression of Best3 mRNA in Mouse Cultured Astrocytes

The results of the experiments are presented in **Figure 4**. To confirm that Best3 is altered in astrocytes after injury we investigated mRNA expression for Best3 in cultured astrocytes after inducing ER stress by TG. Before inducing ER stress the "−6" variant was dominating. ER stress caused an increase in expression of total Best3 and both its splice variants (**Figures 4A–C**). The increase in the long "+6" splice variant was the most pronounced ($P < 0.01$; **Figure 4B**). Nestin also increased after TG ($P < 0.01$; **Figure 4D**), and CHOP, as an ER-stress marker, was dramatically upregulated ($P < 0.001$; **Figure 4E**).

Best3 Protein Expression Analysis by Western Blot

Protein analysis by western blot was performed in brain tissue using ARP50108_P050 antibody and in astrocyte culture by Bst-301AP. It revealed Best3-related protein bands in the range of 55–80 kDa (**Figure 5**). In homogenates of parts of cortex from each hemisphere, typically Best3 staining revealed a pair of bands with molecular weight differing by approximately 2–3 kDa, which might correspond to the predicted difference between "+6" and "−6" splice variants of Best3. As there is no antibody specifically recognizing splice variants of Best3, we calculated the density of both bands together in our analysis.

Lighter pairs of bands at about 65 kDa could often be seen. The appearance of these additional bands likely might be related to the homogenization protocol, by which possibly posttranslational modifications or tightly bound proteins, for example a protein phosphatase (Marmorstein et al., 2002) could be partially removed. It is interesting to note that in cultured astrocytes the Best3-related band had a weight of approximately 52–55 kDa, closer to the theoretically predicted weight for "+6" and "−6" splice variants of Best3. Whether the lower molecular weight in cultured cells relates to a lack of modifications/associations remains to be determined.

Quantification of western blot results showed downregulation of Best3 protein expression in brain cortex and hippocampus after HI ($P < 0.05$) and in cultured mouse astrocytes in ER stress ($P < 0.001$; **Figure 5**), although this was not apparent in the cytoplasmic fraction of the brain tissue after HI injury ($P > 0.05$). The same result was observed whether Best3-related protein bands were normalized to total protein (**Figure 5**) or to GAPDH (data not shown).

DISCUSSION

Best3 protein has previously not been described in the brain, and there are only a few reports where Best3 mRNA was detected in the whole adult mouse brain, although without identification of the cells expressing it (Krämer et al., 2004; Srivastava et al., 2008), and only weakly detected in the normal adult human brain (Stöhr et al., 2002). We show for the first time that Best3 protein and mRNA are expressed in normal and injured brain in newborn mouse pups and in a term infant with white matter gliosis.

Our main focus in this study was to investigate Best3 in cell injury as recent studies suggest a novel role for Best3 in apoptosis and ER-stress. In our mouse experiments we describe for the first time a subpopulation of nestin-positive astrocytes appearing after the HI injury, which expresses Best3 and can be visualized primarily in the penumbra-like area (**Figure 1a**). These cells have an astrocyte morphology, are positive for GFAP, a classic marker of astrocytes (**Figures 1b,d**) and for nestin (**Figures 1a,c**), and do not co-express neuronal or microglial markers. Under normal conditions nestin expression in the brain is more characteristic for progenitor cells than for astrocytes. We cannot exclude the possibility that some of the Best3-positive cells were neural progenitor cells, yet we did not see Best3 expression in the uninjured brain. However, the possibility that progenitor cell proliferation, triggered by injury, contributes to the Best3 expression cannot be ruled out. After injury a subpopulation of activated astrocytes start expressing nestin (Gilyarov, 2008), and these cells have been suggested to be in an early stage of activation preceding hypertrophic changes (Cho et al., 2013). Functionally, these cells have been shown to be proliferating astrocytes that have a positive influence on tissue recovery (Suzuki et al., 2012). The appearance of nestin+/GFAP+ cells has been described in the neonatal rat brain after HI, and these cells are suggested to be

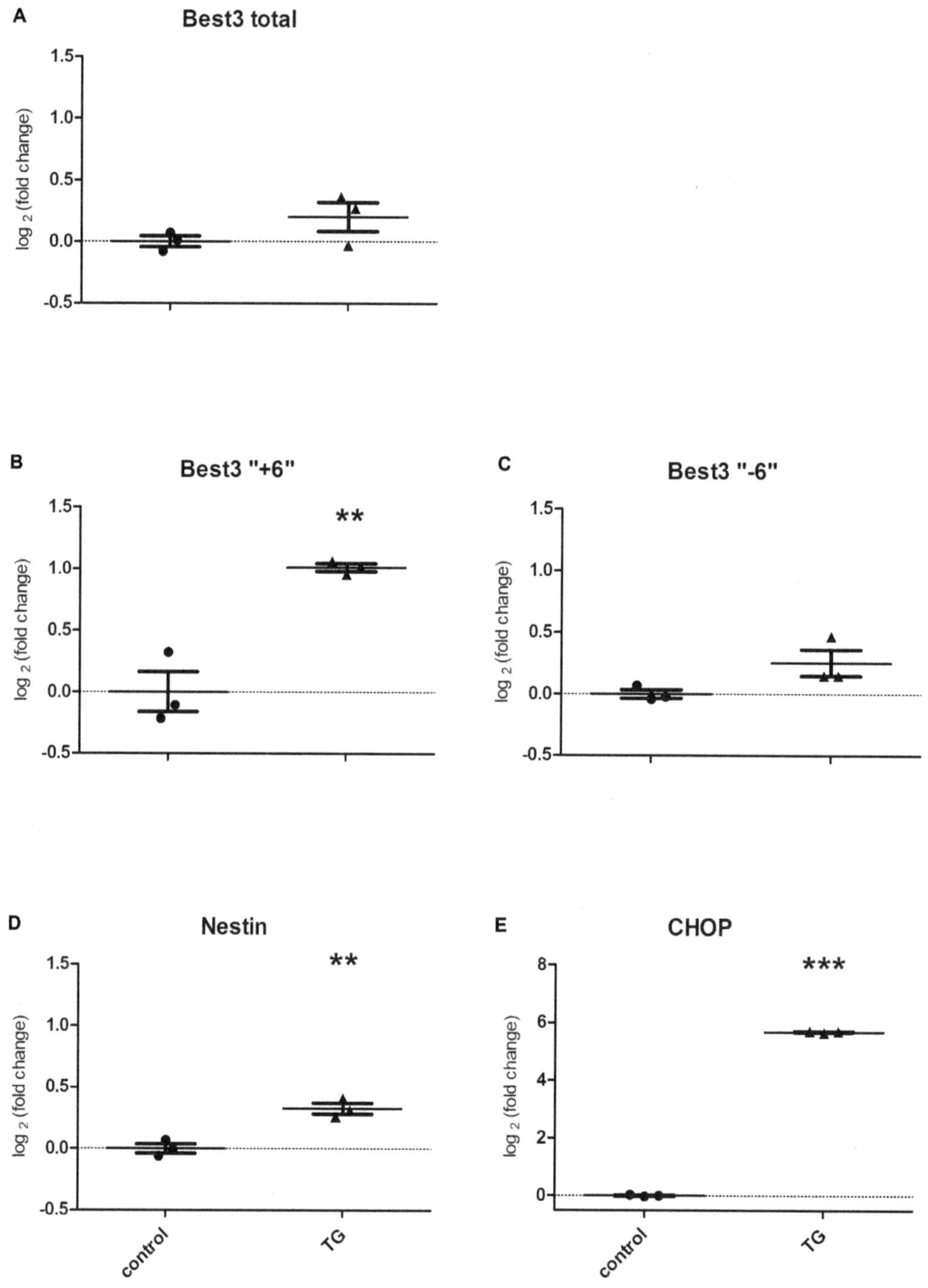

FIGURE 4 | Best3 mRNA is expressed in the primary culture of mouse astrocytes. TG caused very small changes in total Best3 **(A)** and in its short splice variant expression **(C)**, but induced a noticeable increase in expression of the long "+6" splice variant of Best3 **(B)**. TG-treated cells showed a pronounced ER-stress **(E)** and increase in nestin expression **(D)**. $^{**}P < 0.01$, $^{***}P < 0.001$ *t*-test control vs. treatment.

in a transition state from nestin-positive radial glia into GFAP-expressing mature astrocytes (Sizonenko et al., 2008). Mouse astrocytes in primary culture in the present study showed a similar pattern of Best3 protein expression as after HI *in vivo*: partial overlap with GFAP and high degree of co-expression with nestin (**Figures 1e,f**). These results confirm the presence of Best3 in astrocytes, and the pronounced expression of both nestin and Best3 in the majority of cells suggests that astrocytes in culture are to a large extent in an activated state.

We also show that Best3 is expressed in astrocytes in the human term neonatal brain with neuropathology as a result of an acute event leading to intrauterine death (**Figures 1g,h**).

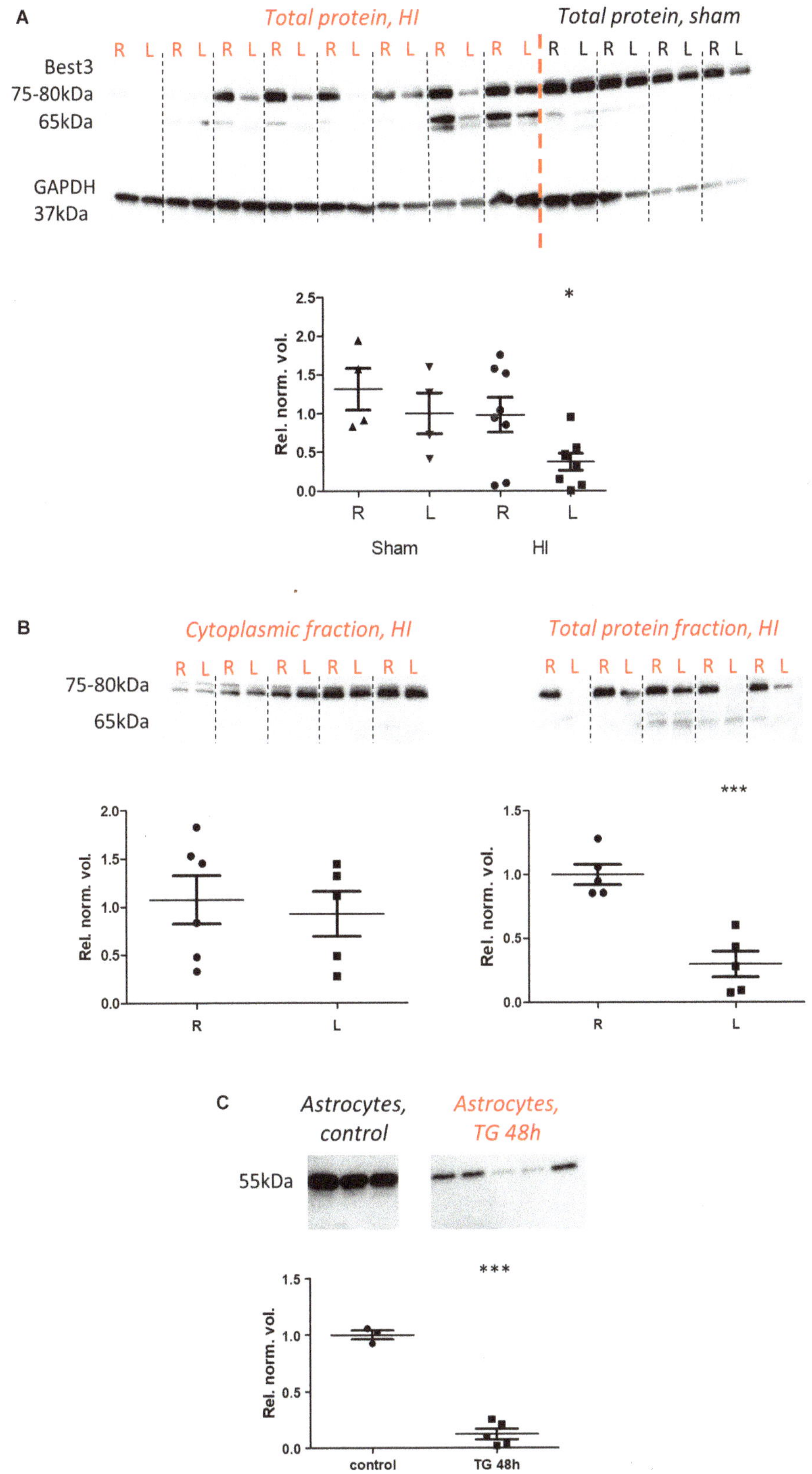

FIGURE 5 | Best3 protein is downregulated in mouse brain tissue and cultured mouse astrocytes after injury. Western blot analysis of brain tissue **(A,B)** and cultured astrocytes **(C)**. Brain specimens from right uninjured (R) and left injured (L) hemispheres were alternately placed on the gels in **(A,B)**; the same was done for

(Continued)

FIGURE 5 | Continued
sham-operated animals **(A)**. Two neighboring R and L lanes belong to the same animal. In total protein samples from brain **(A)** at approximately 75–80 kDa two bands with close molecular weights could be detected; their density was summarized in the analysis. These bands were reduced in injury. Additional lighter pairs of bands could be observed at approximately 65 kDa. The result of subcellular fractionation of brain tissue is shown in **(B)**, where two bands of approximately 75–80 kDa were detected in the cytoplasmic fraction as well as in the total protein fraction. The content of Best3 in the cytoplasm did not change significantly in injury, while Best3 in the total protein fraction was downregulated. In cultured astrocytes **(C)** treatment with thapsigargin for 48 h (TG 48 h) also caused downregulation of Best3. *$P < 0.05$ by two-way ANOVA and estimated marginal means; ***$P < 0.001$ *t*-test R vs. L or treated vs. untreated cells. A total of 18 pups (14 HI, 4 sham) were used; for details see section "Materials and Methods."

This indicates the relevance of our observations in mice to situations with brain injury in humans. This term neonate very likely had injury to brain cells as a result of different traumatic events leading to death. As a result, the brain tissue shows signs of pronounced gliosis, in particular strong activation of astrocytes, and it was interesting to see expression of Best3 in this clinical case. Best3-positive cells were reminiscent of activated astrocytes by their morphology and developed cell processes. Based on the morphology we can suggest that Best3 can be expressed in a subpopulation of activated astrocytes in situations of neuropathology in neonates. The specific relevance of this discovery to hypoxic-ischemic brain injury in neonates, however, is not determined, and a more detailed study of the co-localization of Best3 with various cell markers is required to characterize the Best3-positive human cells.

In the HI model exposure to hypoxia alone does not induce brain injury, while its combination with ischemia causes appearance of an infarct area and cell apoptosis (Hedtjärn et al., 2002). Total Best3 mRNA was upregulated early after HI in both hemispheres. This change thus is related either to hypoxemia or to some influence of the injury on both hemispheres, whether neural or humoral. Interestingly, the rise in Best3 mRNA lasted longer in the uninjured hemisphere. Whether this relates to that hemisphere coping with the hypoxemia, and the other one succumbing, remains to be investigated.

The alternative splicing of Best3 mRNA after the HI injury in mouse brain was also analyzed. In mouse Best3 mRNA exons 2, 3, and 6 can be spliced out in different combinations in different organs, and the whole brain homogenate from the adult mouse was reported to have two splice variants "−2−3+6" and "−2−3−6", but not the full-length mRNA (Krämer et al., 2004). Similar results were obtained in our PCR analysis of Best3 splicing in the brains of neonatal mice (**Figure 2**), and the composition of splice variants was similar in contralateral non-injured and ipsilateral injured brain hemispheres. However, there is also recent data on possible splicing of the C-terminal region of Best3 mRNA and protein in mouse myoblasts (Wu et al., 2016). If this is the case also in brain, the "+6" and "−6" variants seen in our experiments could represent more than one transcript each. A more detailed analysis of alternative splicing of Best3 in situations with brain injury may therefore require RNA sequencing.

In contrast to total Best3, expression of the long "+6" splice variant changed in an injury-related manner, it was downregulated in the injured hemisphere in parallel with developing ER stress, but it was upregulated on the non-injured side (**Figure 3**). The short "−6" was less injury-dependent and was mostly upregulated in both hemispheres. These changes in splicing started already at 6 h after HI, and it is interesting to note that the changes in expression of both splice variants showed biphasic dynamics: the values always tended to transiently return to control levels 24 h after the injury.

Increased expression of the transcription factor CHOP and nestin mRNA was present in the injured hemisphere only (**Figure 3**) suggesting pro-apoptotic ER stress in this tissue (Xu et al., 2005), although the degree of apoptosis was not examined in the present study. In non-injured brain tissue CHOP and nestin were actually downregulated after HI, which might be related to compensatory changes in blood flow and is an interesting observation for future investigation.

In mouse astrocyte cell culture (**Figure 4**) direct induction of strong ER stress by blocking the SERCA pump showed, together with a dramatic increase in CHOP expression, also a tendency for total Best3 mRNA to increase as well as mRNA for both its splice variants, with the most pronounced change in "+6" splice variant expression in contrast to the injury in the brain tissue, where "+6" variant was downregulated. This may indicate that different origins of ER stress can influence Best3 expression differently, but it could also show that cultured astrocytes, being already in an activated state, respond to ER stress differently from astrocytes *in vivo*.

Our results of Best3 mRNA expression show that it is important to study not only the total expression of the gene, but also to analyze individual splice variants, as such proteins can have different functions. Alternative splicing of mRNA can be changed by cell injury and inflammation, and this phenomenon is well described for the protein family Bcl2 (Bcl2, Bcl2L1, Bax, and other), which can act as pro- or antiapoptotic proteins depending on their splicing (Glasgow et al., 2001; Akgul et al., 2004; Miura et al., 2012). A change in the ratio between the antiapoptotic long Bcl-xL and the proapoptotic short Bcl-xS splice variants of one of the members of this family, Bcl2L1 (also called BclX), was also described in neonatal HI injury (Xiao et al., 2012). The results of the present work and of our previous studies (Golubinskaya et al., 2015) reveal a new protein, Best3, alternative splicing of which changes in the situation of tissue injury.

Analysis of Best3 protein expression by western blot showed that the general expression of Best3 protein in brain cortex and hippocampus was reduced after HI injury, and yet in our IHC experiments Best3 appeared in a specific cell population around the injured area. This data suggests that the western blot shows the overall expression in all cell types of the brain and cannot detect an increase in a small sub-population of

Best3-positive astrocytes. At the same time expression of Best3 protein was strongly reduced in cultured astrocytes after 48 h with thapsigargin treatment. Both HI injury and thapsigargin treatment caused ER stress, judging from the increase in CHOP. The Best3 protein was downregulated in cultured cells during ER stress, which calls into question whether Best3 is actually involved in resolving the ER-stress response in astrocytes. On the other hand, the severity of ER stress may differ between the brain astrocytes in HI and thapsigargin-treated cultured astrocytes, where thapsigargin presumably is a much stronger inducer of ER stress or induces ER stress by different mechanisms. Another reason may be that ER stress as such may cause downregulation of Best3 protein, whereas signals related to tissue injury and coming from other types of the cells cause upregulation of Best3 in astrocytes close to the injured area. It is also interesting to note that Best3 protein levels did not change significantly in the cytoplasmic fraction of brain cortex, suggesting the reduction in protein must occur in other compartments of the cells.

In summary, our study demonstrates expression of Best3 in a nestin-positive subpopulation of astrocytes in neonatal mouse brain after hypoxic-ischemic injury, with a general suppression of its expression in the cortex as a whole. Best3 also shows localized expression in astrocyte-like cells in human neonatal brain with pathologies. Analysis of alternative splicing for Best3 mRNA in mouse brain after HI injury showed that even if total expression of Best3 mRNA may not show much change, its splice variants respond differently and thus might have different roles in development of injury in brain tissue. The shorter splice variants are unlikely to function as ion channels (Srivastava et al., 2008) although they may have both intracellular and membrane localization. Their function is so far unknown. If Best3 actually functions as a regulator of apoptosis, it is possible that this property is associated with one variant as it is with Bcl-X, however, this is highly speculative and needs further investigation. Best3 expression in astrocytes near injury in the neonatal brain is a novel and important finding. As a marker for a certain cell population it can help understanding mechanisms of brain injury, where glial cells play an important role. A definitive determination of the role for Best3 in pathophysiology hinges upon the development of a knock-out model.

AUTHOR CONTRIBUTIONS

VG, HG, CM, and HN designed the study. VG, RV, and JW-A collected the data. VG, RV, JW-A, CM, and HN analyzed the data. VG, CM, and HN drafted the manuscript. All authors revised and approved the manuscript.

FUNDING

This study was supported by grants from Vetenskapsrådet (2012-2992), CM, http://www.vr.se, Swedish state under the agreement between the Swedish Government and the county councils, the ALF-agreement (ALFGBG 432291), CM, http://www.fou.nu/is/alfgbg, Leducq Foundation (DSRR_P34404), CM, https://www.fondationleducq.org, Swedish Brain Foundation (FO2014-008), CM, http://www.hjarnfonden.se, Torsten Söderberg Foundation (M98/15), CM, http://www.torstensoderbergsstiftelse.se, Åhlén Foundation (CM and HN) http://www.ahlen-stiftelsen.se/index.html, Stiftelsen Wilhelm och Martina Lundgrens Vetenskapsfond (VG, CM, and HN) http://www.wmlundgren.se, Stiftelsen Fru Mary von Sydows, född Wijk, donationsfond (VG) http://www.maryvonsydowstiftelsen.se, Svenska Frimurare Barnhusdirektionen i Göteborg (VG) https://www.frimurarorden.se/loger/tredje-fordelningen/gota-provinsialloge/caritas. The funders had no role in study design, data collection and analysis, decision to publish, or preparation of the manuscript.

ACKNOWLEDGMENTS

We thank the families who consented to the "Postmortem MRI study" and our colleagues in the Perinatal Pathology Services at St Thomas' Hospital.

REFERENCES

Akgul, C., Moulding, D. A., and Edwards, S. W. (2004). Alternative splicing of Bcl-2-related genes: functional consequences and potential therapeutic applications. *Cell. Mol. Life Sci.* 61, 2189–2199. doi: 10.1007/s00018-004-4001-7

Blomgren, K., Zhu, C., Wang, X., Karlsson, J.-O., Leverin, A.-L., Bahr, B. A., et al. (2001). Synergistic activation of caspase-3 by m-calpain after neonatal hypoxia-ischemia a mechanism of "pathological apoptosis"? *J. Biol. Chem.* 276, 10191–10198. doi: 10.1074/jbc.M007807200

Chavez-Valdez, R., Flock, D. L., Martin, L. J., and Northington, F. J. (2016). Endoplasmic reticulum pathology and stress response in neurons precede programmed necrosis after neonatal hypoxia-ischemia. *Int. J. Dev. Neurosci.* 48, 58–70. doi: 10.1016/j.ijdevneu.2015.11.007

Cho, J. M., Shin, Y. J., Park, J. M., Kim, J., and Lee, M. Y. (2013). Characterization of nestin expression in astrocytes in the rat hippocampal CA1 region following transient forebrain ischemia. *Anat. Cell Biol.* 46, 131–140. doi: 10.5115/acb.2013.46.2.131

Cox, B., and Emili, A. (2006). Tissue subcellular fractionation and protein extraction for use in mass-spectrometry-based proteomics. *Nat. Protoc.* 1, 1872–1878. doi: 10.1038/nprot.2006.273

de Vellis, J., Ghiani, C. A., Wanner, I. B., and Cole, R. (2010). "Preparation of normal and reactive astrocyte cultures," in *Protocols for Neural Cell Culture Springer Protocols Handbooks*, ed. L. C. Doering (New York, NY: Humana Press), 193–215.

DeGracia, D. J., and Montie, H. L. (2004). Cerebral ischemia and the unfolded protein response. *J. Neurochem.* 91, 1–8. doi: 10.1111/j.1471-4159.2004.02703.x

Duran, C., Thompson, C. H., Xiao, Q., and Hartzell, H. C. (2010). Chloride channels: often enigmatic, rarely predictable. *Annu. Rev. Physiol.* 72, 95–121. doi: 10.1146/annurev-physiol-021909-135811

Ek, C. J., D'Angelo, B., Baburamani, A. A., Lehner, C., Leverin, A.-L., Smith, P. L., et al. (2015). Brain barrier properties and cerebral blood flow in neonatal mice exposed to cerebral hypoxia-ischemia. *J. Cereb. Blood Flow Metab.* 35, 818–827. doi: 10.1038/jcbfm.2014.255

Gilyarov, A. V. (2008). Nestin in central nervous system cells. *Neurosci. Behav. Physiol.* 38, 165–169. doi: 10.1007/s11055-008-0025-z

Glasgow, J. N., Qiu, J., Rassin, D., Grafe, M., Wood, T., and Perez-Pol, J. R. (2001). Transcriptional regulation of the BCL-X gene by NF-kappaB is an element of hypoxic responses in the rat brain. *Neurochem. Res.* 26, 647–659. doi: 10.1023/A:1010987220034

Golubinskaya, V., Elvin, J., Ebefors, K., Gustafsson, H., Mallard, C., Nyström, J., et al. (2015). Bestrophin-3 is differently expressed in normal and injured mouse glomerular podocytes. *Acta Physiol.* 214, 481–496. doi: 10.1111/apha.12516

Han, K. S., Woo, J., Park, H., Yoon, B. J., Choi, S., and Lee, C. J. (2013). Channel-mediated astrocytic glutamate release via Bestrophin-1 targets synaptic NMDARs. *Mol. Brain* 6:4. doi: 10.1186/1756-6606-6-4

Hedtjärn, M., Leverin, A.-L., Eriksson, K., Blomgren, K., Mallard, C., and Hagberg, H. (2002). Interleukin-18 involvement in hypoxic–ischemic brain injury. *J. Neurosci.* 22, 5910–5919. doi: 10.1523/JNEUROSCI.22-14-05910.2002

Jiang, L., Liu, Y., Ma, M. M., Tang, Y. B., Zhou, J. G., and Guan, Y. Y. (2013). Mitochondria dependent pathway is involved in the protective effect of bestrophin-3 on hydrogen peroxide-induced apoptosis in basilar artery smooth muscle cells. *Apoptosis* 18, 556–565. doi: 10.1007/s10495-013-0828-4

Johnson, G. G., White, M. C., Wu, J.-H., Vallejo, M., and Grimaldi, M. (2014). The deadly connection between endoplasmic reticulum, Ca^{2+}, protein synthesis, and the endoplasmic reticulum stress response in malignant glioma cells. *Neuro Oncol.* 16, 1086–1099. doi: 10.1093/neuonc/nou012

Krämer, F., Stöhr, H., and Weber, B. H. (2004). Cloning and characterization of the murine Vmd2 RFP-TM gene family. *Cytogenet. Res.* 105, 107–114. doi: 10.1159/000078016

Lee, S., Yoon, B. E., Berglund, K., Oh, S. J., Park, H., Shin, H. S., et al. (2010). Channel-mediated tonic GABA release from glia. *Science* 330, 790–796. doi: 10.1126/science.1184334

Lee, W. K., Chakraborty, P. K., Roussa, E., Wolff, N. A., and Thevenod, F. (2012). ERK1/2-dependent bestrophin-3 expression prevents ER-stress-induced cell death in renal epithelial cells by reducing CHOP. *Biochim. Biophys. Acta* 1823, 1864–1876. doi: 10.1016/j.bbamcr.2012.06.003

Lehotský, J., Urban, P., Pavlíková, M., Tatarková, Z., Kaminska, B., and Kaplán, P. (2009). Molecular mechanisms leading to neuroprotection/ischemic tolerance: effect of preconditioning on the stress reaction of endoplasmic reticulum. *Cell. Mol. Neurobiol.* 29, 917–925. doi: 10.1007/s10571-009-9376-4

Leonard, A., Paton, A. W., El-Quadi, M., Paton, J. C., and Fazal, F. (2014). Preconditioning with endoplasmic reticulum stress ameliorates endothelial cell inflammation. *PLoS One* 9:e110949. doi: 10.1371/journal.pone.0110949

Lund, S., Christensen, K. V., Hedtjärn, M., Mortensen, A. L., Hagberg, H., Falsig, J., et al. (2006). The dynamics of the LPS triggered inflammatory response of murine microglia under different culture and in vivo conditions. *J. Neuroimmunol.* 180, 71–87. doi: 10.1016/j.jneuroim.2006.07.007

Marmorstein, L. Y., McLaughlin, P. J., Stanton, J. B., Yan, L., Crabb, J. W., and Marmorstein, A. D. (2002). Bestrophin interacts physically and functionally with protein phosphatase 2A. *J. Biol. Chem.* 277, 30591–30597. doi: 10.1074/jbc.M204269200

Matchkov, V. V., Larsen, P., Bouzinova, E. V., Rojek, A., Boedtkjer, D. M., Golubinskaya, V., et al. (2008). Bestrophin-3 (vitelliform macular dystrophy 2-like 3 protein) is essential for the cGMP-dependent calcium-activated chloride conductance in vascular smooth muscle cells. *Circ. Res.* 103, 864–872. doi: 10.1161/CIRCRESAHA.108.178517

Miura, K., Fujibuchi, W., and Unno, M. (2012). Splice variants in apoptotic pathway. *Exp. Oncol.* 34, 212–217.

Oh, S. J., Han, K. S., Park, H., Woo, D. H., Kim, H. Y., Traynelis, S. F., et al. (2012). Protease activated receptor 1-induced glutamate release in cultured astrocytes is mediated by Bestrophin-1 channel but not by vesicular exocytosis. *Mol. Brain* 5:38. doi: 10.1186/1756-6606-5-38

Oh, S.-J., and Lee, C. J. (2017). Distribution and function of the bestrophin-1 (Best1) channel in the brain. *Exp. Neurobiol.* 26, 113–121. doi: 10.5607/en.2017.26.3.113

Park, H., Oh, S. J., Han, K. S., Woo, D. H., Park, H., Mannaioni, G., et al. (2009). Bestrophin-1 encodes for the Ca^{2+}-activated anion channel in hippocampal astrocytes. *J. Neurosci.* 29, 13063–13073. doi: 10.1523/JNEUROSCI.3193-09.2009

Rice, J. E. III, Vannucci, R. C., and Brierley, J. B. (1981). The influence of immaturity on hypoxic-ischemic brain damage in the rat. *Ann. Neurol.* 9, 131–141. doi: 10.1002/ana.410090206

Sheldon, R. A., Sedik, C., and Ferriero, D. M. (1998). Strain-related brain injury in neonatal mice subjected to hypoxia-ischemia. *Brain Res.* 810, 114–122. doi: 10.1016/S0006-8993(98)00892-0

Singh, K., Han, K., Tilve, S., Wu, K., Geller, H. M., and Sack, M. N. (2018). Parkin targets NOD2 to regulate astrocyte endoplasmic reticulum stress and inflammation. *Glia* 66, 2427–2437. doi: 10.1002/glia.23482

Sizonenko, S. V., Camm, E. J., Dayer, A., and Kiss, J. Z. (2008). Glial responses to neonatal hypoxic-ischemic injury in the rat cerebral cortex. *Int. J. Dev. Neurosci.* 26, 37–45. doi: 10.1016/j.ijdevneu.2007.08.014

Song, W., Yang, Z., and He, B. (2014). Bestrophin 3 ameliorates TNFα-induced inflammation by inhibiting NF-κB activation in endothelial cells. *PLoS One* 9:e111093. doi: 10.1371/journal.pone.0111093

Srivastava, A., Romanenko, V. G., Gonzalez-Begne, M., Catalan, M. A., and Melvin, J. E. (2008). A variant of the Ca^{2+}-activated Cl channel Best3 is expressed in mouse exocrine glands. *J. Membr. Biol.* 222, 43–54. doi: 10.1007/s00232-008-9098-4

Stöhr, H., Marquardt, A., Nanda, I., Schmid, M., and Weber, B. H. (2002). Three novel human VMD2-like genes are members of the evolutionary highly conserved RFP-TM family. *Eur. J. Hum. Genet.* 10, 281–284. doi: 10.1038/sj.ejhg.5200796

Supramaniam, V., Vontell, R., Srinivasan, L., Wyatt-Ashmead, J., Hagberg, H., and Rutherford, M. (2013). Microglia activation in the extremely preterm human brain. *Pediatr. Res.* 73, 301–309. doi: 10.1038/pr.2012.186

Suzuki, T., Sakata, H., Kato, C., Connor, J. A., and Morita, M. (2012). Astrocyte activation and wound healing in intact-skull mouse after focal brain injury. *Eur. J. Neurosci.* 36, 3653–3664. doi: 10.1111/j.1460-9568.2012.08280.x

Vannucci, S. J., and Hagberg, H. (2004). Hypoxia-ischemia in the immature brain. *J. Exp. Biol.* 207, 3149–3154. doi: 10.1242/jeb.01064

Vontell, R., Supramaniam, V., Thornton, C., Wyatt-Ashmead, J., Mallard, C., Gressens, P., et al. (2013). Toll-like receptor 3 expression in glia and neurons alters in response to white matter injury in preterm infants. *Dev. Neurosci.* 35, 130–139. doi: 10.1159/000346158

Vontell, R., Supramaniam, V., Wyatt-Ashmead, J., Gressens, P., Rutherford, M., Hagberg, H., et al. (2015). Cellular mechanisms of toll-like receptor-3 activation in the thalamus are associated with white matter injury in the developing brain. *J. Neuropathol. Exp. Neurol.* 74, 273–285. doi: 10.1097/NEN.0000000000000172

Wu, L., Sun, Y., Ma, L., Zhu, J., Zhang, B., Pan, Q., et al. (2016). A C-terminally truncated mouse Best3 splice variant targets and alters the ion balance in lysosome-endosome hybrids and the endoplasmic reticulum. *Sci. Rep.* 6:27332. doi: 10.1038/srep27332

Xiao, Q., Ford, A. L., Xu, J., Yan, P., Lee, K. Y., Gonzales, E., et al. (2012). Bcl-x pre-mRNA splicing regulates brain injury after neonatal hypoxia-ischemia. *J. Neurosci.* 32, 13587–13596. doi: 10.1523/JNEUROSCI.2617-12.2012

Xu, C., Bailly-Maitre, B., and Reed, J. C. (2005). Endoplasmic reticulum stress: cell life and death decisions. *J. Clin. Invest.* 115, 2656–2664. doi: 10.1172/JCI26373

Zhu, C., Wang, X., Xu, F., Bahr, B. A., Shibata, M., Uchiyama, Y., et al. (2005). The influence of age on apoptotic and other mechanisms of cell death after cerebral hypoxia–ischemia. *Cell Death Differ.* 12, 162–176. doi: 10.1038/sj.cdd.4401545

9

UNICORN Babies: Understanding Circulating and Cerebral Creatine Levels of the Preterm Infant: An Observational Study Protocol

*Mary J. Berry[1,2], Melissa Schlegel[1,2], Greg M. Kowalski[3], Clinton R. Bruce[3], Damien L. Callahan[4], Miranda L. Davies-Tuck[5], Hayley Dickinson[5], Angus Goodson[2], Angie Slocombe[2], Rod J. Snow[3], David W. Walker[6] and Stacey J. Ellery[5]**

[1]Department of Paediatrics and Child Health, University of Otago, Wellington, New Zealand, [2]Capital and Coast District Health Board, Wellington, New Zealand, [3]School of Exercise Sciences, Institute for Physical Activity and Nutrition, Deakin University, Geelong, VIC, Australia, [4]Centre for Cellular and Molecular Biology, School of Life and Environmental Science, Deakin University, Melbourne, VIC, Australia, [5]The Ritchie Centre, Hudson Institute of Medical Research, and Department of Obstetrics and Gynaecology, Monash University, Clayton, VIC, Australia, [6]School of Health and Biomedical Sciences, RMIT University, Melbourne, VIC, Australia

***Correspondence:**
Stacey J. Ellery
stacey.ellery@hudson.org.au

Creatine is an essential metabolite for brain function, with a fundamental role in cellular (ATP) energy homeostasis. It is hypothesized that preterm infants will become creatine deplete in the early postnatal period, due to premature delivery from a maternal source of creatine and a limited supply of creatine in newborn nutrition. This potential alteration to brain metabolism may contribute to, or compound, poor neurological outcomes in this high-risk population. Understanding Creatine for Neurological Health in Babies (UNICORN) is an observational study of circulating and cerebral creatine levels in preterm infants. We will recruit preterm infants at gestational ages 23^{+0}–26^{+6}, 27^{+0}–29^{+6}, 30^{+0}–32^{+6}, 33^{+0}–36^{+6}, and a term reference group at 39^{+0}–40^{+6} weeks of gestation, with 20 infants in each gestational age group. At birth, a maternal capillary blood sample, as well as a venous cord blood sample, will be collected. For preterm infants, serial infant plasma (heel prick), urine, and nutrition samples [total parenteral nutrition (TPN), breast milk, or formula] will be collected between birth and term "due date." Key fetomaternal information, including demographics, smoking status, and maternal diet, will also be collected. At term corrected postnatal age (CPA), each infant will undergo an MRI/^{1}H-MRS scan to evaluate brain structure and measure cerebral creatine content. A general movements assessment (GMA) will also be conducted. At 3 months of CPA, infants will undergo a second GMA as well as further neurodevelopmental evaluation using the Developmental Assessment of Young Children – Second Edition (DAYC-2) assessment tool. The primary outcome measures for this study are cerebral creatine content at CPA and plasma and urine creatine and guanidinoacetate (creatine precursor) concentrations in the early postnatal period. We will also determine associations between (1) creatine levels at term CPA and neurodevelopmental outcomes (MRI, GMA, and DAY-C); (2) dietary creatine intake and circulating and cerebral creatine content; and (3) creatine levels and maternal characteristics. Novel approaches are needed to try and improve preterm-associated brain injury. Inclusion of creatine in preterm nutrition may better support *ex utero* brain development through improved cerebral cellular energy availability during a period of significant brain growth and development.

Ethics Ref: HDEC 18/CEN/7 New Zealand.

ACTRN: ACTRN12618000871246.

Keywords: premature, nutrition, brain metabolism, cellular energy, neurodevelopment

INTRODUCTION

The global incidence of preterm birth (delivery prior to 37 completed weeks of gestation) is reported to be ~11% (Blencowe et al., 2013). Advances in perinatal care mean that increasing numbers of infants born even at extremes of gestational age (extreme preterm: <28 weeks of gestational age) survive beyond the neonatal period (Davidoff et al., 2006; Mohangoo et al., 2011; Lawn et al., 2013). Additionally, within resource-rich neonatal care settings, the age of human viability continues to fall with increasing survival rates at even 22 and 23 weeks of gestational age. However, this increase in survival has not been coupled with a reduction in long-term morbidity. Neurodevelopmental disorders, including those of executive function, psychiatric, and behavioral sequelae (Blencowe et al., 2013), are more prevalent in those born preterm than at term, with increasing risk, the lesser the gestational age at birth (Crump et al., 2010; Johnson et al., 2010).

The etiology of brain injury in preterm infants is complex and often unexplained. Historically, intraventricular hemorrhage (IVH) with resultant disruption of brain tissue and formation of macrocystic lesions was associated with global developmental delay. With the improvements in perinatal care, high grade IVH and/or periventricular leukomalacia (PVL) has become far less common, and standard cranial ultrasound or magnetic resonance imaging (MRI) examination usually do not demonstrate gross structural lesions (Penn et al., 2016). In Australia and New Zealand, the rate of high grade IVH in infants born prior to 32 weeks' gestation declined from 8% to just over 4% in the period between 2004 and 2013 (Chow et al., 2013). As such, longitudinal studies now indicate that a large percentage of children born preterm have neurodevelopmental problems in the absence of structural brain abnormalities detected with conventional imaging (Constable et al., 2008; Mullen et al., 2011; Aeby et al., 2013). These data suggest that conventional prognostication based on measures of cerebral structure is poorly discriminatory and will not always identify infants at risk of neurodevelopmental morbidity. We, and others, propose that our focus should be widened to explore the role of altered brain metabolism in the pathophysiology of preterm brain injury and neurodevelopmental disability (Koob et al., 2016).

Creatine is a metabolite essential for brain development and energy metabolism (Braissant et al., 2007). It is an amino acid derivative that fuels the creatine kinase circuit; a phosphagen system that mitigates temporal imbalances in energy (ATP) supply and demand (Wallimann et al., 1992). *Via* the creatine kinase circuit, creatine and its phosphorylated derivative (phosphocreatine, PCr) shuttle high-energy phosphate groups from the mitochondria into the cytosol, for the regeneration of ATP from ADP (Ellington, 2001). The creatine kinase isoforms required to run the circuit are found in the cerebellum, choroid plexus, hippocampal granular layer, and pyramidal cells of the brain (Hemmer et al., 1994) and are involved in maintaining ATP homeostasis in the central nervous system (CNS) from early in embryonic development through to adulthood (Braissant et al., 2001; Braissant et al., 2007).

Both creatine and phosphocreatine are spontaneously broken down into creatinine at a rate of ~1.7%/day (Brosnan and Brosnan, 2007). Thus, there is a requirement to replenish creatine and PCr stores on a daily basis. Creatine can be obtained from the diet and is also endogenously synthesized *de novo*. Synthesis involves the production of guanidinoacetate (GAA) from arginine and glycine, in a reaction catalyzed by arginine:glycine aminotransferase (AGAT) that occurs predominately in the kidney and pancreas. GAA is then methylated by guanidinoacetate N-methyltransferase (GAMT), mainly in the liver, to produce creatine. Once synthesized or absorbed, creatine is transported into cells *via* the sodium-dependent SLC6A8 creatine transporter (Wyss and Kaddurah-Daouk, 2000). Creatine is able to cross the blood-brain barrier (Ohtsuki et al., 2002), and the brain itself also has some inherent capacity to synthesize creatine, with both AGAT and GAMT expressed by neurons, astrocytes, and oligodendrocytes (Braissant et al., 2001; Tachikawa et al., 2004; Nakashima et al., 2005). Despite the importance of creatine for brain growth and development, the relative importance of cerebral creatine derived from systemic rather than local synthesis has not yet been established.

In utero fetal magnetic resonance spectroscopy (^{1}H-MRS) studies indicate cerebral creatine accretion occurs from 18 to 40 weeks of gestation (Evangelou et al., 2015). Postnatal studies have also clearly identified that an increase in cerebral creatine concentration occurs during the first 3 months of life (Blüml et al., 2012; Blüml et al., 2014). The importance of a maternal source of creatine for the developing fetus and the continued postnatal accretion of cerebral creatine is made evident by those infants diagnosed with inherited creatine deficiency syndromes. These infants typically raise no concerns antenatally; however, as postnatal creatine levels fall, they become progressively more symptomatic with altered neurological state

(Almeida et al., 2006) and complex neurological symptoms including impaired psychomotor development, seizures, and cognitive impairment (Battini et al., 2006).

In adults, creatine is acquired *via* the diet and *de novo* synthesis, with each contributing ~50% (Brosnan and Brosnan, 2007). However, in infancy, due to low levels of creatine in human breast milk and commercial formulas, a term infant most likely synthesizes between 64 and 93% of their daily creatine requirements (Edison et al., 2013). The age at which a fetus/newborn develops the capacity to synthesize creatine is currently unknown, but it requires sufficient renal, hepatic, and cerebral maturity to express the enzymes necessary for creatine synthesis. Evaluation of AGAT and GAMT expression in the rat embryo found that AGAT was expressed in isolated cells of the CNS from 0.6 gestation; however, widespread expression of AGAT and rudimentary GAMT expression were not apparent before 0.8 gestation (Braissant et al., 2005). Our own studies in the precocial spiny mouse found that the fetal kidney and liver do not express AGAT and GAMT before 0.9 gestation, an age and maturation equivalent to ~35 weeks' human gestation (Ireland et al., 2009). Taken together, these observations raise compelling questions about progressive creatine depletion in preterm infants, and whether this complication of nutritional compromise predisposes or compounds their risk of altered cerebral metabolism and thus long-term neurodevelopmental disability.

To date, a number of small observational studies have identified perturbations in creatine homeostasis in preterm infants (Blüml et al., 2014; Koob et al., 2016). Koob et al. (2016) reported that at term CPA creatine concentrations in the centrum semiovale of infants born preterm (born 29.1 ± 2 weeks) were reduced compared to those born at term (Koob et al., 2016). In addition, Lage et al. (2013) found that by hospital discharge, preterm infants had higher urinary GAA and reduced urinary creatine excretion, suggesting differences in systemic creatine synthesizing capacity. This was particularly apparent in their very preterm group (28–29 weeks) (Lage et al., 2013).

No studies have characterized longitudinal changes in creatine metabolism among preterm infants or the association between cerebral creatine content and neurodevelopmental outcomes. Further to this, no studies have monitored systemic creatine levels (both circulating and excreted) in a single preterm population nor have they assessed nutritional creatine availability for preterm infants fed with total parenteral nutrition (TPN), preterm infant formulas, or breast milk.

We hypothesize that following preterm birth, peripheral and cerebral creatine levels will fall, so that at term CPA, preterm infants will have relative systemic and cerebral creatine deficiency. Furthermore, this reduction in creatine bioavailability will jeopardize normal brain metabolism and development, ultimately predisposing the infant to neurodevelopmental dysfunction.

The overall aim of this study is to assess whether preterm infants become creatine deplete in the early postnatal period, by measuring the preterm infants' circulating and excreted levels of creatine and GAA and comparing these measures to cerebral creatine content, as determined by ^{1}H-MRS, at term corrected age. This study will correlate preterm creatine levels with neurological outcomes using MRI, general movements assessment (GMA), and the Developmental Assessment of Young Children – Second Edition (DAYC-2) Test (Novak et al., 2017). This study will also establish the levels of creatine provided through dietary intake during the days and weeks after preterm birth. Results of this study may support the use of creatine supplementation as standard nutritional care of the preterm infant, in order to improve neurodevelopmental function in this vulnerable population.

Specific Aims

1. Compare cerebral, plasma, and urine creatine and GAA content between preterm and term infants at CPA.
2. Describe preterm infant plasma and urine creatine and GAA concentrations and creatine:GAA ratio in the early postnatal period.
3. Describe associations between cerebral creatine content, plasma, and urine creatine concentrations with maternal and infant characteristics at CPA.
4. Compare creatine, GAA, arginine, glycine, and methionine concentrations in standard preterm nutrition, including TPN, preterm infant formulas, and breast milk.
5. Determine whether dietary source of creatine (TPN, formula, or breast milk) is related to plasma or urine creatine concentrations in the early postnatal period.
6. Describe associations between cerebral creatine content and blood and urine creatine concentrations with neurological outcomes (GMA, MRI, and DAYC-2) at CPA and at 3 months of corrected postnatal age.

METHOD/DESIGN

Study Design

Prospective, single-center, observational study.

Study Setting

Neonatal Intensive Care Unit and Postnatal Wards, Capital Coast District Hospital Board (CCDHB), Wellington, New Zealand.

Primary Outcome Measures

1. Cerebral creatine content at term CPA
2. Plasma (bi-weekly) and urine (weekly) creatine and GAA levels from birth until hospital discharge and at CPA
3. Creatine, GAA, and amino acid levels in infant nutrition (TPN, formula, or breast milk) supplied from birth until discharge and at CPA

Secondary Outcome Measures

1. Global injury score from MRI at term CPA
2. General movement assessment score at term CPA and 3 months of CPA
3. DAYC-2 assessment score at 3 months of CPA

Study Population

Inclusion Criteria

1. Preterm infants receiving care within the Neonatal Intensive Care Unit at CCDHB or healthy term infants at 39–40 weeks' gestation from low-risk pregnancies delivered at CCDHB.

Exclusion Criteria

1. Babies with major congenital, genetic, or chromosomal abnormalities known to affect neurodevelopmental outcomes
2. Hypoxic ischemic encephalopathy
3. Inborn (proven or suspected) errors of metabolism
4. Fetal growth restriction (birth weight < 10th percentile on customized percentiles)

Recruitment

We will recruit infants at gestational ages 23^{+0}–26^{+6}, 27^{+0}–29^{+6}, 30^{+0}–32^{+6}, 33^{+0}–36^{+6}, and 39^{+0}–40^{+6} weeks. We will aim to capture 20 infants at each time point (with equal numbers of males and females). Eligible infants will be identified based on gestational age at delivery and consideration of inclusion and exclusion criteria. Pregnant women will be approached at presentation to Delivery Suite to discuss study participation. If consent is obtained, the mother and infant will be recruited to the study and the consulting obstetric, midwifery, neonatal, and nursing team advised of their involvement. Where pre-delivery consent is not obtained due to rapidity of labor and/or other clinical factors, cord blood will be collected preemptively, and retrospective consent and maternal blood sample sought within 24 h of delivery. If the parents do not wish to participate, the cord blood sample will be disposed of using routine clinical biological waste disposal systems and no further study samples collected.

Sample and Data Collection

Blood, Urine, and Nutrition Sampling

A schematic overview of the sampling regime for each participant is outlined in **Figure 1**. At the time of birth, we will use a finger prick to collect ~120 μl of maternal whole blood using a capillary tube. A 2-ml venous cord blood sample will also be collected from which a ~120 μl sample will be obtained using a capillary tube. Then, while infants are receiving care in the NICU, or on postnatal wards, and at follow-up appointments, the following samples will be collected. Sample frequency will be dictated by gestational age at birth.

Blood sampling: A blood sample will be collected biweekly. We will perform a heel prick to collect ~120 μl of whole blood using a capillary tube. All blood samples (cord, maternal, or infant) will be transferred to a Hemaspot™ SE blood separation device to facilitate collection of the cell-free blood fraction (referred to throughout as plasma for clarity) from a small volume of whole blood. Hemaspots are allowed to dry at room temperature before being stored at −20°C for future analysis.

Urine sampling: Around the same time as the blood collection, and on each alternate week, we will place some gauze into the infant's nappy to facilitate a spot urine collection. Once obtained, this sample will be transferred to an Eppendorf tube and stored at −80°C for future analysis.

Nutrition sampling: A 200 μl sample of the nutrition (TNP, formula, and breast milk) being fed to each infant at the time of the blood and urine sampling will be collected. If in powdered form (formula), this will be reconstituted following standard practices. All samples will be transferred into an Eppendorf tube and stored at −80°C for future analysis.

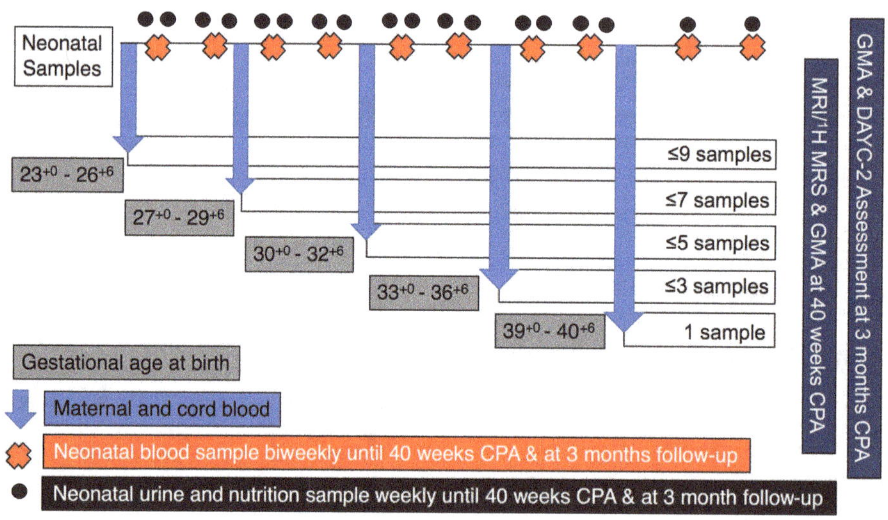

FIGURE 1 | Schematic representation of UNICORN sampling regime. Samples of neonatal blood, urine, and nutrition will be collected weekly or bi-weekly for the duration of the infants stay in hospital. Magnetic resonance imaging (MRI) and magnetic resonance spectroscopy (^{1}H-MRS) will be performed at term corrected postnatal age (CPA). Infants will also undergo a general movements assessment (GMA) at CPA and at 3 months CPA. At the follow-up appointment at 3 months CPA, further neurological assessment will be completed using the Developmental Assessment of Young Children – Second Edition (DAYC-2) assessment tool.

Monitoring and Data Collection

The following covariates/potential confounders will be collected as part of this study:

Maternal characteristics and birth outcomes data:

- Maternal age
- Comorbidities/factors (preeclampsia, gestational diabetes, chorioamnionitis, IVF)
- Country of birth
- Dietary preferences (omnivorous, vegetarian, vegan)
- Smoking status
- Parity
- Gravity
- Mode of delivery
- Placental weight

Infant characteristics:

- Gestational age
- Sex
- Birth weight
- Ethnicity
- Weight and corrected postnatal age at the time of each sample collection
- Presence of postnatal infection (blood culture positive and/or treatment with systemic antibiotics for >24 h) or necrotizing enterocolitis (Modified Bells Classification Grade II-III determined by the treating Pediatric Surgeon at time of diagnosis).
- Feeding schedule prior to each sample collection (<24 h)
- Venous hemoglobin and hematocrit count prior to blood sample collection

MRI/^{1}H-MRS Data Acquisition

At 40 weeks of corrected postnatal age (CPA), each participant will undergo a MRI/^{1}H-MRS scan. MR examinations will be performed on a Siemens 3T Skyra using a 16-channel dedicated pediatric head coil. Infants will be examined without sedation using a "feed and wrap" technique according to standard institutional practice. In brief, infants are brought to the MRI unit, fed, and swaddled comfortably while being monitored with continuous pulse oximetry before being placed in the MRI scanner. Standard, size appropriate, hearing protection will be used for all infants. Sequences will be performed to demonstrate brain anatomy and will include T1 3D 1 mm volumetric, T2 1 mm 3D volumetric scans, T2 TSE FLAIR, and T1SE MTC sequences. These sequences will also contribute to the analysis of any detected brain pathology. T2 SWI axial images will be performed to show calcification and blood products. Sequences for the detection of vascular injury and infarction will include diffusion sequences (b value = 2000), resting BOLD, and arterial spin labeling. ^{1}H-MRS will provide chemical spectra of the brain to further analyze brain pathology and measurement of cerebral creatine content. For MR spectroscopy, the voxel will be placed over the white matter underlying the central sulcus within the centrum semiovale and spectra acquired with a long echo time (TE 135 ms) (Koob et al., 2016).

Neurodevelopmental Observations

At term CPA, prior to the MRI/^{1}H-MRS scan, an experienced neurodevelopmental therapist will record a 5-minute video of the infant to conduct a general movements assessment (GMA); a validated tool to noninvasively identify neurological issues, which may lead to cerebral palsy and other developmental disabilities (Spittle et al., 2018). Infants are placed in a supine position, with minimal clothing to allow freedom of movement. The video will be taken when the infant is fully alert, but not directly interacting with parents, healthcare providers, or receiving stimulus from any external sources.

At 3 months of CPA, we will request participants meet again with a developmental therapist. At this appointment, information about general health (including weight gain trajectories, feeding habits, and number of visits to a GP) will be recorded. A questionnaire about developmental milestones at 3 months of age (developed by the American Academy of Pediatrics) will be completed, as well as a Developmental Assessment of Young Children – Second Edition (DAYC-2) Test, a validated tool to identify children with possible developmental delay in the following domains: cognition, communication, social-emotional development, physical development, and adaptive behavior (Saleh and Smadi, 2017). A 5-minute video of the infant will also be recorded to allow for a second GMA to be completed.

Sample and Data Analysis

Creatine, GAA, and Amino Acid Analysis

Creatine, GAA, arginine, glycine, and methionine will be measured in biological and nutrition samples *via* LC-MS/MS, according to the methods of (Tran et al., 2014), with slight modification (Tran et al., 2014). Briefly, a 6-mm hole punch of the "cell-free" plasma fraction of the Hemaspot™, 7 µl of urine, nutrition, or unlabeled standard, will be transferred to 1.5-ml safety lock Eppendorf tubes. 200 µl of methanol containing 10 µM 2,2-d_3 Creatine (Sigma), 2.5 µM 2,2-d_2 GAA (Sigma), and 2.5 µM of Labeled Amino Acid Standard Set A (Cambridge Isotope Laboratories Inc.) internal standards is added to each tube. Samples are sonicated for 5 min then vortexed for 20 min, before being centrifuged at 20,000× g for 5 min to pellet any precipitate or filter paper at the bottom of the tube. Supernatant (~170 µl) is transferred into 250-µl glass inserts placed in 2-ml glass vials (Agilent), followed by evaporation to complete dryness in a speed vacuum (Labconco, Kansas, MO, USA). After drying, the GAA and creatine carboxyl groups are derivatized (butylated) by the addition of 100 µl of 3 M butanol-HCL followed by incubation at 60°C for 30 min. After cooling to room temperature, excess butanol-HCL is evaporated under speed vacuum, after which the dry residue is resuspended in 200 µl of methanol: water (1:1 v/v) solution prior to LC-MS/MS analysis. The external standards consist of an eight sample serial dilution series of known concentration range (0–25 µM unlabeled GAA and 0–100 µM unlabeled creatine).

The LC-MS/MS system is composed of a vacuum degasser, binary pumps, column oven, and a temperature-controlled autosampler (Shimadzu, Nexera® UPLC). This will be interfaced with a triple quadrupole mass spectrometer (Shimadzu, LCMS-8030) with electrospray ionization. The LC column (Agilent

–2.1 × 100 mm, 1.8 μm C18 Zorbax Eclipse plus) will be maintained at 30°C and elution carried out with a binary gradient mobile phase at a flow rate of 0.4 ml min^{-1}. Mobile phase A will contain water with 0.1% formic acid, and mobile phase B will contain acetonitrile with 0.1% formic acid. The initial mobile phase composition will be 5% B, which is ramped linearly to 50% B over 6 min followed by a 2-min column wash at 100% B, with the column finally undergoing re-equilibration at 5% B for 3 min, thus yielding a total runtime of 11 min. The first 1 min is diverted to waste. The following ESI source conditions will be used: nebulizer gas flow rate 3 L min^{-1}, desolvation line temperature at 250°C, heater block temperature 400°C, and drying gas flow rate of 15 L min^{-1}. The MS will be operated in positive ionization with multiple reaction monitoring (MRM). The collision energy, Q1 and Q3 pre-bias voltages for the MRM transitions have been optimized using authentic creatine and GAA standards (SIGMA) *via* the automatic optimisation software (Labsolutions, Shimadzu), with optimal collision energy for creatine and GAA for the instrument being −15 eV. The precursor and product ion transitions were creatine 188.2–90 *m/z*, d_3-Creatine 191.2–93 *m/z*, GAA 174.2–101.1 *m/z*, and d_2-GAA 176.1–103.1 *m/z*. The sample and standard injection volume will be 5 μl. Peak areas will be determined using Lab solutions post-run browser software (Shimadzu). The creatine, GAA and amino acid concentrations of blood spots, urine, or nutrition samples will be calculated *via* linear regression of the serially diluted external (unlabeled) standard series using the isotope dilution technique.

MRI/^{1}H-MRS

MRI images will be scored according to the Kidokoro assessment tool (Kidokoro et al., 2013). Briefly, cerebral white matter, cortical gray matter, deep gray matter, and cerebellar abnormalities will be independently graded, and then the scores combined to calculate a single global brain injury score. The assessor will also note the presence of hemorrhage or cystic lesions throughout the brain. Hemorrhagic lesions will be graded using the Papile classification system (Papile et al., 1978) and cystic lesions characterized as periventricular leukomalacia, periventricular hemorrhagic infarction, or other (Barkovich, 2000).

Metabolic ratios from ^{1}H-MRS spectra obtained with a TE of 135 ms will be calculated as previously described, with water used as an internal reference to normalize metabolite signal intensities (Koob et al., 2016).

Neurodevelopmental Observations

Motor function will be assessed by a developmental therapist trained in GMA and blinded to the clinical history of the infant. At term CPA, infants will be assessed on withering movements, which should include complex movements of the arms, legs, neck, and trunk. Poor withering movements include rigid or chaotic movements that lack fluency and coordination (Spittle et al., 2013) and are predictive of adverse neurodevelopmental outcomes. At 3 months of CPA, infants will be assessed on fidgety movements, which appear as small continual movements of limbs in all directions. Poor quality fidgety movements include larger amplitude and jerking movements (Spittle et al., 2013) and are again predictive of later outcomes. Infants will be scored independently at each postnatal age.

At 3-month CPA, infants' development will also be reviewed using the DAYC-2 assessment tool (Saleh and Smadi, 2017). An overall score from the five domains tested (cognition, communication, social-emotional development, physical development, and adaptive behavior) will be generated for each infant. Collectively, MRI, GMA, and DAYC-2 scores will be used to assess the potential risk of poor neurological outcomes, based on early diagnosis strategies for cerebral palsy (Novak et al., 2017).

Sample Size

This study will be the first observational study of creatine homeostasis in the preterm infant that encompasses plasma, urine, nutrition, and cerebral creatine measures across time. As the outcomes are mainly descriptive, no formal power calculation has been performed. However, ^{1}H-MRS results reported by Koob et al. (2016) showed comparison of 13 preterm vs term infants allowed for measurement of a statistically significant (−17%) reduction in cerebral creatine content in preterm infants at CPA ($tCr/H_20 \times 10^{-3}$; term 0.12 ± 0.1 vs preterm 0.10 ± 0.1). This same study had a 20–25% failure rate in obtaining accurate MRI/^{1}H-MRS measurements at CPA (Koob et al., 2016). Taking these data into consideration and a potential loss to follow-up at 3-month of 20%, we aim to capture 20 infants in each gestational group.

Statistical Analysis

Characteristics of the population will be tabulated, along with appropriate descriptive statistics of the study sample. Continuous data will be assessed for normality and expressed as means and standard deviations or median and interquartile range as appropriate. Categorical data will be expressed as counts and proportions. Average creatine content from nutrition per week for each baby in the early postnatal period will be calculated.

Differences in creatine and GAA measures (^{1}H-MRS, plasma or urine) between infants born preterm and those born at term will be assessed at CPA using a t-test or Mann-Whitney U test as appropriate. The correlation between gestational age at birth and creatine and GAA measures at CPA will also be determined using a Spearman or Pearson correlation. Preterm infant plasma and urine creatine and GAA concentrations and creatine:GAA ratio in the early postnatal period will be described and plotted. Associations between cerebral creatine content, plasma and urine creatine concentrations with maternal, and infant characteristics at CPA will be determined using Spearman or Pearson correlations for continuous data (maternal age, gestational age, birth weight, parity, gravity, placental weight) or a t-test or Mann-Whitney U test for categorical data (infant sex, mode of delivery, maternal comorbidities, country of birth, ethnicity, and dietary preferences), as appropriate. Differences in creatine, GAA, and amino acid content of nutrition sources (TNP, formula or breast milk) will be determined using a one-way ANOVA or Kruskal-Wallis H test as appropriate. The association between creatine, GAA, and amino acid content of nutrition sources (TNP, formula or breast milk) and infant plasma and urine creatine at CPA will be assessed using a Spearman or Pearson correlation as appropriate. Finally, the association between cerebral creatine content, plasma creatine levels, and the ratio of plasma:cerebral creatine at CPA with GMA, MRI global injury, and DAYC-2 scores will be determined using linear regression at both CPA and at 3 months' corrected postnatal age. Potential confounders such as gestational age and maternal and infant characteristics will be assessed, along with collinearity, prior to performing multivariable linear regression.

DISCUSSION

Both creatine and the creatine kinase circuit are critical for brain metabolism (Braissant et al., 2011). It is hypothesized that preterm infants will become creatine deplete in the early postnatal period, due to premature delivery from a maternal source of creatine *in utero,* limited capacity for endogenous synthesis postnatally, and a limited supply of creatine in newborn nutrition. This creatine depletion may alter cerebral creatine metabolism, contributing to or compounding the risk of neurological disability in this population.

We anticipate that preterm babies will have altered creatine homeostasis and reduced creatine accretion in the early postnatal period compared to an infant of the same postconceptional age. Whether or not relative creatine deficiency is associated with neurological deficit will be a secondary outcome of this study. As the results are mainly descriptive and a formal power calculation could not be completed, there is the possibility that sample size may become a limitation for some of the proposed analyses in this observational study. However, the data obtained will enable calculation of effect size for future studies. If our overall hypothesis is supported, this observational study will inform a future randomized control trial of infant dietary creatine supplementation following premature birth, with the aim of improving brain metabolism during a key stage of development and thereby reducing the burden of neurodevelopmental disability in this high-risk population.

AUTHOR CONTRIBUTIONS

MB, SE, HD, and DW conceptualized the study. MS is a research nurse coordinating recruitment, sample collection, and data management. AG was involved in ethics development and study design. GK, CB, DC, and RS developed the LC-MS/MS protocol for creatine and metabolite assessment. AS developed the MR data acquisition protocol. MD-T designed the statistical approaches to the study. MB and SE wrote the manuscript. All authors contributed to the drafting of the manuscript.

FUNDING

The authors would like to acknowledge funding support from the Cerebral Palsy Alliance (PG2715) and Rebecca L Cooper Medical Research Foundation (10624) for the completion of this study.

REFERENCES

Aeby, A., De Tiège, X., Creuzil, M., David, P., Balériaux, D., Van Overmeire, B., et al. (2013). Language development at 2 years is correlated to brain microstructure in the left superior temporal gyrus at term equivalent age: a diffusion tensor imaging study. *Neuroimage* 78, 145–151. doi: 10.1016/j.neuroimage.2013.03.076

Almeida, L. G. S., Rosenberg, E. H., Verhoeven, N. M., Jakobs, C., and Salomons, G. S. (2006). Are cerebral creatine deficiency syndromes on the radar screen? *Future Neurol.* 1, 637–649. doi: 10.2217/14796708.1.5.637

Barkovich, A. J. (2000). Brain and spine injury in infancy and childhood. *J. Pediatr. Neurol.* 30, 157–250.

Battini, R., Alessandri, M., Leuzzi, V., Moro, F., Tosetti, M., Bianchi, M., et al. (2006). Arginine:glycine amidinotransferase (AGAT) deficiency in a newborn: early treatment can prevent phenotypic expression of the disease. *J. Pediatr.* 148, 828–830. doi: 10.1016/j.jpeds.2006.01.043

Blencowe, H., Cousens, S., Chou, D., Oestergaard, M., Say, L., Moller, A. -B., et al. (2013). Born too soon: the global epidemiology of 15 million preterm births. *Reprod. Health* 10:S2. doi: 10.1186/1742-4755-10-S1-S2

Blüml, S., Wisnowski, J. L., Nelson, M. D. Jr., Paquette, L., Gilles, F. H., Kinney, H. C., et al. (2012). Metabolic maturation of the human brain from birth through adolescence: insights from in vivo magnetic resonance spectroscopy. *Cereb. Cortex* 23, 2944–2955. doi: 10.1093/cercor/bhs283

Blüml, S., Wisnowski, J. L. Nelson, M. D. Jr., Paquette, L., and Panigrahy, A. (2014). Metabolic maturation of white matter is altered in preterm infants. *PLoS One* 9:E85829. doi: 10.1371/journal.pone.0085829

Braissant, O., Bachmann, C., and Henry, H. (2007). "Expression and function of AGAT, GAMT and CT1 in the mammalian brain" in *Creatine and creatine kinase in health and disease.* Subcellular Biochemistry. eds. G. S. Salomons, and M. Wyss vol 46, (Dordrecht: Springer). doi: 10.1007/978-1-4020-6486-9_4

Braissant, O., Henry, H., Béard, E., and Uldry, J. (2011). Creatine deficiency syndromes and the importance of creatine synthesis in the brain. *Amino Acids* 40, 1315–1324. doi: 10.1007/s00726-011-0852-z

Braissant, O., Henry, H., Loup, M., Eilers, B., and Bachmann, C. (2001). Endogenous synthesis and transport of creatine in the rat brain: an in situ hybridization study. *Mol. Brain Res.* 86, 193–201. doi: 10.1016/S0169-328X(00)00269-2

Braissant, O., Henry, H., Villard, A. -M., Speer, O., Wallimann, T., and Bachmann, C. (2005). Creatine synthesis and transport during rat embryogenesis: spatiotemporal expression of AGAT, GAMT and CT1. *BMC Dev. Biol.* 5:9. doi: 10.1186/1471-213X-5-9

Brosnan, J., and Brosnan, M. (2007). Creatine: endogenous metabolite, dietary, and therapeutic supplement. *Annu. Rev. Nutr.* 27, 241–261. doi: 10.1146/annurev.nutr.27.061406.093621

Chow, S., Le Marsney, R., Hossain, S., Haslam, R., and Lui, K. (2013). *Report Of The Australian And New Zealand Neonatal Network 2012.* Sydney: Anznn.

Constable, R. T., Ment, L. R., Vohr, B. R., Kesler, S. R., Fulbright, R. K., Lacadie, C., et al. (2008). Prematurely born children demonstrate white matter microstructural differences at 12 years of age, relative to term control subjects: an investigation of group and gender effects. *Pediatrics* 121, 306–316. doi: 10.1542/peds.2007-0414

Crump, C., Winkleby, M. A., Sundquist, K., and Sundquist, J. (2010). Preterm birth and psychiatric medication prescription in young adulthood: a Swedish national cohort study. *Int. J. Epidemiol.* 39, 1522–1530. doi: 10.1093/ije/dyq103

Davidoff, M. J., Dias, T., Damus, K., Russell, R., Bettegowda, V. R., Dolan, S., et al. (2006). Changes in the gestational age distribution among us singleton births: impact on rates of late preterm birth, 1992 to 2002. *Semin. Perinatol.* 30, 8–15. doi: 10.1053/j.semperi.2006.01.009

Edison, E. E., Brosnan, M. E., Aziz, K., and Brosnan, J. T. (2013). Creatine and guanidinoacetate content of human milk and infant formulas: implications for creatine deficiency syndromes and amino acid metabolism. *Br. J. Nutr.* 110, 1075–1078. doi: 10.1017/S000711451300010X

Ellington, W. R. (2001). Evolution and physiological roles of phosphagen systems. *Annu. Rev. Physiol.* 63, 289–325. doi: 10.1146/annurev.physiol.63.1.289

Evangelou, I. E., Du Plessis, A. J., Vezina, G., Noeske, R., and Limperopoulos, C. (2015). Elucidating metabolic maturation in the healthy fetal brain using 1h-mr spectroscopy. *Am. J. Neuroradiol.* doi: 10.3174/ajnr.A4512

Hemmer, W., Zanolla, E., Furter-Graves, E. M., Eppenberger, H. M., and Wallimann, T. (1994). Creatine kinase isoenzymes in chicken cerebellum: specific localization of brain-type creatine kinase in Bergmann glial cells and muscle-type creatine kinase in Purkinje neurons. *Eur. J. Neurosci.* 6, 538–549. doi: 10.1111/j.1460-9568.1994.tb00298.x

Ireland, Z., Russell, A., Wallimann, T., Walker, D. and Snow, R. (2009). Developmental changes in the expression of creatine synthesizing enzymes and creatine transporter in a precocial rodent, the spiny mouse. *BMC Dev. Biol.* 9, 39–50. doi: 10.1186/1471-213X-9-39

Johnson, S., Hollis, C., Kochhar, P., Hennessy, E., Wolke, D., and Marlow, N. (2010). Psychiatric disorders in extremely preterm children: longitudinal finding at age 11 years in the epicure study. *J. Am. Acad. Child Adolesc. Psychiatry* 49, 453–463.e1. doi: 10.1016/j.jaac.2010.02.002

Kidokoro, H., Neil, J., and Inder, T. (2013). New MR imaging assessment tool to define brain abnormalities in very preterm infants at term. *Am. J. Neuroradiol.* doi: 10.1681/ASN.2012080783

Koob, M., Viola, A., Le Fur, Y., Viout, P., Ratiney, H., Confort-Gouny, S., et al. (2016). Creatine, glutamine plus glutamate, and macromolecules are decreased in the central white matter of premature neonates around term. *PLoS One* 11:E0160990. doi: 10.1371/journal.pone.0160990

Lage, S., Andrade, F., Prieto, J. A., Asla, I., Rodríguez, A., Ruiz, N., et al. (2013). Arginine-guanidinoacetate-creatine pathway in preterm newborns: creatine biosynthesis in newborns. *J. Pediatr. Endocrinol. Metab.* 26, 53–60. doi: 10.1515/jpem-2012-0293

Lawn, J. E., Davidge, R., Paul, V. K., Von Xylander, S., De Graft Johnson, J., Costello, A., et al. (2013). Born too soon: care for the preterm baby. *Reprod. Health* 10:S5. doi: 10.1186/1742-4755-10-S1-S5

Mohangoo, A. D., Buitendijk, S. E., Szamotulska, K., Chalmers, J., Irgens, L. M., Bolumar, F., et al. (2011). Gestational age patterns of fetal and neonatal mortality in Europe: results from the Euro-Peristat project. *PLoS One* 6:E24727. doi: 10.1371/journal.pone.0024727

Mullen, K. M., Vohr, B. R., Katz, K. H., Schneider, K. C., Lacadie, C., Hampson, M., et al. (2011). Preterm birth results in alterations in neural connectivity at age 16 years. *NeuroImage* 54, 2563–2570. doi: 10.1016/j.neuroimage.2010.11.019

Nakashima, T., Tomi, M., Tachikawa, M., Watanabe, M., Terasaki, T., and Hosoya, K. I. (2005). Evidence for creatine biosynthesis in Müller glia. *Glia* 52, 47–52. doi: 10.1002/glia.20222

Novak, I., Morgan, C., Adde, L., Blackman, J., Boyd, R. N., Brunstrom-Hernandez, J., et al. (2017). Early, accurate diagnosis and early intervention in cerebral palsy: advances in diagnosis and treatment. *JAMA Pediatr.* 171, 897–907. doi: 10.1001/jamapediatrics.2017.1689

Ohtsuki, S., Tachikawa, M., Takanaga, H., Shimizu, H., Watanabe, M., Hosoya, K. -I., et al. (2002). The blood-brain barrier creatine transporter is a major pathway for supplying creatine to the brain. *J. Cereb. Blood Flow Metab.* 22, 1327–1335. doi: 10.1097/01.WCB.0000033966.83623.7D

Papile, L. -A., Burstein, J., Burstein, R., and Koffler, H. (1978). Incidence and evolution of subependymal and intraventricular hemorrhage: a study of infants with birth weights less than 1,500 Gm. *J. Pediatr.* 92, 529–534. doi: 10.1016/S0022-3476(78)80282-0

Penn, A. A., Gressens, P., Fleiss, B., Back, S. A., and Gallo, V. (2016). Controversies in preterm brain injury. *Neurobiol. Dis.* 92, 90–101. doi: 10.1016/j.nbd.2015.10.012

Saleh, R. M. A., and Smadi, J. M. (2017). The efficacy of arabic version of the developmental assessment of young children second edition (Dayc-2) scale in detecting developmental delay among Jordanian children aged birth to 71 months. *Int. Educ. Stud.* 10, 113–132. doi: 10.5539/ies.v10n4p113

Spittle, A. J., Morgan, C., Olsen, J. E., Novak, I., and Cheong, J. L. (2018). Early diagnosis and treatment of cerebral palsy in children with a history of preterm birth. *Clin Perinatol.* doi: 10.1111/jpc.14149

Spittle, A. J., Spencer-Smith, M. M., Cheong, J. L., Eeles, A. L., Lee, K. J., Anderson, P. J., et al. (2013). General movements in very preterm children and neurodevelopment at 2 and 4 years. *Pediatr. Peds.* 45. doi: 10.1016/j.clp.2018.05.011

Tachikawa, M., Fukaya, M., Terasaki, T., Ohtsuki, S., and Watanabe, M. (2004). Distinct cellular expressions of creatine synthetic enzyme gamt and creatine kinases UCK-MI And CK-B suggest a novel neuron–glial relationship for brain energy homeostasis. *Eur. J. Neurosci.* 20, 144–160. doi: 10.1111/j.1460-9568.2004.03478.x

Tran, C., Yazdanpanah, M., Kyriakopoulou, L., Levandovskiy, V., Zahid, H., Naufer, A., et al. (2014). Stable isotope dilution microquantification of creatine metabolites in plasma, whole blood and dried blood spots for pharmacological studies in mouse models of creatine deficiency. *Clin. Chim. Acta* 436, 160–168. doi: 10.1016/j.cca.2014.05.007

Wallimann, T., Wyss, M., Brdiczka, D., Nicolay, K., and Eppenberger, H. (1992). Intracellular compartmentation, structure and function of creatine kinase isoenzymes in tissues with high and fluctuating energy demands: the 'phosphocreatine circuit' for cellular energy homeostasis. *Biochem. J.* 281, 21–40. doi: 10.1042/bj2810021

Wyss, M., and Kaddurah-Daouk, R. (2000). Creatine and creatinine metabolism. *Physiol. Rev.* 80, 1107–1213. doi: 10.1152/physrev.2000.80.3.1107

10

The Relationship Between Clinical Imaging and Neurobehavioral Assessment in Posthemorrhagic Ventricular Dilation of Prematurity

Rebecca A. Dorner[1,2], Bruno P. Soares[2,3], Shenandoah Robinson[2,4], Marilee C. Allen[1,2], Jamie Perin[5] and Vera Joanna Burton[6,7]*

[1] Neonatology, Johns Hopkins Hospital, Baltimore, MD, United States, [2] Neurosciences Intensive Care Nursery, Johns Hopkins Hospital, Baltimore, MD, United States, [3] Pediatric Radiology and Pediatric Neuroradiology, Johns Hopkins Hospital, Baltimore, MD, United States, [4] Pediatric Neurosurgery, Johns Hopkins Hospital, Baltimore, MD, United States, [5] Biostatistics, Epidemiology, and Data Management Core, Johns Hopkins Hospital, Baltimore, MD, United States, [6] Neurology and Developmental Medicine, Kennedy Krieger Institute, Baltimore, MD, United States, [7] Department of Neurology, The Johns Hopkins School of Medicine, Baltimore, MD, United States

***Correspondence:**
Rebecca A. Dorner
rdorner1@jhmi.edu

Introduction: Neonatal intraventricular hemorrhage (IVH) and subsequent posthemorrhagic ventricular dilation and hydrocephalus of prematurity are associated with brain injury and neurodevelopmental impairment in the preterm population. Neuroimaging assesses cerebral injury and guides neurosurgical intervention; however, the relationship of head ultrasound (HUS) and magnetic resonance imaging (MRI) parameters to neonatal exams in this group has not been well described. The NICU Network Neurobehavioral Scale (NNNS) is a reproducible, highly reliable battery with motor and cognitive domain scores.

Objective: To evaluate the relationship between neonatal neurobehavioral findings on the NNNS and measures of ventricular dilation and associated brain injury on HUS and MRI.

Materials and Methods: Neonates with IVH and ventricular dilatation with and without posthemorrhagic hydrocephalus were enrolled. NNNS exams were performed at approximately term age equivalent. HUS indices were measured on the last HUS before initial neurosurgical procedure or that with worst ventriculomegaly if no intervention. The posterior fossa was assessed with MRI at term. Descriptive statistics including medians, interquartile ranges, means, and percentages were performed. Correlations were estimated using Pearson's method.

Results: 28 patients had NNNS and HUS, and 18 patients also had an MRI. Ventricle size measures for the cohort were significantly above normal. Motor and cognitive subscores on the NNNS exam varied from established baseline scores for postmenstrual age. Children who required neurosurgical intervention had higher ventricle/brain ratios and worse NNNS habituation scores. Ventricle sizes were modestly correlated with motor abnormalities (0.24–0.59); larger anterior horn width correlated with nonoptimal reflexes, hypertonicity and hypotonicity. Ventricle sizes were modestly correlated with cognitive scores (−0.44 to 0.27); larger ventricular index correlated with worse attention. Periventricular hemorrhagic infarction correlated with worse habituation.

Conclusion: For this cohort of preterm infants with IVH, surgical intervention for posthemorrhagic hydrocephalus correlated with both larger degrees of ventriculomegaly and worse NNNS exams. Findings on both HUS and MRI correlated with motor and cognitive abnormalities on neonatal neurobehavioral exam, suggesting that larger neonatal ventricle sizes and white matter injury have detectable correlates on exam. The NNNS exam provides important additional information when assessing posthemorrhagic ventricular dilation and hydrocephalus of prematurity.

Keywords: intraventricular hemorrhage, prematurity, ventriculomegaly, hydrocephalus, development, neuroimaging

BACKGROUND

Despite advances in neonatal care, intraventricular hemorrhage (IVH) remains a serious complication of prematurity occurring in up to 30% of premature infants. It is estimated that one-third to half of infants with severe IVH (grades 3 or 4) develop posthemorrhagic ventricular dilatation (Alan et al., 2012; Robinson, 2012). Approximately 10% of all neonates with IVH and 20% of infants with severe IVH will need surgical intervention due to posthemorrhagic hydrocephalus (Alan et al., 2012; Robinson, 2012). Preterm children with posthemorrhagic ventricular dilatation, and especially posthemorrhagic hydrocephalus requiring surgical intervention, are at high risk for future neurodevelopmental challenges. Abnormal motor outcomes include a spectrum from cerebral palsy to minor neuromotor dysfunction/developmental coordination disorder (Spittle and Orton, 2014). Other areas of neurodevelopment impacted include: intellectual disability, fine motor coordination problems, memory and executive function deficits, chronic pain, behavior problems, depression and anxiety, attention deficit/hyperactivity disorder and cortical visual impairment (Ment et al., 1999; Brouwer et al., 2008; Roze et al., 2009; Goldstein et al., 2013; Guzzetta et al., 2013; Tsai et al., 2014; Holwerda et al., 2016). Despite these risks, limited data is available regarding observable neurologic abnormalities in the neonatal period in children with ventriculomegaly and hydrocephalus.

The NNNS, or NICU Network Neurobehavioral Scale, is a standardized assessment tool used to measure neurologic integrity and organization (i.e., active and passive tone, reflexes), behavioral and state regulation, and stress/abstinence (Lester et al., 2004). It has strong psychometric qualities and good validity in the assessment of motor and cognitive deficits in the newborn period (Noble and Boyd, 2012) and normative values are available (Tronick et al., 2004). Administration of the exam requires certification after formal instruction and reliability testing. The examination consists of 45 administration and 70 observation items. Summary scores are created for 13 neurobehavioral domains including: habituation, attention, handling, quality of movement, regulation, nonoptimal reflexes, asymmetrical reflexes, stress/abstinence, arousal, hypertonicity, hypotonicity, excitability, and lethargy (Tronick et al., 2004). See **Table 1** for descriptions of each summary score (Tronick et al., 2004). NNNS performance at various time points including birth, term age equivalent, and time of neonatal admission discharge, have been independently correlated with later developmental outcomes in children with a variety of high-risk conditions, including neonatal abstinence syndrome(for which it was originally developed) (Lester et al., 2004), premature and low birthweight babies (Lester et al., 2011; El-Dib et al., 2012), term babies with fetal risk factors (Appleton et al., 2016) and more recently children with hypoxic ischemic encephalopathy (Massaro et al., 2015). Importantly, the NNNS is especially equipped to assess early cognitive function and state regulation. Regulation and adaptation to negative stimuli in the NNNS can begin to predict behavioral regulation, "a higher function that would be missed by other routine neurological examinations" (Lester et al., 2011).

There are no studies in the literature on NNNS exams in children with posthemorrhagic hydrocephalus of prematurity. The NNNS may help caregivers better understand the infant by providing information about early cognitive and motor function. Additionally, exams can be used serially to recognize subtle changes indicative of worsening neurologic status to guide neuroprotective and rehabilitative interventions.

The aim of our study was to evaluate the association between quantitative measures of neurobehavioral performance in the neonatal period with current gold standard measures of cerebral injury, head ultrasound imaging (HUS) and adjunctive magnetic resonance imaging (MRI). We hypothesized that children with more ventricular dilation, white matter injury, and those requiring intervention for posthemorrhagic hydrocephalus would have worse neonatal neurobehavioral assessments in cognitive and motor domains. Neonatal neurobehavioral exams, if associated with both imaging and later developmental milestones, could function as a bridge between commonly-performed imaging and early milestone attainment.

Abbreviations: AHW, anterior horn width; BPD, Bronchopulmonary dysplasia; HUS, Head ultrasound; IVH, Intraventricular hemorrhage; MRI, Magnetic Resonance Imaging; NEC, Necrotizing Enterocolitis; NICU, Neonatal Intensive Care Unit; NNNS, NICU Network Neurobehavioral Scale; PVHI, Periventricular hemorrhagic infarction; RI, Resistive Index; ROP, Retinopathy of Prematurity; TOD, Thalamooccipital Distance; V/B Ratio, Ventricular/Brain Ratio; VI, Ventricular Index; VPS, Ventriculoperitoneal shunt; VSGS, Ventriculosubgaleal shunt.

TABLE 1 | NNNS summary score descriptions (Tronick et al., 2004).

MOTOR SUBSCORES	
Excitability	Measure of high levels of motor, state and physiologic reactivity; sum of items for excitable behaviors
Lethargy	Measure of low levels of motor, state and physiologic reactivity; sum of items for lethargic behaviors
Nonoptimal reflexes	Any nonoptimal response to reflex excitation; sum of items for nonoptimal reflexes
Asymmetric reflexes	Any asymmetric response to reflex excitation; sum of items for asymmetric reflexes
Hypertonicity	Hypertonic response in arms, legs, trunk, or in general tone, sum of items for hypertonic indicators
Hypotonicity	Hypotonic response in arms, legs, trunk, or in general tone, sum of items for hypotonic indicators
Quality of movement	Measurement of motor control including smoothness, maturity, lack of startles and tremors; mean of items recoded for good motor control
COGNITIVE SUBSCORES	
Habituation	Response decrement to repeated auditory and visual stimuli; mean of items
Attention	Response to animate and inanimate auditory and visual stimuli; mean of items
Handling	Handling strategies used during orientation to maintain alert state; mean number of strategies needed
Regulation	Capacity to organize motor activity, physiology, and state during the examination and to respond to cuddling, consoling, and negative stimuli; mean of items recoded for good regulation
Arousal	Level of arousal including state and motor activity during the examination; mean of items for high arousal
Stress/abstinence	Mean amount of observed stress signs

MATERIALS AND METHODS

Recruitment for this prospective cohort study was conducted from July 1, 2016–July 31, 2018. Eligible patients were preterm infants born in this time frame with IVH and ventricular dilatation, with or without posthemorrhagic hydrocephalus. Babies were either in-born or referred to the Johns Hopkins Hospital Level IIIB and IIIC neonatal intensive care units. Infants were excluded if they had suspected or confirmed genetic anomalies. Infants were identified via neurodevelopmental consultation from the Neurosciences Intensive Care Nursery or by request of the clinical team as part of our routine practice for infants with IVH and ventricular dilatation. After NNNS examination was performed for clinical purposes, parents were approached to consent to join the research cohort. Clinically obtained standard-of-care neuroimaging were recorded in addition to NNNS exam results (see **Figure 1**). Twenty-Eight eligible infants were enrolled in this time frame, including 88% (16/18) of infants admitted with posthemorrhagic hydrocephalus.

Baseline demographics and comorbidities, including IVH grade, sepsis, necrotizing enterocolitis (NEC), bronchopulmonary dysplasia (BPD) severity (Jobe and Bancalari, 2001) and retinopathy of prematurity (ROP), were recorded (**Table 2**). Covariates included postmenstrual age at time of NNNS, HUS, and MRI.

NNNS exams were performed at the closest time point to term age equivalent, ideally no sooner than 34 weeks or less than 10 days from any surgical procedure. Although NNNS exams can be performed in infants from 30 to 48 weeks, we wanted to compare our infant exams to well-established norms at term age equivalent. We chose no sooner than 10 days after a procedure, neurosurgical or otherwise, as we found that with any less time infants were excessively irritable. Per exam criteria, NNNS scores were only performed in medically stable infants with the agreement of the treating medical team. NNNS summary scores were grouped into motor and cognitive categories. Motor subscores include hypertonicity, hypotonicity, excitability, lethargy, nonoptimal reflexes, asymmetrical reflexes, and quality of movement. Cognitive subscores include habituation, attention, handling, regulation, stress/abstinence, and arousal.

The last HUS prior to surgical intervention was selected for measurements as it typically represents the most severe ventricular dilation. If not requiring surgical intervention, the HUS with worst ventriculomegaly was selected. A pediatric neuroradiologist (B.P.S) blinded to clinical course measured the following HUS indices of ventricular size: left and right ventricular index (VI), anterior horn width (AHW), thalamooccipital distance (TOD), and ventricle/brain (V/B) ratio. The left (L) is recorded for each sided measurement for brevity as there was no significant difference amongst right- and left- sided values. Doppler resistive indices (RI) in the anterior cerebral artery, both with and without gentle manual pressure on the transducer, as well as presence of periventricular hemorrhagic infarction (PVHI) and cystic changes were evaluated. The posterior fossa was assessed with MRI; the degree of fourth ventricle dilatation was qualitatively scored (0- none; 1-mild, fourth ventricle compresses vermis only; 2-moderate, compresses dorsal brainstem; 3-severe, compresses ventral brainstem against clivus; 4- massive, fourth ventricle extends superiorly to supratentorial compartment), and the anterior-posterior diameter of the cerebellum from the fastigial point to the posterior vermis (pyramid) was measured. Due to the anatomical distortion of brain parenchyma in the majority of the patients, we were not able to complete typical preterm MRI scoring systems such as the Kidokoro system (Kidokoro et al., 2013). For example, due to the severity of fourth ventricle dilation, cerebellar height and transcerebellar diameter were unable to be completed for the majority of patients. Additionally, HUS measurements of ventricular size agreed with MRI measures, and the sample size of MRIs was more limited than HUS. For this reason, the majority of our statistics analyze HUS measures, with the exception of the fourth ventricle size and anterior-posterior diameter of the cerebellum by MRI. Descriptive statistics including medians, interquartile ranges (IQRs), means, and percentages were used to summarize the cohort. Correlations were estimated using Pearson's method. All analyses were conducted in R version 3.5.0 (R Core Development Team, 2018).

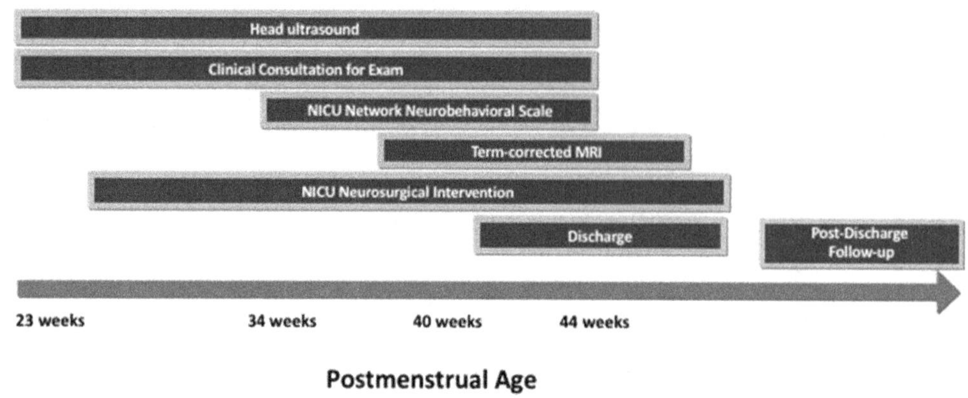

FIGURE 1 | Cohort Timeline of Clinical Milestones, NNNS exam, and Neuroimaging.

RESULTS

In total, 28 patients were consented and had the NNNS and HUS performed. Of these 28, 18 patients had the NNNS, HUS and MRI performed. Average gestational age at birth was 27.1(range 23.4–34.2) weeks and average birthweight 1,115 (range 500–3816) g (**Table 2**). Mean postmenstrual age (PMA) at the time of the HUS was 32.2 weeks, NNNS exam was 37.2 weeks, and MRI was 39.5 weeks (**Table 2**). Ventricle size measures for the cohort were significantly above normal (**Table 3**). Motor and cognitive subscores on the NNNS exam (**Table 4**) varied from established baseline scores for term-corrected age (Lester and Tronick, 2004; Lester et al., 2011; Appleton et al., 2016). The only significant difference between infants with and without MRI was that babies with MRIs were more likely to have a 5 min APGAR score less than 7 (59 vs. 10%, $p = 0.018$).

Significant associations between imaging parameters and NNNS motor and cognitive subscores are summarized in **Figure 2**.

Abnormal radiology measures were associated with other abnormal radiology markers. Ventricle size measures (VI, AHW, TOD, and V/B ratio) were positively associated with one another (**Figure 2**). This is important as many studies have used different measurements to define ventriculomegaly (Sondhi et al., 2008; Maunu et al., 2011; Brouwer et al., 2012; Dorner et al., 2018). Larger AHW (but not other ventricle size measures) and larger fourth ventricle sizes were associated with smaller anterior-posterior diameter of the cerebellum (**Figure 2**). PVHI and cystic changes were associated; the odds ratio between PVHI and cystic changes was infinite (95% CI: 7.22—Infinity, $p = < 0.001$).

Features on both the HUS and NNNS exam were associated with receipt of neurosurgical intervention, where intervention was defined as either ventriculosubgaleal shunt (VSGS) placement or ventriculoperitoneal shunt (VPS) placement (**Table 5**). Fifty-Seven Percent of the cohort (16/28) required shunt placement; 2 patients required a VSGS, 11 had an initial VSGS followed by a VPS, and 3 patients had a VPS alone. Children receiving neurosurgical intervention were more likely to have larger ventricle sizes; means of ventricular size for those receiving neurosurgical intervention versus those not receiving intervention were statistically different as measured by: TOD (45.42 mm vs. 27.67, respectively, $p = < 0.001$), AHW (23.85 vs. 11.53 mm, respectively, $p = 0.001$), VI (24.62 vs. 14.20, respectively, $p = 0.001$), and V/B Ratio (0.615 vs. 0.378, respectively, $p = 0.022$) (**Table 5**). Neurosurgical intervention was most strongly associated with V/B ratio, with a correlation coefficient of 0.78 (**Figure 2**). The NNNS habituation subscore (response decrement to repeated auditory and visual stimuli) was the only additional parameter that differed between those infants receiving intervention and not receiving intervention (**Table 5**). Doppler RI values, with and without compression, did not correlate with receiving surgery.

Ventricle sizes were modestly correlated with motor abnormalities on NNNS exam (estimated correlations −0.72 to 0.39, **Figure 2**). Larger AHW sizes on HUS were associated with higher scores for nonoptimal reflexes (number of nonoptimal responses to reflex elicitation, such as excessive clonus), hypotonicity (number of hypotonic responses in arm, legs, trunk, or general tone) and hypertonicity (number of hypertonic responses in arm, legs, trunk, or general tone). Correlations between AHW and hypertonicity, hypotonicity, and nonoptimal reflexes subscores from the NNNS exam were: 0.59 (95% CI: 0.09–0.70, $p = 0.018$), 0.24 (95% CI: 0.08–0.70, $p = 0.018$), and 0.44 (95% CI: 0.08–0.70, $p = 0.018$), respectively (**Figure 2**).

Ventricle sizes were modestly inversely correlated with cognitive scores on NNNS exam as well (estimated correlations from −0.44 to 0.27, **Figure 2**). NNNS attention was negatively correlated with VI, where a larger VI was related to a lower average NNNS attention score (−0.06, 95% CI: −0.70 to −0.04, $p = 0.034$).

Of the 16 children in the cohort requiring intervention for posthemorrhagic hydrocephalus, 8 had antecedent Grade 3 IVH and 8 had PVHI (formerly called Grade 4 IVH). Presence of PVHI was associated with decreased or inadequate habituation to stimuli; the mean (standard deviation) for habituation for those with PVHI was 5.41 (1.75) and for no PVHI was 7.73 (1.18), $p = 0.012$.

TABLE 2 | Characteristics of 28 Preterm Neonates with IVH with and without Hydrocephalus ($n = 28$).

Mean gestational age at birth	27.2 weeks (range: 23.4–34.2 weeks)
Mean birthweight	1,130 g (500–3,816 g)
Mean PMA at NNNS	37.2 weeks (32.4–45.1 weeks)
Number of exams performed in PMA category	<34 weeks: 3 34.0–34.6 weeks: 5 35.0–35.6 weeks: 3 36.0–36.6 weeks: 4 37+ weeks: 13
Mean PMA at HUS	37.2 weeks (25.6–41.3 weeks)
Mean PMA at MRI	39.5 weeks (33.5–49.2 weeks)
Sex	16 (57%) male, 12 (43%) female
Ethnicity	9 (32%) African-American, 16(57%) Caucasian, 1(4%) Asian, 2 (7%) Hispanic
Adequate prenatal betamethasone*	18 (64%)
Grade of Intraventricular hemorrhage	Grade 1: 4 (14%) Grade 2: 3 (11%) Grade 3: 11 (39%) Grade 4 (PVHI): 10 (36%)
Moderate/severe BPD+	29 (68%)
Severe ROP (Stage 3 or surgical intervention/biologic medication)	7(25%)
Necrotizing enterocolitis (NEC)^	2 patients Stage 3B, 1 patient Stage 3B after spontaneous intestinal perforation, 1 patient Stage 1B
Treated for culture positive or negative sepsis	20 (71%)
5-min Apgar <7	11(39%)

PMA, Postmenstrual Age.
**Completed 24 h in-utero after second dose.*
+Per NICHD criteria (Jobe and Bancalari, 2001); moderate BPD as O_2 for ≥28 days plus treatment with <30% FiO_2 at 36 weeks' PMA and severe BPD as O_2 for ≥ 28 days plus ≥ 30% FiO_2 and/or positive pressure at 36 weeks' PMA.
^Modified bell staging criteria for NEC (Lee and Polin, 2003).

There was clustering of NNNS exam findings in preterm children with IVH. In terms of motor development, those with abnormally high levels of motor, state, and physiologic reactivity (higher excitability scores) were more likely to have abnormal movement (quality of movement score), less regulation, and higher stress/abstinence and arousal scores. Those with low levels of activity, or lethargy, were more hypotonic, and exhibited lower attention and arousal scores. Interestingly, hypotonicity was correlated with hypertonicity (correlation 0.46, 95% CI: 0.11–0.71, $p = 0.014$) and both were correlated with nonoptimal reflexes: (hypertonicity—0.71, 95% CI: 0.46–0.86, $p = 0.00$) and (hypotonicity—0.45, 95% CI: 0.10–0.71, $p = 0.015$) (**Figure 2**).

NNNS scores were also associated with medical morbidities. Infants with severe ROP had higher NNNS Excitability [average (SD) 4.6 (1.9) vs. 2.3 (1.9), $p = 0.006$). Severe BPD was also associated with higher nonoptimal reflexes [5.4 (1.9) for those with BPD, 3.6 (1.6) without, $p = 0.027$] and lower movement [3.7 (0.8) for those with BPD and 4.7 (0.6) without, $p = 0.003$].

Of note, BPD does not confound the relationship of non-optimal reflexes with AHW; the mean AHW for infants without BPD is 14.4 mm and with moderate/severe BPD was 18.2, $p = 0.308$. No NNNS items were independently associated with Sepsis or NEC.

DISCUSSION

This is the first study to analyze the relationship between HUS and MRI imaging with neonatal neurobehavioral exams in posthemorrhagic ventricular dilation and hydrocephalus of prematurity. It is also the first to describe the range of NNNS findings in this group. Our patient population had severe ventriculomegaly, with means for all ventricular size measurements on HUS far above norms for age. As intended, the NNNS exams were performed around term equivalent age (average 37.3 weeks) in the attempt to correlate with published norms for term babies (Tronick et al., 2004). MRIs were also performed at term age equivalent (39.5 weeks), but only fourth ventricle dilation and anterior-posterior diameter of the cerebellum were analyzed due to technical challenges and lack of standardization of MRI reads for posthemorrhagic ventricular dilatation.

For this cohort of 28 preterm infants, the degree of ventriculomegaly—using precise imaging parameters such as V/B ratio and AHW—correlated with surgical intervention, as expected. This suggests that decisions regarding intervention are made either on the basis of ventricular size alone or due to changes in ventricular size in combination with the clinical course. Importantly, different radiologic measurements of the lateral ventricles were all related to each other, suggesting that the choice of ventricular measurement may be less important than choosing a standard measure. Specific ventricular measurements may be superior, however, for different purposes. In this study, intervention had the highest association with V/B ratio, AHW with NNNS motor subscores and the VI with NNNS cognitive subscores. The NNNS cognitive exam, specifically the habituation subscore, also correlated with receipt of surgical intervention. The relationship of intervention and NNNS exam suggests that posthemorrhagic hydrocephalus and/or intervention itself may create a detectable signal of reactivity.

In this participant group, V/B ratio best correlated with receipt of intervention. V/B ratios > 0.35 on ultrasound have been associated with smaller cerebrum and cerebellar volumes on term-corrected MRI (Govaert and de Vries, 1997). Decreased cerebral and cerebellar parenchymal volumes are associated with lower cognitive and language scores, abnormal motor outcome and processing speed (Nosarti et al., 2008; Maunu et al., 2009). Smaller cerebellar size, which has previously been shown to correlate with worse future cognitive outcomes (de Vries et al., 2019), was associated both with larger AHW and more fourth ventricle dilatation in our population.

Higher AHWs were associated with worse motor exams, specifically a higher number of nonoptimal reflexes and more hypotonicity. An increase in AHW has been suggested to be a more sensitive marker for early worsening of hydrocephalus and is seen subjectively as rounding of the frontal horns (Brouwer et al., 2010). Both lower (>6 mm) and higher (>10mm) AHW

TABLE 3 | Head ultrasound and magnetic resonance imaging parameters.

Measure	Number patients	Cohort median (IQR)	**Normal** (Sondhi et al., 2008; Brouwer et al., 2010, 2012; Maunu et al., 2011; Graca et al., 2013; Kidokoro et al., 2013)
Ventricular index (mm)	28	21.00 (10.75–24.25)	10–13
Anterior horn width (mm)	28	19.00 (8.50–24.25)	Less than 3
Thalamooccipital distance (mm)	28	40.00 (23.75–45.25)	5–25
Ventricle/brain ratio	28	0.52 (0.32–0.60)	Less than 0.35
Resistive Index (with pressure)	28	0.87 (0.78–0.93)	0.5–0.8
Resistive Index (without pressure)	28	0.81 (0.75–0.89)	0.5–0.8
AP diameter cerebellum (mm)	18	14.00 (10.25–17.25)	22–24
4th ventricle dilatation (qualitative score)*	18	1.00 (0.00–1.75)	0
	Number patients	**Observed (%)**	
PVHI (present)	28	10 (36%)	None
Cystic changes (present)	28	8 (29%)	None

PVHI, Periventricular Hemorrhagic Infarction.
**4th ventricle dilatation: 0-none, 1- compresses vermis, 2-compresses dorsal brainstem, 3-compresses ventral brainstem against clivus, 4- to supratentorial compartment.*

size cutoffs for surgical intervention have been used (Leijser et al., 2018; de Vries et al., 2019). The fact that early AHW dilatation correlates to exam findings in the neonatal period provides an opportunity to follow this parameter in a more multifaceted way.

Ventricle sizes and white matter injury were associated with worst neonatal cognitive assessment scores. Children with larger ventricles had lower attention scores; larger VI measurements were negatively correlated with the NNNS attention cognitive subscore. Attention is the ability to pay attention to salient stimuli in the environment. Additionally, PVHI, present in 10 of our children, correlated with decreased habituation to stimuli. Habituation is the ability to stop responding to (i.e., to ignore) repetitive stimuli. An inability to inhibit a response is one of the earliest measures of executive function and is well-developed by 6–7 months of age in typically developing infants (Diamond et al., 1994). In general, the children with larger VI and with PVHI were more irritable and responded more continuously to noxious stimuli, at the expense of paying attention to important stimuli such as a face or voice. It is possible that difficulty with attention and habituation in this early time frame are signs of later difficulty with inhibition and attention and a marker for later executive dysfunction (Diamond et al., 1994). Executive function and attention difficulties are well described in the hydrocephalus population (Holwerda et al., 2016). This early internal disorganization and over-responsiveness may be early markers of such difficulties.

Fourth ventricle dilatation on MRI was not associated with changes in NNNS exam (**Table 5**). While this attempt to evaluate fourth ventricle dilatation did not correlate with neonatal exams, this parameter has not yet been adequately assessed in this population. Further data are needed to understand the impact of fourth ventricular dilatation and on exams and outcomes.

We also saw informative patterns in the NNNS exam. Both ends of the arousal spectrum were seen; abnormally high excitability, stress and arousal score subgroups were present as were lethargy, hypotonia, and lower attention and arousal scores.

TABLE 4 | NICU Network Neurobehavioral Scale (NNNS) measurements.

	Cohort mean (SD)	Standardized relative to typical scores	Typical mean* (SD)
MOTOR SUBSCORES			
Excitability	3.43 (2.32)	−0.59 (−1.06 to 0.84)	4.23 (2.10)
Lethargy	4.79 (2.18)	−0.72 (−1.02 to −0.02)	6.32 (3.24)
Nonoptimal reflexes	4.96 (1.97)	0.39 (−0.18 to 0.97)	4.32 (1.73)
Asymmetric reflexes	1.41 (1.55)	−0.70 (−1.45 to 0.05)	1.93 (1.33)
Hypertonicity	0.29 (0.53)	−0.27 (−0.27 to 0.69)	0.07 (0.26)
Hypotonicity	0.64 (0.73)	−0.07 (−0.72 to 0.59)	0.55 (0.76)
Quality of movement	3.95 (0.86)	0.24 (−0.30 to 1.10)	3.81 (0.78)
COGNITIVE SUBSCORES			
Habituation	6.77 (1.82)	−0.80 (−2.26 to 0.08)	7.91 (1.14)
Attention	5.25 (1.16)	0.26 (−0.84 to 0.81)	5.30 (1.04)
Handling	0.47 (0.22)	0.85 (0.16 to 1.32)	0.27 (0.27)
Regulation	4.95 (0.74)	−0.28 (−0.74 to 0.67)	5.0 (0.82)
Arousal	3.63 (0.91)	−0.81 (−1.43 to 0.16)	4.16 (0.81)
Stress/ Abstinence	0.19 (0.05)	0.80 (0.20 to 1.50)	0.15 (0.05)

**, per Maternal Lifestyle Study (Lester et al., 2011).*
SD, Standard deviation.

These groups were not mutually exclusive; indeed, many children scored high on both lethargy and excitability, meaning during the exam they were often either too sleepy or too irritable. Both result in a failure to interact and pay attention to informative stimuli. Along the same lines, hypotonicity within our cohort was correlated with hypertonicity (correlation 0.46, 0.11–0.71, $p = 0.014$) and both were correlated with nonoptimal reflexes: (hypertonicity- 0.71, 0.46–0.86, $p = 0.00$) and (hypotonicity- 0.45 (0.10–0.71, $p = 0.015$). These patterns fit what we often see as a

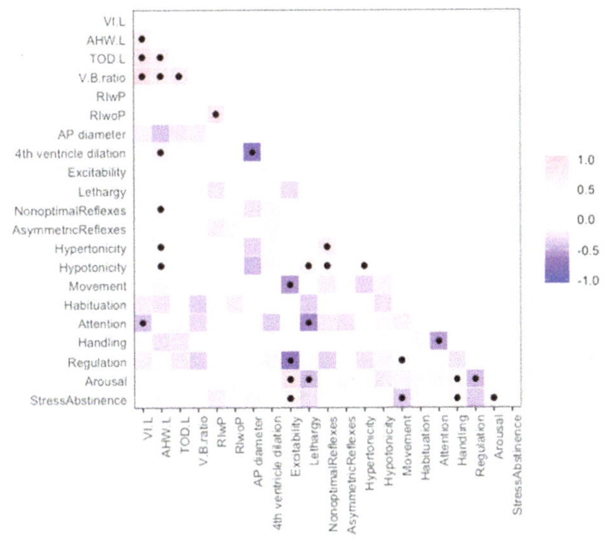

FIGURE 2 | Correlations among ventricular size measurements and NNNS motor and cognitive subscores, where pink indicates positive correlation and purple negative correlation. Significant correlations with $p < 0.05$ are marked with a black dot.

concerning pattern in ventricular dilatation; axial hypotonia and poor head control with high appendicular tone in the extremities. Together, these patterns of extreme reactions reflect a limited ability of the injured brain to regulate responses.

It is important to consider that ventricular dilatation and hydrocephalus are not isolated in preterm infants; the relationship of HUS and MRI measures to NNNS scores may be influenced by comorbidities. We found that severe ROP and moderate/severe BPD were associated with abnormalities in NNNS items regardless of ventricular size. Severe ROP was associated with higher NNNS excitability scores and moderate/severe BPD was associated with more nonoptimal reflexes and lower movement scores. Although both moderate/severe BPD and AHW were both associated with worse non-optimal reflexes, on further analysis BPD did not confound the relationship of non-optimal reflexes with AHW. It will be important in the future to consider both effects from hydrocephalus and comorbid conditions to better describe the contribution of hydrocephalus to neurodevelopmental delay.

Our data suggests that ventricular size is associated with neonatal exam as larger ventricle sizes were related to poorer scores on both motor and cognitive sections of the NNNS exam. The observed modest correlations are not unexpected; likely other factors in the infant's clinical course might also affect exam performance. Given that aspects of the neonatal neurobehavioral exam are associated with ventricular size measurements, our data suggests that exam and imaging may provide complementary and additive information on existing neurodevelopmental status.

There are limitations to the present study. Although a large portion of infants with posthemorrhagic hydrocephalus were captured, not all consecutive admissions to the NICU with IVH

TABLE 5 | Means of HUS and MRI parameters, NNNS subscales by infants with and without neurosurgical intervention for hydrocephalus.

Feature	Mean (SD) or *N* (%) for infants who received intervention ($n = 16$)	Mean (SD) or *N* (%) for infants with no intervention ($n = 12$)	Test for difference (p*)
VI (mm)	23.88 (5.48)	12.58 (5.62)	<0.001*
AHW (mm)	22.88 (6.01)	9.75 (11.54)	0.003*
TOD (mm)	43.90 (9.00)	25.25 (14.95)	0.001*
V/B ratio	0.60 (0.08)	0.34 (0.08)	<0.001*
RI w/P	0.87 (0.11)	0.85 (0.10)	0.532
RI w/o P	0.83 (0.10)	0.79 (0.08)	0.209
AP diameter cerebellum (mm)	11.62 (7.43)	16.40 (3.65)	0.089
4th ventricle dilatation (mm)	1.31 (1.25)	0.60 (0.55)	0.116
PVHI (present)	8 (50%)	2 (17%)	0.114
Cystic changes (present)	7 (44%)	1 (8%)	0.088
Excitability	2.92 (1.98)	3.81 (2.54)	0.303
Lethargy	4.17 (1.70)	5.25 (2.44)	0.177
Nonoptimal reflexes	4.42 (1.51)	5.38 (2.22)	0.185
Asymmetric reflexes	1.17 (1.64)	1.60 (1.50)	0.487
Hypertonicity	0.17 (0.39)	0.38 (0.62)	0.286
Hypotonicity	0.50 (0.67)	0.75 (0.77)	0.371
Movement	4.06 (0.93)	3.87 (0.82)	0.569
Habituation	7.72 (1.68)	5.93 (1.57)	0.039*
Attention	5.50 (0.94)	5.08 (1.29)	0.359
Handling	0.54 (0.20)	0.43 (0.23)	0.217
Regulation	5.18 (0.76)	4.76 (0.71)	0.160
Arousal	3.46 (0.81)	3.75 (0.98)	0.403
Stress/abstinence	0.21 (0.05)	0.18 (0.06)	0.253

**Significance determined by Student's t-test or by Fisher's exact test for categorical factors.*

and some ventricular dilatation completed a NNNS evaluation; this may introduce selection bias. The average postmenstrual age at NNNS examination was 37.2 weeks, but some infants had exams earlier, as seen in **Table 2**. The nature of our NICUs are such that convalescing preterm infants, even after neurosurgery, are often transferred to lower acuity locations. As such, some infants were examined before term-corrected age due to imminent discharge. The impact of postnatal age on the NNNS is unclear in this study; previous studies have shown that postmenstrual age has an effect on NNNS subscores (Spittle et al., 2016). Additionally, given our small sample size, inclusion and analysis of all potential covariates was not feasible and we could not evaluate the cumulative impact of measured co-morbidities, such as NEC, on NNNS scores. Adequately powered larger samples are needed to address this important issue.

CONCLUSION

In summary, for this cohort of 28 preterm infants with IVH and ventricular dilatation, surgical intervention was associated with degree of ventriculomegaly, using precise imaging parameters, as well as NNNS exam. Findings on both HUS and MRI imaging correlated with motor and cognitive abnormalities on neonatal neurobehavioral exam. These results suggest that larger neonatal ventricle sizes and white matter injury have detectable correlates on exam in this population. The NNNS exam may be additive with imaging in assessment of a common form of neonatal hydrocephalus. Importantly, the NNNS is identifying deficits at term equivalence, and even earlier, during a preterm infant's NICU stay. This risk identification is much earlier than typical neurodevelopmental exams done in follow-up care. This can allow for better developmental care during the NICU as changes can be made to the environment and rehabilitative interventions begun as soon as neurobehavioral deficits are identified (Mahoney and Cohen, 2005; Symington and Pinelli, 2006; King et al., 2008; Als and McAnulty, 2011; Fucile et al., 2011). It will be important to achieve longer-term follow-up in these infants to determine if these findings correlate with later neurodevelopmental disability.

AUTHOR CONTRIBUTIONS

RD and VB conceived of and designed the study, performed exams, supervised data entry and analysis, analyzed and interpreted data, and wrote and edited manuscript. BS performed neuroimaging analysis. BS, JP, SR, and MA analyzed data and edited manuscript.

ACKNOWLEDGMENTS

We would like to thank Veena Billioux for her help with statistical work conceptualizing this project. This project was supported by the Thomas Wilson Sanitarium for Children of Baltimore City awarded to RD and MA and the NIH T32 Training Grant (T32HL125239-03) awarded to RD.

REFERENCES

Alan, N., Manjila, S., Minich, N., Bass, N., Cohen, A. R., Walsh, M., et al. (2012). Reduced ventricular shunt rate in very preterm infants with severe intraventricular hemorrhage: an institutional experience. *J. Neurosurg. Pediatr.* 10, 357–364. doi: 10.3171/2012.7.PEDS11504

Als, H., and McAnulty, G. B. (2011). The Newborn Individualized Developmental Care and Assessment Program (NIDCAP) with Kangaroo Mother Care (KMC): comprehensive care for preterm infants. *Curr. Women Health Rev.* 7, 288–301. doi: 10.2174/157340411796355216

Appleton, A. A., Murphy, M. A., Koestler, D. C., Lesseur, C., Paquette, A. G., Padbury, J. F., et al. (2016). Prenatal programming of infant neurobehaviour in a healthy population. *Paediatr. Perinat. Epidemiol.* 30, 367–375. doi: 10.1111/ppe.12294

Brouwer, A., Groenendaal, F., van Haastert, I. L., Rademaker, K., Hanlo, P., and de Vries, L. (2008). Neurodevelopmental outcome of preterm infants with severe intraventricular hemorrhage and therapy for post-hemorrhagic ventricular dilatation. *J. Pediatr.* 152, 648–654. doi: 10.1016/j.jpeds.2007.10.005

Brouwer, M. J., de Vries, L. S., Groenendaal, F., Koopman, C., Pistorius, L. R., Mulder, E. J., et al. (2012). New reference values for the neonatal cerebral ventricles. *Radiology* 262, 224–233. doi: 10.1148/radiol.11110334

Brouwer, M. J., de Vries, L. S., Pistorius, L., Rademaker, K. J., Groenendaal, F., and Benders, M. J. (2010). Ultrasound measurements of the lateral ventricles in neonates: why, how and when? A systematic review. *Acta Paediatr.* 99, 1298–1306. doi: 10.1111/j.1651-2227.2010.01830.x

de Vries, L. S., Groenendaal, F., Liem, K. D., Heep, A., Brouwer, A. J., van 't Verlaat, E., et al. (2019). Treatment thresholds for intervention in posthaemorrhagic ventricular dilation: a randomised controlled trial. *Arch. Dis. Childh. Fetal Neonatal Ed.* 104, F70–F75. doi: 10.1136/archdischild-2017-314206

Diamond, A., Werker, J. F., and Lalonde, C. (1994). "Toward understanding commonalities in the development of object search, detour navigation, categorization, and speech perception," in *Human Behavior and the Developing Brain*, eds G. Dawson and K. W. Fischer (New York, NY: Guilford Press), 380–426.

Dorner, R. A., Burton, V. J., Allen, M. C., Robinson, S., and Soares, B. P. (2018). Preterm neuroimaging and neurodevelopmental outcome: a focus on intraventricular hemorrhage, post-hemorrhagic hydrocephalus, and associated brain injury. *J. Perinatol.* 38, 1431–1443. doi: 10.1038/s41372-018-0209-5

El-Dib, M., Massaro, A. N., Glass, P., and Aly, H. (2012). Neurobehavioral assessment as a predictor of neurodevelopmental outcome in preterm infants. *J. Perinatol.* 32, 299–303. doi: 10.1038/jp.2011.100

Fucile, S., Gisel, E. G., McFarland, D. H., and Lau, C. (2011). Oral and non-oral sensorimotor interventions enhance oral feeding performance in preterm infants. *Dev. Med. Child Neurol.* 53, 829–835. doi: 10.1111/j.1469-8749.2011.04023.x

Goldstein, R. F., Cotten, C. M., Shankaran, S., Gantz, M. G., and Poole, W. K. (2013). Influence of gestational age on death and neurodevelopmental outcome in premature infants with severe intracranial hemorrhage. *J. Perinatol.* 33, 25–32. doi: 10.1038/jp.2012.91

Govaert, P., and de Vries, L. S. (1997). *An Atlas of Neonatal Brain Sonography.* London: Mac Keith Press.

Graca, A. M., Geraldo, A. F., Cardoso, K., and Cowan, F. M. (2013). Preterm cerebellum at term age: ultrasound measurements are not different from infants born at term. *Pediatr. Res.* 74, 698–704. doi: 10.1038/pr.2013.154

Guzzetta, A., Fiori, S., Scelfo, D., Conti, E., and Bancale, A. (2013). Reorganization of visual fields after periventricular haemorrhagic infarction: potentials and limitations. *Dev. Med. Child Neurol.* 55(Suppl. 4), 23–26. doi: 10.1111/dmcn.12302

Holwerda, J. C., Van Braeckel, K., Roze, E., Hoving, E. W., Maathuis, C. G. B., Brouwer, O. F., et al. (2016). Functional outcome at school age of neonatal post-hemorrhagic ventricular dilatation. *Early Hum. Dev.* 96, 15–20. doi: 10.1016/j.earlhumdev.2016.02.005

Jobe, A. H., and Bancalari, E. (2001). Bronchopulmonary dysplasia. *Am. J. Respir. Crit. Care Med.* 163, 1723–1729. doi: 10.1164/ajrccm.163.7.2011060

Kidokoro, H., Neil, J. J., and Inder, T. E. (2013). New MR imaging assessment tool to define brain abnormalities in very preterm infants at term. *Am. J. Neuroradiol.* 34, 2208–2214. doi: 10.3174/ajnr.A3521

King, G., Currie, M., Bartlett, D. J., Strachan, D., Tucker, M. A., and Willoughby, C. (2008). The development of expertise in paediatric rehabilitation therapists: the roles of motivation, openness to experience, and types of caseload experience. *Aust. Occup. Ther. J.* 55, 108–122. doi: 10.1111/j.1440-1630.2007.00681.x

Lee, J. S., and Polin, R. A. (2003). Treatment and prevention of necrotizing enterocolitis. *Semin. Neonatol.* SN8, 449–459. doi: 10.1016/S1084-2756(03)00123-4

Leijser, L. M., Miller, S. P., van Wezel-Meijler, G., Brouwer, A. J., Traubici, J., van Haastert, I. C., et al. (2018). Posthemorrhagic ventricular dilatation in preterm infants: when best to intervene? *Neurology* 90, e698–e706. doi: 10.1212/WNL.0000000000004984

Lester, B. M., Miller, R. J., Hawes, K., Salisbury, A., Bigsby, R., Sullivan, M. C., et al. (2011). Infant neurobehavioral development. *Semin. Perinatol.* 35, 8–19. doi: 10.1053/j.semperi.2010.10.003

Lester, B. M., and Tronick, E. Z. (eds) (2004). *NICU Network Neurobehavioral Scale, (NNNS) Manual*. Baltimore, MD: Paul H. Brookes Pub. Co.

Lester, B. M., Tronick, E. Z., and Brazelton, T. B. (2004). The neonatal intensive care unit network neurobehavioral scale procedures. *Pediatrics* 113 (3 Pt 2), 641–667.

Mahoney, M. C., and Cohen, M. I. (2005). Effectiveness of developmental intervention in the neonatal intensive care unit: implications for neonatal physical therapy. *Pediatr. Phys. Ther.* 17, 194–208.

Massaro, A. N., Evangelou, I., Brown, J., Fatemi, A., Vezina, G., McCarter, R., et al. (2015). Neonatal neurobehavior after therapeutic hypothermia for hypoxic ischemic encephalopathy. *Early Hum. Dev.* 91, 593–599. doi: 10.1016/j.earlhumdev.2015.07.008

Maunu, J., Lehtonen, L., Lapinleimu, H., Matomaki, J., Munck, P., Rikalainen, H., et al. (2011). Ventricular dilatation in relation to outcome at 2 years of age in very preterm infants: a prospective Finnish cohort study. *Dev. Med. Child Neurol.* 53, 48–54. doi: 10.1111/j.1469-8749.2010.03785.x

Maunu, J., Parkkola, R., Rikalainen, H., Lehtonen, L., Haataja, L., and Lapinleimu, H. (2009). Brain and ventricles in very low birth weight infants at term: a comparison among head circumference, ultrasound, and magnetic resonance imaging. *Pediatrics* 123, 617–626. doi: 10.1542/peds.2007-3264

Ment, L. R., Vohr, B., Allan, W., Westerveld, M., Katz, K. H., Schneider, K. C., et al. (1999). The etiology and outcome of cerebral ventriculomegaly at term in very low birth weight preterm infants. *Pediatrics* 104(2 Pt 1), 243–248. doi: 10.1542/peds.104.2.243

Noble, Y., and Boyd, R. (2012). Neonatal assessments for the preterm infant up to 4 months corrected age: a systematic review. *Dev. Med. Child Neurol.* 54, 129–139. doi: 10.1111/j.1469-8749.2010.03903.x

Nosarti, C., Giouroukou, E., Healy, E., Rifkin, L., Walshe, M., Reichenberg, A., et al. (2008). Grey and white matter distribution in very preterm adolescents mediates neurodevelopmental outcome. *Brain* 131 (Pt 1), 205–217. doi: 10.1093/brain/awm282

R Core Development Team (2018). *R: A Language, and Environment for Statistical Computing*. The R Foundation for Statistical Computing.

Robinson, S. (2012). Neonatal posthemorrhagic hydrocephalus from prematurity: pathophysiology and current treatment concepts. *J. Neurosurg. Pediatr.* 9, 242–258. doi: 10.3171/2011.12.PEDS11136

Roze, E., Van Braeckel, K. N., van der Veere, C. N., Maathuis, C. G., Martijn, A., and Bos, A. F. (2009). Functional outcome at school age of preterm infants with periventricular hemorrhagic infarction. *Pediatrics* 123, 1493–1500. doi: 10.1542/peds.2008-1919

Sondhi, V., Gupta, G., Gupta, P. K., Patnaik, S. K., and Tshering, K. (2008). Establishment of nomograms and reference ranges for intra-cranial ventricular dimensions and ventriculo-hemispheric ratio in newborns by ultrasonography. *Acta Paediatr.* 97, 738–744. doi: 10.1111/j.1651-2227.2008.00765.x

Spittle, A. J., and Orton, J. (2014). Cerebral palsy and developmental coordination disorder in children born preterm. *Semin. Fetal Neonatal Med.* 19, 84–89. doi: 10.1016/j.siny.2013.11.005

Spittle, A. J., Walsh, J., Olsen, J. E., McInnes, E., Eeles, A. L., Brown, N. C., et al. (2016). Neurobehaviour and neurological development in the first month after birth for infants born between 32-42 weeks' gestation. *Early Hum. Dev.* 96, 7–14. doi: 10.1016/j.earlhumdev.2016.02.006

Symington, A., and Pinelli, J. (2006). Developmental care for promoting development and preventing morbidity in preterm infants. *Cochr. Datab. Syst. Rev.* CD001814. doi: 10.1002/14651858.CD001814.pub2

Tronick, E. Z., Olson, K., Rosenberg, R., Bohne, L., Lu, J., and Lester, B. M. (2004). Normative neurobehavioral performance of healthy infants on the neonatal intensive care unit network neurobehavioral scale. *Pediatrics* 113(3 Pt 2), 676–678.

Tsai, A. J., Lasky, R. E., John, S. D., Evans, P. W., and Kennedy, K. A. (2014). Predictors of neurodevelopmental outcomes in preterm infants with intraparenchymal hemorrhage. *J. Perinatol.* 34, 399–404. doi: 10.1038/jp.2014.21

11

Cognitive Development Trajectories in Preterm Children with very Low Birth Weight Longitudinally Followed Until 11 Years of Age

Sofia Ryytty Stålnacke[1], Mesfin Tessma[2], Birgitta Böhm[1†] and Eric Herlenius[1†]*

[1] *Department of Women's and Children's Health, Karolinska Institutet, Karolinska University Hospital, Stockholm, Sweden,*
[2] *Department of Learning, Informatics, Management and Ethics – LIME, Karolinska Institutet, Stockholm, Sweden*

Correspondence:
Eric Herlenius
eric.herlenius@ki.se

†Shared last authorship

Background: There is a high prevalence of cognitive dysfunction in very low birthweight (500–1250 g) infants (VLBW). Understanding long-term risk factors associated with cognitive development in preterm children requires longitudinal characterization. Thus, follow-up evaluations, including identification of risks and resilience influences–are important to promote health and cognitive abilities of children born preterm.

Aim: To examine changes in cognitive development from birth until 11 years of age in preterm children with very low birthweight.

Methods: 24 VLBW infants, at the Karolinska University Hospital, Stockholm, were assessed with regards to cognitive functioning at three times during development at 18 months, 5 and 11 years of age using standardized tests. Longitudinal data were analyzed using Generalized Estimating Equation (GEE) univariate and multivariate models.

Results: The follow-up rate was 100%. Level of cognitive functioning at 18 months and at 11 years was similar. Females had higher cognitive scores than males at all three timepoints. We found that intraventricular hemorrhage (IVH) and prolonged invasive ventilatory support (>7 days) had a negative effect on cognitive functioning. Higher levels of parental education had a favorable influence on cognitive functioning over time.

Conclusion: Level of cognitive development at 18 months was highly predictive of level of cognitive function at 11 years of age and differences in assessment scores between male and female VLBW infants persisted. Additional longitudinal studies, performed before school entry and across childhood, are needed to further elucidate the cognitive trajectories of preterm children.

Keywords: preterm (birth), development, cognitive stability, medical complications, academic achievements

INTRODUCTION

Pre-term birth is associated with dysfunctional development of vital organs and increased risk of cognitive impairment later in life. Some problems appear during the first weeks of life and can be successfully treated, whilst others have a permanent influence on the development. Brain injury such as intraventricular hemorrhage (IVH) and periventricular leukomalacia (PVL) are associated with a high risk of neurodevelopmental disability (Volpe, 1980; Volpe et al., 2011). Preventing brain injury by supporting the respiratory control systems in the preterm infant is crucial. Apnea of prematurity can prolong the need for invasive ventilatory support and bronchopulmonary dysplasia, which are both associated with neurodevelopmental impairment (Janvier et al., 2004; Hofstetter et al., 2008; Doyle and Anderson, 2009). The degree of prematurity and the presence of comorbidities of more than one harmful factor influence the severity of developmental deficiencies in cognitive functioning, as well as in academic achievements (Schmidt et al., 2015). Inflammation has emerged as a critical contributor to both normal development and injury outcome in the immature brain (Hagberg et al., 2015). Neonatal factors found to predict a lower adulthood IQ include: respiratory distress syndrome, IVH, mechanical ventilation, mobility problems, parenteral nutrition, low to middle socioeconomic status of parents, and poor parent-infant relationship (Breeman et al., 2017). Furthermore, a range of perinatal vulnerability factors have been associated with male sex supporting the concept that male sex is an important biological risk factor in extremely preterm infants. Future prospects for preterm children are of utmost interest for parents, pediatric medicine, schools, and society (Moore et al., 2012; Aylward, 2014).

The results of cognitive assessments in children who were born very (week 28–32) or extremely (<week 28) preterm, range from severe and mild levels of intellectual disability to cognitive levels above average. The prevalence for severe cognitive delay is higher in populations of very (Murray et al., 2014) and extremely premature children (Johnson et al., 2009). Though the majority of preterm children perform within normal range of general cognitive functioning, as a group they perform 0.5–1 SD below that of full term children (Bohm et al., 2002; Rose et al., 2011; Luttikhuizen dos Santos et al., 2013; Linsell et al., 2018). Specific cognitive functions such as attention, working memory, and processing speed are also often delayed (Rose et al., 2012; Murray et al., 2014).

Early developmental assessment of cognition from 18 to 24 months post term age (corrected for prematurity) tend to be stable in preterm children with average cognitive development, but future cognitive functioning seems harder to predict when children are performing 1 to 2 SD below expectation, especially in VLBW infants (Roberts et al., 2010; Luttikhuizen dos Santos et al., 2013; Wong et al., 2016).

There is strong evidence that parental education acts as a predictor for cognitive development in preterm children (Bohm et al., 2002; Breeman et al., 2017). In addition, parental level of education, employment and income have additionally shown independent, and additive effects on cognitive gain across preschool years (Manley et al., 2015; Beauregard et al., 2018). Cognitive outcome after preterm birth is heterogeneous, and group level analyses may disguise individual variability in development.

Thus, long-term studies that address individual patterns and explore trajectories in cognitive development are emerging (Stalnacke et al., 2015; Wong et al., 2016; Mangin et al., 2017). A significant number of children born very preterm or VLBW experience difficulties in school. To be able to reduce the long-term risks associated with VLBW birth, an improved understanding of the mechanisms and risk factors placing these children at risk of cognitive delay and dysfunction is necessary. Identifying factors affecting the predictive accuracy of early neurodevelopmental assessments and individual trajectories of overall, as well as specific, cognitive function is important in order to enable earlier support and intervention.

Aim

The aim of the present study was to investigate trajectories of cognitive functioning at the age of 18 months, 5 and 11 years in a Swedish cohort of preterm children with very low birth-weight (500–1250 g). The concordance over time in different aspects of cognition were studied as well as the differences within the cohort predicted by sex, preterm birth factors, medical risk factors, and parental level of education.

MATERIALS AND METHODS

The Swedish cohort is part of an international multisite follow-up study, the Caffeine for Apnea of Prematurity trial (CAP), a randomized and placebo-controlled study of the safety and efficacy of neonatal Caffeine citrate (Methylxanthines), for management and/or prevention of apnea in premature children with a birth-weight of 500–1250 g (Schmidt, 2005; Schmidt et al., 2011). Information about the random assignment is confidential to members of the double-blind CAP trial. Therefore, effects of drug treatment are not evaluated in this study.

Participants

The present Swedish cohort consists of 24 VLBW infants, born at the Karolinska University Hospital between 2001–2004. They were enrolled in the study during the first week after birth and received caffeine therapy or placebo, until it was no longer needed during the neonatal period (Schmidt et al., 2006). The characteristics of the preterm infants and parental education is presented in **Table 1**.

Ethics Statement

The study was performed in accordance with European Community guidelines. The regional ethics committees at the Karolinska Institutet and Stockholm County approved the study (2012/1401). Informed written consent was obtained from the parents. Feedback to parents was communicated after assessments.

Procedure

Follow-up in terms of medical, motor, and cognitive assessment was performed three times. The cognitive assessment was performed by clinical psychologists at 18–24 months and at the 5th and 11th years of age. The assessment at 18 months, at 5 years as well as at 11 years were corrected for preterm birth. Child and parent ratings of behavior was collected at 11 years: Presentation of motor assessments and behavior ratings have been planned for in the near future.

TABLE 1 | Characteristics of preterm infants and parents' educational level, Swedish CAP cohort.

Variables	Descriptive statistics
Infants Characteristics, *n* = 24	
Birth weight, mean (SD), g	981 (167)
Gestational age, mean (SD), week	27 (1.1)
Female, no. (%)	10 (42)
Very preterm (28–29 weeks), no. (%)	6 (25)
Extremely preterm (<28 weeks), no. (%)	18 (75)
SGA, no. (%)	8 (33)
Singleton birth, no. (%)	20 (83)
Respiratory support <8 days no. (%)	7 (25)
Invasive ventilatory support <6 days no. (%)	13 (54)
Invasive ventilatory support >7 days no. (%)	4 (17)
Medical complications	
CLD, no. (%)	4 (17)
BPD, no. (%)	7 (29)
IVH, no. (%)	5 (21)
ROP, grade >3, treated, no. (%)	4 (17)
ROP, grade 1–2, no. (%)	3 (13)
Sepsis, no. (%)	16 (67)
Parental Education Level, at 11 years (*n* = 48)	
Less than elementary school level yes, no. (%)	2 (4)
High school, yes, no. (%)	21 (45)
Diploma, yes, no. (%)	11(23)
Bachelor/masters, yes, no. (%)	11(23)
PhD, yes, no. (%)	2 (4)

Respiratory support (Invasive and non-invasive ventilatory support combined) <8 days. CLD = chronic lung disease, BPD = bronchopulmonary dysplasia, IVH = intraventricular hemorrhage, ROP = retinopathy of prematurity.

Tests and Measures

General cognitive development/functioning was estimated at the three assessments points, with the second edition of the Bayley Scales of Infant Development, (BSID-II), mental development index (MDI), WPPSI-III full scale index (FSIQ), and WISC-IV full scale index (FSIQ), respectively. A validated WISC-IV-short form was used (Crawford et al., 2010) in exchange for WASI-II and DLS Swedish Reading and Spelling tests replaced the corresponding sub-tests from WRAT-4. Standard scores on cognitive indexes have a mean of 100 and standard deviation (SD) of 15, with higher scores indicating a higher level of cognitive development/functioning (Bayley, 1993; David, 2006, 2007). Tests and measures evaluated in the study are presented in **Table 2**.

Statistical Methods

Descriptive statistics are presented either as means, SD, and medians (ranges) for continuous data, or as frequencies or percentages for categorical variables.

For continuous variables the paired *t* test was used to examine within subject changes between two assessment time points and the independent *t* test was applied to examine difference between males and females. The Mann-Whitney test was employed when there was a violation of the assumptions of normality and equal variance.

Based on the three indexes, BSID-II (MDI), WPPSI-III (FSIQ), and WISC-IV (FSIQ) a standardized cognitive scale was created (-2 to $+2$). The Friedman ANOVA was performed to compare the three scales considering the ordinal property of the outcome variable. *Post hoc* analysis with Wilcoxon signed-rank tests was conducted with a Bonferroni correction applied since the overall Friedman ANOVA was significant.

We employed Generalized Estimating Equation (GEE) to analyze the change over time and to examine the fixed effects of male/female sex. A time x sex interaction term was introduced in the model to examine heterogeneity effect. GEE was also performed to control for potential confounders. Explanatory variables were selected based on clinical relevance, earlier research findings and univariate GEE models. Upon completion of the univariate analyses, we selected variables for the multivariate analyses including factors judged to be potential confounders. We have also employed Linear mixed model (LMM) to examine the relationship between the response

TABLE 2 | Cognitive test during follow up.

Age	Test methods	Measures
18 month	BSID-II, Bayley scales of infant development – second edition	Mental development index (MDI)
5 year	WPPSI-III, Wechsler's Preschool and Primary Scale of Intelligence - Third edition	Full scale IQ (FSIQ): verbal function (VI) visual function (PI) and processing speed (SI)
5 and 11 year	Beery -Buktenica Developmental Test of Visual-Motor Integration (VMI) – sixth edition	Visuomotor integration (VMI), visual perception (VP) and fine motor coordination (FMC)
11 year	WISC-IV, Wechsler's Intelligence Scale for Children – fourth edition, short form	Full scale IQ (FSIQ): 7 subtests. Verbal function index (VI): subtests similarities and vocabulary. Performance index (PI): subtests block design and matrix reasoning. Index speed of process (SI): subtests coding and symbol search. Working memory: subtest digit span
	RCFT: rey complex figure test and recognition trial	Copy score and Recall score
	TEA-Ch; test of everyday attention for children	Selective (subtest sky search), sustained (subtest score), divided (subtest sky search dt) and shifting (subtest creature)
	WRAT-4: the wide range achievement test	Mathematics (numerical operations)
	DLS for school year 4–6; diagnostic material for reading and writing. Swedish tests	Spelling 36 words and Reading 47 words

IQ score as numerical continuous outcome variable and clinical and demographic explanatory variables. Both GEE and LMM simultaneously examine the relationship between each predictor and the outcome variable and the relationship between changes in the predictors and changes in the dependent variable. The dependent variable cognitive level was coded as −2, −1, 0, 1, and 2 for each timepoint, based on the standardized cognitive level which represent severe delay (≤ = 70), moderate delay (71–85), normal (86–114), high (115–130), and superior (≥131) cognitive levels, respectively. Categorical explanatory variables were coded depending on their level. If only two levels existed, the reference category was the category with the higher code number: The variable sex was coded as female = 1 and male = 2, thus male was the reference category. The categorical variable "educational level" constituted six levels, which were coded as 1 = less than elementary, 2 = elementary, 3 = high school, 4 = diploma, 5 = university degree (Bachelor or Masters), and 6 = Ph.D. holder. Less than elementary was the reference category. IVH was coded as 0 = no IVH, 1 = Grade 1, 2 = Grade 2; grade 2 was the reference category. Time was coded as 1 = 18 months, 2 = 5 years, and 3 = 11 years (the reference category). Level of respiratory support was coded as: 0 = Invasive (endotracheal tube *in situ*) and non-invasive (continuous positive airway pressure- CPAP) ventilatory support combined <8 days, 1 = mild (combined ventilatory support >8 days but invasive ventilatory support ≤6 days) and 2 = prolonged (invasive ventilatory support >6 days). The results of GEE are presented as estimate (regression coefficient), standard error (SE), Wald Chi-square value and *p*-value. Results of LMM are included in **Supplementary Table 1**. SPSS version 25.0 (IBM, NY, United States) was used for all data analyses and Statistica 13 for case profile graphical presentation. The level of significance was specified as $p = 0.05$.

RESULTS

All 24 children in the Swedish cohort participated in all three assessments, thus the follow up was 100%. **Table 1** shows the characteristics of preterm birth, medical and social background factors for the complete group as well as separated for by sex. At the 5-year and 11-year assessment, no child was deaf, blind or had cerebral palsy. Preterm medical risk variables that were considered to have too few participants to be included in further analyses are not shown in the tables. The level of the cognitive index score at the three assessment points for each gender are summarized in **Figure 1**. **Table 2** shows all tests, including abbreviations, cognitive, and academic measures for the Swedish CAP cohort. The test results are summarized in **Table 3**. The mean test score of the study subjects is presented by sex, maternal education level, paternal education level, and IVH (**Figures 2A–D**, respectively). The independent sample *t*-test was employed to compare means for between group differences and the paired *t*-test for within-subject change (**Table 4**).

Cognitive Level Through Development

Friedman test revealed a statistically significant difference in the standardized cognitive index over time, $\chi^2 = 18.7$, df = 2, $p < 0.001$. *Post hoc* analysis with Wilcoxon signed-rank tests was conducted with a Bonferroni correction applied, resulting in a significance level set at $p = 0.017$. We observed a statistically significant difference between Bayley-II MDI (at 18 months) and WPPSI-III FSIQ (at 5 years) ($p = 0.001$) and between WPPSI-III FSIQ (at 5 years) and WISC-IV FSIQ (at 11 years) ($p = 0.002$). However, we did not observe significant differences between BSID-II MDI and WISC-IV FSIQ ($Z = -1.67$, $p = 0.096$). WISC-FI was significantly related to WISC-SI, Mathematics SS, sex, and IVH (**Supplementary Table 1**). LMM also revealed that time was a statistically significant predictor of cognitive score. We observed a statistically significant difference between WPPSI-III FSIQ (at 5 years) and WISC-IV FSIQ at 11 years ($p = 0.02$). However, we did not observe a significant difference between BSID-II MDI and WISC-IV FSIQ ($p = 0.79$).

The univariate and multivariable General Estimating Equation (GEE) analysis were carried out and are presented in **Tables 5, 6** respectively. Sex was observed to be a predictor of standardized

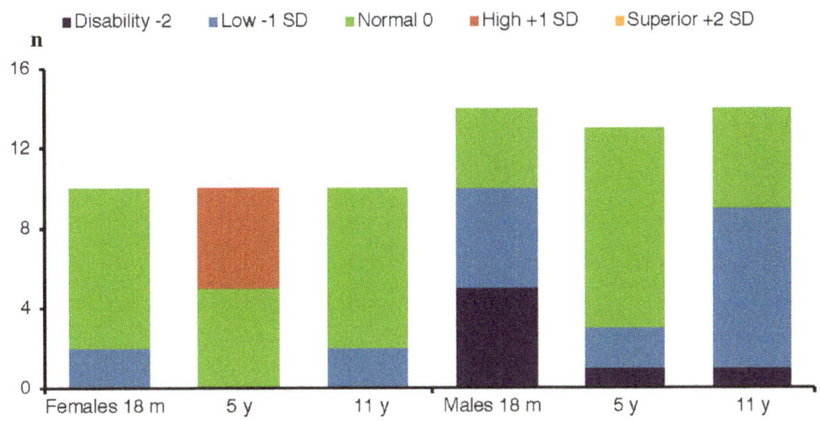

FIGURE 1 | Cognitive level for females and males at three assessment points. Cognitive index scores standardized in levels. Index score <70 = disability/severe delay. 71–85 = low/moderate delay. 86–115 = normal/average. 116–130 = high. <131 = superior. Assessment at 18 months, 5 and 11 years of age, 10 female and 14 male preterm VLBW children.

TABLE 3 | Test results for the Swedish cohort.

Tests	Swedish data: *N* = 24 mean (SD)	Female *N* = 10 mean (SD)	Male *N* = 14 mean (SD)	Total *N* = 24 min.– max. Results
BSID-II MDI **18 months**	85.7 (17.0)	97.8 (15.1)	77.1 (12.7)	55 – 114
WPPSI-III FSIQ **5 year** (full scale)	102.0 (16.6)	110.4 (14.6)	95.9 (15.7)	57 – 128
WPPSI-III VI (verbal)	98.1 (17.8)	107.0 (15.9)	91.8 (16.8)	47 – 137
WPPSI-III PI (visual)	97.3 (12.9)	100.8 (11.8)	94.7 (13.4)	70 – 120
WPPSI-III SI (speed)	79.0 (12.8)	87.9 (12.6)	72.6 (8.7)	46 – 114
WISC-IV FSIQ **11 year**	86.9 (13.4)	95.1 (12.8)	81.0 (10.8)	56 – 113
WISC-IV VI (verbal)	89.0 (15.0)	98.9 (14.8)	86.2 (11.3)	70 – 122
WISC-IV PI (visual)	95.5 (12.0)	101.2 (12.9)	91.4 (9.8)	77 – 121
WISC-IV SI (speed)	89.4 (14.1)	95.6 (12.4)	84.9 (13.8)	55 – 116
Beery VMI **5 year** (copying**)**	96.3 (16.8)	102.9 (21.7)	91.6 (10.8)	70 – 132
VMI VP (perception)	105.9 (23.6)	111.1 (23.7)	102.1 (23.7)	45 – 132
VMI FMC (fine-motor control)	92.4 (21.0)	101.3 (21.7)	86.1 (18.8)	45 – 130
Beery VMI **11 year** (copying)	90.5 (15.1)	98.4 (10.4)	84.9 (15.7)	62 – 115
VMI VP (perception)	96.0 (17.3)	100.9 (16.1)	92.5 (17.7)	45 – 113
VMI FMC (fine-motor control)	87.8 (15.7)	95.1 (15.3)	82.6 (14.3)	45 – 114
WRAT-4, Mathematic	81.2 (16.4)	86.7 (16.4)	77.3 (9.7)	16 – 40
Reading 47 words; %	80.0 (21.0)	87.9 (14.1)	74.4 (23.7)	4 – 47
Spelling 36; stanine	3.3 (1.9)	4.4 (1.7)	2.5 (1.7)	3 – 32
TEA-Ch: selective att.	7.6 (3.3)	9.1 (3.3)	6.5 (2.9)	2 – 13
TEA-Ch: sustained	7.1 (2.1)	8.1 (2.2)	6.4 (1.8)	4 – 13
TEA-Ch: divided	5.3 (2.4)	5.4 (2.8)	5.2 (2.2)	1 – 10
TEA-Ch: shifting	9.3 (3.3)	10.2 (3.4)	8.6 (3)	3 – 13
WISC-IV digit span, forward	5.0 (1.0)	5.2 (1.3)	4.9 (0.8)	3 – 7
WISC-IV digit span, backward	3.6 (0.9)	3.8 (1.0)	3.4 (0.8)	2 – 6
RCFT, copy	24.3 (9.6)	28.8 (5.8)	21.1 (10.6)	3 – 36
RCFT, delayed recall	11.7 (7.9)	13.9 (5.0)	10.0 (9.4)	0 – 25.5

cognitive score. Female sex was positively associated with standardized score in all multivariable models, **Table 6.** Univariate GEE revealed that the likelihood of having a higher cognitive score was positively related to time at 5 years ($B = 1.58$, Wald Chi-square = 10.8, $p = 0.001$) with 11 years as a reference. However, when the dependent variable was the standardized Z score, GEE revealed that the likelihood of having a higher Z cognitive score was positively related to time (Wald Chi square 18.7, df = 2, $p < 0.001$). Higher Z score value was positively related to time at 5 years ($B = 2.1$, Wald Chi-square = 12.9, df = 1, $p < 0.001$) with 11 years as a reference.

General Estimating Equation showed that IVH was a predictor of standardized cognitive score. In addition, level of respiratory support was a significant predictor of standardized cognitive score in the univariate ($p = 0.03$) and multivariable GEE analysis when controlling for sex and time in the latter analysis ($p = 0.04$). SGA and BPD were not statistically significant in either univariate and multivariable GEE analyses, when controlled for sex and time, **Tables 5, 6.**

Univariate GEE analysis revealed a positive relationship between parental education levels and the standardized score (**Table 5**). Both maternal and paternal educational levels were positively associated with the standardized score in all multivariable models when controlling for sex and time (**Supplementary Table 2**). We did not observe interactions between time and other clinical and demographic factors in all used multivariable models.

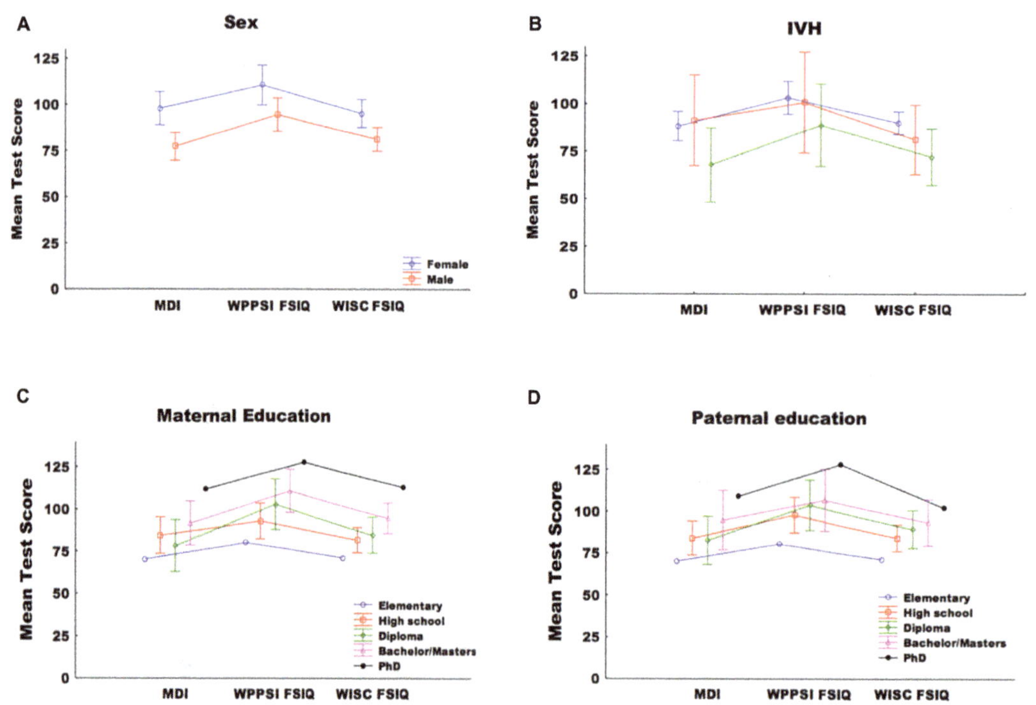

FIGURE 2 | (A) Mean test score by sex and test type. **(B)** Mean test score by IVH and test type. **(C)** Mean test score by maternal educational level and test type, **(D)** mean test score by paternal educational level and test type. Mental development index (MDI), WPPSI-III Full scale index (FSIQ), and WISC-IV Full scale index (FSIQ) 18 month, 5 and 11 years, respectively. Data is presented as mean + SEM.

TABLE 4 | Results of the paired and independent *t* tests of the Swedish cohort.

Scale	Mean difference (95% CI)	*P*-value
Paired *t* test		
2 VMI SS – VMI SS	−5.5 (−9.8, −1.3)	0.01
2 VMI VP – VMI VP	−10.1 (−17.0, −3.2)	<0.01
2 VMI Motor – VMI motor	−5.2 (−11.6, 1.1)	0.1
WISC VI – WPPSI VI	−13.1 (−17.3, −8.8)	<0.001
WISC PI – WPPSI PI	−8.8 (−12.6, −4.9)	<0.001
WISC SI – WPPSI S	10.4 (5.8, 15.6)	<0.001
Independent *t* test (female – male)		
2VMI SS	13.5 (1.6, 25.3)	0.03
2VMI VP	0.03 (−0.4, 0.5)	0.42
2VMI FMC	13.1 (0.5, 25.7)	0.04
WPPSI FSIQ	14.6 (1.6, 27.7)	0.03
WPPSI VI (verbal)	16.0 (1.1, 30.8)	0.04
WPPSI PI (visual)	6.5 (−4.9, 18.0)	0.25
WPPSI SI (speed)	17.2 (−4.9, 27.2)	<0.001
WISC FSIQ	14.1 (4.1, 24.1)	<0.01
WISC VI (verbal)	12.6 (1.7, 23.7)	0.03
WISC PI (visual)	9.8 (0.2, 19.3)	<0.05
WISC SI (speed)	10.7 (−0.7, 22.1)	0.17

Mean differences, 95% confidence interval (CI) and p-values for paired t and independent t tests.

The independent *t*-test revealed that there was statistically significant score differences in between the sexes for many items indicating higher score for girls compared to boys (**Table 4**). The paired mean differences were also statistically significant for most items (**Table 4**).

TABLE 5 | Results of GEE univariate analysis with parameter estimates, standard errors and Wald Chi square for the cohort for the dependent variable cognitive level.

Variable	B	SE	Wald Chi-square	*P*-value
Sex = Female	2.25	0.79	8.14	0.004
Time			16.2	<0.001
Time = 18 months	−0.41	0.31	1.78	0.18
Time = 5 years	1.58	0.48	10.8	0.001
SGA = 0	1.1	0.72	2.34	0.12
BPD = 0	−0.12	0.67	0.03	0.86
IVH			8.6	0.01
IVH = 0	2.4	0.93	6.45	0.01
IVH = 1	2.9	1.00	8.43	0.004
Maternal education*				
University	5.5	0.86	40.6	<0.001
Bachelor/masters	3.4	0.83	16.5	<0.001
Diploma	1.7	0.42	16.3	<0.001
Elementary	1.9	0.72	7.2	0.007
Paternal education*				
University	5.3	0.91	34.1	<0.001
Bachelor/masters	2.9	0.92	10.1	0.001
Diploma	3.8	0.59	41.6	<0.001
High School	2.2	0.42	27.4	<0.001
Elementary	1.9	0.67	7.8	0.005
Respiratory# support level				
Level = 0	1.7	0.70	5.5	0.019
Level = 1	1.6	0.65	5.8	0.015

**Reference: less than elementary. #Reference: respiratory support = level 2 (invasive ventilatory support >6 days).*

Cognitive Functioning and Academic Achievement at 11 Years of Age

Data analyses revealed broad confidence intervals for results of specific cognitive measures (TEA-Ch, RCFT, and WISC-IV digit span) at 11 years of age. WISC-IV SI was found significantly lower than WISC-IV FSIQ at 11 years ($p \leq 0.001$). Measures of academic achievement showed sex difference in Mathematic WRAT-4 ($p = 0.04$) and Spelling DLS measures ($p = 0.01$), favoring girls. We did not observe differences in reading ability.

DISCUSSION

This prospective cohort study has three assessment points of cognitive development and a follow-up rate of 100%, which adds stability to the results and bolster our conclusions. We found that, male sex and parental education had a significant impact on cognitive test results. This concurs with previous studies but the present data further underline the effect of sex and parental education in long term cognitive and academic outcomes (Bohm et al., 2002; Linsell et al., 2015, 2018; Mangin et al., 2017). IVH was identified as a strong predictor of cognitive outcome, and so was the cumulative duration of invasive ventilatory support. This is in accordance with recent studies, e.g., (Breeman et al., 2017). However, other medical complications (ROP, CLD/BPD, SGA, and sepsis) did not contribute to the explained variance. Sex differences were seen in all tests given, with females acquiring higher scores than males. Parental education was on average high in both mothers and fathers and all levels significantly influenced the cognitive outcome in the multivariate analyses.

The GEE is an appropriate statistical method to fit a marginal model for longitudinal data analysis since we have repeated measures over time. We measured 24 children at three time points with three different cognitive tests to examine their cognitive development/functioning. The repeated measurements thus provides a multivariate response of similar individuals. GEE is a common approach to longitudinal data based on population-averaged (marginal) approach. The GEE models the average response over the subpopulation sharing a common value of the predictors, as a function of the predictors (Liang and Zeger, 1986).

Cognitive z-scores from −2 to +2 are represented in this Swedish cohort of VLBW infants. GEE showed that the cognitive results were similar at 18 months and 11 years of age. We found the results to be important since predictability of early assessments varies. Robust findings based on meta-analyses and single studies imply that the predictability for later cognitive functioning in pre-school and school-aged children vary, from moderate in very preterm to poor in extremely preterm infants. In contrast, several studies of cognitive outcome between pre-school and middle-school age as well as adolescence,

TABLE 6 | Results of GEE multivariable analysis with parameter estimates, standard errors and Wald Chi square for the cohort for the dependent variable cognitive level.

Variable	B	SE	Wald Chi-square	*P*-value
Model 1 with SGA				
SGA	0.82	0.76	1.2	0.28
Sex = female	2.51	0.91	7.51	0.006
Time = 18 months	−0.70	0.42	2.81	0.09
Time = 5 years	1.88	0.49	15.0	<0.001
Model 2 with IVH				
IVH = 0	1.6	1.08	2.12	0.14
IVH = 1	3.6	1.07	11.2	0.001
Sex = female	2.76	1.00	7.6	0.006
Time = 18 months	−0.75	0.47	2.5	0.11
Time = 5 years	2.01	0.52	14.7	<0.001
Model 3* Maternal education				
University	5.1	1.26	16.4	<0.001
Bachelor/masters	3.6	0.97	13.8	<0.001
Diploma	1.9	0.68	7.81	0.005
Elementary	1.5	0.90	2.8	0.094
Sex = female	2.68	0.96	7.77	0.005
Time = 18 months	−0.77	0.45	2.86	0.09
Time = 5 years	1.51	0.84	3.21	0.07
Model 4* Paternal Education				
University	4.51	1.22	12.1	<0.001
Bachelor/Masters	1.93	0.95	4.0	0.047
Diploma	2.43	1.25	3.78	
High school	2.60	0.72	13.4	<0.001
Elementary	1.74	0.78	4.91	0.027
Sex = female	2.53	1.26	3.93	0.047
Time = 18 months	−0.78	0.48	2.71	0.10
Time = 5 years	2.04	0.54	14.3	<0.001
Model 5 Respiratory support#				
Level = 0	3.15	1.25	6.3	0.012
Level = 1	2.35	1.25	3.5	0.06

**Reference: less than elementary; #Reference: respiratory support = level 2. The multivariable models include the variables sex and time with the interaction.*

report stability in cognitive development (Stalnacke et al., 2015; Mangin et al., 2017).

Summarizing other studies of cognitive development from infancy to adolescence is challenging due to methodological deficiencies. Outcome studies often have only one or two assessment points, lack of a control group, loss to follow up, and a varied application of standardized test norms and statistical methodologies, rendering the conclusions of these studies hard to compare (Wong et al., 2016). Based on our study design and results we find it important to take into account that time points and time between cognitive assessments can affect findings in cognitive follow-up of preterm children. Of equal importance are longitudinal studies, and maintaining high retention throughout follow-up (Doyle and Anderson, 2018). Recently, the longitudinal EPI Cure study showed that cognitive test score in infancy and early childhood reflect early adult outcomes (Linsell et al., 2018).

The cognitive results at 5 years of age were markedly higher compared to cognitive levels at both 18 months and 11 years of age, which requires an account of potential methodological issues in the performance of said test. The Swedish WPPSI-III norms are based on British norms and validated in a limited sample of Swedish children (David, 2006). Thus, the high results at 5 years of age might be due to an incomplete Swedish validation of the British WPPSI-III norms. Test construction, validity and reliability issues of cognitive assessment in preterm children can have an impact on cognitive results and are also addressed in other studies (Luttikhuizen dos Santos et al., 2013; Spencer-Smith et al., 2015). The results are similar at 18 months and 11 years, both at individual and group level. Thus, the apparent increase at the 5-year assessment are likely due to test norm differences. Nevertheless, the heterogeneous nature of cognitive outcomes in individuals emphasize the importance of long-term follow-up and monitoring of infants born VLBW (Manley et al., 2015; Beauregard et al., 2018).

We know little about the developmental pace regarding different aspects of cognition, especially for preterm children, with their risk of suboptimal neurocognitive development/cognition. There is still considerable debate and uncertainty with regards to whether very preterm children grow into or out of their cognition problems (Mangin et al., 2017). Our and other long-term studies, that address individual patterns and explore trajectories in cognitive development, indicate that cognitive test scores in infancy and early childhood may reflect cognition and academic performance during early school years (Stalnacke et al., 2015; Wong et al., 2016; Mangin et al., 2017; Linsell et al., 2018). Notably, cognitive trajectories may differ. Recently, several distinct language trajectories were revealed, in very preterm and full term infants examined at 2, 5, 7, and 13 years (Nguyen et al., 2018). This and our study underline the importance of monitoring cognition in children born very preterm before school entry and across childhood.

The process of cognitive maturation is complex, multidimensional and influenced by genetic predisposition, environmental factors and experience (Fuster, 2005) and ruptures in development (Anderson, 2001; Anderson et al., 2008). Effects on brain development (Haynes et al., 2011; Volpe et al., 2011) and coherent alternated cognitive trajectories (Mangin et al., 2017) are found in preterm children (Thompson et al., 2018). Comparing the cognitive results at 5 years and 11 years of age indicated both stability and change in the cohort. Level of verbal intelligence (VI) was significantly lower at 11 years and so was the visuo-constructive measure (Beery VMI). Perceptual intelligence (PI) was found to be stable. Processing speed (SI) was higher at 11 years. The visuo-constructive measure (Beery VMI) was significantly lower at 11 years. Declining results and differences between cognitive functions may be affected by specific deficits especially in executive functions. In our study it was not possible to draw a conclusion from executive tests at 11 years since the single specific cognitive measures, TEA-Ch, RCFT, and Digit Span, had broad confidence intervals and in combination with the effect of the cohort size could lead to random results. Problems with attention, working memory and processing speed are significantly more present among preterm children and tend to emerge during development (Rose et al., 2011, 2012; Murray et al., 2014). Deficits in attention and processing speed are identified as important abilities contributing to lower level of cognitive intelligence in preterm children (Rose et al., 2009, 2011, 2012). Cognitive functioning in preterm children is of great importance for school performance. Results in academic achievement are of special interest, as they will show any issues that may be a problem in school. Our test battery included mathematics, reading and spelling. Mathematics were significantly correlated to FSIQ at 11 years (r = 0.77) and WISC PI, WISC SI, and IVH-2 were found to significantly explain most of the variance (R^2 = 0.64) of the dependent variable Mathematics.

Sex differences were seen in all tests given, with females acquiring higher scores than males. Except for the VMI visual perception (VP) and fine motor coordination, this was also consistent between the two assessment points. Females also performed higher in academics, mathematics and spelling. Male sex is known to be a disadvantage with regards to mortality, morbidity and incidence of brain injury in preterm children (Marlow et al., 2005; Hintz et al., 2006; Skiold et al., 2014). The major type of brain injury involves cerebral white matter and the principal cellular target is the developing oligodendrocytes (Volpe et al., 2011). Neonatal white matter abnormalities are associated with cognitive impairment across childhood (Mangin et al., 2017). The view of male sex as a risk factor for cognitive development varies. Extremely premature boys have an increased risk of lower cognitive outcome (Linsell et al., 2018) and of developing severe cognitive disability (Marlow et al., 2005). However, in very preterm children the difference based on male sex decreases with age and environmental factors become more significant (Linsell et al., 2015; Mangin et al., 2017). The present results are in line with previous as well as recent studies (Doyle et al., 2015; Linsell et al., 2018; Thompson et al., 2018) and underlines the importance of considering sex in the potential cognitive developmental of preterm infants. Structural asymmetries and sexual brain dimorphism already exist at 1 month after birth in healthy term infants (Dean et al., 2018). In general, males have larger total brain volume and volumes differ by sex in regionally specific brain regions. We speculate that the different rates of maturation between the sexes renders the male brain, and hence male sex, a risk factor for long term cognitive outcome especially in VLBW preterm infants. Some of the underlying mechanisms for sex differences found, are delayed myelinization in preterm males, lower white matter volumes in males and differences in cerebral white matter microstructure compared to preterm females (Constable et al., 2008; Skiold et al., 2014).

We cannot exclude the effect of neonatal caffeine therapy from our findings. However, no adverse long-term effects of caffeine on development have been shown in the CAP studies, e.g., (Schmidt et al., 2006, 2017; Mürner-Lavanchy et al., 2018). The CAP-trial indicated a positive developmental trend in cognitive scores, between 18 months and 5 years of age, independent of treatment. Thus, our data are consistent with the results from this larger cohort (Schmidt et al., 2012). However, in the present cohort, the data and trajectories suggest that the increase was temporary and likely due to test norm differences. Nevertheless, cognitive results in our cohort indicate similar levels between 18 months and 11 years of age. Thus, on a group level, this does not support the suggestion that cognitive outcomes for preterm VLBW infants may improve throughout childhood (Ment et al., 2003). However, they are in line with, and underscore previous findings with regards to the importance of IVH, level of ventilatory support, sex as well as parental education for the long-term cognitive and academic outcomes (Doyle et al., 2015). These data emphasize the importance of early and repeated individual assessment enabling early intervention as well as adequate support during early childhood into adolescence, especially for those with cognitive delay and at risk for cognitive decline (Stalnacke et al., 2015; Mangin et al., 2017).

A strength of the present study is the 100% follow-up rate. The small group size is a limitation, which is why all medical variables and possible background variables could not be included in the model. The specific cognitive measures at 11 years of age, were found to have broad confidence intervals and thus in combination with the effect of cohort size these results could be random.

In summary analyzing measures of cognitive development across time better clarify changes and risk factors. We suggest long-term study designs, with more than two assessment points and with a substantial time between follow-up. It is possible to explore trajectories of cognitive function in a small cohort, when the cohort remains the same. Exploring individual patterns of cognition and brain development, as well as the underlying mechanisms associated with these, is necessary to increase knowledge about the maturation of preterm children. Cognitive development extends well beyond adolescence; and thus future follow-up should continue beyond 11 years. Early identification of children in need of support to promote development is an imperative necessity, especially for those with cognitive delay and at risk for cognitive decline.

AUTHOR CONTRIBUTIONS

EH and BB conceptualized and designed the study. EH, SS, and BB acquired the data and revised the manuscript. All authors analyzed the data, drafted a significant portion of the manuscript or figures, and accepted the final version of the manuscript.

FUNDING

This study was supported by the Swedish Research Council (2009-3724 and 2016-0111), the Stockholm County Council (ALF projects 2012-0465 and 20140011), the Karolinska Institutet, and grants from the Swedish Brain (2015-0020), Axel Tielman (2015-00220 and 2018-00418), Freemasons Children's House, Astrid Lindgren Children's Hospital and Swedish National Heart and Lung (2015-0558) Foundations. The funding sources of the study had no role in the study design, data collection, analysis, interpretation, or writing of the results of this study, or in the decision to submit.

ACKNOWLEDGMENTS

We acknowledge research nurse Lena Legnevall for providing technical assistance and psychologist Anette Holm and Stephanie Cullberg-Sundén for assisting with the testing procedures. We thank Dr. Louise Steinhoff and Ph.D. Wiktor Phillips for English language assistance and Prof. Peter J. Anderson for discussion and advice. We are indebted to the CAP investigators who made this study possible and importantly the children and their families who participated in this follow-up study.

REFERENCES

Anderson, V. (2001). *Developmental Neuropsychology: A Clinical Approach*. Hove: Psychology Press.

Anderson, V., Jacobs, R., and Anderson, P. (2008). *Executive Functions And The Frontal Lobes: A Lifespan Perspective*. Didcot: Taylor & Francis.

Aylward, G. P. P. A. (2014). Neurodevelopmental outcomes of infants born prematurely. *J. Dev. Behav. Pediatr.* 35, 394–407. doi: 10.1097/01.DBP.0000452240.39511.d4

Bayley, N. (1993). *Bayley Scales of Infant Development*, 2nd Edn. San Antonio, TX: The Psychological Corporation.

Beauregard, J. L., Drews-Botsch, C., Sales, J. M., Flanders, W. D., and Kramer, M. R. (2018). Does socioeconomic status modify the association between preterm birth and children's early cognitive ability and kindergarten academic achievement in the United States? *Am. J. Epidemiol.* 187, 1704–1713. doi: 10.1093/aje/kwy068

Bohm, B., Katz-Salamon, M., Institute, K., Smedler, A. C., Lagercrantz, H., and Forssberg, H. (2002). Developmental risks and protective factors for influencing cognitive outcome at 5 1/2 years of age in very-low-birthweight children. *Dev. Med. Child Neurol.* 44, 508–516. doi: 10.1111/j.1469-8749.2002.tb00321.x

Breeman, L. D., Jaekel, J., Baumann, N., Bartmann, P., and Wolke, D. (2017). Neonatal predictors of cognitive ability in adults born very preterm: a prospective cohort study. *Dev. Med. Child Neurol.* 59, 477–483. doi: 10.1111/dmcn.13380

Constable, R. T., Ment, L. R., Vohr, B. R., Kesler, S. R., Fulbright, R. K., Lacadie, C., et al. (2008). Prematurely born children demonstrate white matter microstructural differences at 12 years of age, relative to term control subjects: an investigation of group and gender effects. *Pediatrics* 121, 306–316. doi: 10.1542/peds.2007-0414

Crawford, J. R., Anderson, V., Rankin, P. M., and Macdonald, J. (2010). An index-based short-form of the WISC-IV with accompanying analysis of the reliability and abnormality of differences. *Br. J. Clin. Psychol.* 49, 235–258. doi: 10.1348/014466509X455470

David, W. (2006). *Wechsler Preschool and Primary Scale of Intelligence*, 2nd Edn. Stockholm: Harcourt Assessment.

David, W. (2007). *Wechsler Intelligence Scale for Children*, 4th Edn. Stockholm: Harcourt Assessment.

Dean, D. C., Planalp, E. M., Wooten, W., Schmidt, C. K., Kecskemeti, S. R., Frye, C., et al. (2018). Investigation of brain structure in the 1-month infant. *Brain Struct. Funct.* 223, 1953–1970. doi: 10.1007/s00429-017-1600-2

Doyle, L. W., and Anderson, P. J. (2009). Long-term outcomes of bronchopulmonary dysplasia. *Semin. Fetal Neonatal Med.* 14, 391–395. doi: 10.1016/j.siny.2009.08.004

Doyle, L. W., and Anderson, P. J. (2018). Stability of general cognition in children born extremely preterm as they grow older: good or bad news? *Arch. Dis. Child Fetal Neonatal Educ.* 103, F299–F300. doi: 10.1136/archdischild-2017-313987

Doyle, L. W., Cheong, J. L., Burnett, A., Roberts, G., Lee, K. J., Anderson, P. J., et al. (2015). Biological and social influences on outcomes of extreme-preterm/low-birth weight adolescents. *Pediatrics* 136, e1513–e1520. doi: 10.1542/peds.2015-2006

Fuster, J. M. (2005). *Cortex and Mind*. Oxford: Oxford University Press. doi: 10.1093/acprof:oso/9780195300840.001.0001

Hagberg, H., Mallard, C., Ferriero, D. M., Vannucci, S. J., Levison, S. W., Vexler, Z. S., et al. (2015). The role of inflammation in perinatal brain injury. *Nat. Rev. Neurol.* 11, 192–208. doi: 10.1038/nrneurol.2015.13

Haynes, R. L., Xu, G., Folkerth, R. D., Trachtenberg, F. L., Volpe, J. J., and Kinney, H. C. (2011). Potential neuronal repair in cerebral white matter injury in the human neonate. *Pediatr. Res.* 69, 62–67. doi: 10.1203/PDR.0b013e3181ff3792

Hintz, S. R., Kendrick, D. E., Vohr, B. R., Kenneth Poole, W., Higgins, R. D., and Nichd Neonatal Research Network. (2006). Gender differences in neurodevelopmental outcomes among extremely preterm, extremely-low-birthweight infants. *Acta Paediatr.* 95, 1239–1248. doi: 10.1080/08035250600599727

Hofstetter, A. O., Legnevall, L., Herlenius, E., and Katz-Salamon, M. (2008). Cardiorespiratory development in extremely preterm infants: vulnerability to infection and persistence of events beyond term-equivalent age. *Acta Paediatr.* 97, 285–292. doi: 10.1111/j.1651-2227.2007.00618.x

Janvier, A., Khairy, M., Kokkotis, A., Cormier, C., Messmer, D., and Barrington, K. J. (2004). Apnea is associated with neurodevelopmental impairment in very low birth weight infants. *J. Perinatol.* 24, 763–768. doi: 10.1038/sj.jp.7211182

Johnson, S., Fawke, J., Hennessy, E., Rowell, V., Thomas, S., Wolke, D., et al. (2009). Neurodevelopmental disability through 11 years of age in children born before 26 weeks of gestation. *Pediatrics* 124, e249–e257. doi: 10.1542/peds.2008-3743

Liang, K.-Y., and Zeger, S. L. (1986). Longitudinal data analysis using generalized linear models. *Biometrika* 73, 13–22. doi: 10.1093/biomet/73.1.13

Linsell, L., Johnson, S., Wolke, D., O'reilly, H., Morris, J. K., Kurinczuk, J. J., et al. (2018). Cognitive trajectories from infancy to early adulthood following birth before 26 weeks of gestation: a prospective, population-based cohort study. *Arch. Dis. Child.* 103, 363–370. doi: 10.1136/archdischild-2017-313414

Linsell, L., Malouf, R., Morris, J., Kurinczuk, J. J., and Marlow, N. (2015). Prognostic factors for poor cognitive development in children born very preterm or with very low birth weight: a systematic review. *JAMA Pediatr.* 169, 1162–1172. doi: 10.1001/jamapediatrics.2015.2175

Luttikhuizen dos Santos, E. S., De Kieviet, J. F., Konigs, M., Van Elburg, R. M., and Oosterlaan, J. (2013). Predictive value of the Bayley scales of infant development on development of very preterm/very low birth weight children: a meta-analysis. *Early Hum. Dev.* 89, 487–496. doi: 10.1016/j.earlhumdev.2013.03.008

Mangin, K. S., Horwood, L. J., and Woodward, L. J. (2017). Cognitive development trajectories of very preterm and typically developing children. *Child Dev.* 88, 282–298. doi: 10.1111/cdev.12585

Manley, B. J., Roberts, R. S., Doyle, L. W., Schmidt, B., Anderson, P. J., Barrington, K. J., et al. (2015). Social variables predict gains in cognitive scores across the preschool years in children with birth weights 500 to 1250 grams. *J. Pediatr.* 166, 870–876.e2. doi: 10.1016/j.jpeds.2014.12.016

Marlow, N., Wolke, D., Bracewell, M. A., and Samara, M. (2005). Neurologic and developmental disability at six years of age after extremely preterm birth. *N. Engl. J. Med.* 352, 9–19. doi: 10.1056/NEJMoa041367

Ment, L. R., Vohr, B., Allan, W., Katz, K. H., Schneider, K. C., Westerveld, M., et al. (2003). Change in cognitive function over time in very low-birth-weight infants. *JAMA* 289, 705–711. doi: 10.1001/jama.289.6.705

Moore, T., Hennessy, E. M., Myles, J., Johnson, S. J., Draper, E. S., Costeloe, K. L., et al. (2012). Neurological and developmental outcome in extremely preterm children born in England in 1995 and 2006: the EPICure studies. *BMJ* 345:e7961. doi: 10.1136/bmj.e7961

Mürner-Lavanchy, I. M., Doyle, L. W., Schmidt, B., Roberts, R. S., Asztalos, E. V., Costantini, L., et al. (2018). Neurobehavioral outcomes 11 years after neonatal caffeine therapy for apnea of prematurity. *Pediatrics* 141:e20174047. doi: 10.1542/peds.2017-4047

Murray, A. L., Scratch, S. E., Thompson, D. K., Inder, T. E., Doyle, L. W., Anderson, J. F., et al. (2014). Neonatal brain pathology predicts adverse attention and processing speed outcomes in very preterm and/or very low birth weight children. *Neuropsychology* 28, 552–562. doi: 10.1037/neu0000071

Nguyen, T. N., Spencer-Smith, M., Haebich, K. M., Burnett, A., Scratch, S. E., Cheong, J. L. Y., et al. (2018). Language trajectories of children born very preterm and full term from early to late childhood. *J. Pediatr.* 202, 81–91e1. doi: 10.1016/j.jpeds.2018.06.036

Roberts, G., Anderson, P. J., Doyle, L. W., and Victorian Infant Collaborative Study Group. (2010). The stability of the diagnosis of developmental disability between ages 2 and 8 in a geographic cohort of very preterm children born in 1997. *Arch. Dis. Child.* 95, 786–790. doi: 10.1136/adc.2009.160283

Rose, S. A., Feldman, J. F., and Jankowski, J. J. (2009). Information processing in toddlers: continuity from infancy and persistence of preterm deficits. *Intelligence* 37, 311–320. doi: 10.1016/j.intell.2009.02.002

Rose, S. A., Feldman, J. F., Jankowski, J. J., and Van Rossem, R. (2011). Basic information processing abilities at 11 years account for deficits in IQ associated with preterm birth. *Intelligence* 39, 198–209. doi: 10.1016/j.intell.2011.03.003

Rose, S. A., Feldman, J. F., Jankowski, J. J., and Van Rossem, R. (2012). Information processing from infancy to 11 years: continuities and prediction of IQ. *Intelligence* 40, 445–457. doi: 10.1016/j.intell.2012.05.007

Schmidt, B. (2005). Methylxanthine therapy for apnea of prematurity: evaluation of treatment benefits and risks at age 5 years in the international caffeine for apnea of prematurity (CAP) trial. *Biol. Neonate* 88, 208–213. doi: 10.1159/000087584

Schmidt, B., Anderson, P. J., Doyle, L. W., Dewey, D., Grunau, R. E., Asztalos, E. V., et al. (2012). Survival without disability to age 5 years after neonatal caffeine therapy for apnea of prematurity. *JAMA* 307, 275–282. doi: 10.1001/jama.2011.2024

Schmidt, B., Roberts, R. S., Anderson, P. J., Asztalos, E. V., Costantini, L., Davis, P. G., et al. (2017). Academic performance, motor function, and behavior 11 years after neonatal caffeine citrate therapy for apnea of prematurity: an 11-year follow-up of the CAP randomized clinical trial. *JAMA Pediatr.* 171, 564–572. doi: 10.1001/jamapediatrics.2017.0238

Schmidt, B., Roberts, R. S., Davis, P. G., Doyle, L. W., Asztalos, E. V., Opie, G., et al. (2015). Prediction of late death or disability at age 5 years using a count of 3 neonatal morbidities in very low birth weight infants. *J. Pediatr.* 167, 982–986.e2. doi: 10.1016/j.jpeds.2015.07.067

Schmidt, B., Roberts, R. S., Davis, P., Doyle, L. W., and Steering Committee of the Caffeine for Apnea of Prematurity (CAP) Trial. (2011). Archimedes: does caffeine treatment for apnoea of prematurity improve neurodevelopmental outcome in later life? *Arch Dis Child.* 96:784. doi: 10.1136/adc.2010.206698

Schmidt, B., Roberts, R. S., Davis, P., Doyle, L. W., Barrington, K. J., Ohlsson, A., et al. (2006). Caffeine therapy for apnea of prematurity. *N. Engl. J. Med.* 354, 2112–2121. doi: 10.1056/NEJMoa054065

Skiold, B., Alexandrou, G., Padilla, N., Blennow, M., Vollmer, B., and Aden, U. (2014). Sex differences in outcome and associations with neonatal brain morphology in extremely preterm children. *J. Pediatr.* 164, 1012–1018. doi: 10.1016/j.jpeds.2013.12.051

Spencer-Smith, M. M., Spittle, A. J., Lee, K. J., Doyle, L. W., and Anderson, P. J. (2015). Bayley-III cognitive and language scales in preterm children. *Pediatrics* 135, e1258–e1265. doi: 10.1542/peds.2014-3039

Stalnacke, J., Lundequist, A., Bohm, B., Forssberg, H., and Smedler, A. C. (2015). Individual cognitive patterns and developmental trajectories after preterm birth. *Child Neuropsychol.* 21, 648–667. doi: 10.1080/09297049.2014.958071

Thompson, D. K., Kelly, C. E., Chen, J., Beare, R., Alexander, B., Seal, M. L., et al. (2018). Early life predictors of brain development at term-equivalent age in infants born across the gestational age spectrum. *Neuroimage* 185, 813–824. doi: 10.1016/j.neuroimage.2018.04.031

Volpe, J. J. (1980). Evaluation of neonatal periventricular-intraventricular hemorrhage. A major advance. *Am. J. Dis. Child* 134, 1023–1025. doi: 10.1001/archpedi.1980.02130230003001

Volpe, J. J., Kinney, H. C., Jensen, F. E., and Rosenberg, P. A. (2011). Reprint of "the developing oligodendrocyte: key cellular target in brain injury in the premature infant". *Int. J. Dev. Neurosci.* 29, 565–582. doi: 10.1016/j.ijdevneu.2011.07.008

Wong, H. S., Santhakumaran, S., Cowan, F. M., Modi, N., and Medicines for Neonates Investigator Group. (2016). Developmental assessments in preterm children: a meta-analysis. *Pediatrics* 138:e20160251. doi: 10.1542/peds.2016-0251

12

Mesenchymal Stromal Cell Derived Extracellular Vesicles Reduce Hypoxia-Ischemia Induced Perinatal Brain Injury

Claudia Sisa[1], Sharad Kholia[2], Jordan Naylor[1], Maria Beatriz Herrera Sanchez[3], Stefania Bruno[2], Maria Chiara Deregibus[3], Giovanni Camussi[2], Jameel M. Inal[4], Sigrun Lange[5] and Mariya Hristova[1]**

[1] Perinatal Brain Protection and Repair Group, EGA Institute for Women's Health, University College London, London, United Kingdom, [2] Department of Medical Sciences, University of Turin, Turin, Italy, [3] 2i3T, Incubator and Technology Transfer, Molecular Biotechnology Center, University of Turin, Turin, Italy, [4] Extracellular Vesicle Research Unit and Bioscience Research Group, School of Life and Medical Sciences, University of Hertfordshire, Hatfield, United Kingdom, [5] Tissue Architecture and Regeneration Research Group, School of Life Sciences, University of Westminster, London, United Kingdom

***Correspondence:**
Sigrun Lange
S.lange@westminster.ac.uk
Mariya Hristova
m.hristova@ucl.ac.uk*

Background: Neonatal hypoxic-ischemic (HI) insult is a leading cause of disability and death in newborns, with therapeutic hypothermia being the only currently available clinical intervention. Thus there is a great need for adjunct and novel treatments for enhanced or alternative post-HI neuroprotection. Extracellular vesicles (EVs) derived from mesenchymal stromal/stem cells (MSCs) have recently been shown to exhibit regenerative effects in various injury models. Here we present findings showing neuroprotective effects of MSC-derived EVs in the Rice–Vannucci model of severe HI-induced neonatal brain insult.

Methods: Mesenchymal stromal/stem cell-derived EVs were applied intranasally immediately post HI-insult and behavioral outcomes were observed 48 h following MSC-EV treatment, as assessed by negative geotaxis. Brains were thereafter excised and assessed for changes in glial responses, cell death, and neuronal loss as markers of damage at 48 h post HI-insult.

Results: Brains of the MSC-EV treated group showed a significant decrease in microglial activation, cell death, and percentage tissue volume loss in multiple brain regions, compared to the control-treated groups. Furthermore, negative geotaxis test showed improved behavioral outcomes at 48 h following MSC-EV treatment.

Conclusion: Our findings highlight the clinical potential of using MSC-derived EVs following neonatal hypoxia-ischaemia.

Keywords: hypoxia, ischaemia, extracellular vesicles, mesenchymal stromal/stem cells, microglia, neuroprotection

INTRODUCTION

Neonatal hypoxic-ischaemic (HI) brain injury is a major contributing factor to cerebral palsy and other neurological disabilities and is estimated to occur in 3 in 1000 live births in the Western world and even at higher frequency in less developed countries (Perlman, 2006; Kurinczuk et al., 2010). Oxygen deprivation has been identified as a major cause of brain injury both in term and preterm babies (Wu and Colford, 2000; Hagberg et al., 2002; Mallard et al., 2003). While 15–20% of affected neonates will die postnatally, it has been found that in surviving babies 5–10% will develop persistent motor deficiencies. Furthermore, 20–50% will suffer from sensory or cognitive abnormalities; for example approximately 15% of cerebral palsy cases are due to severe neonatal HI (Hack et al., 1992; Vohr et al., 2000; Volpe, 2012; Lee et al., 2013).

Following HI insult, changes in cellular transcription, mitochondrial function, *de novo* protein synthesis and post-translational modifications all play pivotal roles (Culman et al., 2007; Pirianov et al., 2007; Yi et al., 2007). In experimental murine models of HI, implications have for example been shown for epigenetic mechanisms (Kumral et al., 2012; Lange et al., 2014), pH changes (Kendall et al., 2011b; Uria-Avellanal and Robertson, 2014), cytokines (Kendall et al., 2011a), transcription factors (Hristova et al., 2016), and protein kinases (Thei et al., 2018). Reperfusion injury and associated reactive oxygen species, together with persistent inflammation, are also a significant contributor to brain damage in neonates following HI insult (Rocha-Ferreira and Hristova, 2016). Following positive outcomes in clinical studies of hypothermia (Wyatt et al., 2007), cooling brain or whole body to 33°C (moderate hypothermia) is currently the only strategy with a demonstrated clinical benefit. In full-term infants with moderate to severe HI, cooling significantly improves survival and disability by 11% (Shankaran et al., 2012; Jacobs et al., 2013; Azzopardi et al., 2014). Importantly, as cooling is not always effective, with 40% of treated infants still suffering neurodevelopmental disabilities, recent studies have underscored the importance of combining hypothermia with safe adjunct therapies for more substantial neuroprotection. In addition, as hypothermia equipment is not readily available worldwide, novel safe and easy to apply treatments are of pivotal importance.

Mesenchymal stromal/stem cells (MSCs) have gained popularity over the years for their potential to implement regenerative medical treatment to damaged tissues of the body (Uccelli et al., 2008; Bruno et al., 2009; Gatti et al., 2011; Bruno et al., 2012; Lee et al., 2012; Tan et al., 2014; Collino et al., 2015; Heldring et al., 2015). Stem cells participate in the maintenance of homeostasis and restoration of tissues after injury through secretion of soluble factors and extracellular vesicles (EVs). EVs (exosomes and microvesicles) are 30–1000 nm lipid bilayer-enclosed structures which are released from parental cells and participate in cell-to-cell signaling processes. EVs have been shown to transport various biologically active molecules such as proteins, mRNAs, miRNAs, lncrRNAs, DNA, and lipids to target cells (Inal et al., 2012; Yeo et al., 2013; György et al., 2015; Bruno et al., 2017; Tricarico et al., 2017; van Niel et al., 2018). These molecules can act on various cell types by signaling proliferative and/or regenerative pathways including angiogenesis, cell proliferation, and immune tolerance (Deregibus et al., 2007; Camussi et al., 2010; Ranghino et al., 2012; de Jong et al., 2014; Robbins and Morelli, 2014; Lamichhane et al., 2015; Kholia et al., 2016; Merino-González et al., 2016; Zhang et al., 2016). Anti-inflammatory factors are one key group of molecules released by MSCs that are important in mediating repair and include interleukin 1 receptor agonist (IL-1ra) (Prockop and Oh, 2012), interleukin 10 (IL-10) (Németh et al., 2009), TNF-α-stimulated gene-6 (TSG6) (Drago et al., 2013; English, 2013; Madrigal et al., 2014), prostaglandin (PG) E2 (Prockop and Oh, 2012; Drago et al., 2013; English, 2013; Németh et al., 2009), and indoleamine 2,3-dioxygenase (IDO) (Meisel et al., 2004; Croitoru-Lamoury et al., 2011; Kang et al., 2012; Lin et al., 2012; Rong et al., 2012).

Recent studies have suggested that EVs released from MSCs may be more important than the actual stem cells themselves in mediating tissue-protective effects due to the therapeutic factors secreted by EVs, including anti-inflammatory mediators, cytokines and growth factors, as well as microRNAs (Collino et al., 2015; Vallabhaneni et al., 2015; Bruno et al., 2017).

Studies in regenerative models, using total EVs or separate applications of either 100K EVs (population enriched with exosomes) or 10K EVs (population enriched with microvesicles), have led to indicate that 100K EVs provide the bulk of pro-regenerative effects, although when total EVs were used it was found that 10K EVs do not interfere negatively with 100K EVs function (Bruno et al., 2017). Other studies have found that the application of total EVs was more effective than using isolated vesicle populations of 100K EVs or 10K EVs, respectively (Wen et al., 2016). Variations in these findings have not been fully explained yet but may possibly be due to differing target tissues.

HI studies using MSCs as putative treatment, have found that these stem cells have neuroprotective potential (van Velthoven et al., 2010; Kim et al., 2012; Donega et al., 2014; Park et al., 2015; Ahn et al., 2016; Corcelli et al., 2018) and the therapeutic time window was shown to be further extended when combining MSC treatment with hypothermia (Ahn et al., 2018). Furthermore, a potential for using stem cell derived EVs was recently shown in an ovine HI study, using intravenous administration of MSC-derived EVs following transient umbilical cord occlusion *in utero*, which lead to improved brain function following MSC-EV treatment (Ophelders et al., 2016).

As intranasal administration has shown to be more efficient compared to intravenous administration in experimental HI models, due to direct transport to the CNS and bypassing peripheral elimination (Merkus and van den Berg, 2007; Hanson and Frey, 2008), we thus aimed in the present study at assessing whether intranasal administration of MSC-EVs following HI-insult would have neuroprotective effects. We used the Rice-Vannucci neonatal mouse model, which involves permanent unilateral common carotid artery occlusion followed by severe (1 h) hypoxia (Vannucci and Vannucci, 1997).

Here we provide evidence that compared to control-treated littermates, the brains of animals treated intranasally with MSC-derived EVs, immediately following HI insult, show significant neuroprotection and reduced neuroinflammation, as well as improved behavioral outcome, when assessed at 48 h post-treatment.

MATERIALS AND METHODS

Animals and Procedures

All animal experiments and care protocols were approved by the UK Home Office (PPL 70/8784) and UCL Animal Welfare and Ethical Review Board, carried out according to the United Kingdom Animals (Scientific Procedures) Act 1986. The ARRIVE guidelines were followed. Operations were performed at post-natal day 9 (P9) on C57/BI6 mice (Charles River, United Kingdom), bred in house, using a modification of the Rice-Vannucci model of neonatal HI as previously described (Hristova et al., 2010; Lange et al., 2014; Rocha-Ferreira et al., 2018). The parental animals were bred in an environment providing 12 h light/dark cycle and food and water *ad libitum*. The HI procedure was carried out as follows: P9 mice (males and females) were anesthetized using isoflurane (5% induction, 1.5% maintenance). Permanent occlusion of the left common carotid artery was established with 8/0 polypropylene sutures followed by wound closure with tissue glue. The pups were recovered at 36°C and then were returned to the dam for 2 h, whereafter they were placed in a 36°C hypoxic chamber for 60 min, in humidified 10% oxygen/90% nitrogen at 3 L/min. Immediately following hypoxic exposure, the animals were randomly allocated to HI, EV- or PBS-treatment group. The experimental (EV) group (n = 15) received one intranasal dose of 6 μL of EVs (100KTOT-EV; 1.25 × 10^9 particles/dose) in PBS, obtained from human bone marrow derived MSCs (Poietics hMSC, Cat no: PT-2501, Lot no: 0000446319, Lonza, Switzerland) and prepared according to Bruno et al. (2017). In brief, total EVs were isolated from characterized MSC cultures (Bruno et al., 2009), which were positive for the typical MSC markers (CD105, CD29, CD73, CD44, and CD90). The total EVs were collected from the supernatants of MSCs, cultured in fetal calf serum (FCS)-depleted RPMI medium, overnight. The EVs were a pool of 5 EV isolations with each isolation comprised of 10 flasks with a passage number ranging from P3 to P5 progressively. Cell debris and apoptotic bodies were removed by centrifugation at 3000 g for 20 min and thereafter total EVs were isolated by ultracentrifugation for 2 h at 100,000 g at 4°C and stored at −80°C until used. Details on EV characterization by nanoparticle tracking analysis (NTA, Nanosight, Malvern, United Kingdom), electron microscopy, FACS analysis and Western blotting for MSC-EV specific markers are shown in **Supplementary Figure S1**. EV payload characterization of proteomic and genomic content of these EVs was previously published in Bruno et al. (2017). The control treated groups received either 6 μL intranasal phosphate-buffered saline (PBS) (n = 14; vehicle only group) or no intervention (n = 16; HI only group). The pups where returned to the dam and left for 48 h before behavioral assessment and subsequent histological analysis of extracted brains. All animals (both males and females) from all litters were used in the experiments. Following the HI protocol the mums and pups were observed and scored for welfare of neonatal rodents (Lloyd et al., 2000). All pups were taken care of by the mums and achieved overall scores 0–1.

Post-natal day 9 mice were used in this particular experiment as they most closely resemble term neonates (Mallard and Vexler, 2015) and also possess injury responses phenotypically similar to white and gray matter damage, such as tissue loss, microglia-mediated immunity, cell-death-mediated apoptosis, astrogliosis, and neurobehavioral alterations (Vannucci and Vannucci, 1997). The hypoxic chamber conditions were 10% oxygen/90% nitrogen according to previously described protocols (Rocha-Ferreira et al., 2018). Differences between male and female mice were not taken into account and male and female pups were combined in the analysis, as testosterone levels in mice are similar in both genders at this age (P9–P11) (Clarkson and Herbison, 2016).

Tissue Sample Preparation

For histological assessment, animals were sacrificed 48 h post-HI insult with an intraperitoneal injection of pentobarbitone and perfusion with 30 mL of 4% paraformaldehyde in PBS. Brains were extracted and fixed in 4% paraformaldehyde in PBS at 4°C for 1 h, followed by cryoprotection in 30% sucrose dissolved in phosphate buffer (PB) for 24 h. Thereafter brains were frozen on dry ice, sectioned by cryostat into sequential 40 μm sections and stored at −80°C until histological analysis.

Histological Analysis

Coronal brain sections were compared between animals receiving MSC-derived EVs and control-treated animals (PBS-vehicle or HI only), for microglial activation, cell death, and infarct size. Tissue sections were scored blindly by two independent observers.

Microglial Activation Assessment

Tissue staining was performed according to established protocols as previously described (Hristova et al., 2010; Lange et al., 2014; Rocha-Ferreira et al., 2018). In brief, cryosections were thawed and rehydrated in distilled water, spread onto glass slides coated with 0.5% gelatine under a dissecting microscope, dried for 10 min, fixed in 4% formaldehyde in 100 mM PB for 5 min, treated with acetone (50, 100, 50%: 2 min each), 0.1% bovine serum albumin (PB/BSA) and washed twice in PB. The sections were pre-incubated with 5% goat serum (Sigma, St. Louis, MO, United States) in PB for 30 min and incubated overnight at 4°C with an antibody against αMβ2 integrin (Serotec, Oxford, United Kingdom) 1/5000. The sections were then washed in PB/BSA, PB, PB, PB/BSA (2 min each), incubated with biotin-labeled anti-rat IgG (Vector Laboratories, Inc., Burlingame, CA, United States) and visualized with Avidin-Biotinylated peroxidase Complex (ABC, Vector Laboratories, Inc.) and diaminobenzidine/hydrogen peroxide (DAB) stain. Sections were processed through alcohol and xylene and mounted with DEPEX (Sigma). Per animal, five cryosections (400 μm apart) of each brain were stained. Semi-quantitative scores for microglial activation were obtained as follows: 0 = no activation; 1 = focal activation; 2 = mild phagocytic activation affecting <50% of the region, thus showing diffuse activation with occasional phagocytic macrophages; 3 = phagocytic activation affecting > 50% of the region, thus showing widespread activation with predominant phagocytic macrophages; 4 = total phagocytic activation (Rocha-Ferreira et al., 2015, 2018; Hristova et al., 2016). Microglial activation was scored for the following brain regions: cortex, pyriform cortex, hippocampus, striatum, thalamus, and external capsule. These regions were selected based on known selective vulnerability as a result of increased metabolic rate (Martin et al., 1997; Barkovich et al., 1998; Johnston et al., 2001, 2002; Volpe, 2001; McQuillen et al., 2003; Castillo, 2007; Leisman et al., 2014; Schmidt-Kastner, 2015).

TUNEL Staining

For assessment of changes in cell death, brain tissue sections were stained at 400 μm intervals for DNA fragmentation using terminal deoxynucleotidyl transferase dUTP nick end labeling (TUNEL) according to the manufacturer's instructions (Roche, United Kingdom). Cell death was quantified by averaging the numerical count of TUNEL-positive nuclei in three representative optical fields in each brain region, comparing EV-treated versus control-treated brains.

Infarct Volume Measurement

Infarct volume was measured by Nissl stain in five coronal sections at 400 μm intervals from each forebrain, stained with cresyl violet (VWR, United Kingdom). The Optimas 6.5 imaging analysis software (Bothell, WA, United States) was used to calculate the surviving brain tissue in each brain region as percentage between experimental and control side to estimate reduction in infarct size following EV treatment compared to control groups, according to previously described methods (Kendall et al., 2006).

Behavioral Assessment by Negative Geotaxis

The negative geotaxis test, assessing the labyrinthine reflex which reflects the strength and co-ordination of neonatal mice, was used for behavioral analysis in EV treated and control-treated or non-treated groups at 48 h post insult, before sacrificing the animals for brain extraction and subsequent histological assessment. The order of testing of the animals within the litters was randomly assigned. The mice were placed in the center of a 45° incline board with their heads facing downwards. The time for the animal to make a 180° turn to face upward and begin to move up the hill was recorded. Time was capped at 30 s. If the animal failed to complete the task by this time, 30 s was the recorded outcome. Each animal attempted this task three times and these values were averaged per animal (Rocha-Ferreira et al., 2018). The animal numbers tested per group were as follows: MSC-EV treated: n = 10; PBS-control treated: n = 10; and HI-untreated control: n = 13.

Statistical Analysis

Statistical analysis was carried out with GraphPad Prism 7 (La Jolla, CA, United States), using brain region as the repeated measure for the following statistical analyses: The same six forebrain regions (cortex, pyriform cortex, hippocampus, striatum, thalamus, external capsule) were used for each outcome and each assay. Only the TUNEL data-set passed the D'Agostino and Pearson normality test. Normalized data (only one data set: TUNEL-thalamus) were analyzed using the one-way ANOVA test and the Tukey's multiple comparisons test.

It is likely that with repeated measures such as these the observations from a single subject are correlated, therefore the first stage of the analysis included the observations from all the regions tested in a single mixed model with a random subject effect, to produce an estimate of the treatment effect and associated inference that accounts for the correlations in the data arising from the repeated measures. Further *post hoc* Tukey's multiple comparisons test was carried out to assess evidence for subregional differences, $p < 0.05$. Other regional data sets, being non-normalized data, were analyzed using the Kruskal–Wallis test and the Dunn's multiple comparisons test. For each outcome, the overall effect from the mixed linear model is reported, followed by the results from the individual regional *post hoc* tests. All data is presented as means and standard error of the mean (SEM) for each group. Group sizes (n = 15 EV, n = 14 PBS, n = 16 HI), were based on power calculations for test power >0.80 and significance <0.05. Statistical significance was determined for p-value <0.05.

Statistical significance in the negative geotaxis behavioral testing was assessed through Kruskal–Wallis with Dunn's multiple comparison test, as the data was non-normally distributed. Normal distribution was assessed using Shapiro–Wilk normality test. The data is presented as individual values and median ± interquartile bars.

RESULTS

Intranasal Application of MSC-Derived EVs Decreases Microglial Activation in HI

Microglial activation (AlphaM), as assessed through αMβ2 integrin immunoreactivity, was significantly reduced in the EV-treated, compared to control PBS-treated groups overall (Kruskal–Wallis test p = 0.0168, Dunn's multiple comparison test p = 0.0175) with subregional differences in cortex (p = 0.0319), hippocampus (p = 0.0392), and striatum (p = 0.0376) (**Figure 1**). Only a trend toward reduction, but not reaching significance, was observed in the other brain regions (**Figure 1**). Combining all six regions, using the Kruskal–Wallis test, the mean AlphaM scores varied significantly between treatment groups (p = 0.0168) (**Figure 1**).

Intranasal Application of MSC-Derived EVs Decreases HI-Mediated Cell Death

Intranasal application of MSC-derived EVs significantly reduced TUNEL+ cell death in cortex and external capsule (**Figure 2**). Using the Kruskal–Wallis test, the mean ipsilateral TUNEL+ cell counts per representative area in the cortex varied significantly between treatment groups (EV: 12.86; PBS: 26.09; HI: 32.82;

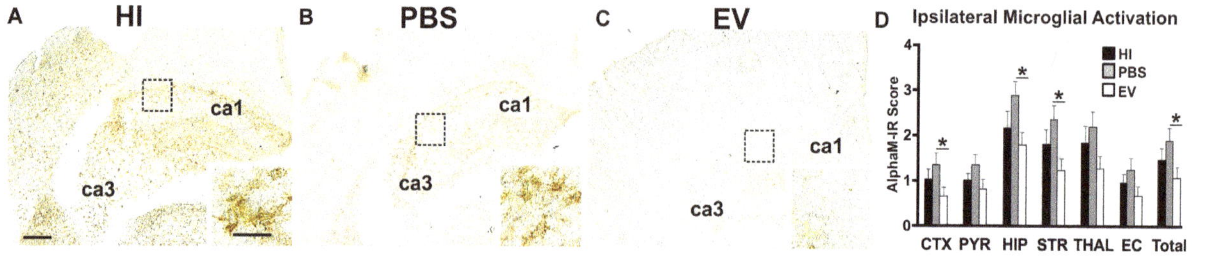

FIGURE 1 | Intranasal application of MSC-derived EVs, immediately following HI, significantly reduces microglial activation after 48 h. **(A–C)** Ipsilateral overview of early microglial activation in EV- and control treated animals. Note the strong microglial activation in the HI **(A)** and PBS-treated **(B)** groups with αM+ cells showing phagocytic morphology at high magnification (**A,B** – inserts, hippocampus), compared to the EV-treated brains exhibiting a ramified phenotype (**C** – insert). The ca1 and ca3 areas of hippocampus are indicated for reference. **(D)** Intranasal EV treatment significantly reduced ipsilateral microglial activation score (**D**, Mean + SEM) overall compared to control-treated groups (PBS or HI) (Kruskal–Wallis test, $p = 0.0168$; Dunn's test EV vs. PBS $^*p = 0.0175$) with significant individual decrease in cortex (Kruskal–Wallis test, $p = 0.0371$; Dunn's test EV vs. PBS $^*p = 0.0319$), hippocampus (Kruskal–Wallis test, $p = 0.0451$; Dunn's test EV vs. PBS $^*p = 0.0392$), striatum (Kruskal–Wallis test, $p = 0.0442$; Dunn's test EV vs. PBS $^*p = 0.0376$). CTX, cerebral iscocortex; PYR, pyriform cortex; HIP, hippocampus; STR, striatum, Thal, thalamus; EC, external capsule. Scale bars: **A–C** = 150 μm; inserts = 15 μm.

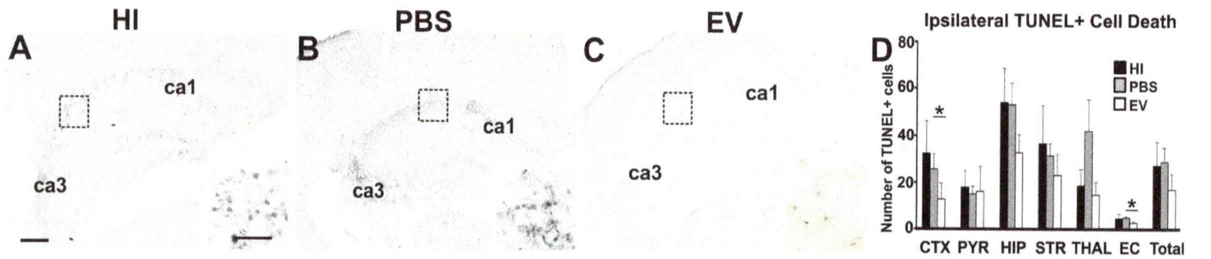

FIGURE 2 | Intranasal application of MSC-derived EVs, immediately following HI, significantly reduces TUNEL+ cell death after 48 h. **(A–C)** Histochemical overview of TUNEL+ cell death in the ipsilateral forebrain of HI **(A)**, PBS- **(B)**, and EV-treated **(C)** animals. Note the typical pyknotic nuclear morphology of the TUNEL+ cells observed in the HI and PBS groups (**A,B** – inserts, hippocampus) and the lack of such cells in the EV-treated group (**C** – insert). The ca1 and ca3 areas of hippocampus are indicated for reference. **(D)** Quantification of the number of TUNEL+ cells per 20× eye-field (Mean + SEM). Compared to HI and PBS-treated control animals, Intranasal EV treatment significantly reduced ipsilateral TUNEL+ cell death in cortex (Kruskal–Wallis test, $p = 0.0305$; Dunn's test EV vs. PBS $^*p = 0.0320$) and external capsule (Kruskal–Wallis test, $p = 0.0131$; Dunn's test EV vs. PBS $^*p = 0.0117$). CTX, cerebral iscocortex; PYR, pyriform cortex; HIP, hippocampus; STR, striatum; Thal, thalamus; EC, external capsule. Scale bars: **A–C** = 150 μm; inserts = 15 μm.

$p = 0.0305$). Using the Dunn's multiple comparisons test, significant decrease was found in EV-treated compared to the PBS treated control group ($p = 0.0320$).

The mean ipsilateral TUNEL+ cell counts per representative area in the external capsule varied significantly between treatment groups (Kruskal–Wallis test, EV: 2.125; PBS: 4.556; HI: 4.09; $p = 0.0131$). Dunn's multiple comparisons test showed significant decrease in the TUNEL+ cell counts in the EV-treated compared to control PBS-treated group ($p = 0.0117$) (**Figure 2**).

Intranasal Application of MSC-Derived EVs Decreases HI-Mediated Volume Loss

Intranasal EV-treatment resulted in significant reduction of tissue loss as assessed through NISSL staining, compared to control treated littermates overall (Kruskal–Wallis test, $p = 0.0453$), as well as in pyriform cortex, thalamus, and external capsule (**Figure 3**).

The mean ipsilateral volume loss in the pyriform cortex varied significantly between treatment groups (Kruskal-Wallis test, EV: 16.13%; PBS: 25.5%; HI: 19.63%; $p = 0.0273$). Dunn's multiple comparisons test showed significant decrease in the EV-treated compared to the PBS-treated groups ($p = 0.0219$). The mean ipsilateral volume loss in the thalamus varied significantly between treatment groups (Kruskal-Wallis test, EV: 17.53%; PBS: 23.43%; HI: 30.44%; $p = 0.0445$). Dunn's multiple comparisons test showed significant reduction in the EV-treated compared to HI groups ($p = 0.0348$). The mean ipsilateral volume loss in the external capsule varied significantly between treatment groups (Kruskal–Wallis test, EV: 10.8%; PBS: 25.21%; HI: 21.63%; $p = 0.0114$). Dunn's multiple comparisons test showed significant decrease in the EV-treated compared to the PBS-treated control groups ($p = 0.0126$) (**Figure 3**).

Intranasal Application of MSC-Derived EVs Improves Behavioral Outcomes

Intranasal administration of MSC-derived EVs significantly improved behavioral outcomes using the negative geotaxis test at 48 h (postnatal day 11, P11) postneonatal HI insult compared to control-treated animals (**Figure 4**). The Kruskal-Wallis test showed significant variation in the mean-time in seconds between treatment groups ($p = 0.0151$). Dunn's

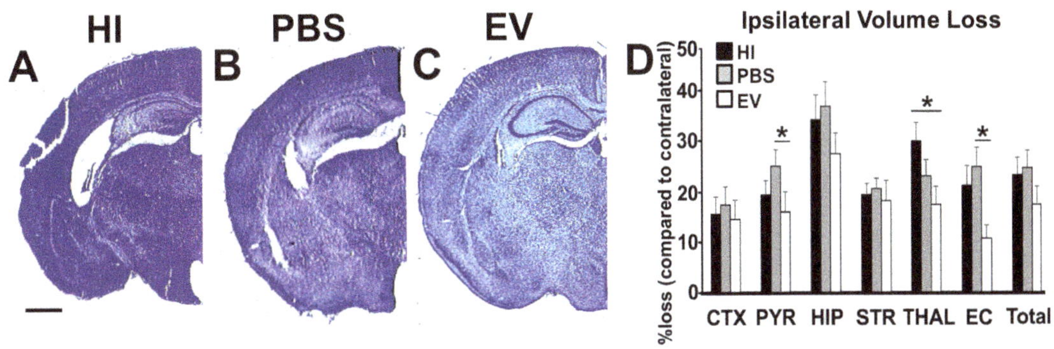

FIGURE 3 | Intranasal application of MSC-derived EVs, immediately following HI, significantly reduces tissue loss after 48 h. Ipsilateral forebrain Nissl staining (Cresyl-Violet, at rostral parietal level) of HI **(A)**, PBS- **(B)**, and EV-treated **(C)** animals and quantification of ipsilateral brain tissue volume loss **(D)** at 48 h following HI-insult. Intranasal EV treatment reduced volume loss (Mean + SEM) compared to HI and PBS-treated littermates (Kruskal–Wallis test, $p = 0.0453$) with significant, individual decrease in pyriform cortex (Kruskal–Wallis test, $p = 0.0273$; Dunn's test EV vs. PBS $^*p = 0.0219$), thalamus (Kruskal–Wallis test, $p = 0.0445$; Dunn's test EV vs. HI $^*p = 0.0348$), and external capsule (Kruskal–Wallis test, $p = 0.0114$; Dunn's test EV vs. PBS $^*p = 0.0126$). CTX, cerebral iscocortex; PYR, pyriform cortex; HIP, hippocampus; STR, striatum; Thal, thalamus; EC, external capsule. Scale bars: **A–C** = 470 μm.

multiple comparisons test showed significant decrease of the time necessary for change of orientation in the EV-treated compared to the HI-alone group ($p = 0.0114$) (**Figure 4**).

DISCUSSION

Our study shows evidence for neuroprotective effects of MSC-derived EVs via intranasal administration following neonatal HI brain injury, using the Rice–Vannucci mouse model in P9 mice. Intranasal treatment with MSC-derived EVs, immediately after severe (1 h) hypoxia following unilateral carotid artery occlusion, significantly reduced microglial activation, cell death, and tissue loss in the various brain regions tested, compared to brains in control-treated or untreated groups. In addition, compared to control littermates, intranasal EV treatment significantly improved short term behavioral outcomes as assessed through negative geotaxis.

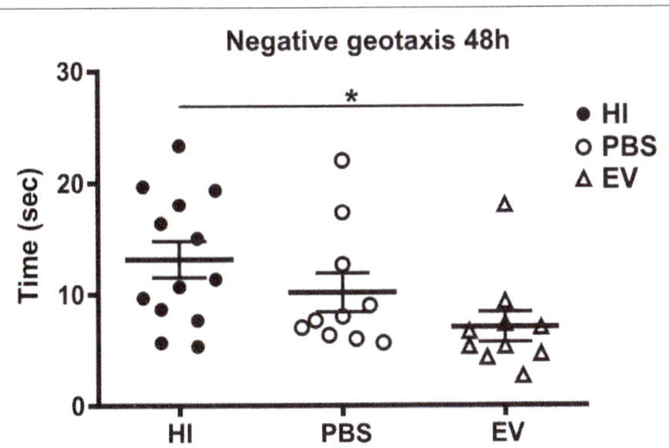

FIGURE 4 | Intranasal application of MSC-derived EVs, immediately following HI reduces the time required to change orientation in negative geotaxis following neonatal HI at 48 h (postnatal day 11). Intranasal treatment with MSC-derived EVs immediately following HI significantly reduces the time necessary for change of orientation compared to HI and PBS-treated littermate controls (Kruskal–Wallis test, $p = 0.0151$, Dunn's test EV vs. HI $^*p = 0.0114$).

Microglial activation was significantly reduced in cortex, hippocampus and striatum, while reduction in cell death was found in cortex and external capsule in the EV-treated group. Tissue volume loss was significantly reduced in pyriform cortex, thalamus and external capsule in the EV-treated group. Assessing all brain regions, the total brain regional means were also significantly decreased for microglial activation and tissue volume loss in the EV-treated groups.

These results are in line with findings from previous studies, showing differential vulnerability of certain brain regions to injury (Rocha-Ferreira and Hristova, 2016). HI injury at term, as modeled in this study, tends to damage the entire brain, most notably gray matter in cortex, hippocampus, and/or thalamus (Alexander et al., 2014).

Damage to the cortex, as well as to the thalamus and striatum (Lubics et al., 2005) have been associated with sensorimotor deficits in animal models of HI (Mercuri and Barnett, 2003; Mercuri et al., 2004; Martinez-Biarge et al., 2011). HI damage in the hippocampus and associated projections to the cortex have been shown to result in disrupted memory function and spatial processing (Aylward, 2005). Significant reductions in hippocampus volume have been shown to reduce long-term reference memory, short-term working memory (Ikeda et al., 2001) and impact the necessary role of the hippocampus in spatial navigation and recollection (Packard and McGaugh, 1996; White and McDonald, 2002). The dorsal striatum, namely the nucleus accumbens, may impact non-spatial navigation, and learning (Packard and Knowlton, 2002; White and McDonald, 2002), thus damage to this structure may account for the non-spatial memory deficits seen for example in HI injured rats (Alexander et al., 2014). Fronto-striato-thalamic circuitry damage from HI injury may lead to deficits in attention, executive function, and activity modulation (Aylward, 2005). As studies have shown anxiety-like behavior in mice following HI injury (Sanches et al., 2013), it has been hypothesized that HI injury may be associated with susceptibility to other pathologies such as attention-deficit hyperactivity disorder (ADHD), autism and schizophrenia, as the hippocampus and striatum are associated with related cognitive functions (DeLong, 1992; Lou, 1996; Dilenge et al., 2001; Van Petten, 2004; de Haan et al., 2006).

The results of the present study, emphasize the clinical potential of MSC-derived EVs for neuroprotection following neonatal HI injury and are in line with studies using MSC treatment in neonatal HI murine models (van Velthoven et al., 2010, 2012; Kim et al., 2012; Donega et al., 2014) as well as MSC-derived EVs treatment in an ovine neonatal HI model (Ophelders et al., 2016). The use of EVs as therapeutic vesicles is thus of great clinical interest. Previous HI studies using whole MSCs have found neuroprotective potential for these stem cells (van Velthoven et al., 2010; Donega et al., 2014; Park et al., 2015; Ahn et al., 2016; Corcelli et al., 2018) and the therapeutic time window was shown to be extended when combining MSC treatment with hypothermia (Ahn et al., 2018).

As there may be practical drawbacks of using whole MSCs in clinic, the use of MSC-derived EVs has been gaining increased interest. Neuroprotective effects were for example shown in a recent HI study following intravenous administration of MSC-derived EVs in an ovine model of transient umbilical cord occlusion *in utero*, with improved brain function and reduction of the number and duration of seizures following treatment (Ophelders et al., 2016). It has been shown that intravenous MSC delivery to the brain is hampered by the blood brain barrier (BBB) and results in a tendency of the MSCs to accumulate in other organs, such as the lungs (Lappalainen et al., 2008; Fischer et al., 2009). Intra-arterial administration can deliver high numbers of MSCs to the brain (Lappalainen et al., 2008; Li et al., 2010; Pendharkar et al., 2010), however, this method also has high incidences of mortality and impaired cerebral blood flow in rat HI models (Walczak et al., 2008; Pendharkar et al., 2010). Attempts to increase cell delivery by disrupting the BBB can leave the animal susceptible to infection or toxins (Burgess et al., 2011). Intranasal administration has shown to be superior to intravenous administration in experimental HI models due to direct transport to the CNS through intranasal drug delivery (Merkus and van den Berg, 2007) via the olfactory and trigeminal neural pathways, which innervate the nasal cavity and create a direct pathway to the CNS (Hanson and Frey, 2008). Thus in this study we delivered MSC-derived EVs intranasally, as this method is more efficient and far less invasive than intracranial, intravenous or intraarterial deliveries and avoids inactivation by the gastrointestinal and hepatic first-pass metabolism (Hanson et al., 2013; Djupesland et al., 2014; Kozlovskaya et al., 2014). The MSC-derived EVs used in this study are well characterized (Collino et al., 2015; Bruno et al., 2017; GEO GSE59958; **Supplementary Figure S1**) and have previously shown to regenerative potential in murine acute renal injury models (Bruno et al., 2012; Bruno et al., 2017).

In the current study, we assessed the neuroprotective effects of MSC-derived EVs following intranasal administration after a HI-insult. We observed significant neuroprotective effects and improved short-term behavioral outcomes. This bodes well for future applications of MSC-derived EVs, or EVs derived from other stem cells, following neonatal HI and may also be translatable to other types of neurotrauma. Tracing of MSC-derived EVs, using PKH26 (Long et al., 2017), would further provide information on the exact fate of intranasally delivered EVs to specific brain-regions and such tracing of EV fate is indeed planned by our group, alongside assessment on longer-term outcomes following MSC-EV treatment. The application of stem-cell derived EVs in combination with hypothermia, for an extended therapeutic time window, should also be explored. The preparation of the EVs is relatively inexpensive and simple, but for successful translation into the clinic strict quality control of MSC cultures and well characterized MSC-derived EVs will be required. Overall our data suggests that intranasal application of MSC-derived EVs following neonatal HI insult has neuroprotective effects and thus possesses potential as clinical treatment for neonatal HI brain damage.

AUTHOR CONTRIBUTIONS

CS and MH carried out the animal experiments. SK, MHS, SB, MD, GC, and JI prepared and characterized the MSC-EVs. CS, JN, and MH generated the histological and behavioral data. All authors contributed to data analysis and read and approved the final manuscript. SL and MH co-designed the study and wrote the manuscript.

FUNDING

This work was supported in parts by the BBSRC LIDo, UCLB Apolo PoC, the UCL graduate school and a University of Westminster Start-Up Grant. The funding bodies had no role in the design of the study, analysis, interpretation of data, or writing the manuscript.

SUPPLEMENTARY MATERIAL

FIGURE S1 | Characterization of the MSC-derived EVs used in the current study for intranasal application following HI. **(A)** Nanosight analysis showing EVs in the size range of 30–1000 nm. **(B)** Electron microscopy showing purified MSC-derived EVs, the scale bar represents 0.5 μm. **(C)** FACS analysis verifying the presence of the following MSC-EV specific markers: CD105, CD44, CD73, CD29, CD63, and CD81. **(D)** Western blotting showing MSC-EV specific markers CD63 and CD9.

REFERENCES

Ahn, S. Y., Chang, Y. S., and Park, W. S. (2016). Stem cells for neonatal brain disorders. *Neonatology* 109, 377–383. doi: 10.1159/000444905

Ahn, S. Y., Chang, Y. S., Sung, D. K., Sung, S. I., and Park, W. S. (2018). Hypothermia broadens the therapeutic time window of mesenchymal stem cell transplantation for severe neonatal hypoxic ischemic encephalopathy. *Sci. Rep.* 8:7665. doi: 10.1038/s41598-018-25902-x

Alexander, M., Garbus, H., Smith, A. L., Rosenkrantz, T. S., and Fitch, R. H. (2014). Behavioral and histological outcomes following neonatal HI injury in a preterm (P3) and term (P7) rodent model. *Behav. Brain Res.* 259, 85–96. doi: 10.1016/j.bbr.2013.10.038

Aylward, G. P. (2005). Neurodevelopmental outcomes of infants born prematurely. *J. Dev. Behav. Pediatr.* 26, 427–440. doi: 10.1097/00004703-200512000-00008

Azzopardi, D., Strohm, B., Marlow, N., Brocklehurst, P., Deierl, A., Eddama, O., et al. (2014). Effects of hypothermia for perinatal asphyxia on childhood outcomes. *N. Engl. J. Med.* 371, 140–149. doi: 10.1056/NEJMoa1315788

Barkovich, A. J., Hajnal, B. L., Vigneron, D., Sola, A., Partridge, J. C., Allen, F., et al. (1998). Prediction of neuromotor outcome in perinatal asphyxia: evaluation of MR scoring systems. *AJNR Am. J. Neuroradiol.* 19, 143–149.

Bruno, S., Grange, C., Collino, F., Deregibus, M. C., Cantaluppi, V., Biancone, L., et al. (2012). Microvesicles derived from mesenchymal stem cells enhance survival in a lethal model of acute kidney injury. *PLoS One* 7:e33115. doi: 10.1371/journal.pone.0033115

Bruno, S., Grange, C., Deregibus, M. C., Calogero, R. A., Saviozzi, S., Collino, F., et al. (2009). Mesenchymal stem cell-derived microvesicles protect against acute tubular injury. *J. Am. Soc. Nephrol.* 20:1053. doi: 10.1681/ASN.2008070798

Bruno, S., Tapparo, M., Collino, F., Chiabotto, G., Deregibus, M. C., Soares Lindoso, R., et al. (2017). Renal regenerative potential of different extracellular vesicle populations derived from bone marrow mesenchymal stromal cells. *Tissue Eng. Part A* 23, 1262–1273. doi: 10.1089/ten.TEA.2017.0069

Burgess, A., Ayala-Grosso, C. A., Ganguly, M., Jordão, J. F., Aubert, I., and Hynynen, K. (2011). Targeted delivery of neural stem cells to the brain using MRI-guided focused ultrasound to disrupt the blood-brain barrier. *PLoS One* 6:e27877. doi: 10.1371/journal.pone.0027877

Camussi, G., Deregibus, M. C., and Tetta, C. (2010). Paracrine/endocrine mechanism of stem cells on kidney repair: role of microvesicle-mediated transfer of genetic information. *Curr. Opin. Nephrol. Hypertens.* 19, 7–12. doi: 10.1097/MNH.0b013e328332fb6f

Castillo, M. (2007). Selective vulnerability and the cerebellum in neonates. *AJNR Am. J. Neuroradiol.* 28, 20–21.

Clarkson, J., and Herbison, A. E. (2016). Hypothalamic control of the male neonatal testosterone surge. *Philos. Trans. R. Soc. London B Biol. Sci.* 371:20150115. doi: 10.1098/rstb.2015.0115

Collino, F., Bruno, S., Incarnato, D., Dettori, D., Neri, F., Provero, P., et al. (2015). AKI recovery induced by mesenchymal stromal cell-derived extracellular vesicles carrying MicroRNAs. *J. Am. Soc. Nephrol.* 26, 2349–2360. doi: 10.1681/ASN.2014070710

Corcelli, M., Hawkins, K., Vlahova, F., Hunjan, A., Dowding, K., De Coppi, P., et al. (2018). Neuroprotection of the hypoxic-ischemic mouse brain by human CD117+CD90+CD105+ amniotic fluid stem cells. *Sci. Rep.* 8:2425. doi: 10.1038/s41598-018-20710-9

Croitoru-Lamoury, J., Lamoury, F. M. J., Caristo, M., Suzuki, K., Walker, D., Takikawa, O., et al. (2011). Interferon-γ regulates the proliferation and differentiation of mesenchymal stem cells via activation of indoleamine 2,3 dioxygenase (IDO). *PLoS One* 6:e14698. doi: 10.1371/journal.pone.0014698

Culman, J., Zhao, Y., Gohlke, P., and Herdegen, T. (2007). PPAR-gamma: therapeutic target for ischemic stroke. *Trends Pharmacol. Sci.* 28, 244–249. doi: 10.1016/j.tips.2007.03.004

de Haan, M., Wyatt, J. S., Roth, S., Vargha-Khadem, F., Gadian, D., and Mishkin, M. (2006). Brain and cognitive-behavioural development after asphyxia at term birth. *Dev. Sci.* 9, 350–358. doi: 10.1111/j.1467-7687.2006.00499.x

de Jong, R., Houtgraaf, J. H., Samiei, S., Boersma, E., and Duckers, H. J. (2014). Intracoronary stem cell infusion after acute myocardial infarction: a meta-analysis and update on clinical trials. *Circ. Cardiovasc. Interv.* 7, 156–167. doi: 10.1161/CIRCINTERVENTIONS.113.001009

DeLong, G. R. (1992). Autism, amnesia, hippocampus, and learning. *Neurosci. Biobehav. Rev.* 16, 63–70. doi: 10.1016/S0149-7634(05)80052-1

Deregibus, M. C., Cantaluppi, V., Calogero, R., Lo Iacono, M., Tetta, C., Biancone, L., et al. (2007). Endothelial progenitor cell derived microvesicles activate an angiogenic program in endothelial cells by a horizontal transfer of mRNA. *Blood* 110, 2440–2448. doi: 10.1182/blood-2007-03-078709

Dilenge, M. E., Majnemer, A., and Shevell, M. I. (2001). Long-term developmental outcome of asphyxiated term neonates. *J. Child Neurol.* 16, 781–792. doi: 10.1177/08830738010160110201

Djupesland, P. G., Messina, J. C., and Mahmoud, R. A. (2014). The nasal approach to delivering treatment for brain diseases: an anatomic, physiologic, and delivery technology overview. *Ther. Deliv.* 5, 709–733. doi: 10.4155/tde.14.41

Donega, V., Nijboer, C. H., van Tilborg, G., Dijkhuizen, R. M., Kavelaars, A., and Heijnen, C. J. (2014). Intranasally administered mesenchymal stem cells promote a regenerative niche for repair of neonatal ischemic brain injury. *Exp. Neurol.* 261, 53–64. doi: 10.1016/j.expneurol.2014.06.009

Drago, D., Cossetti, C., Iraci, N., Gaude, E., Musco, G., Bachi, A., et al. (2013). The stem cell secretome and its role in brain repair. *Biochimie* 95, 2271–2285. doi: 10.1016/j.biochi.2013.06.020

English, K. (2013). Mechanisms of mesenchymal stromal cell immunomodulation. *Immunol. Cell Biol.* 91, 19–26. doi: 10.1038/icb.2012.56

Fischer, U. M., Harting, M. T., Jimenez, F., Monzon-Posadas, W. O., Xue, H., Savitz, S. I., et al. (2009). Pulmonary passage is a major obstacle for intravenous stem cell delivery: the pulmonary first-pass effect. *Stem Cells Dev.* 18, 683–692. doi: 10.1089/scd.2008.0253

Gatti, S., Bruno, S., Deregibus, M. C., Sordi, A., Cantaluppi, V., Tetta, C., et al. (2011). Microvesicles derived from human adult mesenchymal stem cells protect against ischaemia-reperfusion-induced acute and chronic kidney injury. *Nephrol. Dial Transplant.* 26:1474. doi: 10.1093/ndt/gfr015

György, B., Hung, M. E., Breakefield, X. O., and Leonard, J. N. (2015). Therapeutic applications of extracellular vesicles: clinical promise and open questions. *Annu. Rev. Pharmacol. Toxicol.* 55, 439–464. doi: 10.1146/annurev-pharmtox-010814-124630

Hack, M., Breslau, N., Aram, D., Weissman, B., Klein, N., and Borawski-Clark, E. (1992). The effect of very low birth weight and social risk on neurocognitive abilities at school age. *J. Dev. Behav. Pediatr.* 13, 412–420. doi: 10.1097/00004703-199212000-00005

Hagberg, H., Peebles, D., and Mallard, C. (2002). Models of white matter injury: comparison of infectious, hypoxic-ischaemic, and excitotoxic insults. *Ment. Retard. Dev. Disabil. Res. Rev.* 8, 30–38. doi: 10.1002/mrdd.10007

Hanson, L. R., Fine, J. M., Svitak, A. L., and Faltesek, K. A. (2013). Intranasal administration of CNS therapeutics to awake mice. *J. Vis. Exp.* 74:4440. doi: 10.3791/4440

Hanson, L. R., and Frey, W. H. (2008). Intranasal delivery bypasses the blood-brain barrier to target therapeutic agents to the central nervous system and treat neurodegenerative disease. *BMC Neurosci.* 9(Suppl. 3):S5. doi: 10.1186/1471-2202-9-S3-S5

Heldring, N., Mager, I., Wood, M. J. A., and Le Blanc, K. (2015). Therapeutic potential of multipotent mesenchymal stromal cells and their extracellular vesicles. *Hum. Gene Ther.* 26:506. doi: 10.1089/hum.2015.072

Hristova, M., Cuthill, D., Zbarsky, V., Acosta-Saltos, A., Wallace, A., Blight, K., et al. (2010). Activation and deactivation of periventricular white matter phagocytes during postnatal mouse development. *Glia* 58, 11–28. doi: 10.1002/glia.20896

Hristova, M., Rocha-Ferreira, E., Fontana, X., Thei, L., Buckle, R., Christou, M., et al. (2016). Inhibition of Signal Transducer and Activator of Transcription 3 (STAT3) reduces neonatal hypoxic-ischaemic brain damage. *J. Neurochem.* 136, 981–994. doi: 10.1111/jnc.13490

Ikeda, T., Mishima, K., Yoshikawa, T., Iwasaki, K., Fujiwara, M., Xia, Y. X., et al. (2001). Selective and long-term learning impairment following neonatal hypoxic-ischemic brain insult in rats. *Behav. Brain Res.* 118, 17–25. doi: 10.1016/S0166-4328(00)00287-4

Inal, J. M., Ansa-Addo, E. A., Stratton, D., Kholia, S., Antwi-Baffour, S. S., Jorfi, S., et al. (2012). Microvesicles in health and disease. *Arch. Immunol. Ther. Exp.* 60, 107–121. doi: 10.1007/s00005-012-0165-2

Jacobs, S. E., Berg, M., Hunt, R., Tarnow-Mordi, W. O., Inder, T. E., and Davis, P. G. (2013). Cooling for newborns with hypoxic ischaemic encephalopathy.

Cochrane Database Syst. Rev. 1: CD003311. doi: 10.1002/14651858.CD0 03311.pub3

Johnston, M. V., Nakajima, W., and Hagberg, H. (2002). Mechanisms of hypoxic neurodegeneration in the developing brain. *Neuroscientist* 8, 212–220. doi: 10.1177/1073858402008003007

Johnston, M. V., Trescher, W. H., Ishida, A., and Nakajima, W. (2001). Neurobiology of hypoxicischemic injury in the developing brain. *Pediatr. Res.* 49, 735–741. doi: 10.1203/00006450-200106000-00003

Kang, J. W., Koo, H. C., Hwang, S. Y., Kang, S. K., Ra, J. C., Lee, M. H., et al. (2012). Immunomodulatory effects of human amniotic membrane-derived mesenchymal stem cells. *J. Vet. Sci.* 13, 23–31. doi: 10.4142/jvs.2012.13.1.23

Kendall, G. S., Hristova, M., Horn, S., Dafou, D., Acosta-Saltos, A., Almolda, B., et al. (2011a). TNF gene cluster deletion abolishes lipopolysaccharide-mediated sensitization of the neonatal brain to hypoxic ischemic insult. *Lab. Invest.* 91, 328–341. doi: 10.1038/labinvest.2010.192

Kendall, G. S., Hristova, M., Zbarsky, V., Clements, A., Peebles, D. M., Robertson, N. J., et al. (2011b). Distribution of pH changes in mouse neonatal hypoxic-ischaemic insult. *Dev. Neurosci.* 33, 505–518. doi: 10.1159/000333850

Kendall, G. S., Robertson, N. J., Iwata, O., Peebles, D., and Raivich, G. (2006). N-methylisobutyl-amiloride ameliorates brain injury when commenced before hypoxia ischemia in neonatal mice. *Pediatr. Res.* 59, 227–231. doi: 10.1203/01.pdr.0000196805.68082.22

Kholia, S., Ranghino, A., Garnieri, P., Lopatina, T., Deregibus, M. C., Rispoli, P., et al. (2016). Extracellular vesicles as new players in angiogenesis. *Vascul. Pharmacol.* 86, 64–70. doi: 10.1016/j.vph.2016.03.005

Kim, E. S., Ahn, S. Y., Im, G. H., Sung, D. K., Park, Y. R., Choi, S. H., et al. (2012). Human umbilical cord blood-derived mesenchymal stem cell transplantation attenuates severe brain injury by permanent middle cerebral artery occlusion in newborn rats. *Pediatr. Res.* 72, 277–284. doi: 10.1038/pr.2012.71

Kozlovskaya, L., Abou-Kaoud, M., and Stepensky, D. (2014). Quantitative analysis of drug delivery to the brain via nasal route. *J. Control Release* 189, 133–140. doi: 10.1016/j.jconrel.2014.06.053

Kumral, A., Tuzun, F., Tugyan, K., Ozbal, S., Yılmaz, O., Yesilirmak, C. D., et al. (2012). Role of epigenetic regulatory mechanisms in neonatal hypoxic-ischemic brain injury. *Early Hum. Dev.* 89, 165–173. doi: 10.1016/j.earlhumdev.2012.09.016

Kurinczuk, J. J., White-Koning, M., and Badawi, N. (2010). Epidemiology of neonatal encephalopathy and hypoxic-ischaemic encephalopathy. *Early Hum. Dev.* 86, 329–338. doi: 10.1016/j.earlhumdev.2010.05.010

Lamichhane, T. N., Sokic, S., Schardt, J. S., Raiker, R. S., Lin, J. W., and Jay, S. M. (2015). Emerging roles for extracellular vesicles in tissue engineering and regenerative medicine. *Tissue Eng. Part B Rev.* 21, 45–54. doi: 10.1089/ten.TEB.2014.0300

Lange, S., Rocha-Ferreira, E., Thei, L., Mawjee, P., Bennett, K., Thompson, P. R., et al. (2014). Peptidylarginine deiminases: novel drug targets for prevention of neuronal damage following hypoxic ischemic insult (HI) in neonates. *J. Neurochem.* 130, 555–562. doi: 10.1111/jnc.12744

Lappalainen, R. S., Narkilahti, S., Huhtala, T., Liimatainen, T., Suuronen, T., Närvänen, A., et al. (2008). The SPECT imaging shows the accumulation of neural progenitor cells into internal organs after systemic administration in middle cerebral artery occlusion rats. *Neurosci. Lett.* 440, 246–250. doi: 10.1016/j.neulet.2008.05.090

Lee, A. C. C., Kozuki, N., Blencowe, H., Vos, T., Bahalim, A., Darmstadt, G. L., et al. (2013). Intrapartum-related neonatal encephalopathy incidence and impairment at regional and global levels for 2010 with trends from 1990. *Pediatr. Res.* 74(Suppl. 1), 50–72. doi: 10.1038/pr.2013.206

Lee, C., Mitsialis, S. A., Aslam, M., Vitali, S. H., Vergadi, E., Konstantinou, G., et al. (2012). Exosomes mediate the cytoprotective action of mesenchymal stromal cells on hypoxia-induced pulmonary hypertension. *Circulation* 126:2601. doi: 10.1161/CIRCULATIONAHA.112.114173

Leisman, G., Braun-Benjamin, O., and Melillo, R. (2014). Cognitive-motor interactions of the basal ganglia in development. *Front. Syst. Neurosci.* 8:16. doi: 10.3389/fnsys.2014.00016

Li, L., Jiang, Q., Ding, G., Zhang, L., Zhang, Z. G., Li, Q., et al. (2010). Effects of administration route on migration and distribution of neural progenitor cells transplanted into rats with focal cerebral ischemia, an MRI study. *J. Cereb. Blood Flow Metab.* 30, 653–662. doi: 10.1038/jcbfm.2009.238

Lin, W., Oh, S. K. W., Choo, A. B. H., and George, A. J. T. (2012). Activated T cells modulate immunosuppression by embryonic-and bone marrow-derived mesenchymal stromal cells through a feedback mechanism. *Cytotherapy* 14, 274–284. doi: 10.3109/14653249.2011.635853

Lloyd, M., Wolfensohn, S., and Thornton, P. (2000). "Quantitative assessment of welfare in experimental animals: the development and use of scoring systems," in *Proceedings of the 3rd World Congress on Alternatives and Animal Use in the Life Science: Progress in the Reduction, Refinement and Replacement of Animal Experimentation*, eds M. Balls, A.-M. van Zeller, and M. E. Halder (Amsterdam: Elsevier Science), 1107–1117.

Long, Q., Upadhya, D., Hattiangady, B., Kim, D. K., An, S. Y., Shuai, B., et al. (2017). Intranasal MSC-derived A1-exosomes ease inflammation, and prevent abnormal neurogenesis and memory dysfunction after status epilepticus. *Proc. Natl. Acad. Sci. U.S.A.* 114, E3536–E3545. doi: 10.1073/pnas.1703920114

Lou, H. C. (1996). Etiology and pathogenesis of attention-deficit hyperactivity disorder (ADHD): significance of prematurity and perinatal hypoxic-haemodynamic encephalopathy. *Acta Paediatr.* 85, 1266–1271. doi: 10.1111/j.1651-2227.1996.tb13909.x

Lubics, A., Reglodi, D., Tamás, A., Kiss, P., Szalai, M., Szalontay, L., et al. (2005). Neurological reflexes and early motor behavior in rats subjected to neonatal hypoxic-ischemic injury. *Behav. Brain Res.* 157, 157–165. doi: 10.1016/j.bbr.2004.06.019

Madrigal, M., Rao, K. S., and Riordan, N. H. (2014). A review of therapeutic effects of mesenchymal stem cell secretions and induction of secretory modification by different culture methods. *J. Transl. Med.* 12:260. doi: 10.1186/s12967-014-0260-8

Mallard, C., and Vexler, Z. S. (2015). Modeling ischemia in the immature brain: how translational are animal models? *Stroke* 46, 3006–3011. doi: 10.1161/STROKEAHA.115.007776

Mallard, C., Welin, A. K., Peebles, D., Hagberg, H., and Kjellmer, I. (2003). White matter injury following systemic endotoxemia or asphyxia in the fetal sheep. *Neurochem. Res.* 28, 215–223. doi: 10.1023/A:1022368915400

Martin, L. J., Brambrink, A., Koehler, R. C., and Traystman, R. J. (1997). Primary sensory and forebrain motor systems in the newborn brain are preferentially damaged by hypoxia-ischemia. *J. Comp. Neurol.* 377, 262–285. doi: 10.1002/(SICI)1096-9861(19970113)377:2<262::AID-CNE8>3.0.CO;2-1

Martinez-Biarge, M., Diez-Sebastian, J., Kapellou, O., Gindner, D., Allsop, J. M., Rutherford, M. A., et al. (2011). Predicting motor outcome and death in term hypoxic-ischemic encephalopathy. *Neurology* 76, 2055–2061. doi: 10.1212/WNL.0b013e31821f442d

McQuillen, P. S., Sheldon, R. A., Shatz, C. J., and Ferriero, D. M. (2003). Selective vulnerability of subplate neurons after early neonatal hypoxia-ischemia. *J. Neurosci.* 23, 3308–3315. doi: 10.1523/JNEUROSCI.23-08-03308.2003

Meisel, R., Zibert, A., Laryea, M., Göbel, U., Däubener, W., and Dilloo, D. (2004). Human bone marrow stromal cells inhibit allogeneic T-cell responses by indoleamine 2,3-dioxygenasemediated tryptophan degradation. *Blood* 103, 4619–4621. doi: 10.1182/blood-2003-11-3909

Mercuri, E., Barnett, A., Rutherford, M., Guzzetta, A., Haataja, L., Cioni, G., et al. (2004). Neonatal cerebral infarction and neuromotor outcome at school age. *Pediatrics* 113, 95–100. doi: 10.1542/peds.113.1.95

Mercuri, E., and Barnett, A. L. (2003). Neonatal brain MRI and motor outcome at school age in children with neonatal encephalopathy: a review of personal experience. *Neural Plast.* 10, 51–57. doi: 10.1155/NP.2003.51

Merino-González, C., Zuñiga, F. A., Escudero, C., Ormazabal, V., Reyes, C., Nova-Lamperti, E., et al. (2016). Mesenchymal stem cell-derived extracellular vesicles promote angiogenesis: potencial clinical application. *Front. Physiol.* 7:24. doi: 10.3389/fphys.2016.00024

Merkus, F. W. H. M., and van den Berg, M. P. (2007). Can nasal drug delivery bypass the bloodbrain barrier: questioning the direct transport theory. *Drugs R. D.* 8, 133–144. doi: 10.2165/00126839-200708030-00001

Németh, K., Leelahavanichkul, A., Yuen, P. S. T., Mayer, B., Parmelee, A., Doi, K., et al. (2009). Bone marrow stromal cells attenuate sepsis via prostaglandin E(2)-dependent reprogramming of host macrophages to increase their interleukin-10 production. *Nat. Med.* 15, 42–49. doi: 10.1038/nm.1905

Ophelders, D. R. M. G., Wolfs, T. G. A. M., Jellema, R. K., Zwanenburg, A., Andriessen, P., Delhaas, T., et al. (2016). Mesenchymal stromal cell-derived extracellular vesicles protect the fetal brain after hypoxia-ischemia. *Stem Cells Transl. Med.* 5, 754–763. doi: 10.5966/sctm.2015-0197

Packard, M. G., and Knowlton, B. J. (2002). Learning and memory functions of the Basal Ganglia. *Annu. Rev. Neurosci.* 25, 563–593. doi: 10.1146/annurev.neuro.25.112701.142937

Packard, M. G., and McGaugh, J. L. (1996). Inactivation of hippocampus or caudate nucleus with lidocaine differentially affects expression of place and response learning. *Neurobiol. Learn. Mem.* 65, 65–72. doi: 10.1006/nlme.1996.0007

Park, W. S., Sung, S. I., Ahn, S. Y., Yoo, H. S., Sung, D. K., Im, G. H., et al. (2015). Hypothermia augments neuroprotective activity of mesenchymal stem cells for neonatal hypoxic-ischemic encephalopathy. *PLoS One* 10:e0120893. doi: 10.1371/journal.pone.0120893

Pendharkar, A. V., Chua, J. Y., Andres, R. H., Wang, N., Gaeta, X., Wang, H., et al. (2010). Biodistribution of neural stem cells after intravascular therapy for hypoxic-ischemia. *Stroke* 41, 2064–2070. doi: 10.1161/STROKEAHA.109.575993

Perlman, J. M. (2006). Intervention strategies for neonatal hypoxic-ischemic cerebral injury. *Clin. Ther.* 28, 1353–1365. doi: 10.1016/j.clinthera.2006.09.005

Pirianov, G., Brywe, K. G., Mallard, C., Edwards, A. D., Flavell, R. A., Hagberg, H., et al. (2007). Deletion of the c-Jun N-terminal kinase 3 gene protects neonatal mice against cerebral hypoxic-ischaemic injury. *J. Cereb. Blood Flow Metab.* 27, 1022–1032. doi: 10.1038/sj.jcbfm.9600413

Prockop, D. J., and Oh, J. Y. (2012). Mesenchymal stem/stromal cells (MSCs): role as guardians of inflammation. *Mol. Ther.* 20, 14–20. doi: 10.1038/mt.2011.211

Ranghino, A., Cantaluppi, V., Grange, C., Vitillo, L., Fop, F., Biancone, L., et al. (2012). Endothelial progenitor cell-derived microvesicles improve neovascularization in a murine model of hindlimb ischemia. *Int. J. Immunopathol. Pharmacol.* 25, 75–85. doi: 10.1177/039463201202500110

Robbins, P. D., and Morelli, A. E. (2014). Regulation of immune responses by extracellular vesicles. *Nat. Rev. Immunol.* 14, 195–208. doi: 10.1038/nri3622

Rocha-Ferreira, E., and Hristova, M. (2016). Plasticity in the neonatal brain following hypoxic-ischaemic injury. *Neural Plast.* 2016:4901014. doi: 10.1155/2016/4901014

Rocha-Ferreira, E., Phillips, E., Francesch-Domenech, E., Thei, L., Peebles, D. M., Raivich, G., et al. (2015). The role of different strain backgrounds in bacterial endotoxin-mediated sensitization to neonatal hypoxic-ischemic brain damage. *Neuroscience* 311, 292–307. doi: 10.1016/j.neuroscience.2015.10.035

Rocha-Ferreira, E., Vincent, A., Bright, S., Peebles, D. M., and Hristova, M. (2018). The duration of hypothermia affects short-term neuroprotection in a mouse model of neonatal hypoxic ischaemic injury. *PLoS One* 13:e0199890. doi: 10.1371/journal.pone.0199890

Rong, L.-J., Chi, Y., Yang, S.-G., Chen, D.-D., Chen, F., Xu, S.-X., et al. (2012). Effects of interferon-γ on biological characteristics and immunomodulatory property of human umbilical cord-derived mesenchymal stem cells. *Zhongguo Shi Yan Xue Ye Xue Za Zhi* 20, 421–426.

Sanches, E. F., Arteni, N. S., Nicola, F., Boisserand, L., Willborn, S., and Netto, C. A. (2013). Early hypoxia-ischemia causes hemisphere and sex-dependent cognitive impairment and histological damage. *Neuroscience* 237, 208–215. doi: 10.1016/j.neuroscience.2013.01.066

Schmidt-Kastner, R. (2015). Genomic approach to selective vulnerability of the hippocampus in brain ischemia-hypoxia. *Neuroscience* 309, 259–279. doi: 10.1016/j.neuroscience.2015.08.034

Shankaran, S., Pappas, A., McDonald, S. A., Vohr, B. R., Hintz, S. R., Yolton, K., et al. (2012). Childhood outcomes after hypothermia for neonatal encephalopathy. *N. Engl. J. Med.* 366, 2085–2092. doi: 10.1056/NEJMoa1112066

Tan, C. Y., Lai, R. C., Wong, W., Dan, Y. Y., Lim, S. K., and Ho, H. K. (2014). Mesenchymal stem cell-derived exosomes promote hepatic regeneration in drug-induced liver injury models. *Stem Cell Res. Ther.* 5:76. doi: 10.1186/scrt465

Thei, L., Rocha-Ferreira, E., Peebles, D., Raivich, G., and Hristova, M. (2018). Extracellular signal-regulated kinase 2 has duality in function between neuronal and astrocyte expression following neonatal hypoxic-ischaemic cerebral injury. *J. Physiol.* doi: 10.1113/JP275649 [Epub ahead of print].

Tricarico, C., Clancy, J., and D'Souza-Schorey, C. (2017). Biology and biogenesis of shed microvesicles. *Small GTPases* 8, 220–232. doi: 10.1080/21541248.2016.1215283

Uccelli, A., Moretta, L., and Pistoia, V. (2008). Mesenchymal stem cells in health and disease. *Nat. Rev. Immunol.* 8, 726–736. doi: 10.1038/nri2395

Uria-Avellanal, C., and Robertson, N. J. (2014). Na+/H+ exchangers and intracellular pH in perinatal brain injury. *Transl. Stroke Res.* 5, 79–98. doi: 10.1007/s12975-013-0322-x

Vallabhaneni, K. C., Penfornis, P., Dhule, S., Guillonneau, F., Adams, K. V., Mo, Y. Y., et al. (2015). Extracellular vesicles from bone marrow mesenchymal stem/stromal cells transport tumor regulatory microRNA, proteins, and metabolites. *Oncotarget* 6:4953. doi: 10.18632/oncotarget.3211

van Niel, G., D'Angelo, G., and Raposo, G. (2018). Shedding light on the cell biology of extracellular vesicles. *Nat. Rev. Mol. Cell Biol.* 19, 213–228. doi: 10.1038/nrm.2017.125

Van Petten, C. (2004). Relationship between hippocampal volume and memory ability in healthy individuals across the lifespan: review and meta-analysis. *Neuropsychologia* 42, 1394–1413. doi: 10.1016/j.neuropsychologia.2004.04.006

van Velthoven, C. T. J., Kavelaars, A., and Heijnen, C. J. (2012). Mesenchymal stem cells as a treatment for neonatal ischemic brain damage. *Pediatr. Res.* 71, 474–481. doi: 10.1038/pr.2011.64

van Velthoven, C. T. J., Kavelaars, A., van Bel, F., and Heijnen, C. J. (2010). Mesenchymal stem cell treatment after neonatal hypoxic-ischemic brain injury improves behavioral outcome and induces neuronal and oligodendrocyte regeneration. *Brain Behav. Immun.* 24, 387–393. doi: 10.1016/j.bbi.2009.10.017

Vannucci, R. C., and Vannucci, S. J. (1997). A model of perinatal hypoxic-ischemic brain damage. *Ann. N. Y. Acad. Sci.* 835, 234–249. doi: 10.1111/j.1749-6632.1997.tb48634.x

Vohr, B. R., Wright, L. L., Dusick, A. M., Mele, L., Verter, J., Steichen, J. J., et al. (2000). Neurodevelopmental and functional outcomes of extremely low birth weight infants in the National Institute of Child Health and Human Development Neonatal Research Network, 1993-1994. *Pediatrics* 105, 1216–1226. doi: 10.1542/peds.105.6.1216

Volpe, J. J. (2001). Perinatal brain injury: from pathogenesis to neuroprotection. *Ment. Retard. Dev. Disabil. Res. Rev.* 7, 56–64. doi: 10.1002/1098-2779(200102)7:1<56::AID-MRDD1008>3.0.CO;2-A

Volpe, J. J. (2012). Neonatal encephalopathy: an inadequate term for hypoxic-ischemic encephalopathy. *Ann. Neurol.* 72, 156–166. doi: 10.1002/ana.23647

Walczak, P., Zhang, J., Gilad, A. A., Kedziorek, D. A., Ruiz-Cabello, J., Young, R. G., et al. (2008). Dual-modality monitoring of targeted intraarterial delivery of mesenchymal stem cells after transient ischemia. *Stroke* 39, 1569–1574. doi: 10.1161/STROKEAHA.107.502047

Wen, S., Dooner, M., Cheng, Y., Papa, E., Del Tatto, M., Pereira, M., et al. (2016). Mesenchymal stromal cell-derived extracellular vesicles rescue radiation damage to murine marrow hematopoietic cells. *Leukemia* 30, 2221–2231. doi: 10.1038/leu.2016.107

White, N. M., and McDonald, R. J. (2002). Multiple parallel memory systems in the brain of the rat. *Neurobiol. Learn. Mem.* 77, 125–184. doi: 10.1006/nlme.2001.4008

Wu, Y. W., and Colford, J. M. Jr. (2000). Chorioamnionitis as a risk factor for cerebral palsy: a meta analysis. *JAMA* 284, 1417–1424. doi: 10.1001/jama.284.11.1417

Wyatt, J. S., Gluckman, P. D., Liu, P. Y., Azzopardi, D., Ballard, R., Edwards, A. D., et al. (2007). Determinants of outcomes after head cooling for neonatal encephalopathy. *Pediatrics* 119, 912–921. doi: 10.1542/peds.2006-2839

Yeo, R. W. Y., Lai, R. C., Zhang, B., Tan, S. S., Yin, Y., Teh, B. J., et al. (2013). Mesenchymal stem cell: an efficient mass producer of exosomes for drug delivery. *Adv. Drug Deliv. Rev.* 65, 336–341. doi: 10.1016/j.addr.2012.07.001

Yi, J. H., Park, S. W., Kapadia, R., and Vemuganti, R. (2007). Role of transcription factors in mediating post-ischemic cerebral inflammation and brain damage. *Neurochem. Int.* 50, 1014–1027. doi: 10.1016/j.neuint.2007.04.019

Zhang, S., Chu, W. C., Lai, R. C., Lim, S. K., Hui, J. H. P., and Toh, W. S. (2016). Exosomes derived from human embryonic mesenchymal stem cells promote osteochondral regeneration. *Osteoarthr. Cartil.* 24, 2135–2140. doi: 10.1016/j.joca.2016.06.022

13

Emergent Prophylactic, Reparative and Restorative Brain Interventions for Infants Born Preterm with Cerebral Palsy

Megan Finch-Edmondson [1,2], *Catherine Morgan* [1,2], *Rod W. Hunt* [3,4,5,6] *and Iona Novak* [1,2*]

[1] *The Discipline of Child and Adolescent Health, The Children's Hospital at Westmead Clinical School, The University of Sydney Medical School, Sydney, NSW, Australia,* [2] *Cerebral Palsy Alliance Research Institute, The University of Sydney, Sydney, NSW, Australia,* [3] *Department of Neonatal Medicine, The Royal Children's Hospital, Melbourne, VIC, Australia,* [4] *Department of Paediatrics, University of Melbourne, Melbourne, VIC, Australia,* [5] *Neonatal Research, Murdoch Children's Research Institute, Melbourne, VIC, Australia,* [6] *Department of Obstetrics and Gynaecology, Monash University, Melbourne, VIC, Australia*

Correspondence:
Iona Novak
inovak@cerebralpalsy.org.au

Worldwide, an estimated 15 million babies are born preterm (<37 weeks' gestation) every year. Despite significant improvements in survival rates, preterm infants often face a lifetime of neurodevelopmental disability including cognitive, behavioral, and motor impairments. Indeed, prematurity remains the largest risk factor for the development of cerebral palsy. The developing brain of the preterm infant is particularly fragile; preterm babies exhibit varying severities of cerebral palsy arising from reductions in both cerebral white and gray matter volumes, as well as altered brain microstructure and connectivity. Current intensive care therapies aim to optimize cardiovascular and respiratory function to protect the brain from injury by preserving oxygenation and blood flow. If a brain injury does occur, definitive diagnosis of cerebral palsy in the first few hours and weeks of life is difficult, especially when the lesions are subtle and not apparent on cranial ultrasound. However, early diagnosis of mildly affected infants is critical, because these are the patients most likely to respond to emergent treatments inducing neuroplasticity via high-intensity motor training programs and regenerative therapies involving stem cells. A current controversy is whether to test universal treatment in all infants at risk of brain injury, accepting that some patients never required treatment, because the perceived potential benefits outweigh the risk of harm. Versus, waiting for a diagnosis before commencing targeted treatment for infants with a brain injury, and potentially missing the therapeutic window. In this review, we discuss the emerging prophylactic, reparative, and restorative brain interventions for infants born preterm, who are at high risk of developing cerebral palsy. We examine the current evidence, considering the timing of the intervention with relation to the proposed mechanism/s of action. Finally, we consider the development of novel markers of preterm brain injury, which will undoubtedly lead to improved diagnostic and prognostic capability, and more accurate instruments to assess the efficacy of emerging interventions for this most vulnerable group of infants.

Keywords: preterm, brain injury, cerebral palsy, neuroplasticity, neuroprotection, neuro-regeneration, neuro-repair

PREMATURITY

Prematurity remains the leading cause of morbidity and mortality in childhood within the developed world. Global rates of prematurity range from 5 to 18% of all births (Blencowe et al., 2012). In 2015, 9% of all Australian births occurred <37 weeks' gestational age, giving a burden of prematurity of around 27,000 babies (AIHW, 2017). The incidence of babies born extremely prematurely (22–27^{+6} weeks' gestation) is lower, however over 3,000 Australian babies were born very preterm (<30 weeks' gestation) during the same period (AIHW, 2017). Advances in neonatal intensive care ensure that 85% of these very preterm infants survive, but 55% survive with neurobehavioral impairments, 22% with intellectual disability and 7% with cerebral palsy (Aarnoudse-Moens et al., 2009). In the long term it is estimated that their lifetime cost to the health economy will exceed $200 million (Access Economics, 2008).

Current Usual Care for Preterm Infants

Usual care of the preterm infant in the Neonatal Intensive Care Unit (NICU) environment is generally highly protocolized and whilst some variation in practice exists between units, the basic "recipe" is the same (Malcolm, 2014). Almost without exception preterm infants with surfactant deficiency receive exogenous surfactant, with the expectation that reduced severity of lung disease will minimize hypoxia and fluctuations in blood pressure (Polin and Carlo, 2014). Oxygen saturations are targeted to around 90–95%, with a recent increase in our understanding that both hypoxia and hyperoxia increase the risk of cerebral and other end organ injury (Askie et al., 2017). Mean blood pressure is targeted to the gestational age at birth in weeks, and fluctuations in blood pressure are avoided where possible, through judicious use of fluid following assessment of fluid status by clinical indicators such as urine output, perfusion and in some centers, ultrasound measures (Kenner et al., 1998). Where there is any risk of infection/inflammation, there is generally a low threshold for the use of broad spectrum antibiotics to cover against the common bacteria that pose a risk to the preterm infant, most notably Group B streptococcus and *Escherichia coli* (Simonsen et al., 2014). The most premature and smallest infants are at most risk of organ damage, however a recent study has demonstrated that even those infants born in the late premature phase are at risk of neurodevelopmental impairments (Cheong et al., 2017). The goal of all of these therapies collectively is to maintain adequate and steady perfusion and oxygenation of the brain to avoid inflammation and brain injury, but none specifically target either neuroprotection or neural repair.

Brain Injury in Preterm Infants

Brain Injury Diagnostics

Historically, cerebral injury during the perinatal period until term corrected age was detected with cranial ultrasound (cUS). However, the sensitivity and specificity of this imaging modality is variable between operators. cUS remains in common use because of its clinical utility with imaging possible at the bedside, and lower costs compared to magnetic resonance imaging (MRI). With cUS, it is possible to detect common patterns of severe preterm brain injury, such as intraventricular hemorrhage (IVH) and periventricular leukomalacia (PVL), however subtle lesions can be indiscernible (Hintz et al., 2007). Serial cUS is therefore widely used for screening, however approximately one third of preterm infants diagnosed with cerebral palsy may not have lesions identified by cUS (Beaino et al., 2010). The accuracy of cUS to predict long term disability is enhanced when scans are taken sequentially until term-equivalent age, and are then combined with MRI to detect and classify the presence of white matter injury (Martinez-Biarge et al., 2016). MRI provides better anatomical detail and has the sensitivity to detect subtle white matter injury that may not be discernible on ultrasound. However, in experienced hands cUS can still be reliable in the detection of cerebral injury, and whilst MRI provides modest benefit to injury detection (Leijser et al., 2008; Edwards et al., 2018), its cost and availability preclude its routine use in some centers.

White Matter Injury

With increasing use of MRI, a more insidious cerebral insult—*diffuse white matter injury* has been recognized. Damage to the white matter is the most common type of preterm brain injury with severity ranging from mild to severe (Inder et al., 2003). In white matter injury, the preoligodendrocytes are "arrested" in their development, preventing full maturation and thus myelination (Ferriero, 2016). In addition, recurrent infection and long term ventilation exacerbate neuronal and axonal damage (Khwaja and Volpe, 2008), and results in a higher likelihood of white matter injury (Smilga et al., 2018).

Cystic PVL is a condition in which cystic cavitations develop in the periventricular white matter, and their extent can be graded from grade 1 to 3 (classification by De Vries et al., 1992). PVL has been associated with spastic cerebral palsy, with severity of impairment influenced by the location and extent of the lesions (De Vries et al., 2011). With increasing use of MRI and detection of more subtle white matter injury, the term PVL has been applied to non-cystic diffuse white matter injury (Khwaja and Volpe, 2008). Non-cystic PVL is characterized by microscopic focal necroses which generally evolve to form glial scars (Khwaja and Volpe, 2008). The prevalence of cystic PVL has been declining for some time (Van Haastert et al., 2011), and non-cystic PVL now accounts for the majority of cerebral white matter injury observed in premature infants (Khwaja and Volpe, 2008).

Inder et al. showed that cerebral injury in premature infants typically manifests as diffuse white matter atrophy, ventriculomegaly, immature gyral development, and enlarged subarachnoid space (Inder et al., 2003). In addition, this group (Inder et al., 2005) have shown that white matter injury results in reductions in volumes of deep nuclear gray matter and cortical gray matter as well as disturbed white matter microstructure (Cheong et al., 2009).

In addition to these abnormalities, children born prematurely experience interruptions to their third trimester brain development, growth and gyration, and arrested development of the oligodendrocyte cell lineage which disrupts myelination and brain connectivity development (Back et al., 2001). Recent research has demonstrated that preterm infants are at greater risk of: (a) neurodevelopmental difficulties at 2 years (Woodward et al., 2006); (b) motor deficit at 4 years (Spittle et al., 2011); and (c) a range of functional outcomes at 7 years (Anderson et al., 2017). Moreover, preterm birth is a risk factor for lower IQ and poorer educational performance (Cheong et al., 2013). Doyle et al. have shown that biological influences on cerebral structure in early postnatal life have a greater influence on long term outcome than subsequent early childhood environmental factors (Doyle et al., 2015).

Intraventricular Hemorrhage

IVH is bleeding inside the lateral ventricles and occurs in up to 45% of extremely preterm-, and 30% of very preterm- infants (Mukerji et al., 2015). IVH is graded from mild (grade 1) to severe (grade 4), according to a grading system first described by Papile in 1978, and is based on the amount of bleeding into the ventricle, the presence of ventricular dilatation and involvement of the surrounding white matter (Papile et al., 1978). The presence of IVH poses a risk of subsequent post hemorrhagic ventricular dilatation, the risk of which increases from 5% with grade 1 IVH to over 80% with grade 4 (Murphy et al., 2002).

Risks of neurodisability and mortality increase with increasing grades of IVH in a similar fashion. Most studies report a higher likelihood of cerebral palsy with increasing severity of IVH (Mukerji et al., 2015). Beaino et al. reported significantly increased odds ratios of cerebral palsy at 5-years when comparing grade 4 to no IVH (Beaino et al., 2010). Contrastingly, cerebral palsy following grade 3 IVH is variably reported, but the likelihood is higher when post hemorrhagic ventricular dilatation occurs. Although bilateral IVH is common, parenchymal lesions are typically restricted to one side, and thus often lead to unilateral spastic cerebral palsy (De Vries et al., 2011).

CEREBRAL PALSY

Brain injury detected in the newborn period is predictive of cerebral palsy (Linsell et al., 2016). White matter injury, chiefly PVL, and IVH are commonly reported in preterm infants later diagnosed with cerebral palsy (Kidokoro et al., 2014).

Cerebral palsy is an overarching term used to describe a group of disorders of movement and posture that occur due to damage to the developing brain during pregnancy, around the time of birth, or in the first 28 days of life. In many countries post-neonatal brain injury up until 2 years of age (such as stroke or near-drowning) is also included in the definition of cerebral palsy. Registry data in many parts of the world provides useful information about the cerebral palsy prevalence, type and topography related to gestational age. In Australia about 43% of people with cerebral palsy were born preterm, however this proportion is likely to be higher in the United States where a greater proportion of babies are born preterm (7% in Australia vs. 10% in the US) (Martin et al., 2018). Recently published register data shows that the incidence of cerebral palsy in preterm and term populations is starting to fall in high-income countries (1.4–2.1/1,000 live births) (Galea et al., 2018). Moreover, the percentage of children with moderate to severe disability is also declining (Galea et al., 2018).

It has been well established that the rate of cerebral palsy in preterm survivors is inversely related to gestational age (Himpens et al., 2008). A more recent review by Linsell et al. found that gestational age surprisingly did not predict cerebral palsy although included studies were 32 weeks or below (Linsell et al., 2016). It appears that after 27 weeks, rates of cerebral palsy drop off quite quickly. All subtypes of cerebral palsy can result from preterm brain injury although milder subtypes are most common.

Types of Cerebral Palsy

Cerebral palsy can be classified by the type of movement disorder or the parts of the body that are affected. The most common type is spastic cerebral palsy accounting for about 85% of all cerebral palsy (ACPR Group, 2018). Dyskinetic cerebral palsy accounts for 7%, with ataxic and hypotonic cerebral palsy accounting for a combined further 7% (ACPR Group, 2018). Infants with cerebral palsy who are born preterm (<37 weeks') are most likely to have bilateral cerebral palsy, with a diplegic pattern more common than quadriplegia (44 vs. 19%), while unilateral cerebral palsy is diagnosed in about 28% of preterm babies with cerebral palsy (Towsley et al., 2011; Reid et al., 2014; ACPR Group, 2018). Where PVL is cystic and widespread, spastic quadriplegia is the most common outcome (Novak et al., 2017). In these more severe cases it is not just the white matter that is involved but also the other cerebral structures e.g., deep nuclear gray matter, leading to the description "encephalopathy of prematurity" (Volpe, 2009).

Comorbidities

The risk for comorbidities with cerebral palsy is very high, and for the most part correlates with severity of the brain injury and physical disability. Common and disabling comorbidities and co-occurring functional impairments with cerebral palsy include: chronic pain (3 in 4); intellectual disability (1 in 2); hip displacement (1 in 3); epilepsy (1 in 4); behavior disorders (1 in 4); nonverbal (1 in 4); sleep disorders (1 in 5); vision impairment (1 in 10); and hearing impairment (1 in 25) (Novak et al., 2012).

Early Detection of Cerebral Palsy

Although preterm infants are at increased risk of cerebral palsy (Spittle et al., 2018), a diagnosis of cerebral palsy has traditionally not been made until 12–24 months, unless a severe disability was clearly evident in the neonatal intensive care period (ACPR Group, 2018). An international clinical guideline, based upon systematic review evidence, indicates cerebral palsy can now be accurately identified in children as young as 12-weeks corrected age (Novak et al., 2017). Since no biomarkers yet exist for cerebral palsy, the guideline recommends using a combination of standardized assessment tools. The results of these tests should triangulate, with all the tests pointing in the direction of high-risk for cerebral palsy. If the test results are incongruent, the child may have another disability that is not cerebral palsy. The tools with the best psychometric properties for accurately predicting cerebral palsy by 3-months corrected age include: (1) Prechtl's General Movements Assessment (a video-based observation of the infant's spontaneous movement, scored for quality of movement) (98% sensitivity); (2) term-age equivalent MRI indicating damage to the motor areas of the brain (86–89% sensitivity); and (3) the Hammersmith Infant Neurological Examination (a scored neurological physical examination, with risk cut points determined from large sample studies) (90% sensitivity) (Novak et al., 2017). The results of these assessments should be carefully and compassionately communicated to the child's parents. Early diagnosis enables referral to early intervention to improve the child's outcomes, prevent secondary complications and protect parental mental health (Novak et al., 2017).

EMERGENT INTERVENTIONS

There is a wide range of therapeutic interventions that have been proposed and are currently being tested to promote neurological repair in both infants and adults. Wherever possible, in this review, we present data generated from preclinical and clinical studies specifically utilizing preterm models and/or targeting premature populations. Where there is little published evidence, we have cast our net wider to include studies focusing on related neurological conditions such as adult stroke, traumatic brain injury and neurodegenerative conditions. Caution is warranted when interpreting the utility of interventions that are effective in adults back to the preterm infant, as the preterm baby is not simply a small adult, and their physiology often times contradicts the adult literature. Nevertheless, the results of some of these studies may be found to be relevant for preterm brain injury, and thus we see value in reviewing these studies, when there is little preterm-specific evidence available. In **Table 1** we provide a summary of the interventions covered in this review, their mechanism of action, the current phase of research translation, route and timing of administration, plus, potential advantages and controversies to overcome through research. In addition, the timing of administration for known effective and emergent therapies for preterm infants is further illustrated in **Figure 1**.

Biological and Pharmacological Therapies

Cell-Based Therapy

Cell therapies offer great promise for treating neurological diseases and are emerging as a new paradigm in human medicine (Trounson and Dewitt, 2016). The mechanisms by which candidate cell therapies might work for brain injury include (1) anti-inflammatory mechanisms: attenuation of the inflammatory immune response to brain injury via a reduction in the release of excitotoxins, cytotoxins, and reactive oxygen species; (2) trophic mechanisms: to promote cell survival via release of neurotrophic factors to induce endogenous cell migration, proliferation and differentiation and/or promote angiogenesis; and (3) regenerative mechanisms: replacement of damaged brain tissue by engraftment, proliferation and differentiation of transplanted cells (reviewed in Novak et al., 2016). Different types of cells have been proposed, including: amnion epithelial cells (AECs); mesenchymal stromal/stem cells (MSCs); umbilical cord blood (UCB), and neural progenitor/neural stem cells (NSCs) (Novak et al., 2016), each with different advantages and disadvantages that must be considered when contemplating therapeutic application. Substantial preclinical evidence now exists to support the conduct of human trials evaluating efficacy of various cell therapies for perinatal brain injury (reviewed by Fleiss et al., 2014).

There are ethical complexities and controversies to be considered when conducting clinical trials of stem cells in newborns with perinatal brain injury. First, these children have a lot to gain but also a lot to lose from an adverse event. Thus, human ethics committees often favor "first in human" studies to be conducted in adult populations where the patient can consent, rather than consent being obtained by proxy from a parent. Hence there have been no clinical trials in preterm infants where the cells have been delivered in the acute newborn period. Second, not all preterm babies have a disability. Accurate determination of which patients will have a normal outcome and which patients will have a disability can take months, and even years for subtle literacy problems in reading and writing to be apparent. Therefore, the dilemma exists about timing of stem cell treatment for preterm infants. Should universal treatments be applied to all preterm patients in the newborn period given that the risks of disability are high, and the newborn period is the optimal therapeutic window in terms of an effect in the acute phase? Or should we wait and provide targeted therapies once the children with definite long-term disability can be identified, all the while lowering the potential treatment effect size from late intervention in the chronic phase of brain injury? Third, the mechanism of action should match the clinical indication. Cells that have anti-inflammatory and trophic properties (i.e., AECs, MSCs, and UCB) will theoretically will be of most benefit during the acute period of neuroinflammation, if neuro-repair is sought. If administered in the chronic phase, smaller gains may still be possible via trophic effects and the emerging evidence that inflammation persists into the tertiary phase of injury (Fleiss and Gressens, 2012). Contrastingly, cells that have regenerative capacity (i.e., NSCs) are a better therapeutic target for chronic stage injury. Fourth the origin of the cells can be controversial for some. AEC, MSC, and UCB cells can be obtained using morally uncomplicated methods: AECs are obtained from placental tissue under maternal consent, UBC from cords with maternal consent, and MSCs are available in off-the-shelf commercial formats or can be obtained autologously from bone marrow harvesting with patient consent. NSCs cannot be safely obtained from adult donors and therefore need to be obtained with consent from embryonic or fetal sources, or grown autologously from induced pluripotent cells.

Given the challenges of designing stem cell trials for preterm infants, there are limited published studies. However, Rudnicki et al. assessed the safety and feasibility of autologous UCB for extremely preterm (<32 weeks') neonates who developed anemia due to prematurity (Rudnicki et al., 2015). In this trial, infants received an intravenous transfusion of 15 mL/kg of body weight of either autologous UCB ($n = 5$) or allogeneic red blood cells ($n = 9$; control group), administered on average 3.2 and 7.8 days after birth for UCB and red blood cells, respectively. Results from this small study group indicated that autologous UCB transplantation in preterm newborns was generally safe and well

TABLE 1 | Potential therapeutic agents and research progress.

Agent	Mechanism of action	Sub-population of patients that might be treatment responsive	Research phase for preterm brain injury				Route of administration	Timing of administration	Advantages	Disadvantages/ controversies
			Preclinical	Phase 1	Phase 2	Phase 3				
Cell therapy|amnion epithelial cells (AEC) Cells obtained from the placenta	Anti-inflammatory and trophic TARGET = Motor, cognitive, behavioral and respiratory gains	• BPD	✓	✓	✗	✗	IV	If 28-weeks GA and still requiring O2 at 36-weeks GA	• Proven safe for newborns in BPD Phase 1 trial (Lim et al., 2018) • Easily obtained from placenta • Morally uncomplicated source of cells • Low immunogenicity • Can be stored for later use • Can be isolated and expanded to treat multiple patients • Crosses the BBB	• Unknown if it is better to administer AECs as a universal treatment for all preterm births at risk of disability, in the very acute phase OR whether to wait until a disability can be diagnosed and then offer a targeted AEC treatment later after injury
		• All preterm births as a universal neuro-protectant	✓	✗	✓	✗	IV	3 doses in the first week of life		
Cell therapy|mesenchymal stem cells (MSC) Multipotent adult stem cells, found in bone marrow and umbilical cord tissue and blood	Anti-inflammatory and trophic TARGET = Motor and cognitive gains	• CP >6-months of age, of all sub-types and causal pathways	✓	✓	✓	✗	IV and intrathecal from autologous source, bone marrow derived	Tested late in the tertiary phase of injury. Autologous MSC doses of 1–2 $\times 10^7$	• Proven safe in humans • Can be obtained autologously from bone marrow or umbilical cord • Available in off-the-shelf commercial formats for emergency and high/multi-dose administration • Low immunogenicity • Can be stored for later use • Can be isolated and expanded • Short survival following transfusion, lowering the risk of adverse events • Some MSCs may cross the BBB	• Unknown if the cells might be more efficacious when transplanted stereotactically to increase the concentration of cells crossing the BBB • Unknown if the cells might be more efficacious when transplanted in combination with other stem cell types with longer duration effects
		• IVH	✓	✓	✗	✗	Intra-cerebroventricular injection	Within 7 days of IVH		
		• Perinatal stroke	✓	✗	✗	✗	Intranasal and intra-arterial	On day 1 of injury		

(Continued)

TABLE 1 | Continued

Agent	Mechanism of action	Sub-population of patients that might be treatment responsive	Research phase for preterm brain injury				Route of administration	Timing of administration	Advantages	Disadvantages/ controversies
			Preclinical	Phase 1	Phase 2	Phase 3				
									• Bone marrow derived MSCs shown to be more effective than bone marrow mononuclear cells in a clinical trial for CP (Liu et al., 2017)	
Cell therapy|neural stem cells (NSC) Stem cells that make the 3 types of brain cells	Regenerative, anti-inflammatory and trophic TARGET = Cure or Motor and cognitive gains in tertiary phase injury	• CP 1 year old and up, of all sub-types and causal pathways	✓	✓	✓	✗	Intracranial, stereotactically placed neurosurgically	Unknown, may be effective in the tertiary phase of injury as a cure	• Regenerative capabilities • Shown to be safe in human trials when transplanted with immunosuppression • Can be stored for later use • One donor's cells can be expanded to treat multiple patients	• Must be obtained from embryos, fetal or iPSC sources, as it is unsafe for adults to donate • Neurosurgical administration required
Cell therapy|umbilical cord blood (UCB) Umbilical cord blood rich in an array cell types including stem cell populations	Anti-inflammatory and trophic TARGET = Motor and cognitive gains in late tertiary phase treatment; disability-free survival in primary and secondary phase treatment	• CP 1 year old and up, of all sub-types and causal pathways	✓	✓	✓	✗	IV (Autologous and allogeneic)	Tested late in the tertiary phase of injury. Autologous UCB doses >2 × 10^7/kg produced better results (Sun et al., 2017)	• Proven safe in humans • Easily obtained from umbilical cords • Morally uncomplicated source of cells • Source can be autologous or allogeneic and can be HLA matched • Can be stored for later use • Theoretically can be expanded	• Difficult to collect and reinfuse autologous cords in an emergency birth with HI injury • Unknown risks of autologous reinfusion for genetic and/or infection causal pathways to CP, i.e., could the injury be worsened? • Preterm infants have small low volume cords with a different cell make-up to term cords, and therefore autologous infusions may have less therapeutic value
		• HI injury	✓	✓	✓	✗	IV (autologous)	After 6 h of injury and initiation of hypothermia. Multiple doses in the first week of life		
		• All preterm births as a universal neuro-protectant	✓	✗	✗	✗	IV (allogeneic)	Unknown		

(Continued)

TABLE 1 | Continued

Agent	Mechanism of action	Sub-population of patients that might be treatment responsive	Research phase for preterm brain injury				Route of administration	Timing of administration	Advantages	Disadvantages/ controversies
			Preclinical	Phase 1	Phase 2	Phase 3				
										• Efficacy appears higher with higher HLA matching, meaning large, diverse cord banks are needed • Need for off-the-shelf expanded products for emergency and/or high-dose/repeat treatments • Unknown GVHD risk from combining allogeneic cords to deliver high/multi-dose treatments • Unknown effect of delayed cord clamping on cord volumes and efficacy
Extracellular vesicles (EVs) Membrane fragments released from cells (exosomes and microvesicles) with neuroprotective effects	Anti- inflammatory, restoring myelination and cell microstructure TARGET = Cognitive gains	• Preterm stroke • HI injury	✓	✗	✗	✗	IV	Unknown, but presumably in the primary and secondary phases of injury	• Safer alternative to stem cells • Can be stored for later use • Collected in large volumes • Administered off-the-shelf • Low immunogenicity • Can transport cargo • Crosses the BBB	• Autologous preterm derived EVs may lack sufficient aerobic potential to be therapeutic and therefore allogeneic term equivalent sources may be required
Erythropoietin (EPO) Natural red blood cell hormone with neuroprotective effects. Also manufactured synthetically enabling dose titration	Anti-inflammatory, anti-excitotoxic, anti-oxidant, trophic, plus enhanced neurogenesis and angiogenesis	• IVH • Hemorrhagic parenchymal infarction • HI injury	✓	✓	✓	✓	IV	3 doses of 1,000 U/kg of EPO in the first week of life, during the secondary and tertiary phases of injury (Wu et al., 2012)	• Proven safe in neonates • Administered off-the-shelf • Can be administered in the tertiary phase of injury	• Cost • Refrigeration requirements • Lack of standardization between international products

(Continued)

TABLE 1 | Continued

Agent	Mechanism of action	Sub-population of patients that might be treatment responsive	Research phase for preterm brain injury				Route of administration	Timing of administration	Advantages	Disadvantages/ controversies
			Preclinical	Phase 1	Phase 2	Phase 3				
	TARGET = Cognitive (and motor) gains									• Some infants will be discharged from NICU before all 3-doses can be administered
Melatonin Natural hormone that regulates circadian rhythm. Also manufactured synthetically enabling dose titration	Anti-inflammatory and anti-apoptotic TARGET = Motor and cognitive gains	• IUGR	✓	✓	✓	✗	Oral (Maternal)	Antenatal 3x daily 10 mg, from baseline until birth	• Administered off-the-shelf • Low cost • Proven safe in humans	• Large sample sizes required to run Phase 3 public health trials, powered to detect a protective benefit
		• HI injury	✓	✓	✗	✗	Enteral	0.5–3-5 mg/kg dose escalation in first 6 h of life		
Creatine Natural diet compound that builds muscle, with neuroprotective effects	Anti-excitotoxic and anti-apoptotic TARGET = Disability-free survival from HI injury	• Mothers with pre-eclampsia, cervical incompetence, placental abruption, placental previa, IUGR	✓	✗	✗	✗	Oral diet supplementation (Maternal)	Antenatal, especially during the 3rd trimester of pregnancy	• Proven safe in humans • Straightforward bioavailability • Administered off-the-shelf • Low cost • Simple and feasible intervention for patients to adhere to • Manufactured synthetically enabling dose titration • May have the added benefit of reducing labor pains	• Large sample sizes required to run Phase 3 public health trials, powered to detect a protective benefit
		• TBI as proof of concept for HI injury	✓	✓	✓	✗	Oral	0.4 g/kg daily for 6-months duration		
Granulocyte-colony stimulating factor (G-CSF) hematopoietic growth factor	Stimulate neural stem and progenitor cell production TARGET = Motor gains	• CP 2-10 years old, all sub-types and causal pathways	✓	✓	✓	✗	IV	10 µg/kg for 5 days. Should be used >60 h after injury	• Appears safe	• Unclear if there is a clinical benefit

(Continued)

TABLE 1 | Continued

Agent	Mechanism of action	Sub-population of patients that might be treatment responsive	Research phase for preterm brain injury				Route of administration	Timing of administration	Advantages	Disadvantages/ controversies
			Preclinical	Phase 1	Phase 2	Phase 3				
Thyroxine Thyroid hormone	Normalization of thyroid levels as a neuroprotectant TARGET = Disability free survival	• Hypothyroxinemia • IVH	✓	✓	✓	✓	IV	Birth to 42-days	• Proposed reduced mortality • Proposed improved brain structure	• Clinical trials indicated improved long-term neurodevelopmental outcomes but these results are not supported in a meta-analysis
Minocycline Broad-spectrum antibiotic	Inhibition of microglial activation TARGET = Motor and cognitive gains	• HI injury	✓	✗	✗	✗	IV	Before and after injury	• Promising preclinical data indicating a reduction in white matter damage	• Conflicting results in human studies of other adult degenerative neurological disorders, with some studies showing harm • Timing of administration affects the result
Epidermal growth factor (EGF) Growth factor	Regulation of NSC migration, proliferation and oligodendrocyte differentiation to increase myelination TARGET = Motor gains	• Focal demyelination • HI injury • IVH	✓	✗	✗	✗	Overexpression of EGF receptor in oligodendrocytes Intranasal Intra-cerebroventricular injection	Before and after injury Immediately after injury 3 doses at 24, 72 and 120 h post-IVH	• Preliminary preclinical data indicating increased myelination and functional recovery	• Cost • Can induce neurotoxicity • Might promote tumor growth and progression
Diazoxide Vasodilator	Prevention of hypoglycemia TARGET = Motor and cognitive gains	• HI injury	✓	✗	✗	✗	Intraperitoneal	Daily during induction of HI injury	• Well established safety profile (from other indications) • Rapid acting • Inhibits the secretion of insulin	• Does not cross the BBB but affects circulation • May cause hypotension • Fluid retention
Nanoparticles Microscopic particles including dendrimers (branched molecules that can be tailored to store and transport materials)	Drug or gene transporter TARGET = Motor gains; reduction in rates of preterm birth	• HI injury • Infection and PVL	✓	✗	✗	✗	IV	Unknown, but presumably in the primary, secondary and tertiary phases of injury when inflammation is present	• Can transport cargo, including anti-inflammatory agents • Crosses the BBB • Targets abnormal microglia and astrocyte activity • Low immunogenicity	• High manufacturing costs • Potential toxicity

(Continued)

TABLE 1 | Continued

Agent	Mechanism of action	Sub-population of patients that might be treatment responsive	Research phase for preterm brain injury				Route of administration	Timing of administration	Advantages	Disadvantages/ controversies
			Preclinical	Phase 1	Phase 2	Phase 3				
Gene Therapy Delivery of DNA as a drug	Anti-excitotoxic to excessive glutamate via gene delivery of BDNF TARGET = Motor gains via protection of white matter volume loss	• PVL	✓	✗	✗	✗	Intracerebellar	Research indicates in the primary and secondary phases of injury (Gressens et al., 1997)	• Unknown	• Prolonged administration required because precise timing of the insult is usually unknown • Neurosurgical administration required
Parent attachment training Teaching parents to read and respond sensitively to their infant's cues	Experience dependent plasticity	• IVH • PVL	✓	✓	✓	✗	Parent Education Manual guidance	1 h weekly	• Lasting benefits to cognition	• Heterogeneous, under powered samples • Limited effect on motor skills (Nelson et al., 2001; Ohgi et al., 2004)
NIDCAP A low stress and low stimuli NICU environment that mimics the uterine environment	Experience dependent plasticity	• IVH • PVL • Stroke • HIE	✓	✓	✓	✓	Adapted environment e.g., low lighting and noise	24/7	• Possible short term protection of brain structure	• No long term benefits conferred (Ohlsson and Jacobs, 2013)
SPEEDI Parent coaching and environmental enrichment	Experience dependent plasticity Parent Education	• IVH • WMI • HIE • Hydrocephalus	✓	✓	✓	✗	Adapted environment e.g., promoting child active learning	21 days + 12 weeks of daily practice	• Improved problem solving (Dusing et al., 2018)	• Heterogeneous, under powered samples
GAME Task-specific motor training, parent coaching and environmental enrichment	Experience dependent plasticity Parent education	• IVH • PVL • Stroke • HIE	✓	✓	✓	✓	Adapted environment Task practice	Daily 45 min of practice by the child (Morgan et al., 2016b)	• Improved motor skills • Improved cognitive skills	• Co-occurring vision impairment may lower the rate of gains

✓ = Yes; ✗ = No; AEC, Amnion epithelial cells; BBB, Blood brain barrier; BDNF, Brain-Derived Neurotrophic Factor; BPD, Bronchopulmonary dysplasia; CP, Cerebral palsy; CIMT, Constraint induced movement therapy; DNA, Deoxyribonucleic acid; EGF, Epidermal growth factor; EPO, Erythropoietin; EVs, Extracellular vesicles; g, grams; GA, Gestational age; GAME, Goals Activity Motor Enrichment; GVHD, Graft vs. host disease; HI, Hypoxic ischemic; HIE, Hypoxic ischemic encephalopathy; HLA, Human Leukocyte Antigens; iPSC, Induced pluripotent stem cell; IUGR, Intrauterine growth restriction; IV, Intravenous; IVH, Intraventricular hemorrhage; kg, kilograms; μg, micrograms; mg, milligrams; MSC, Mesenchymal stem cell; MRI, Magnetic resonance imaging; NICU, Neonatal Intensive Care Unit; NIDCAP, Newborn Individualized Care and Assessment Program; NSC, Neural stem cell; O2, Oxygen; PVL, Periventricular leukomalacia; SPEEDI, Supporting Play Exploration and Early Developmental Intervention; TBI, Traumatic brain injury; U, Units; UCB, Umbilical cord blood; WMI, White Matter Injury.

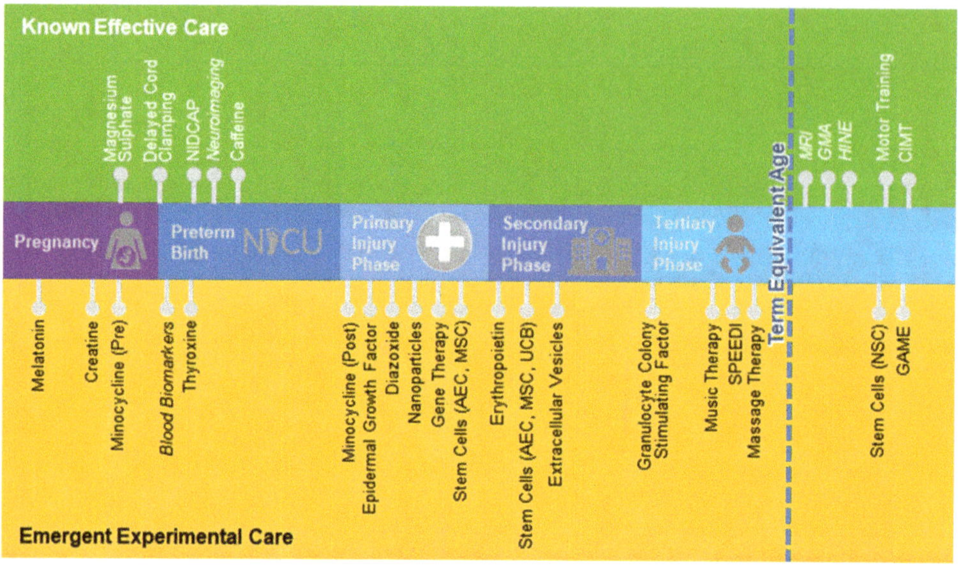

FIGURE 1 | Known effective and emergent treatments and assessments. AEC, Amnion epithelial cells; CIMT, Constraint induced movement therapy; GAME, Goals Activity Motor Enrichment; GMA, General Movements Assessment; HINE, Hammersmith Infant Neurological Examination; MSC, Mesenchymal stem cell; MRI, Magnetic resonance imaging; NICU, Neonatal Intensive Care Unit; NIDCAP, Newborn Individualized Care and Assessment Program; NSC, Neural stem cell; SPEEDI, Supporting Play Exploration and Early Developmental Intervention; UCB, Umbilical cord blood.

tolerated. Recently published, Won Soon Park's team at Samsung Medical Center in South Korea conducted a Phase 1 dose-escalation study of Pneumostem® transplantation in preterm infants with severe IVH (grade 3–4) (NCT02274428) (Ahn et al., 2018). Pneumostem® is a human allogeneic UCB-derived MSC product. Eligible infants were born at 23–34 weeks' gestation, and received cells (5×10^6 cells/kg or 1×10^7 cells/kg) within 7 days of IVH diagnosis. Study results indicated that Pneumostem® transplantation by intracerebroventricular injection was safe; cell transplantation at both doses was not associated with any serious adverse events or dose-limiting toxicity, and there were no cases of mortality in their cohort of 9 infants (Ahn et al., 2018). This is being followed up by a currently-recruiting Phase 2a study to evaluate the efficacy and safety of intraventricular administration of Pneumostem® for treatment of IVH (grade 3–4) in 22 high-risk premature infants (NCT02890953). Participants will be randomized to receive either Pneumostem® or saline control within 28 postnatal days. Outcomes include death, ventricular shunt operation, and ventricular dilatation.

There are now multiple clinical trials underway examining the safety and efficacy of cell therapies (chiefly MSCs and AECs) for other morbidities associated with prematurity, in particular bronchopulmonary dysplasia. It is feasible that these therapies may provide non-specific neuro-protective benefit through reduction of systemic inflammation. These trials should therefore be designed (e.g., length of follow up), and sufficiently powered, to capture any potential neurological benefits of these therapies. As an example, the long-term safety and efficacy follow-up study of Pneumostem® (NCT02023788) in patients who completed the previously mentioned Phase I study (NCT02274428) includes neurological development test outcomes at 5 years (corrected age) comprising the K-ASQ (Korean Ages and Stages Questionnaires) and Bayley Scales of Infant and Toddler Development (Bayley).

Although not specifically targeting preterm infants, the following clinical trials warrant mention. First is the open label trial of 23 term-born neonates (≥35 weeks') with hypoxic ischemic encephalopathy (HIE) who received non-cryopreserved autologous volume- and red blood cell-reduced UCB intravenously (Cotten et al., 2014). Infants received up to four infusions of $1\text{–}5 \times 10^7$ cells/kg, with the first dose as soon as possible after birth, and at 24, 48, and 72 postnatal hours. The authors found that whilst autologous UCB for infants with HIE is feasible, UCB collection at delivery for all "obstetric emergencies" was a challenge that initially resulted in extremely low recruitment rates; they originally intended to recruit 52 HIE infants, however only enrolled 23. They go on to describe how this challenge was overcome by multidisciplinary collaboration. Nevertheless, timely collection of autologous UCB may be a potential barrier for this therapy in certain settings. There are now multiple currently-recruiting Phase 1 and 2 studies of autologous UCB for HIE listed on clinical trial registries. These include the follow-on study (NCT02612155) at Duke University, as well as other studies in the United States (NCT02434965), France (NCT02881970), and China (NCT02551003, NCT03352310). Finally, for a different indication, there is the phase 1/2 open-label study of intranasally administered bone marrow-derived allogeneic MSCs (5×10^7 cells) in term neonates (≥36 weeks') with perinatal arterial stroke (PAIS) (NCT03356821). Referred to as the PASSIoN trial, this study aims to recruit 10 participants for cell administration as soon as possible after confirmation of PAIS (maximum within the first week). PAIS is an important perinatal cause of long-lasting neurodevelopmental problems.

Due to the limited number of published clinical trials of stem cells for perinatal/preterm brain injury, it is not surprising that no systematic reviews have yet been published. However, three reviews with meta-analyses have been conducted analyzing stem cell clinical trials for other indications including two for adult stroke and one for children with cerebral palsy. Interestingly, meta-analysis of the effects of MSCs for ischemic stroke, which included seven studies, indicated no significant difference between stem cell and cell-free treatments (Wang et al., 2016). This was in contrast to the analysis of Chen et al., which revealed stem cell transplantation for patients with ischemic stroke can significantly improve neurological deficits, motor function, daily life quality and functional independence (Chen et al., 2016). This analysis included 18 studies, the majority of which used MSCs ($n = 10$) however neural stem cells ($n = 4$), bone marrow mononuclear cells ($n = 2$), peripheral blood cells ($n = 1$), and umbilical cord MSCs ($n = 1$) were also used (Chen et al., 2016). It is therefore possible that cell types other than MSCs contributed to the larger effect size observed. For children with cerebral palsy, stem cells appeared to induce short-term improvements in gross motor skills, despite the acknowledged limitation of heterogeneous data e.g., cell type, participant age range and cerebral palsy sub-type (Novak et al., 2016). Collectively, these papers conclude that further research, in particular randomized controlled trials (RCTs), using rigorous methodologies, is warranted to determine the optimal stem cell treatments for neurological conditions.

Extracellular Vesicles (EVs)

MSCs, and likely other types of cells, exert their neuro-protective/reparative effects via secretion of extracellular vesicles (EVs), namely exosomes and microvesicles (reviewed by Willis et al., 2017). EVs are small membrane-bound particles with a size of 70–1,000 nm that contain an array of bioactive "cargo" which includes DNA, messenger RNA, microRNA, proteins, and lipids (Willis et al., 2017). EVs offer an attractive option as a novel, cell-free alternative therapy for the treatment of perinatal brain injury, since their use eliminates some of the largest perceived risks of cell therapy: tumorigenic potential of administered live cells, as well as immunologic reactions and/or rejection of transplanted cells. Another benefit of EVs is that they can be easily collected in large quantities and stored for future use (Willis et al., 2017), providing "off-the-shelf" capability for clinical emergencies.

The efficacy of EVs for perinatal brain injury is still being explored in preclinical studies, including a rodent model of inflammation-induced preterm birth with resultant brain damage (Drommelschmidt et al., 2017), and a preterm sheep model of hypoxic-ischemic (HI) brain injury (Ophelders et al., 2016). In rats, MSC-EVs ameliorated inflammation-induced cellular damage, restoring myelination deficits and abnormal microstructure, indicated by reduced fractional anisotropy measured using diffusion tensor MRI, resulting in improved long-term cognitive function assessed using the spatial probe test as an indicator for adaptive memory function (Drommelschmidt et al., 2017). Similarly in sheep, MSC-EVs partially rescued brain function following HI-induced injury, and appeared to mildly protect against hypomyelination (Ophelders et al., 2016). Additionally, there are numerous published studies demonstrating the utility of EVs for adult brain injury, in particular traumatic brain injury (TBI) (Zhang et al., 2015, 2017b; Kim et al., 2016; Li et al., 2017; Williams et al., 2019), and stroke (Otero-Ortega et al., 2018). Together, these studies highlight the potential of EVs for the treatment of brain injury, and more research into their use for neurological conditions is merited. Lessons learned from EV studies using these models may be beneficial for preterm indications.

An important consideration for EV therapy is the source of the EVs and the timing of retrieval. EVs can be derived from different cell types. It seems logical to favor autologous products because, as for cell-based therapies, they are considered safer due to the eliminated risk of immune rejection of the cell product or development of graft-versus-host disease, or transmission of infectious diseases from donor to recipient. Intriguingly, a 2016 study presents evidence that autologous EVs for preterm infants might not be best choice (Panfoli et al., 2016). In this study, exosomes derived from umbilical cord-MSCs of preterm babies (28–30 weeks' gestation) had reduced aerobic potential compared to those derived from term babies (≥37 weeks') (Panfoli et al., 2016). Reduced aerobic potential might affect their ability to rescue the bioenergetics of damaged tissues (i.e., by restoring ATP and NADH levels). Thus, preterm exosomes may have a diminished capacity to provide therapeutic benefit, which may have design implications for EV-therapies in preterm infants.

Interestingly, EVs may also be utilized to deliver gene therapy to target cells. In a series of *in vitro* experiments, Lee et al., used MSCs genetically modified to express fluorescently labeled microRNA-124 to demonstrate that MSCs can deliver microRNA to neural cells via the secretion of exosomes (Lee et al., 2014). MicroRNA-124 was selected because it plays a role in neurogenesis, indeed miRNA-124 is the most abundant miRNA in the brain, which suppresses cell proliferation, promotes neuronal differentiation and neurite outgrowth, and represses astrocytic differentiation (reviewed in Sun et al., 2015). Consistent with this, delivery of microRNA-124 induced neuronal differentiation in targeted neural progenitor cells. This concept has now progressed to clinical trial: a Phase 1 trial will examine the safety and efficacy of allogeneic MSC-derived exosomes "enriched" with microRNA-124 in five adults (40–80 years) with acute ischemic stroke (NCT03384433). MicroRNA-124 enrichment will be achieved via transfection of MSCs. Outcome measures include the incidence of treatment-emergent adverse events and the Modified Rankin Scale to measure change in disability or dependence in daily activities. Other developments in the EV clinical trial space include published studies of chronic kidney disease (Nassar et al., 2016) and graft-vs.-host disease (Kordelas et al., 2014), as well as the currently recruiting study for healing of large and refractory macular holes using MSC-derived exosomes (NCT03437759).

Given the potential advantages of EVs (Hall et al., 2016), this raises an ethical controversy of whether researchers should be progressing predominantly EV- rather than cell-based- therapies.

Studies such as that published by Doeppner et al., which compared the efficacy of human bone marrow-derived MSCs with EVs obtained from the same cells in a rodent model of stroke (Doeppner et al., 2015), are highly valuable. This study showed that EVs were equally effective as cells in promoting neurological recovery and brain remodeling following transient focal cerebral ischemia. More such head-to-head studies are warranted to confirm the utility of EVs for a range of indications. The efficacy of EVs for neuro-regeneration/repair is expected to be limited to situations that involve anti-inflammatory and/or trophic signaling mechanisms; it is unlikely that EVs would be useful when cell engraftment is desired, for example in neural stem cell replacement therapy.

Erythropoietin (EPO)

Originally identified for its role in erythropoiesis, erythropoietin (EPO) was later shown to be neuroprotective in a variety of animal models of neurological conditions including stroke, TBI and multiple sclerosis (MS) (Siren et al., 2009). Unsurprisingly, EPO garnered significant interest as a potential neuroprotectant for preterm infants, and numerous preclinical- and clinical-studies have since been completed. Three recent systematic reviews with meta-analyses of EPO for reducing neurodevelopmental disability in preterm infants have been published. These studies comprised: four RCTs with 297 infants (Zhang et al., 2014), two RCTs and three quasi-RCTs with 233 infants (Wang et al., 2015), and four RCTs with 1,133 infants (Fischer et al., 2017), in the meta-analyses, respectively. Analyses were conducted on mostly non-overlapping trials: seven original studies in total, and all three concluded that EPO treatment improved cognitive outcome in preterm infants. Important to note is that no significant effect was observed for other neurodevelopmental outcomes including cerebral palsy, visual impairment, severe hearing deficit, and necrotizing enterocolitis.

New clinical trials of EPO for preterm infants continue to be launched. A currently recruiting, multicenter, randomized, placebo-controlled study plans to recruit 312 infants (<32 weeks' gestation, ≤1,500 grams) for repeated administration of high-dose EPO within 48 h of birth (NCT02550054). The primary outcomes are neurodevelopmental function at 18 months measured using the Bayley and GMFM-88. Similarly, "EpoRepair" (NCT02076373) is an RCT of repetitive high-dose EPO in 120 preterm infants (23–31 weeks'). Contrastingly however, recruited infants will be those with a diagnosed brain injury (IVH and/or hemorrhagic parenchymal infarction), and neurodevelopmental follow-up using a composite intelligence quotient will be conducted at the longer time-point of 5 years of age (Ruegger et al., 2015). Moreover, the active, though not recruiting Phase 3 Preterm Erythropoietin Neuroprotection "PENUT" Trial (NCT01378273) has enrolled 941 preterm infants specifically in the lower age range of 24–27 weeks' gestation. Infants in this study will likewise receive repeated high-dose EPO initiated soon after birth. The primary endpoint is 24–26 months corrected age, at which neurodevelopmental outcome will be measured using the Bayley (Juul et al., 2015). The selection of extremely low gestational age neonates for the PENUT Trial is significant since in a subgroup analysis reported by Fischer et al., no significant benefit of EPO was seen on cognitive outcome in infants <28 weeks' (Fischer et al., 2017). Whilst the authors acknowledged that the small sample size used for the analysis was a limitation, the results of the PENUT Trial should definitively address the efficacy of EPO for neuroprotection in extremely preterm infants. Of particular note, whilst the EPO regimens of the above listed trials differ, the effect of EPO on cognitive outcome appears to be robust enough to withstand variations in both timing and dose (Fischer et al., 2017). Thus, hopefully the results of these studies will provide conclusive evidence to support change in the clinical practice guidelines for the care of preterm infants.

Melatonin

Melatonin (N-acetyl-5-methoxytryptamin) is a hormone produced by the pineal gland that is responsible for regulating circadian rhythms via activation of specific melatonin receptors. Melatonin also acts as an antioxidant and has demonstrated anti-inflammatory and anti-apoptotic effects (Welin et al., 2007). It is these properties that make melatonin a promising candidate for the treatment of perinatal brain injury in preterm neonates. Accordingly, there is now substantial evidence from animal studies supporting a neuroprotective role of melatonin administered either antenatally, or postnatally after the injurious event (reviewed in Biran et al., 2014; Wilkinson et al., 2016). For example, in a murine model of excitotoxic periventricular white matter injury, which mimics human PVL, melatonin given immediately following intracerebral injection of the glutamatergic analog ibotenate promoted secondary lesion repair, effectively reducing the size of white matter cysts (Husson et al., 2002). Similarly, in a rat model of acute neonatal hemorrhagic brain injury commonly observed in very low birth weight preterm infants, systemic administration of melatonin 1 h after injury normalized brain atrophy and led to improved cognitive and sensorimotor function (Lekic et al., 2011). Moreover, Watanabe et al., demonstrated that antenatal administration of melatonin reduced *in utero* ischemia/reperfusion oxidative brain injury in neonatal rats. Rat pups born to mothers who received melatonin exhibited reduced markers of oxidative stress, had numbers of intact mitochondria comparable to control animals, and had reduced brain damage quantified by protection of hippocampal pyramidal neurons from ischemia/reperfusion-induced degeneration (Watanabe et al., 2012). Likewise, maternal antenatal melatonin reduced brain injury in an ovine model of fetal growth restriction (Miller et al., 2014). In this model, fetal growth restriction was induced surgically by single umbilical artery ligation at 0.7 gestation after which melatonin was administered for the remainder of the pregnancy. Antenatal melatonin rescued oxidative stress, white matter hypomyelination and axonal damage leading to significant functional improvements in neonatal lamb behaviors, in particular suckling (Miller et al., 2014). Collectively, these studies demonstrate the broad utility of melatonin in improving outcomes following perinatal injury from a variety of etiologies. In addition, there is encouraging data on the neuroprotective efficacy of melatonin in a range of related adult conditions including stroke (Watson et al., 2016), TBI (Barlow et al.,

2018), and neurodegenerative diseases (Wongprayoon and Govitrapong, 2017).

The results of these pivotal animal studies have led to pilot clinical trials of either antenatal or postnatal melatonin for neuroprotection of preterm or growth restricted infants. Though few trials have been published to date, a single-arm, open-label study of antenatal oral melatonin administration to 16 women with a growth restricted fetus (diagnosed <34 weeks gestation) was completed in November 2014 (NCT01695070) (Alers et al., 2013). This study is being followed by the 2017-registered "Protect Me Trial" which aims to recruit 292 mothers with a growth restricted fetus for a Phase 2 RCT of daily antenatal melatonin supplementation for improving early childhood neurodevelopmental outcomes at 2-years (ACTRN12617001515381). Trial participants will be stratified according to gestational age (<28 weeks' and 28 to <32 weeks'), and recruitment is anticipated to start in late-2018. For postnatally administered melatonin, a pharmacokinetic study was conducted in which 18 preterm infants (<31 weeks') were administered melatonin intravenously at varying concentrations for up to 6 h (NCT00649961). The objective was to determine the dose required to achieve melatonin blood levels in the preterm infant similar to that of the mother, to guide potential future therapeutic trials. It was found that peak adult melatonin concentration could be achieved by a relatively short (2 h) infusion of low dose (0.1 μg/kg/h) melatonin in preterm infants (Merchant et al., 2013). Using this dosing regime, a Phase 2 RCT (The Mint Study) was conducted to evaluate the neuroprotective effect of melatonin in 58 preterm infants (30 received melatonin and 28 received placebo) (Merchant et al., 2014). No between group difference was shown for the primary outcome, which was a 5% difference in the fractional anisotropy in the white matter measured using MRI at term equivalent age. Similar to the Mint Study, "PREMELIP" aimed to assess the neuroprotective effect of melatonin administered in the immediate prepartum period in very preterm infants (<28 weeks') (NCT02395783). Also designed to measure white matter injury at term equivalent age using MRI as the primary outcome, this study was terminated in 2018 after recruiting 14 participants. No reason was provided by study investigators. Melatonin is also being studied in *term*-born neonatal populations (Aly et al., 2015), however this is beyond the scope of this review.

Creatine

Creatine is a natural compound that is synthesized in the liver, kidney and pancreas, and is also obtained through diet. Creatine's main role is in cellular energy homeostasis; creatine participates in a reversible reaction with creatine kinase to continuously and efficiently replenish ATP (the energy currency of the cell) from ADP, to meet energy demands (Wallimann et al., 1992). There is evidence to suggest that creatine is neuroprotective for the developing perinatal brain (Dickinson et al., 2014b). Specifically, offspring born to pregnant spiny mice fed a creatine-supplemented diet had a significantly increased capacity to survive a hypoxic birth event, and these pups showed improved postnatal weight gain (Ireland et al., 2008). In a follow-up mechanistic study, maternal creatine supplementation protected pups from hypoxia-induced brain lipid peroxidation and apoptosis, hypothesized to be mediated via preservation of mitochondrial function (Ireland et al., 2011). However, no clinical trials of antenatal creatine supplementation to protect against perinatal brain injury have yet been conducted (Dickinson et al., 2014a).

Complexities exist around the practicalities of antenatal creatine administration for neuroprotection of preterm infants. For example, should creatine be administered as a prophylactic to all pregnant women on the off chance that their babies experience birth asphyxia and/or prematurity? Alternatively, the utility of postnatal creatine for neuroprotection of preterm infants who do not experience birth asphyxia is unclear. Creatine has been pilot tested in clinical trial for children with TBI, with daily administration from the day of injury to 6 months post-injury. The results suggested improved memory and functional skills, with reduced intensive care stay (Sakellaris et al., 2006). Thus, creatine could potentially be given postnatally to newborns with encephalopathic brain injury at high-risk of cerebral palsy. Notably, creatinine (the breakdown product of creatine) is excreted by the kidneys, which are known to have reduced function in premature infants (Stritzke et al., 2017). Thus, the effects of administering potentially high therapeutic doses of creatine to preterm infants with reduced kidney function warrants careful consideration and thorough investigation. Creatine is also being studied in adult neurodegenerative diseases (Pastula et al., 2012; Xiao et al., 2014; Bender and Klopstock, 2016), however these are beyond the scope of this review.

Granulocyte-Colony Stimulating Factor (G-CSF)

Granulocyte-colony stimulating factor (G-CSF) is a hematopoietic growth factor that is used clinically in cancer patients diagnosed with neutropenia following chemotherapy, due to its ability to stimulate hematopoietic stem cell mobilization and neutrophil differentiation. G-CSF also exhibits non-hematopoietic neurotrophic functions, with evidence from experimental studies indicating that G-CSF is neuroprotective in stroke, TBI, and neurodegenerative diseases (reviewed by Solaroglu et al., 2007). Despite this, results of studies examining the effect of G-CSF in perinatal brain injury were initially controversial. While two studies of HI injury in neonatal rats showed that G-CSF inhibited neuronal apoptosis to attenuate brain damage (Yata et al., 2007; Kim et al., 2008), Keller et al., found that G-CSF actually increased cortical and white matter lesions in a newborn mouse model of excitotoxic brain injury (Keller et al., 2006). Similarly, in a follow-up study, acute administration of G-CSF led to increased hippocampal brain damage in a murine model of neonatal HI (Schlager et al., 2011). This disparity was explained 5 years later, when it was revealed that the neuroprotective effects of G-CSF are contingent on the timing of administration following the insult (Neubauer et al., 2016). Delayed administration of G-CSF (in combination with stem cell factor or flt3-ligand) at 60 h post-injury, compared to 1 h used previously, conveyed significant neuroprotection against excitotoxic insult (Neubauer et al., 2016). This was consistent with other studies showing G-CSF reduced white matter injury in a sheep model of preterm brain injury (Jellema et al., 2013), and attenuated neuroinflammation and stabilized the blood brain barrier (BBB) following HI (Li et al., 2015). However, it remains unclear why Schlager et al., failed to find any long-term neuroprotective effects of G-CSF after neonatal HI (Schlager et al., 2011).

Thus far, the only clinical trials assessing the neuroreparative potential of G-CSF in pediatric patients has been in children with cerebral palsy (NCT02983708, NCT02866331). In the first study (NCT02983708), G-CSF was given to 57 children with non-severe cerebral palsy for 5 days to mobilize peripheral blood mononuclear cells. These were then collected and re-infused at either 1- or 7-months post-cell collection, in a double-blind, cross-over study (Rah et al., 2017). Neurodevelopmental improvement, above what would normally be expected, was seen in 42% of patients in response to G-CSF treatment. Interestingly, larger improvements in test scores were observed in patients who received delayed cell re-infusion at 7 months, although this was in contrast to the results of the MRI analysis. The authors concluded that further studies are needed to delineate the effect of repeated G-CSF either alone, or in combination with reinfusion of G-CSF-stimulated peripheral blood cells. The second study, a subsequent trial from the same lead investigator, is currently recruiting (NCT02866331). In this study, the efficacy of autologous UCB mononuclear cells and/or repeated G-CSF administration for children with cerebral palsy will be assessed. In addition to these limited pediatric studies, numerous clinical trials of G-CSF for adult stroke have been completed. Meta-analyses of clinical trial data however paint a less-than-convincing picture, with conflicting conclusions (Fan et al., 2015; England et al., 2016; Huang et al., 2017). There has also been substantial interest in G-CSF for ALS, however early phase clinical trials have failed to show efficacy (Cashman et al., 2008; Nefussy et al., 2010; Chio et al., 2011; Duning et al., 2011). This serves as a timely reminder that compelling preclinical results, like creatine for neurodegenerative conditions, does not always translate to clinical benefit.

Thyroid Hormone (Thyroxine)

The thyroid hormones (thyroxine and triiodothyronine) are essential for brain development during fetal and postnatal life (reviewed by Williams, 2008). Preterm infants often exhibit transient low levels of thyroid hormones (hypothyroxinemia) (Rooman et al., 1996), which is thought to be due to immaturity of the hypothalamic-pituitary-thyroid axis. Long-term follow up of very preterm and/or very low birth weight infants revealed that neurologic dysfunction at age 5, and school failure at age nine, significantly correlated with lower neonatal thyroxine levels (Den Ouden et al., 1996). This result has been challenged by another cohort study in which thyroxine levels in the first 6 weeks of life were correlated with cognitive outcome at 7 years of age, and in this study higher thyroxine exposure was associated with poorer cognitive outcome (Scratch et al., 2014). Consequently, thyroxine substitution therapy was proposed to improve neurodevelopmental outcomes in this vulnerable population. Multiple clinical trials have been conducted, however a systematic review failed to find any significant difference in neonatal mortality, morbidity or neurodevelopmental outcomes in preterm infants who received thyroid hormones compared to controls (Osborn and Hunt, 2007). Since then, additional studies have been completed (Suzumura et al., 2011; Ng et al., 2014; Van Wassenaer-Leemhuis et al., 2014), however only Suzumura et al., found any neurodevelopmental benefit of thyroxine supplementation in preterm infants.

The failure of thyroxine substitution therapy to provide neurological benefit at clinical trial may be related to a lack of monocarboxylate transporter 8 (MCT8, also known as SLC16A2) which is required for transport of thyroid hormones across the cell membrane for its action and metabolism (Friesema et al., 2003). MCT8 expression has been shown to decrease following lipopolysaccharide (LPS)-induced systemic inflammation (Wittmann et al., 2015) and severe intrauterine growth restriction (Chan et al., 2014). It is feasible that preterm infants may similarly exhibit a lack of MCT8, thus may be unresponsive to thyroxine substitution. Future preclinical studies should examine whether up-regulation of MCT8 could improve response to thyroxine, and/or investigate use of a thyroxine hormone analog that does not require MCT8 to cross the plasma membrane.

Nevertheless, two new clinical trials of thyroxine for preterm infants have been registered on clinicaltrials.gov, both yet to start recruiting. The first is a Phase 3 study of 1,224 preterm infants (<28 weeks') randomized to receive either continuous infusion of thyroxine plus oral potassium iodide, or placebo, for 42 days (NCT02103998). The primary outcome for this trial is a composite endpoint of cerebral palsy or Bayley score <85 at 36 months' corrected age. The second is a Phase 2 trial which aims to recruit 100 preterm infants (<28 weeks') with a grade 3–4 IVH to determine whether thyroxine treatment can improve brain structure measured using MRI (NCT03390530). Secondary outcomes include infant mortality and neurodevelopmental impairment at 2 years of age.

Minocycline

Minocycline is a semi-synthetic broad-spectrum antibiotic that has been in commercial use for nearly 50 years. It is lipid soluble and can cross the BBB, making it an attractive drug for neurological application. Due to its ability to inhibit microglial activation, minocycline has demonstrated efficacy in various models of adult neurological conditions such as stroke, MS, Parkinson's disease and ALS (Yong et al., 2004; see reviews by Garrido-Mesa et al., 2013). Studies have also shown that minocycline can improve outcomes following perinatal brain injury. For example, minocycline administered 12 h before, and then periodically after LPS exposure, protected against white matter injury, oligodendrocyte loss and abnormal neurobehavioral performance in the neonatal rat (Fan et al., 2005). Similarly, in a preterm rodent model, post-HI treatment with minocycline abolished neuroinflammation and white matter injury (Carty et al., 2008). Notably however, other studies have shown that minocycline actually worsened brain injury in neonatal models (Tsuji et al., 2004; Strahan et al., 2017), although this effect was alleviated when minocycline was administered at a lower dose or later time-point (Strahan et al., 2017). Clearly, dose and timing is very important, and the use of minocycline in pediatric patients warrants careful consideration.

There have been numerous clinical trials conducted of minocycline for various neurological conditions with mixed results. Whilst a 2010 futility study concluded that further investigation of minocycline for Huntington's disease was not warranted (Huntington Study Group Domino Investigators, 2010), data from a recent systematic review indicated efficacy of minocycline in acute stroke patients (Malhotra et al., 2018). Similarly, in a Phase 2 trial for Parkinson's disease, minocycline could not be rejected as futile based on the threshold of a 30% reduction in UPDRS progression (Ninds Net-Pd Investigators., 2006), though no Phase 3 clinical trial has yet been launched. Results are also pending from a dose-escalation study of minocycline for TBI (NCT01058395). Worryingly however, is the finding from a multicenter, randomized Phase 3 trial, that minocycline had a harmful effect on patients with ALS (Gordon et al., 2007). Thus, trials of minocycline, and indeed other neuroprotective agents, should proceed with caution.

Epidermal Growth Factor (EGF)

Epidermal growth factor (EGF), together with its receptor EGFR, is a key mediator of neural progenitor cell proliferation, migration and differentiation (reviewed by Galvez-Contreras et al., 2013). In preclinical studies, overexpression of EGFR shifted neural progenitor cells from a non-migratory- to a migratory-phenotype (Aguirre et al., 2005), and EGF stimulated *in vitro* neural progenitor cell oligodendrogenesis (Aguirre and Gallo, 2007). Importantly, EGFR overexpression enhanced proliferation of neural progenitors and their migration to the lesion following lysolecithin-induced focal demyelination in the mouse brain (Aguirre et al., 2007). This led to accelerated and more extensive remyelination, with more rapid functional recovery (Aguirre et al., 2007). Similarly, in a mouse model of preterm hypoxic brain injury, EGFR overexpression or intranasal administration of heparin-binding EGF decreased oligodendrocyte death, promoted oligodendrocyte-progenitor maturation, and led to improved behavioral recovery of mice assessed using various white matter-dependent sensori-motor tests (Scafidi et al., 2014). Moreover, in rabbits with IVH, intracerebroventricular injection of recombinant human EGF significantly increased myelination, promoted proliferation and maturation of oligodendrocyte-progenitors, and enhanced neurobehavioral recovery (Vinukonda et al., 2016). Thus, EGF is an exciting potential neuroprotective therapeutic.

Diazoxide

Diazoxide is a potassium channel activator that is used as a vasodilator in the treatment of acute hypertension, and to counter hypoglycemia caused by congenital hyperinsulinism in infants. The neuroprotective potential of diazoxide following ischemia/reperfusion injury was first investigated nearly 20 years ago (Domoki et al., 1999). Despite positive findings, the utilization of diazoxide for reducing neuronal injury in the newborn has been slow to progress. Nevertheless, in a series of *in vitro* and *in vivo* experiments, Fogal et al., demonstrated that diazoxide stimulated proliferation of cultured oligodendrocyte-progenitor cells, enhanced myelination of cerebellar-slice fibers, and prevented hypoxia-induced ventriculomegaly and hypomyelination (Fogal et al., 2010). In a follow-up mechanistic study, the authors' showed that diazoxide actually enhanced maturation of oligodendrocytes, rather than increasing oligodendrocyte proliferation, as their previous *in vitro* studies suggested (Zhu et al., 2014). Given the well-established safety profile of diazoxide, and accumulating efficacy data in stroke, further preclinical studies, in other models of perinatal brain injury, are warranted.

Nanoparticle-Targeted Drug Delivery

Nanoparticles for targeted drug delivery are emerging as a promising strategy for the treatment of a range of disorders. Nanoparticle delivery can improve drug bioavailability and targeting, particularly across the BBB. Dendrimers are nanoparticles that have a branching, tree-like structure with a high density of tailorable surface functional groups. Systemically administered hydroxyl-terminated polyamidoamine dendrimers crossed the BBB to localize in activated microglia and astrocytes in the brain of newborn rabbits with cerebral palsy, but not healthy controls (Kannan et al., 2012). Moreover, administration of dendrimers conjugated with the anti-oxidant and anti-inflammatory agent N-acetyl-L-cysteine (NAC; D-NAC), suppressed neuroinflammation and led to a dramatic improvement in motor function. NAC has long been used clinically for acetaminophen poisoning, and has been shown to be an effective treatment for a multitude of psychiatric and neurological conditions including autism, Alzheimer's disease, addiction, schizophrenia, and progressive myoclonic epilepsy (reviewed by Deepmala et al., 2015).

In a mouse model of ischemia-induced neonatal white matter injury, administration of D-NAC suppressed the "detrimental" pro-inflammatory response and increased myelination in regions of white matter injury, indicative of functional recovery (Nance et al., 2015). Furthermore, in a mouse model of perinatal HIE, systemically delivered D-NAC targeted all three types of neural cells involved in brain injury after HI (microglia, neurons, and astrocytes), but only in injured tissue (Nemeth et al., 2017). Importantly, uptake of D-NAC was not significantly altered by exposure to therapeutic hypothermia, suggesting that D-NAC can be used as a combinatorial therapy for the clinical management of HIE (Nemeth et al., 2017). Interestingly, using a mouse model of intrauterine inflammation Lei et al., demonstrated that a single dose of D-NAC, maternally delivered, significantly reduced the rate of preterm birth in pregnant dams exposed to LPS (Lei et al., 2017). Maternal D-NAC treatment altered the placental immune profile, decreased placental T-cell infiltration, and reduced microglial activation. Moreover, D-NAC significantly improved the neuromotor outcomes of LPS-exposed pups (Lei et al., 2017). Whilst the concept of NAC for the prevention of preterm birth is not in itself novel, the high effective dose required for free NAC can induce side-effects of nausea, vomiting, stomatitis, and fever. This publication demonstrates for the first time that low dose NAC delivered via dendrimer-conjugation is effective in reducing preterm birth. Thus, it is feasible that maternally administered D-NAC could be a well-tolerated prophylactic therapy for preterm birth.

Similarly, Chinese researchers have developed a novel catalase-containing nanoparticle that improved outcomes in a rodent stroke model (Zhang et al., 2017a). Catalase is an anti-oxidant and promising neuroprotectant, however its clinical application is hindered by its rapid degradation, immunogenicity and inability to cross the BBB. By modifying catalase containing nanoparticles by (a) cross-linking the polymer to increase drug stability, and (b) adding a peptide tag that is recognized and taken up by infiltrating neutrophils, catalase could effectively piggy-back across the BBB to the target site in the brain (Zhang et al., 2017a). Accordingly, nanoparticle delivery of catalase significantly reduced the infarct volume, mediated by reduced apoptosis, in a mouse model of ischemia/reperfusion injury (Zhang et al., 2017a). It is hypothesized that this technology could be beneficial in any neurological condition characterized by neuroinflammation, including preterm brain injury.

Gene Therapy

Gene therapy is the delivery of DNA as a drug to treat disease; the idea being that the transferred DNA would be stably overexpressed as a protein to provide therapeutic benefit. Gene therapy is being actively studied for a range of adult neurological conditions including Alzheimer's disease, ALS and stroke (reviewed in Choong et al., 2016). In contrast, few studies have examined gene therapy for perinatal brain injury. One example however is the overexpression of brain-derived neurotrophic factor (BDNF) to protect the newborn mouse brain from excitotoxic insult. BDNF has been shown to protect the newborn mouse brain from periventricular white matter lesions (Husson et al., 2005). However, since these lesions progress over several days to weeks, the most effective BDNF therapy should involve prolonged/continual administration. Using the same mouse model of neonatal excitotoxic challenge, Bemelmans et al., demonstrated that lentiviral-mediated gene transfer of BDNF to the newborn mouse brain is feasible and affords significant neuroprotection against excitotoxic insult (Bemelmans et al., 2006). Despite these encouraging findings, no published follow-up study was found during the literature search for this review.

Emergent Combinatorial Therapies

With the discovery of new, efficacious therapies for neuroprotection and repair of the injured preterm brain, we will undoubtedly see the emergence of combinatorial therapies in an attempt to maximize neurodevelopmental outcome. Some emergent combinatorial therapies are already being tested for various neurological conditions in the clinic, e.g., administration of allogeneic UCB plus EPO in three adults with TBI (Min et al., 2013). Moreover, besides the previously mentioned trial for children with cerebral palsy (NCT02866331), UCB plus G-CSF has been used for stroke patients (Shin and Cho, 2016), and adults with either a brain injury, cerebral palsy, Parkinson's disease or ALS (NCT02236065). Interestingly, EPO together with G-CSF has been proposed for adults with neurological diseases (NCT02018406), though the status of this trial is unknown. Unsurprisingly, various other combination therapies are being investigated at the preclinical stage. Recently, genetically engineered UCB mononuclear cells were used to deliver triple gene therapy in a rodent model of stroke (Sokolov et al., 2018). Treatment with minocycline followed by NAC is showing encouraging results for TBI (Sangobowale et al., 2018), and Jantzie et al., is exploring postnatal administration of EPO and melatonin in a rat model of perinatal brain injury caused by extreme preterm birth (Jantzie et al., 2018).

Neuroplasticity-Inducing Rehabilitation

Neuroplasticity

The brain's capacity to recover after injury is what makes early intervention scientifically possible. Neuroplasticity encompasses the ability of the brain to organize/reorganize its circuitry and produce new cells (neurogenesis) and connections (synaptogenesis) (Johnston, 2009). Environmental stimulation (early intervention) protects neurons and promotes the secretion of growth factors in the brain (Vaccarino and Ment, 2004). Neuroplasticity occurs at all ages however the developing brain has greater capacity for change. Both genetic and environmental factors play important roles in neuroplasticity during development.

Critical Periods and Timing

The preclinical work of Kolb and others show that critical periods exist during development in which the brain's capacity to reorganize in response to injury is enhanced while at other times neuroplastic mechanisms can be detrimental (Kolb et al., 2011). A suite of experiments involving various drug therapies and neurotrophic agents has demonstrated the ability of the developing brain to develop new neural networks when treatments were strategically introduced during known critical periods.

Kolb et al. describe three types of neuroplasticity: experience independent (largely genetically determined but modified by both internal and external events), experience dependent plasticity which lasts a lifetime, and experience expectant plasticity (Kolb et al., 2017). This latter type is characterized by a critical period that is moderated by a balance of inhibitory and excitatory inputs that may be chemically modifiable, thus enabling a widening of the critical period.

Environmental enrichment is the most commonly used method of inducing neuroplasticity in animal studies. The harnessing of activity-dependent mechanisms by enriching the housing and social environments of experimental animals has demonstrated improved outcomes after injury in both adult and infant models (Nithianantharajah and Hannan, 2006). The use of enriched environments for animals with perinatal brain injury produces structural brain changes including increased brain volumes as well as improved cognitive, motor and behavioral skill acquisition. Tactile stimulation, or sensory enrichment has been shown in numerous studies to improve cognitive, motor and visual function (Sale et al., 2009; Kolb et al., 2017).

Although activity-dependent plasticity is a lifelong mechanism, the timing of experience and training post injury seems important. A cat model of cerebral palsy showed that early stimulation of the corticospinal tract using forelimb training resulted in functional skill acquisition as well as connectivity, whereas animals who received delayed training did not develop functional use of the affected limb (Friel et al., 2012). Studies in adult stroke patients have also indicated that training close to the time of the infarct leads to better functional skills and structural brain changes (Kleim and Jones, 2008).

Principles of Experience Dependent Neuroplasticity

Kleim and Jones describe activity-dependent neuroplasticity principles that should be applied to rehabilitation programs in humans with brain damage, stressing the importance of active engagement of neural circuits to avoid degradation and enhance function (Kleim and Jones, 2008). Although primarily focused on adult and animal studies these principles (task specificity, repetition, salience, timing, and intensity) also apply to infants with brain damage who need to learn for the first time, rather than re-learn, how to move, think, and communicate. Thus the principles of neuroplasticity along with environmental enrichment strategies should be applied in infant early intervention, with reference to the child's context—most importantly the parent-child relationship. Attachment to a primary caregiver is paramount for early brain development as studies of institutionalized children attest (Fox et al., 2011). Early intervention programs for infants with brain injuries should support not only the parent (Benzies et al., 2013), who are at higher risk of poor mental health (Whittingham et al., 2014) but also provide support to the child-parent relationship in order to maximize outcomes.

Measuring neuroplasticity using advanced imaging techniques is possible in adults post-stroke (Cramer et al., 2011), and increasingly advocated for children with cerebral palsy (Reid et al., 2017). Imaging of cortical thickness and gray matter can identify neuroplastic change (Reid et al., 2015) and has been conducted in very young children with unilateral cerebral palsy post constraint induced movement therapy (Sterling et al., 2013). Transcranial magnetic stimulation can also be used to measure cortical reorganization and is currently being trialed in infants post perinatal stroke (Chen et al., 2017). However, ethical dilemmas exist for this age group since conducting MRI for research purposes require anesthetics to guarantee useable images.

Neuroplasticity-Inducing Rehabilitation Trials

A multitude of early intervention trials have been conducted in cohorts of preterm infants. These interventions may be delivered during the NICU stay (Ustad et al., 2016) or commence post discharge (Spittle et al., 2010). Some intervention studies start during NICU admission and continue for a short period after discharge (Dusing et al., 2015, 2018). Since it is clear that prematurity significantly impacts all developmental domains, in most instances study inclusion is based on gestational age or birthweight. A meta-analysis of controlled trials (random and quasi randomized) demonstrates that cognitive outcomes are significantly improved through early intervention, with effects lasting until school-age (Spittle et al., 2015). Motor outcomes however were only marginally improved in these studies and the clinical significance of the improvement is not clear. This systematic review included any early developmental intervention programs that aimed to improve cognitive or motor outcomes initiated within 12 months post-term age. Types of interventions included physiotherapy, occupational therapy, neurodevelopmental therapy, parent-infant relationship enhancement, infant stimulation, and early education intervention. Thus the included interventions are heterogeneous in terms of content, dose and outcome measurement (Spittle et al., 2015), making it difficult to draw out the key ingredients for beneficial effects. Most approaches focus on training parents to recognize and respond to their infant's cues as well as providing information and guidance to support the infant to meet developmental milestones. Some early intervention approaches are more child focused and delivered by a physiotherapist or occupational therapist (Spittle et al., 2015).

Very few studies target preterm infants with brain injuries and in fact many studies specifically exclude preterm infants with imaging abnormalities. The two small RCTs that specifically targeted preterm infants with cerebral injuries did not find statistically significant between group differences in either motor or cognitive outcomes (Nelson et al., 2001; Ohgi et al., 2004), although short term neurobehavioral benefits were found in one study (Ohgi et al., 2004).

Environmental enrichment

Whilst the impact of prematurity on cerebral brain development has been extensively studied, the impact of the NICU admission itself on the brain is less certain. Painful or stressful stimuli and deprivation can have profound negative effects on brain development. It is difficult to disentangle prematurity and its associated co-morbidities from the life-saving therapies, but also the various "threats" that admission into an intensive care environment provides. The magnitude of these threats is being more accurately quantified, and we now know that the premature infant goes into an environment of light for most of the 24 h cycle (Rodriguez and Pattini, 2016), a relatively noisy environment (Shoemark et al., 2016), and a situation in which painful procedures e.g., heel lances, are common (Brummelte et al., 2012). Reproduction of the *in utero* environment, with low-level sensory input and safety, is not currently possible, however clinician scientists are now beginning to investigate the potential benefit of "normalizing" the environment for the preterm infants, for example by promoting appropriate circadian sleep-wake rhythm cycles and protecting the infant from sensory overload. Length of stay in the NICU is rarely controlled for as a confounder in RCT's, but it is easily quantified and is often used as a short term outcome in trials of neonatal interventions—with reduced length of stay considered as a significant positive outcome, both for the baby, the family, and the health service economist.

Enriching the newborn care environment via the Newborn Individualized Care and Assessment Program (NIDCAP) is an intervention that has been widely adopted (reviewed in Moody et al., 2017). NIDCAP aims to provide an environment with minimal stress that adapts to the needs of the infant through identification and response to infant cues. Though some early trials showed improved brain function and structure in low-risk preterm infants (Als et al., 2004), subsequent studies have generally not reproduced these findings, and meta-analyses do not show significant gains from NIDCAP in the short or long term (Ohlsson and Jacobs, 2013). To date NIDCAP does not appear to prevent or ameliorate brain injury in preterm infants, nor does it do harm. Studies of infant massage (sensory enrichment) have shown positive results in a small sample of preterm infants (Guzzetta et al., 2009), as has music therapy (Lubetzky et al., 2010).

Although early intervention aims to harness naturally occurring neuroplastic mechanisms such as experience-dependent plasticity, a number of interventions that have been studied have involved the infant largely in a passive capacity in a clinic-based environment (Weindling et al., 1996).

Systematic review evidence indicates that a small effect on motor outcomes is gained for infants 0–2 years with brain injuries, when interventions are applied that enrich at least one aspect of the environment (social, motor, sensory, or cognitive) (Morgan et al., 2013). Since this review, two further studies of preterm infants (with and without brain damage) (Dusing et al., 2015, 2018) have shown early promising results in early problem solving skills. "SPEEDI" (Supporting Play Exploration and Early Developmental Intervention) is an intervention where parents are coached and supported to promote daily movement opportunities and environmental enrichment strategies with their infant. Larger trials are underway to explore the importance of timing of the intervention (NCT03518736).

Training motor skills

Traditional physiotherapy for cerebral palsy has been largely a passive experience for the child, however systematic review evidence favors approaches that are goal directed and involve repetitive practice of specific and functional tasks (Novak et al., 2013). Recent systematic reviews of early intervention (from birth to 24 months) for infants with cerebral palsy have not only revealed the lack of rigorous trial data available but also that traditional early intervention is largely ineffective for infants with cerebral palsy (Morgan et al., 2016a). The majority of studies identified in this review did not demonstrate any motor gains for infants with cerebral palsy. However, only half of the included trials began early intervention prior to 6 months of age. Delayed definitive diagnosis of cerebral palsy, after 12 months, has typically meant that a mixed group of "at risk" infants are recruited, leading to underpowered trials. Alternatively, waiting for a confirmed diagnosis prior to recruitment means that infants with cerebral palsy don't receive intervention until the second year of life.

An important study from 1988 randomized 48 infants with spastic diplegia, most of whom were preterm, to receive either a home-based active enrichment intervention ("Learning Games") or Neurodevelopmental Therapy, the most commonly applied physiotherapy intervention (Palmer et al., 1988). Infants randomized to the enrichment intervention were significantly more advanced in motor and cognitive skills after 6 months of intervention as measured using the Bayley.

Evidence for early interventions that involve active motor skill training has been growing slowly over the last 4 years. Two RCTs of GAME (Goals Activity Motor Enrichment; Morgan et al., 2014) intervention in infants aged 3–6 months with or at high risk of cerebral palsy demonstrated improved motor (Morgan et al., 2015, 2016b) and cognitive skills (Morgan et al., 2016b) after a minimum of 3 months intervention, when compared to standard care. GAME is a motor learning intervention that coaches and supports parents to train motor and cognitive skills through play, in an enriched environment. GAME is always delivered in the family home with practice carried out by parents throughout the week between face to face therapy sessions. A large multicenter single blind randomized controlled trial ($n =$ 300) of GAME vs. standard care is currently being undertaken (ACTRN12617000006347).

About 20–30% of preterm infants with cerebral palsy will be diagnosed with unilateral cerebral palsy (Himpens et al., 2008; ACPR Group, 2018). High quality evidence exists for the use of constraint induced movement therapy (CIMT) in children with unilateral cerebral palsy (Novak et al., 2013) and there is early evidence to support the use of a modified version of CIMT for infants. A retrospective study of 72 infants with unilateral cerebral palsy confirmed that children who had received CIMT as an infant (baby-CIMT) were significantly more likely to have superior hand function at age two than those who did not, even when controlling for the type of lesion (Nordstrand et al., 2015). A recently published RCT ($n = 37$) confirmed that infants with unilateral cerebral palsy had better function of their affected hand after 36 h of baby-CIMT than infants who had received the same dose of infant massage (Eliasson et al., 2018). Bimanual therapy, a training intervention that targets using both hands together, is equally effective as CIMT at a matched dose in older children with hemiplegia however trials in infants are not yet published (Sakzewski et al., 2014). A randomized trial comparing baby CIMT with bimanual training is currently underway (Boyd et al., 2017).

While the evidence for early habilitation interventions in infants with cerebral palsy is small it is steadily growing evidenced by the large number of registered clinical trials underway and an increasing focus on earlier detection (Byrne et al., 2017; Novak et al., 2017). Further research is required regarding interventions that can be applied very early (during the NICU) in preterm infants at high risk of cerebral palsy since motor and sensory pathways are still developing at this point. Ideally, combining pharmacological and/or cell based therapies with habilitation interventions to drive experience-dependent plasticity, appears to be the approach that should be targeted by those working with preterm infants with cerebral palsy.

POTENTIAL FUTURE ADVANCES: BIOMARKERS OF PRETERM BRAIN INJURY

An early diagnosis of cerebral palsy at 12-weeks of age corrected is a major step forward, but still falls short of the need to accurately diagnose brain injury and predict the likelihood of disability within hours of injury, so as to instigate novel and conventional protective treatments, such as therapeutic hypothermia in the case of HIE. The race is now on to identify reliable biomarkers of brain injury.

Blood biomarkers are under intense investigation, because the BBB "opens" after injury (Anblagan et al., 2016). This opening is mediated by a number of factors, including disruption of the tight-junction complexes connecting brain endothelial cells, increased production of inflammatory mediators resulting in infiltration of immune cells into the injured site. A permeabilized BBB enables by-products of the injury cascade to be released into the circulatory system (Graham et al., 2018). Several candidate biomarkers have been identified and have been thoroughly appraised in a systematic review (Graham et al., 2018). Candidate biomarkers include: Glial Fibrillary Acidic Protein (GFAP); Neuron-Specific Enolase (NSE); S100B; Ubiquitin Carboxy-Terminal Hydrolase L1 Protein (UCHL1); Cleaved Tau (C-TAU); Microtubule-Associated Protein 2 (MAP2); Myelin Basic Protein (MBP); Spectrin Breakdown Products (SBDP); Brain-Derived Neurotrophic Factor (BDNF); Activin A; Matrix Metalloproteinase-9 (MMP-9); Vascular Endothelial Growth Factor (VEGF); Platelet Derived Growth Factor Receptor b (PDGFRb); Thrombospondin-1 (TSP-1); Tumor Necrosis Factor Alpha (TNF-a); Granulocyte Colony Stimulating Factor (G-CSF); MicroRNA (miRNA); and Exosomes (Graham et al., 2018). These proteins, neurotrophins, factors, inflammatory and metabolic markers are only released peripherally after injury, and are therefore being studied as indicators of the presence of brain injury. Importantly, it is likely that a panel/s of biomarkers will be most useful for identifying infants with neurological injury, and a combination of markers, in addition to existing tools, would provide the greatest diagnostic sensitivity (Yokobori et al., 2013).

In addition to blood biomarkers, neuroimaging techniques including ultrasonography, MRI and electroencephalography (EEG) are crucial tools in the diagnosis and prediction of prognosis following preterm brain injury (Jin et al., 2015). Though current techniques have distinct advantages and disadvantages (e.g., cost, accessibility, sensitivity, need for general anesthetic during MRI), development of advanced techniques such as volumetric MRI, diffusion tensor imaging, metabolic imaging (MR spectroscopy), functional ultrasound (Deffieux et al., 2018) and amplitude-integrated EEG, are transforming the neuroimaging field. Advanced MRI techniques as well as the "Baby Connectome Project" (Howell et al., 2019) are likely to result in the development of improved diagnostic and prognostic markers in addition to novel outcome measures for quantifying neuroplasticity change from intervention.

Importantly, it has been proposed that a combination or panel of biomarkers may provide clues about the type of injury, allowing identification of new treatment paradigms that address the underlying cellular damage mechanisms. In addition, biomarkers may enable clinical triage of combinatory treatments and therefore they offer great promise to the field (Graham et al., 2018).

CONCLUSIONS

Preterm birth is a significant cause of morbidity and mortality for infants, and remains a significant risk factor for cerebral palsy. Encouragingly, there are numerous emerging biological, pharmacological, and rehabilitation interventions for the prevention, minimization, and even reversal of preterm brain injury. Many of these therapies are showing promising signs of efficacy in early-phase clinical trials and preclinical studies. However, as new interventions emerge, so arise various controversies surrounding their implementation, which need to be solved before they can gain acceptance and be widely implemented in the clinic. Finally, the development of reliable biomarkers of preterm brain injury, will enable better detection, diagnosis and prediction of long-term outcomes, which will undoubtedly lead to more efficacious, better-targeted therapies, with improved outcomes for infants born preterm.

AUTHOR CONTRIBUTIONS

MF-E, CM, and IN: conceived the project. MF-E, CM, RH, and IN: drafted the article. All authors were involved in editing and approval of the final manuscript.

REFERENCES

Aarnoudse-Moens, C. S., Weisglas-Kuperus, N., Van Goudoever, J. B., and Oosterlaan, J. (2009). Meta-analysis of neurobehavioral outcomes in very preterm and/or very low birth weight children. *Pediatrics* 124, 717–728. doi: 10.1542/peds.2008-2816

Access Economics (2008). *The Economic Impact of Cerebral Palsy in Australia in 2007.* Report by Access Economics Pty Limited for Cerebral Palsy Australia. Canberra, ACT: Access Economics. Available online at: https://cpaustralia.com.au/media/20379/access_economics_report.pdf

ACPR Group (2018). *Report of the Australian Cerebral Palsy Register, Birth Years 1995–2012.* The Australian Cerebral Palsy Register Group, Australia.

Aguirre, A., Dupree, J. L., Mangin, J. M., and Gallo, V. (2007). A functional role for EGFR signaling in myelination and remyelination. *Nat. Neurosci.* 10, 990–1002. doi: 10.1038/nn1938

Aguirre, A., and Gallo, V. (2007). Reduced EGFR signaling in progenitor cells of the adult subventricular zone attenuates oligodendrogenesis after demyelination. *Neuron Glia Biol.* 3, 209–220. doi: 10.1017/S1740925X08000082

Aguirre, A., Rizvi, T. A., Ratner, N., and Gallo, V. (2005). Overexpression of the epidermal growth factor receptor confers migratory properties to nonmigratory postnatal neural progenitors. *J. Neurosci.* 25, 11092–11106. doi: 10.1523/JNEUROSCI.2981-05.2005

Ahn, S. Y., Chang, Y. S., Sung, S. I., and Park, W. S. (2018). Mesenchymal stem cells for severe intraventricular hemorrhage in preterm infants: phase i dose-escalation clinical trial. *Stem Cells Transl Med.* 7, 847–856. doi: 10.1002/sctm.17-0219

AIHW (2017). *Australia's Mothers and Babies 2015—in Brief. Perinatal Statistics Series No. 33. Cat no. PER 91.* Canberra, ACT: Australian Institute of Health and Welfare.

Alers, N. O., Jenkin, G., Miller, S. L., and Wallace, E. M. (2013). Antenatal melatonin as an antioxidant in human pregnancies complicated by fetal growth restriction–a phase I pilot clinical trial: study protocol. *BMJ Open* 3:e004141. doi: 10.1136/bmjopen-2013-004141

Als, H., Duffy, F. H., Mcanulty, G. B., Rivkin, M. J., Vajapeyam, S., Mulkern, R. V., et al. (2004). Early experience alters brain function and structure. *Pediatrics* 113, 846–857. doi: 10.1542/peds.113.4.846

Aly, H., Elmahdy, H., El-Dib, M., Rowisha, M., Awny, M., El-Gohary, T., et al. (2015). Melatonin use for neuroprotection in perinatal asphyxia: a randomized controlled pilot study. *J. Perinatol.* 35, 186–191. doi: 10.1038/jp.2014.186

Anblagan, D., Pataky, R., Evans, M. J., Telford, E. J., Serag, A., Sparrow, S., et al. (2016). Association between preterm brain injury and exposure to chorioamnionitis during fetal life. *Sci. Rep.* 6, 37932–37932. doi: 10.1038/srep37932

Anderson, P. J., Treyvaud, K., Neil, J. J., Cheong, J. L. Y., Hunt, R. W., Thompson, D. K., et al. (2017). Associations of newborn brain magnetic resonance imaging with long-term neurodevelopmental impairments in very preterm children. *J. Pediatr.* 187, 58.e1–65.e1. doi: 10.1016/j.jpeds.2017.04.059

Askie, L. M., Darlow, B. A., Davis, P. G., Finer, N., Stenson, B., Vento, M., et al. (2017). Effects of targeting lower versus higher arterial oxygen saturations on death or disability in preterm infants. *Cochr. Database Syst. Rev.* 4:Cd011190. doi: 10.1002/14651858.CD011190.pub2

Back, S. A., Luo, N. L., Borenstein, N. S., Levine, J. M., Volpe, J. J., and Kinney, H. C. (2001). Late oligodendrocyte progenitors coincide with the developmental window of vulnerability for human perinatal white matter injury. *J. Neurosci.* 21, 1302–1312. doi: 10.1523/JNEUROSCI.21-04-01302.2001

Barlow, K. M., Esser, M. J., Veidt, M., and Boyd, R. (2018). Melatonin as a treatment after traumatic brain injury: a systematic review and meta-analysis of the pre-clinical and clinical literature. *J. Neurotrauma* doi: 10.1089/neu.2018.5752. [Epub ahead of print].

Beaino, G., Khoshnood, B., Kaminski, M., Pierrat, V., Marret, S., Matis, J., et al. (2010). Predictors of cerebral palsy in very preterm infants: the EPIPAGE prospective population-based cohort study. *Dev. Med. Child Neurol.* 52, e119–e125. doi: 10.1111/j.1469-8749.2010.03612.x

Bemelmans, A. P., Husson, I., Jaquet, M., Mallet, J., Kosofsky, B. E., and Gressens, P. (2006). Lentiviral-mediated gene transfer of brain-derived neurotrophic factor is neuroprotective in a mouse model of neonatal excitotoxic challenge. *J. Neurosci. Res.* 83, 50–60. doi: 10.1002/jnr.20704

Bender, A., and Klopstock, T. (2016). Creatine for neuroprotection in neurodegenerative disease: end of story? *Amino Acids* 48, 1929–1940. doi: 10.1007/s00726-015-2165-0

Benzies, K. M., Magill-Evans, J. E., Hayden, K. A., and Ballantyne, M. (2013). Key components of early intervention programs for preterm infants and their parents: a systematic review and meta-analysis. *BMC Pregnancy Childbirth* 13:S10. doi: 10.1186/1471-2393-13-S1-S10

Biran, V., Phan Duy, A., Decobert, F., Bednarek, N., Alberti, C., and Baud, O. (2014). Is melatonin ready to be used in preterm infants as a neuroprotectant? *Dev Med Child Neurol.* 56, 717–723. doi: 10.1111/dmcn.12415

Blencowe, H., Cousens, S., Oestergaard, M. Z., Chou, D., Moller, A. B., Narwal, R., et al. (2012). National, regional, and worldwide estimates of preterm birth rates in the year 2010 with time trends since 1990 for selected countries: a systematic analysis and implications. *Lancet* 379, 2162–2172. doi: 10.1016/S0140-6736(12)60820-4

Boyd, R. N., Ziviani, J., Sakzewski, L., Novak, I., Badawi, N., Pannek, K., et al. (2017). REACH: study protocol of a randomised trial of rehabilitation very early in congenital hemiplegia. *BMJ Open* 7, 385–396. doi: 10.1136/bmjopen-2017-017204

Brummelte, S., Grunau, R. E., Chau, V., Poskitt, K. J., Brant, R., Vinall, J., et al. (2012). Procedural pain and brain development in premature newborns. *Ann. Neurol.* 71, 385–396. doi: 10.1002/ana.22267

Byrne, R., Noritz, G., and Maitre, N. L. (2017). Implementation of early diagnosis and intervention guidelines for cerebral palsy in a high-risk infant follow-up clinic. *Pediatr Neurol.* 76, 66–71. doi: 10.1016/j.pediatrneurol.2017.08.002

Carty, M. L., Wixey, J. A., Colditz, P. B., and Buller, K. M. (2008). Post-insult minocycline treatment attenuates hypoxia-ischemia-induced neuroinflammation and white matter injury in the neonatal rat: a comparison of two different dose regimens. *Int. J. Dev. Neurosci.* 26, 477–485. doi: 10.1016/j.ijdevneu.2008.02.005

Cashman, N., Tan, L. Y., Krieger, C., Madler, B., Mackay, A., Mackenzie, I., et al. (2008). Pilot study of granulocyte colony stimulating factor (G-CSF)-mobilized peripheral blood stem cells in amyotrophic lateral sclerosis (ALS). *Muscle Nerve* 37, 620–625. doi: 10.1002/mus.20951

Chan, S. Y., Hancox, L. A., Martín-Santos, A., Loubière, L. S., Walter, M. N. M., González, A.-M., et al. (2014). MCT8 expression in human fetal cerebral cortex is reduced in severe intrauterine growth restriction. *J Endocrinol.* 220, 85–95. doi: 10.1530/JOE-13-0400

Chen, C. Y., Georgieff, M., Elison, J., Chen, M., Stinear, J., Mueller, B., et al. (2017). Understanding brain reorganization in infants with perinatal stroke through neuroexcitability and neuroimaging. *Pediatr. Phys. Ther.* 29, 173–178. doi: 10.1097/PEP.0000000000000365

Chen, L., Zhang, G., Khan, A. A., Guo, X., and Gu, Y. (2016). Clinical efficacy and meta-analysis of stem cell therapies for patients with brain ischemia. *Stem Cells Int.* 2016:6129579. doi: 10.1155/2016/6129579

Cheong, J. L., Anderson, P. J., Roberts, G., Burnett, A. C., Lee, K. J., Thompson, D. K., et al. (2013). Contribution of brain size to IQ and educational underperformance in extremely preterm adolescents. *PLoS ONE* 8:e77475. doi: 10.1371/journal.pone.0077475

Cheong, J. L., Doyle, L. W., Burnett, A. C., Lee, K. J., Walsh, J. M., Potter, C. R., et al. (2017). Association between moderate and late preterm birth and neurodevelopment and social-emotional development at age 2 years. *JAMA Pediatr.* 171:e164805. doi: 10.1001/jamapediatrics.2016.4805

Cheong, J. L., Thompson, D. K., Wang, H. X., Hunt, R. W., Anderson, P. J., Inder, T. E., et al. (2009). Abnormal white matter signal on MR imaging is related to abnormal tissue microstructure. *Am. J. Neuroradiol.* 30, 623–628. doi: 10.3174/ajnr.A1399

Chio, A., Mora, G., La Bella, V., Caponnetto, C., Mancardi, G., Sabatelli, M., et al. (2011). Repeated courses of granulocyte colony-stimulating factor in amyotrophic lateral sclerosis: clinical and biological results from a prospective multicenter study. *Muscle Nerve.* 43, 189–195. doi: 10.1002/mus.21851

Choong, C.-J., Baba, K., and Mochizuki, H. (2016). Gene therapy for neurological disorders. *Expert Opin. Biol. Ther.* 16, 143–159. doi: 10.1517/14712598.2016.1114096

Cotten, C. M., Murtha, A. P., Goldberg, R. N., Grotegut, C. A., Smith, P. B., Goldstein, R. F., et al. (2014). Feasibility of autologous cord blood cells for infants with hypoxic-ischemic encephalopathy. *J. Pediatr.* 164, 973–979.e1. doi: 10.1016/j.jpeds.2013.11.036

Cramer, S. C., Sur, M., Dobkin, B. H., O'brien, C., Sanger, T. D., Trojanowski, J. Q., et al. (2011). Harnessing neuroplasticity for clinical applications. *Brain* 134, 1591–1609. doi: 10.1093/brain/awr039

De Vries, L. S., Eken, P., and Dubowitz, L. M. (1992). The spectrum of leukomalacia using cranial ultrasound. *Behav. Brain Res.* 49, 1–6. doi: 10.1016/S0166-4328(05)80189-5

De Vries, L. S., Van Haastert, I. C., Benders, M. J., and Groenendaal, F. (2011). Myth: cerebral palsy cannot be predicted by neonatal brain imaging. *Semin. Fetal Neonatal Med.* 16, 279–287. doi: 10.1016/j.siny.2011.04.004

Deepmala, Slattery, J., Kumar, N., Delhey, L., Berk, M., Dean, O, et al. (2015). Clinical trials of N-acetylcysteine in psychiatry and neurology: a systematic review. *Neurosci. Biobehav. Rev.* 55, 294–321. doi: 10.1016/j.neubiorev.2015.04.015

Deffieux, T., Demene, C., Pernot, M., and Tanter, M. (2018). Functional ultrasound neuroimaging: a review of the preclinical and clinical state of the art. *Curr. Opin. Neurobiol.* 50, 128–135. doi: 10.1016/j.conb.2018.02.001

Den Ouden, A. L., Kok, J. H., Verkerk, P. H., Brand, R., and Verloove-Vanhorick, S. P. (1996). The relation between neonatal thyroxine levels and neurodevelopmental outcome at age 5 and 9 years in a national cohort of very preterm and/or very low birth weight infants. *Pediatr. Res.* 39, 142–145. doi: 10.1203/00006450-199601000-00021

Dickinson, H., Bain, E., Wilkinson, D., Middleton, P., Crowther, C. A., and Walker, D. W. (2014a). Creatine for women in pregnancy for neuroprotection of the fetus. *Cochr Datab Syst Rev.* 12:Cd010846. doi: 10.1002/14651858.CD010846.pub2

Dickinson, H., Ellery, S., Ireland, Z., Larosa, D., Snow, R., and Walker, D. W. (2014b). Creatine supplementation during pregnancy: summary of experimental studies suggesting a treatment to improve fetal and neonatal morbidity and reduce mortality in high-risk human pregnancy. *BMC Pregnancy Childbirth* 14:150. doi: 10.1186/1471-2393-14-150

Doeppner, T. R., Herz, J., Gorgens, A., Schlechter, J., Ludwig, A. K., Radtke, S., et al. (2015). Extracellular vesicles improve post-stroke neuroregeneration and prevent postischemic immunosuppression. *Stem Cells Transl. Med.* 4, 1131–1143. doi: 10.5966/sctm.2015-0078

Domoki, F., Perciaccante, J. V., Veltkamp, R., Bari, F., and Busija, D. W. (1999). Mitochondrial potassium channel opener diazoxide preserves neuronal-vascular function after cerebral ischemia in newborn pigs. *Stroke* 30, 2713–8; discussion, 2718–9. doi: 10.1161/01.STR.30.12.2713

Doyle, L. W., Cheong, J. L., Burnett, A., Roberts, G., Lee, K. J., and Anderson, P. J. (2015). Biological and social influences on outcomes of extreme-preterm/low-birth weight adolescents. *Pediatrics* 136, e1513–e1520. doi: 10.1542/peds.2015-2006

Drommelschmidt, K., Serdar, M., Bendix, I., Herz, J., Bertling, F., Prager, S., et al. (2017). Mesenchymal stem cell-derived extracellular vesicles ameliorate inflammation-induced preterm brain injury. *Brain Behav. Immun.* 60, 220–232. doi: 10.1016/j.bbi.2016.11.011

Duning, T., Schiffbauer, H., Warnecke, T., Mohammadi, S., Floel, A., Kolpatzik, K., et al. (2011). G-CSF prevents the progression of structural disintegration of white matter tracts in amyotrophic lateral sclerosis: a pilot trial. *PLoS ONE* 6:e17770. doi: 10.1371/journal.pone.0017770

Dusing, S. C., Brown, S. E., Van Drew, C. M., Thacker, L. R., and Hendricks-Munoz, K. D. (2015). Supporting play exploration and early development intervention from NICU to home: a feasibility study. *Pediatr. Phys. Ther.* 27, 267–274. doi: 10.1097/PEP.0000000000000161

Dusing, S. C., Tripathi, T., Marcinowski, E. C., Thacker, L. R., Brown, L. F., and Hendricks-Munoz, K. D. (2018). Supporting play exploration and early developmental intervention versus usual care to enhance development outcomes during the transition from the neonatal intensive care unit to home: a pilot randomized controlled trial. *BMC Pediatr.* 18:46. doi: 10.1186/s12887-018-1011-4

Edwards, A. D., Redshaw, M. E., Kennea, N., Rivero-Arias, O., Gonzales-Cinca, N., Nongena, P., et al. (2018). Effect of MRI on preterm infants and their families: a randomised trial with nested diagnostic and economic evaluation. *Arch. Dis. Childh. Fetal* 103, F15–F21. doi: 10.1136/archdischild-2017-313102

Eliasson, A. C., Nordstrand, L., Ek, L., Lennartsson, F., Sjostrand, L., Tedroff, K., et al. (2018). The effectiveness of Baby-CIMT in infants younger than 12 months with clinical signs of unilateral-cerebral palsy; an explorative study with randomized design. *Res. Dev. Disabil.* 72, 191–201. doi: 10.1016/j.ridd.2017.11.006

England, T. J., Sprigg, N., Alasheev, A. M., Belkin, A. A., Kumar, A., Prasad, K., et al. (2016). Granulocyte-colony stimulating factor (G-CSF) for stroke: an individual patient data meta-analysis. *Sci. Rep.* 6:36567. doi: 10.1038/srep36567

Fan, L. W., Pang, Y., Lin, S., Tien, L. T., Ma, T., Rhodes, P. G., et al. (2005). Minocycline reduces lipopolysaccharide-induced neurological dysfunction and brain injury in the neonatal rat. *J. Neurosci. Res.* 82, 71–82. doi: 10.1002/jnr.20623

Fan, Z. Z., Cai, H. B., Ge, Z. M., Wang, L. Q., Zhang, X. D., Li, L., et al. (2015). The efficacy and safety of granulocyte colony-stimulating factor for patients with stroke. *J. Stroke Cerebrovasc. Dis.* 24, 1701–1708. doi: 10.1016/j.jstrokecerebrovasdis.2014.11.033

Ferriero, D. M. (2016). The vulnerable newborn brain: imaging patterns of acquired perinatal injury. *Neonatology* 109, 345–351. doi: 10.1159/000444896

Fischer, H. S., Reibel, N. J., Buhrer, C., and Dame, C. (2017). Prophylactic early erythropoietin for neuroprotection in preterm infants: a meta-analysis. *Pediatrics* 139, 556–566. doi: 10.1542/peds.2016-4317

Fleiss, B., and Gressens, P. (2012). Tertiary mechanisms of brain damage: a new hope for treatment of cerebral palsy? *Lancet Neurol.* 11, 556–566. doi: 10.1016/s1474-4422(12)70058-3

Fleiss, B., Guillot, P. V., Titomanlio, L., Baud, O., Hagberg, H., and Gressens, P. (2014). Stem cell therapy for neonatal brain injury. *Clin. Perinatol.* 41, 133–148. doi: 10.1016/j.clp.2013.09.002

Fogal, B., Mcclaskey, C., Yan, S., Yan, H., and Rivkees, S. A. (2010). Diazoxide promotes oligodendrocyte precursor cell proliferation and myelination. *PLoS ONE* 5:e10906. doi: 10.1371/journal.pone.0010906

Fox, N. A., Almas, A. N., Degnan, K. A., Nelson, C. A., and Zeanah, C. H. (2011). The effects of severe psychosocial deprivation and foster care intervention on cognitive development at 8 years of age: findings from the Bucharest early intervention project. *J. Child Psychol. Psychiatry* 52, 919–928. doi: 10.1111/j.1469-7610.2010.02355.x

Friel, K., Chakrabarty, S., Kuo, H. C., and Martin, J. (2012). Using motor behavior during an early critical period to restore skilled limb movement after damage to the corticospinal system during development. *J. Neurosci.* 32, 9265–9276. doi: 10.1523/JNEUROSCI.1198-12.2012

Friesema, E. C., Ganguly, S., Abdalla, A., Manning Fox, J. E., Halestrap, A. P., and Visser, T. J. (2003). Identification of monocarboxylate transporter 8 as a specific thyroid hormone transporter. *J. Biol. Chem.* 278, 40128–40135. doi: 10.1074/jbc.M300909200

Galea, C., Mcintyre, S., Smithers-Sheedy, H., Reid, S. M., Gibson, C., Delacy, M., et al. (2018). Cerebral palsy trends in Australia (1995–2009): a population-based observational study. *Dev. Med. Child Neurol.* 61, 186–193. doi: 10.1111/dmcn.14011

Galvez-Contreras, A., Quinones-Hinojosa, A., and Gonzalez-Perez, O. (2013). The role of EGFR and ErbB family related proteins in the oligodendrocyte specification in germinal niches of the adult mammalian brain. *Front. Cell. Neurosci.* 7, 337–352. doi: 10.3389/fncel.2013.00258

Garrido-Mesa, N., Zarzuelo, A., and Galvez, J. (2013). Minocycline: far beyond an antibiotic. *Br. J. Pharmacol.* 169, 337–352. doi: 10.1111/bph.12139

Gordon, P. H., Moore, D. H., Miller, R. G., Florence, J. M., Verheijde, J. L., Doorish, C., et al. (2007). Efficacy of minocycline in patients with amyotrophic lateral sclerosis: a phase III randomised trial. *Lancet Neurol.* 6, 1045–1053. doi: 10.1016/S1474-4422(07)70270-3

Graham, E. M., Everett, A. D., Delpech, J. C., and Northington, F. J. (2018). Blood biomarkers for evaluation of perinatal encephalopathy: state of the art. *Curr. Opin. Pediatr.* 30, 199–203. doi: 10.1097/MOP.0000000000000591

Gressens, P., Marret, S., Hill, J. M., Brenneman, D. E., Gozes, I., Fridkin, M., et al. (1997). Vasoactive intestinal peptide prevents excitotoxic cell death in the murine developing brain. *J. Clin. Invest.* 100, 390–397. doi: 10.1172/JCI119545

Guzzetta, A., Baldini, S., Bancale, A., Baroncelli, L., Ciucci, F., Ghirri, P., et al. (2009). Massage accelerates brain development and the maturation of visual function. *J. Neurosci.* 29, 6042–6051. doi: 10.1523/JNEUROSCI.5548-08.2009

Hall, J., Prabhakar, S., Balaj, L., Lai, C. P., Cerione, R. A., and Breakefield, X. O. (2016). Delivery of therapeutic proteins via extracellular vesicles: review and potential treatments for Parkinson's disease, glioma, and schwannoma. *Cell Mol. Neurobiol.* 36, 417–427. doi: 10.1007/s10571-015-0309-0

Himpens, E., Van Den Broeck, C., Oostra, A., Calders, P., and Vanhaesebrouck, P. (2008). Prevalence, type, distribution, and severity of cerebral palsy in relation to gestational age: a meta-analytic review. *Dev. Med. Child Neurol.* 50, 334–340. doi: 10.1111/j.1469-8749.2008.02047.x

Hintz, S. R., Slovis, T., Bulas, D., Van Meurs, K. P., Perritt, R., Stevenson, D. K., et al. (2007). Interobserver reliability and accuracy of cranial ultrasound scanning interpretation in premature infants. *J. Pediatr.* 150, 592–596.e5. doi: 10.1016/j.jpeds.2007.02.012

Howell, B. R., Styner, M. A., Gao, W., Yap, P. T., Wang, L., Baluyot, K., et al. (2019). The UNC/UMN Baby Connectome Project (BCP): an overview of the study design and protocol development. *Neuroimage* 185, 891–905. doi: 10.1016/j.neuroimage.2018.03.049

Huang, X., Liu, Y., Bai, S., Peng, L., Zhang, B., and Lu, H. (2017). Granulocyte colony stimulating factor therapy for stroke: a pairwise meta-analysis of randomized controlled trial. *PLoS ONE* 12:e0175774. doi: 10.1371/journal.pone.0175774

Huntington Study Group Domino Investigators (2010). A futility study of minocycline in Huntington's disease. *Mov. Disord.* 25, 2219–2224. doi: 10.1002/mds.23236

Husson, I., Mesples, B., Bac, P., Vamecq, J., Evrard, P., and Gressens, P. (2002). Melatoninergic neuroprotection of the murine periventricular white matter against neonatal excitotoxic challenge. *Ann. Neurol.* 51, 82–92. doi: 10.1002/ana.10072

Husson, I., Rangon, C. M., Lelievre, V., Bemelmans, A. P., Sachs, P., Mallet, J., et al. (2005). BDNF-induced white matter neuroprotection and stage-dependent neuronal survival following a neonatal excitotoxic challenge. *Cereb. Cortex.* 15, 250–261. doi: 10.1093/cercor/bhh127

Inder, T. E., Warfield, S. K., Wang, H., Huppi, P. S., and Volpe, J. J. (2005). Abnormal cerebral structure is present at term in premature infants. *Pediatrics* 115, 286–294. doi: 10.1542/peds.2004-0326

Inder, T. E., Wells, S. J., Mogridge, N. B., Spencer, C., and Volpe, J. J. (2003). Defining the nature of the cerebral abnormalities in the premature infant: a qualitative magnetic resonance imaging study. *J. Pediatr.* 143, 171–179. doi: 10.1067/S0022-3476(03)00357-3

Ireland, Z., Castillo-Melendez, M., Dickinson, H., Snow, R., and Walker, D. W. (2011). A maternal diet supplemented with creatine from mid-pregnancy protects the newborn spiny mouse brain from birth hypoxia. *Neuroscience* 194, 372–379. doi: 10.1016/j.neuroscience.2011.05.012

Ireland, Z., Dickinson, H., Snow, R., and Walker, D. W. (2008). Maternal creatine: does it reach the fetus and improve survival after an acute hypoxic episode in the spiny mouse (*Acomys cahirinus*)? *Am. J. Obstet. Gynecol.* 198, 431.e1–6. doi: 10.1016/j.ajog.2007.10.790

Jantzie, L. L., Oppong, A. Y., Conteh, F. S., Yellowhair, T. R., Kim, J., Fink, G., et al. (2018). Repetitive neonatal erythropoietin and melatonin combinatorial treatment provides sustained repair of functional deficits in a rat model of cerebral palsy. *Front. Neurol.* 9:233. doi: 10.3389/fneur.2018.00233

Jellema, R. K., Lima Passos, V., Ophelders, D. R., Wolfs, T. G., Zwanenburg, A., De Munter, S., et al. (2013). Systemic G-CSF attenuates cerebral inflammation and hypomyelination but does not reduce seizure burden in preterm sheep exposed to global hypoxia-ischemia. *Exp. Neurol.* 250, 293–303. doi: 10.1016/j.expneurol.2013.09.026

Jin, C., Londono, I., Mallard, C., and Lodygensky, G. A. (2015). New means to assess neonatal inflammatory brain injury. *J. Neuroinflammation* 12:180. doi: 10.1186/s12974-015-0397-2

Johnston, M. V. (2009). Plasticity in the developing brain: implications for rehabilitation. *Dev. Disabil. Res. Rev.* 15, 94–101. doi: 10.1002/ddrr.64

Juul, S. E., Mayock, D. E., Comstock, B. A., and Heagerty, P. J. (2015). Neuroprotective potential of erythropoietin in neonates; design of a randomized trial. *Matern. Health Neonatol. Perinatol.* 1:27. doi: 10.1186/s40748-015-0028-z

Kannan, S., Dai, H., Navath, R. S., Balakrishnan, B., Jyoti, A., Janisse, J., et al. (2012). Dendrimer-based postnatal therapy for neuroinflammation and cerebral palsy in a rabbit model. *Sci. Transl. Med.* 4:130ra46. doi: 10.1126/scitranslmed.3003162

Keller, M., Simbruner, G., Gorna, A., Urbanek, M., Tinhofer, I., Griesmaier, E., et al. (2006). Systemic application of granulocyte-colony stimulating factor and stem cell factor exacerbates excitotoxic brain injury in newborn mice. *Pediatr. Res.* 59, 549–553. doi: 10.1203/01.pdr.0000205152.38692.81

Kenner, C., Lott, J. W., and Flandermeyer, A. A. (eds.). (1998). *Comprehensive Neonatal Care: A physiologic Perspective, 2nd Edn.* Philadelphia, PA: W.B. Saunders.

Khwaja, O., and Volpe, J. J. (2008). Pathogenesis of cerebral white matter injury of prematurity. Archives of disease in childhood. *Fetal Neonatal Edition.* 93, F153–F161. doi: 10.1136/adc.2006.108837

Kidokoro, H., Anderson, P. J., Doyle, L. W., Woodward, L. J., Neil, J. J., and Inder, T. E. (2014). Brain injury and altered brain growth in preterm infants: predictors and prognosis. *Pediatrics* 134, e444–e453. doi: 10.1542/peds.2013-2336

Kim, B. R., Shim, J. W., Sung, D. K., Kim, S. S., Jeon, G. W., Kim, M. J., et al. (2008). Granulocyte stimulating factor attenuates hypoxic-ischemic brain injury by inhibiting apoptosis in neonatal rats. *Yonsei Med. J.* 49, 836–842. doi: 10.3349/ymj.2008.49.5.836

Kim, D. K., Nishida, H., An, S. Y., Shetty, A. K., Bartosh, T. J., and Prockop, D. J. (2016). Chromatographically isolated CD63+CD81+ extracellular vesicles from mesenchymal stromal cells rescue cognitive impairments after TBI. *Proc. Natl. Acad. Sci. U.S.A.* 113, 170–175. doi: 10.1073/pnas.1522297113

Kleim, J. A., and Jones, T. A. (2008). Principles of experience-dependent neural plasticity: implications for rehabilitation after brain damage. *J. Speech Lang. Hear. Res.* 51, S225–S239. doi: 10.1044/1092-4388(2008/018)

Kolb, B., Harker, A., and Gibb, R. (2017). Principles of plasticity in the developing brain. *Dev. Med. Child. Neurol.* 59, 1218–1223. doi: 10.1111/dmcn.13546

Kolb, B., Mychasiuk, R., Williams, P., and Gibb, R. (2011). Brain plasticity and recovery from early cortical injury. *Dev. Med. Child. Neurol.* 53(Suppl 4), 4–8. doi: 10.1111/j.1469-8749.2011.04054.x

Kordelas, L., Rebmann, V., Ludwig, A. K., Radtke, S., Ruesing, J., Doeppner, T. R., et al. (2014). MSC-derived exosomes: a novel tool to treat therapy-refractory graft-versus-host disease. *Leukemia* 28:970. doi: 10.1038/leu.2014.41

Lee, H. K., Finniss, S., Cazacu, S., Xiang, C., and Brodie, C. (2014). Mesenchymal stem cells deliver exogenous miRNAs to neural cells and induce their differentiation and glutamate transporter expression. *Stem Cells Dev.* 23, 2851–2861. doi: 10.1089/scd.2014.0146

Lei, J., Rosenzweig, J. M., Mishra, M. K., Alshehri, W., Brancusi, F., Mclane, M., et al. (2017). Maternal dendrimer-based therapy for inflammation-induced preterm birth and perinatal brain injury. *Sci. Rep.* 7:6106. doi: 10.1038/s41598-017-06113-2

Leijser, L. M., Liauw, L., Veen, S., De Boer, I. P., Walther, F. J., and Van Wezel-Meijler, G. (2008). Comparing brain white matter on sequential cranial ultrasound and MRI in very preterm infants. *Neuroradiology* 50:799. doi: 10.1007/s00234-008-0408-4

Lekic, T., Manaenko, A., Rolland, W., Virbel, K., Hartman, R., Tang, J., et al. (2011). Neuroprotection by melatonin after germinal matrix hemorrhage in neonatal rats. *Acta Neurochir. Suppl.* 111, 201–206. doi: 10.1007/978-3-7091-0693-8_34

Li, L., Mcbride, D. W., Doycheva, D., Dixon, B. J., Krafft, P. R., Zhang, J. H., et al. (2015). G-CSF attenuates neuroinflammation and stabilizes the blood-brain barrier via the PI3K/Akt/GSK-3beta signaling pathway following neonatal hypoxia-ischemia in rats. *Exp. Neurol.* 272, 135–144. doi: 10.1016/j.expneurol.2014.12.020

Li, Y., Yang, Y. Y., Ren, J. L., Xu, F., Chen, F. M., and Li, A. (2017). Exosomes secreted by stem cells from human exfoliated deciduous teeth contribute to functional recovery after traumatic brain injury by shifting microglia M1/M2 polarization in rats. *Stem Cell Res. Ther.* 8:198. doi: 10.1186/s13287-017-0648-5

Lim, R., Malhotra, A., Mockler, J., and Wallace, E. (2018). Allogeneic amniotic epithelial cells for established bronchopulmonary dysplasia in premature, low birthweight infants: a first-in-human safety trial. *Cytotherapy* 20:S21. doi: 10.1016/j.jcyt.2018.02.046

Linsell, L., Malouf, R., Morris, J., Kurinczuk, J. J., and Marlow, N. (2016). Prognostic factors for cerebral palsy and motor impairment in children born very preterm or very low birthweight: a systematic review. *Dev. Med. Child Neurol.* 58, 554–569. doi: 10.1111/dmcn.12972

Liu, X., Fu, X., Dai, G., Wang, X., Zhang, Z., Cheng, H., et al. (2017). Comparative analysis of curative effect of bone marrow mesenchymal stem cell and bone marrow mononuclear cell transplantation for spastic cerebral palsy. *J. Transl. Med.* 15:48. doi: 10.1186/s12967-017-1149-0

Lubetzky, R., Mimouni, F. B., Dollberg, S., Reifen, R., Ashbel, G., and Mandel, D. (2010). Effect of music by Mozart on energy expenditure in growing preterm infants. *Pediatrics.* 125, e24–e28. doi: 10.1542/peds.2009-0990

Malcolm, W. F. (ed.). (2014). *Beyond the NICU: Comprehensive Care of the High-Risk Infant.* New York, NY: McGraw-Hill Professional Publication.

Malhotra, K., Chang, J. J., Khunger, A., Blacker, D., Switzer, J. A., Goyal, N., et al. (2018). Minocycline for acute stroke treatment: a systematic review and meta-analysis of randomized clinical trials. *J. Neurol.* 265, 1871–1879. doi: 10.1007/s00415-018-8935-3

Martin, J., Hamilton, B., Osterman, M., Driscoll, A., and Drake, P. (2018). *Births: Final Data for 2016, National Vital Statistics Reports.* Hyattsville, MD: National Center for Health Statistics.

Martinez-Biarge, M., Groenendaal, F., Kersbergen, K. J., Benders, M. J., Foti, F., Cowan, F. M., et al. (2016). MRI based preterm white matter injury classification: the importance of sequential imaging in determining severity of injury. *PLoS ONE* 11:e0156245. doi: 10.1371/journal.pone.0156245

Merchant, N., Azzopardi, D., Counsell, S., Gressens, P., Dierl, A., Gozar, I., et al. (2014). Melatonin as a novel neuroprotectant in preterm infants – a double blinded randomised controlled trial (mint study). *Arch. Dis. Childhood* 99:A43. doi: 10.1136/archdischild-2014-307384.125

Merchant, N. M., Azzopardi, D. V., Hawwa, A. F., Mcelnay, J. C., Middleton, B., Arendt, J., et al. (2013). Pharmacokinetics of melatonin in preterm infants. *Br. J. Clin. Pharmacol.* 76, 725–733. doi: 10.1111/bcp.12092

Miller, S. L., Yawno, T., Alers, N. O., Castillo-Melendez, M., Supramaniam, V. G., Vanzyl, N., et al. (2014). Antenatal antioxidant treatment with melatonin to decrease newborn neurodevelopmental deficits and brain injury caused by fetal growth restriction. *J. Pineal Res.* 56, 283–294. doi: 10.1111/jpi.12121

Min, K., Song, J., Lee, J. H., Kang, M. S., Jang, S. J., Kim, S. H., et al. (2013). Allogenic umbilical cord blood therapy combined with erythropoietin for patients with severe traumatic brain injury: three case reports. *Restor. Neurol. Neurosci.* 31, 397–410. doi: 10.3233/RNN-120289

Moody, C., Callahan, T. J., Aldrich, H., Gance-Cleveland, B., and Sables-Baus, S. (2017). Early initiation of newborn individualized developmental care and assessment program (NIDCAP) reduces length of stay: a quality improvement project. *J. Pediatr. Nurs.* 32, 59–63. doi: 10.1016/j.pedn.2016.11.001

Morgan, C., Darrah, J., Gordon, A. M., Harbourne, R., Spittle, A., Johnson, R., et al. (2016a). Effectiveness of motor interventions in infants with cerebral palsy: a systematic review. *Dev. Med. Child. Neurol.* 58, 900–909. doi: 10.1111/dmcn.13105

Morgan, C., Novak, I., and Badawi, N. (2013). Enriched environments and motor outcomes in cerebral palsy: systematic review and meta-analysis. *Pediatrics* 132, e735–e746. doi: 10.1542/peds.2012-3985

Morgan, C., Novak, I., Dale, R. C., and Badawi, N. (2015). Optimising motor learning in infants at high risk of cerebral palsy: a pilot study. *BMC Pediatr.* 15:30. doi: 10.1186/s12887-015-0347-2

Morgan, C., Novak, I., Dale, R. C., Guzzetta, A., and Badawi, N. (2014). GAME (Goals - Activity - Motor Enrichment): protocol of a single blind randomised controlled trial of motor training, parent education and environmental enrichment for infants at high risk of cerebral palsy. *BMC Neurol.* 14:203. doi: 10.1186/s12883-014-0203-2

Morgan, C., Novak, I., Dale, R. C., Guzzetta, A., and Badawi, N. (2016b). Single blind randomised controlled trial of GAME (Goals - Activity - Motor Enrichment) in infants at high risk of cerebral palsy. *Res. Dev. Disabil.* 55, 256–267. doi: 10.1016/j.ridd.2016.04.005

Mukerji, A., Shah, V., and Shah, P. S. (2015). Periventricular/intraventricular hemorrhage and neurodevelopmental outcomes: a meta-analysis. *Pediatrics* 136, 1132–1143. doi: 10.1542/peds.2015-0944

Murphy, B. P., Inder, T. E., Rooks, V., Taylor, G. A., Anderson, N. J., Mogridge, N., et al. (2002). Posthaemorrhagic ventricular dilatation in the premature infant: natural history and predictors of outcome. *Arch. Dis. Child Fetal Neonatal Ed.* 87, F37–F41. doi: 10.1136/fn.87.1.F37

Nance, E., Porambo, M., Zhang, F., Mishra, M. K., Buelow, M., Getzenberg, R., et al. (2015). Systemic dendrimer-drug treatment of ischemia-induced neonatal white matter injury. *J. Control Release* 214, 112–120. doi: 10.1016/j.jconrel.2015.07.009

Nassar, W., El-Ansary, M., Sabry, D., Mostafa, M. A., Fayad, T., Kotb, E., et al. (2016). Umbilical cord mesenchymal stem cells derived extracellular vesicles can safely ameliorate the progression of chronic kidney diseases. *Biomater. Res.* 20:21. doi: 10.1186/s40824-016-0068-0

Nefussy, B., Artamonov, I., Deutsch, V., Naparstek, E., Nagler, A., and Drory, V. E. (2010). Recombinant human granulocyte-colony stimulating factor administration for treating amyotrophic lateral sclerosis: a pilot study. *Amyotroph. Lateral. Scler.* 11, 187–193. doi: 10.3109/17482960902933809

Nelson, M. N., White-Traut, R. C., Vasan, U., Silvestri, J., Comiskey, E., Meleedy-Rey, P., et al. (2001). One-year outcome of auditory-tactile-visual-vestibular intervention in the neonatal intensive care unit: effects of severe prematurity and central nervous system injury. *J. Child Neurol.* 16, 493–498. doi: 10.1177/088307380101600706

Nemeth, C. L., Drummond, G. T., Mishra, M. K., Zhang, F., Carr, P., Garcia, M. S., et al. (2017). Uptake of dendrimer-drug by different cell types in the hippocampus after hypoxic-ischemic insult in neonatal mice: Effects of injury, microglial activation and hypothermia. *Nanomedicine* 13, 2359–2369. doi: 10.1016/j.nano.2017.06.014

Neubauer, V., Wegleiter, K., Posod, A., Urbanek, M., Wechselberger, K., Kiechl-Kohlendorfer, U., et al. (2016). Delayed application of the haematopoietic growth factors G-CSF/SCF and FL reduces neonatal excitotoxic brain injury. *Brain Res.* 1634, 94–103. doi: 10.1016/j.brainres.2015.12.058

Ng, S. M., Turner, M. A., Gamble, C., Didi, M., Victor, S., Atkinson, J., et al. (2014). Effect of thyroxine on brain microstructure in extremely premature babies: magnetic resonance imaging findings in the TIPIT study. *Pediatr. Radiol.* 44, 987–996. doi: 10.1007/s00247-014-2911-6

Ninds Net-Pd Investigators. (2006). A randomized, double-blind, futility clinical trial of creatine and minocycline in early Parkinson disease. *Neurology* 66, 664–671. doi: 10.1212/01.wnl.0000201252.57661.e1

Nithianantharajah, J., and Hannan, A. J. (2006). Enriched environments, experience-dependent plasticity and disorders of the nervous system. *Nat. Rev. Neurosci.* 7, 697–709. doi: 10.1038/nrn1970

Nordstrand, L., Holmefur, M., Kits, A., and Eliasson, A. C. (2015). Improvements in bimanual hand function after baby-CIMT in two-year old children with unilateral cerebral palsy: a retrospective study. *Res. Dev. Disabil.* 41–42, 86–93. doi: 10.1016/j.ridd.2015.05.003

Novak, I., Hines, M., Goldsmith, S., and Barclay, R. (2012). Clinical prognostic messages from a systematic review on cerebral palsy. *Pediatrics* 130, e1285–e1312. doi: 10.1542/peds.2012-0924

Novak, I., Mcintyre, S., Morgan, C., Campbell, L., Dark, L., Morton, N., et al. (2013). A systematic review of interventions for children with cerebral palsy: state of the evidence. *Dev. Med. Child Neurol.* 55, 885–910. doi: 10.1111/dmcn.12246

Novak, I., Morgan, C., Adde, L., Blackman, J., Boyd, R. N., Brunstrom-Hernandez, J., et al. (2017). Early, accurate diagnosis and early intervention in cerebral palsy: advances in diagnosis and treatment. *JAMA Pediatr.* 171, 897–907. doi: 10.1001/jamapediatrics.2017.1689

Novak, I., Walker, K., Hunt, R. W., Wallace, E. M., Fahey, M., and Badawi, N. (2016). Concise review: stem cell interventions for people with cerebral palsy: systematic review with meta-analysis. *Stem Cells Transl. Med.* 5, 1014–1025. doi: 10.5966/sctm.2015-0372

Ohgi, S., Fukuda, M., Akiyama, T., and Gima, H. (2004). Effect of an early intervention programme on low birthweight infants with cerebral injuries. *J. Paediatr. Child Health.* 40, 689–695. doi: 10.1111/j.1440-1754.2004.00512.x

Ohlsson, A., and Jacobs, S. E. (2013). NIDCAP: a systematic review and meta-analyses of randomized controlled trials. *Pediatrics* 131, e881–e893. doi: 10.1542/peds.2012-2121

Ophelders, D. R., Wolfs, T. G., Jellema, R. K., Zwanenburg, A., Andriessen, P., Delhaas, T., et al. (2016). Mesenchymal stromal cell-derived extracellular vesicles protect the fetal brain after hypoxia-ischemia. *Stem Cells Transl. Med.* 5, 754–763. doi: 10.5966/sctm.2015-0197

Osborn, D. A., and Hunt, R. W. (2007). Prophylactic postnatal thyroid hormones for prevention of morbidity and mortality in preterm infants. *Cochr. Database Syst. Rev.* 1:Cd005948. doi: 10.1002/14651858.CD005948.pub2

Otero-Ortega, L., Gomez De Frutos, M. C., Laso-Garcia, F., Rodriguez-Frutos, B., Medina-Gutierrez, E., Lopez, J. A., et al. (2018). Exosomes promote restoration after an experimental animal model of intracerebral hemorrhage. *J. Cereb. Blood Flow Metab.* 38, 767–779. doi: 10.1177/0271678X17708917

Palmer, F. B., Shapiro, B. K., Wachtel, R. C., Allen, M. C., Hiller, J. E., Harryman, S. E., et al. (1988). The effects of physical therapy on cerebral palsy. *New Engl. J. Med.* 318, 803–808. doi: 10.1056/NEJM198803313181302

Panfoli, I., Ravera, S., Podesta, M., Cossu, C., Santucci, L., Bartolucci, M., et al. (2016). Exosomes from human mesenchymal stem cells conduct aerobic metabolism in term and preterm newborn infants. *FASEB J.* 30, 1416–1424. doi: 10.1096/fj.15-279679

Papile, L. A., Burstein, J., Burstein, R., and Koffler, H. (1978). Incidence and evolution of subependymal and intraventricular hemorrhage: a study of infants with birth weights less than 1,500 gm. *J. Pediatr.* 92, 529–534. doi: 10.1016/S0022-3476(78)80282-0

Pastula, D. M., Moore, D. H., and Bedlack, R. S. (2012). Creatine for amyotrophic lateral sclerosis/motor neuron disease. *Cochr. Database Syst. Rev.* 12:Cd005225. doi: 10.1002/14651858.CD005225.pub3

Polin, R. A., and Carlo, W. A. (2014). Surfactant replacement therapy for preterm and term neonates with respiratory distress. *Pediatrics* 133:156. doi: 10.1542/peds.2013-3443

Rah, W. J., Lee, Y. H., Moon, J. H., Jun, H. J., Kang, H. R., Koh, H., et al. (2017). Neuroregenerative potential of intravenous G-CSF and autologous peripheral blood stem cells in children with cerebral palsy: a randomized, double-blind, cross-over study. *J. Transl. Med.* 15:16. doi: 10.1186/s12967-017-1120-0

Reid, L. B., Pagnozzi, A. M., Fiori, S., Boyd, R. N., Dowson, N., and Rose, S. E. (2017). Measuring neuroplasticity associated with cerebral palsy rehabilitation: an MRI based power analysis. *Int. J. Dev. Neurosci.* 58, 17–25. doi: 10.1016/j.ijdevneu.2017.01.010

Reid, L. B., Rose, S. E., and Boyd, R. N. (2015). Rehabilitation and neuroplasticity in children with unilateral cerebral palsy. *Nat. Rev. Neurol.* 11, 390–400. doi: 10.1038/nrneurol.2015.97

Reid, S. M., Dagia, C. D., Ditchfield, M. R., Carlin, J. B., and Reddihough, D. S. (2014). Population-based studies of brain imaging patterns in cerebral palsy. *Dev. Med. Child. Neurol.* 56, 222–232. doi: 10.1111/dmcn.12228

Rodriguez, R. G., and Pattini, A. E. (2016). Neonatal intensive care unit lighting: update and recommendations. *Arch. Argent. Pediatr.* 114, 361–367. doi: 10.5546/aap.2016.361

Rooman, R. P., Du Caju, M. V., De Beeck, L. O., Docx, M., Van Reempts, P., and Van Acker, K. J. (1996). Low thyroxinaemia occurs in the majority of very preterm newborns. *Eur. J. Pediatr.* 155, 211–215. doi: 10.1007/BF01953940

Rudnicki, J., Kawa, M. P., Kotowski, M., Michalczyk, B., Ustianowski, P., Czajka, R., et al. (2015). Clinical evaluation of the safety and feasibility of whole autologous cord blood transplant as a source of stem and progenitor cells for extremely premature neonates: preliminary report. *Exp. Clin. Transplant.* 13, 563–572. doi: 10.6002/ect.2015.0081

Ruegger, C. M., Hagmann, C. F., Buhrer, C., Held, L., Bucher, H. U., and Wellmann, S. (2015). Erythropoietin for the repair of cerebral injury in very preterm infants (EpoRepair). *Neonatology* 108, 198–204. doi: 10.1159/000437248

Sakellaris, G., Kotsiou, M., Tamiolaki, M., Kalostos, G., Tsapaki, E., Spanaki, M., et al. (2006). Prevention of complications related to traumatic brain injury in children and adolescents with creatine administration:

an open label randomized pilot study. *J Trauma.* 61, 322–329. doi: 10.1097/01.ta.0000230269.46108.d5

Sakzewski, L., Gordon, A., and Eliasson, A. C. (2014). The state of the evidence for intensive upper limb therapy approaches for children with unilateral cerebral palsy. *J. Child Neurol.* 29, 1077–1090. doi: 10.1177/0883073814533150

Sale, A., Berardi, N., and Maffei, L. (2009). Enrich the environment to empower the brain. *Trends Neurosci.* 32, 233–239. doi: 10.1016/j.tins.2008.12.004

Sangobowale, M., Nikulina, E., and Bergold, P. J. (2018). Minocycline plus N-acetylcysteine protect oligodendrocytes when first dosed 12 hours after closed head injury in mice. *Neurosci. Lett.* 682, 16–20. doi: 10.1016/j.neulet.2018.06.010

Scafidi, J., Hammond, T. R., Scafidi, S., Ritter, J., Jablonska, B., Roncal, M., et al. (2014). Intranasal epidermal growth factor treatment rescues neonatal brain injury. *Nature* 506, 230–234. doi: 10.1038/nature12880

Schlager, G. W., Griesmaier, E., Wegleiter, K., Neubauer, V., Urbanek, M., Kiechl-Kohlendorfer, U., et al. (2011). Systemic G-CSF treatment does not improve long-term outcomes after neonatal hypoxic-ischaemic brain injury. *Exp. Neurol.* 230, 67–74. doi: 10.1016/j.expneurol.2010.11.021

Scratch, S. E., Hunt, R. W., Thompson, D. K., Ahmadzai, Z. M., Doyle, L. W., Inder, T. E., et al. (2014). Free thyroxine levels after very preterm birth and neurodevelopmental outcomes at age 7 years. *Pediatrics* 133, e955–e963. doi: 10.1542/peds.2013-2425

Shin, Y. K., and Cho, S. R. (2016). Exploring erythropoietin and G-CSF combination therapy in chronic stroke patients. *Int. J. Mol. Sci.* 17:463. doi: 10.3390/ijms17040463

Shoemark, H., Harcourt, E., Arnup, S. J., and Hunt, R. W. (2016). Characterising the ambient sound environment for infants in intensive care wards. *J. Paediatr. Child Health* 52, 436–440. doi: 10.1111/jpc.13084

Simonsen, K. A., Anderson-Berry, A. L., Delair, S. F., and Davies, H. D. (2014). Early-onset neonatal sepsis. *Clin. Microbiol. Rev.* 27, 21–47. doi: 10.1128/CMR.00031-13

Siren, A. L., Fasshauer, T., Bartels, C., and Ehrenreich, H. (2009). Therapeutic potential of erythropoietin and its structural or functional variants in the nervous system. *Neurotherapeutics* 6, 108–127. doi: 10.1016/j.nurt.2008.10.041

Smilga, A. S., Garfinkle, J., Ng, P., Andersen, J., Buckley, D., Fehlings, D., et al. (2018). Neonatal infection in children with cerebral palsy: a registry-based cohort study. *Pediatr. Neurol.* 80, 77–83. doi: 10.1016/j.pediatrneurol.2017.11.006

Sokolov, M. E., Bashirov, F. V., Markosyan, V. A., Povysheva, T. V., Fadeev, F. O., Izmailov, A. A., et al. (2018). Triple-gene therapy for stroke: a proof-of-concept *in vivo* study in rats. *Front. Pharmacol.* 9:111. doi: 10.3389/fphar.2018.00111

Solaroglu, I., Jadhav, V., and Zhang, J. H. (2007). Neuroprotective effect of granulocyte-colony stimulating factor. *Front. Biosci.* 12, 712–724. doi: 10.2741/2095

Spittle, A., Orton, J., Anderson, P. J., Boyd, R., and Doyle, L. W. (2015). Early developmental intervention programmes provided post hospital discharge to prevent motor and cognitive impairment in preterm infants. *Cochr. Datab. Syst. Rev.* 11:Cd005495. doi: 10.1002/14651858.CD005495.pub4

Spittle, A. J., Anderson, P. J., Lee, K. J., Ferretti, C., Eeles, A., Orton, J., et al. (2010). Preventive care at home for very preterm infants improves infant and caregiver outcomes at 2 years. *Pediatrics* 126, e171–e178. doi: 10.1542/peds.2009-3137

Spittle, A. J., Cheong, J., Doyle, L. W., Roberts, G., Lee, K. J., Lim, J., et al. (2011). Neonatal white matter abnormality predicts childhood motor impairment in very preterm children. *Dev. Med. Child. Neurol.* 53, 1000–1006. doi: 10.1111/j.1469-8749.2011.04095.x

Spittle, A. J., Morgan, C., Olsen, J. E., Novak, I., and Cheong, J. L. Y. (2018). Early diagnosis and treatment of cerebral palsy in children with a history of preterm birth. *Clin. Perinatol.* 45, 409–420. doi: 10.1016/j.clp.2018.05.011

Sterling, C., Taub, E., Davis, D., Rickards, T., Gauthier, L. V., Griffin, A., et al. (2013). Structural neuroplastic change after constraint-induced movement therapy in children with cerebral palsy. *Pediatrics* 131, e1664–e1669. doi: 10.1542/peds.2012-2051

Strahan, J. A., Walker, W. H. 2nd, Montgomery, T. R., and Forger, N. G. (2017). Minocycline causes widespread cell death and increases microglial labeling in the neonatal mouse brain. *Dev. Neurobiol.* 77, 753–766. doi: 10.1002/dneu.22457

Stritzke, A., Thomas, S., Amin, H., Fusch, C., and Lodha, A. (2017). Renal consequences of preterm birth. *Mol. Cell. Pediatr.* 4:2. doi: 10.1186/s40348-016-0068-0

Sun, J. M., Song, A. W., Case, L. E., Mikati, M. A., Gustafson, K. E., Simmons, R., et al. (2017). Effect of autologous cord blood infusion on motor function and brain connectivity in young children with cerebral palsy: a randomized, placebo-controlled trial. *Stem Cells Transl Med.* 6, 2071–2078. doi: 10.1002/sctm.17-0102

Sun, Y., Luo, Z.-M., Guo, X.-M., Su, D.-F., and Liu, X. (2015). An updated role of microRNA-124 in central nervous system disorders: a review. *Front. Cell. Neurosci.* 9:193. doi: 10.3389/fncel.2015.00193

Suzumura, H., Nitta, A., Tsuboi, Y., Watabe, Y., Kuribayashi, R., and Arisaka, O. (2011). Thyroxine for transient hypothyroxinemia and cerebral palsy in extremely preterm infants. *Pediatr. Int.* 53, 463–467. doi: 10.1111/j.1442-200X.2010.03287.x

Towsley, K., Shevell, M. I., and Dagenais, L. (2011). Population-based study of neuroimaging findings in children with cerebral palsy. *Eur. J. Paediatr. Neurol.* 15, 29–35. doi: 10.1016/j.ejpn.2010.07.005

Trounson, A., and Dewitt, N. D. (2016). Pluripotent stem cells progressing to the clinic. *Nat. Rev. Mol. Cell. Biol.* 17, 194–200. doi: 10.1038/nrm.2016.10

Tsuji, M., Wilson, M. A., Lange, M. S., and Johnston, M. V. (2004). Minocycline worsens hypoxic-ischemic brain injury in a neonatal mouse model. *Exp. Neurol.* 189, 58–65. doi: 10.1016/j.expneurol.2004.01.011

Ustad, T., Evensen, K. A., Campbell, S. K., Girolami, G. L., Helbostad, J., Jorgensen, L., et al. (2016). Early parent-administered physical therapy for preterm infants: a randomized controlled trial. *Pediatrics* 138, F190–F192. doi: 10.1542/peds.2016-0271

Vaccarino, F. M., and Ment, L. R. (2004). Injury and repair in developing brain. *Arch. Dis. Child Fetal Neonatal Ed.* 89, F190–F192. doi: 10.1136/adc.2003.043661

Van Haastert, I. C., Groenendaal, F., Uiterwaal, C. S., Termote, J. U., Van Der Heide-Jalving, M., Eijsermans, M. J., et al. (2011). Decreasing incidence and severity of cerebral palsy in prematurely born children. *J. Pediatr.* 159, 86–91.e1. doi: 10.1016/j.jpeds.2010.12.053

Van Wassenaer-Leemhuis, A., Ares, S., Golombek, S., Kok, J., Paneth, N., Kase, J., et al. (2014). Thyroid hormone supplementation in preterm infants born before 28 weeks gestational age and neurodevelopmental outcome at age 36 months. *Thyroid* 24, 1162–1169. doi: 10.1089/thy.2013.0618

Vinukonda, G., Hu, F., Mehdizadeh, R., Dohare, P., Kidwai, A., Juneja, A., et al. (2016). Epidermal growth factor preserves myelin and promotes astrogliosis after intraventricular hemorrhage. *Glia* 64, 1987–2004. doi: 10.1002/glia.23037

Volpe, J. J. (2009). The encephalopathy of prematurity-brain injury and impaired brain development inextricably intertwined. *Semin. Pediatr. Neurol.* 16, 167–178. doi: 10.1016/j.spen.2009.09.005

Wallimann, T., Wyss, M., Brdiczka, D., Nicolay, K., and Eppenberger, H. M. (1992). Intracellular compartmentation, structure and function of creatine kinase isoenzymes in tissues with high and fluctuating energy demands: the 'phosphocreatine circuit' for cellular energy homeostasis. *Biochem. J.* 281(Pt 1), 21–40. doi: 10.1042/bj2810021

Wang, H., Zhang, L., and Jin, Y. (2015). A meta-analysis of the protective effect of recombinant human erythropoietin (rhEPO) for neurodevelopment in preterm infants. *Cell Biochem. Biophys.* 71, 795–802. doi: 10.1007/s12013-014-0265-1

Wang, Q., Duan, F., Wang, M. X., Wang, X. D., Liu, P., and Ma, L. Z. (2016). Effect of stem cell-based therapy for ischemic stroke treatment: a meta-analysis. *Clin. Neurol. Neurosurg.* 146, 1–11. doi: 10.1016/j.clineuro.2016.04.011

Watanabe, K., Hamada, F., Wakatsuki, A., Nagai, R., Shinohara, K., Hayashi, Y., et al. (2012). Prophylactic administration of melatonin to the mother throughout pregnancy can protect against oxidative cerebral damage in neonatal rats. *J. Matern. Fetal Neonatal. Med.* 25, 1254–1259. doi: 10.3109/14767058.2011.636094

Watson, N., Diamandis, T., Gonzales-Portillo, C., Reyes, S., and Borlongan, C. V. (2016). Melatonin as an antioxidant for stroke neuroprotection. *Cell Transplant.* 25, 883–891. doi: 10.3727/096368915X689749

Weindling, A. M., Hallam, P., Gregg, J., Klenka, H., Rosenbloom, L., and Hutton, J. L. (1996). A randomized controlled trial of early physiotherapy for high-risk infants. *Acta Paediatr.* 85, 1107–1111. doi: 10.1111/j.1651-2227.1996.tb14226.x

Welin, A. K., Svedin, P., Lapatto, R., Sultan, B., Hagberg, H., Gressens, P., et al. (2007). Melatonin reduces inflammation and cell death in white matter in the mid-gestation fetal sheep following umbilical cord occlusion. *Pediatr. Res.* 61, 153–158. doi: 10.1203/01.pdr.0000252546.20451.1a

Whittingham, K., Boyd, R. N., Sanders, M. R., and Colditz, P. (2014). Parenting and prematurity: understanding parent experience and preferences for support. *J. Child Family Stud.* 23, 1050–1061. doi: 10.1007/s10826-013-9762-x

Wilkinson, D., Shepherd, E., and Wallace, E. M. (2016). Melatonin for women in pregnancy for neuroprotection of the fetus. *Cochr Datab Syst Rev.* 3:Cd010527. doi: 10.1002/14651858.CD010527.pub2

Williams, A. M., Dennahy, I. S., Bhatti, U. F., Halaweish, I., Xiong, Y., Chang, P., et al. (2019). Mesenchymal stem cell-derived exosomes provide neuroprotection and improve long-term neurologic outcomes in a swine model of traumatic brain injury and hemorrhagic shock. *J. Neurotrauma.* 36, 54–60. doi: 10.1089/neu.2018.5711

Williams, G. R. (2008). Neurodevelopmental and neurophysiological actions of thyroid hormone. *J. Neuroendocrinol.* 20, 784–794. doi: 10.1111/j.1365-2826.2008.01733.x

Willis, G. R., Kourembanas, S., and Mitsialis, S. A. (2017). "Therapeutic applications of extracellular vesicles: perspectives from newborn medicine," in *Extracellular Vesicles: Methods and Protocols,* editors W. P. Kuo, and S. Jia (New York, NY: Springer New York), 409–432. doi: 10.1007/978-1-4939-7253-1_34

Wittmann, G., Szabon, J., Mohácsik, P., Nouriel, S. S., Gereben, B., Fekete, C., et al. (2015). Parallel regulation of thyroid hormone transporters OATP1c1 and MCT8 during and after endotoxemia at the blood-brain barrier of male rodents. *Endocrinology* 156, 1552–1564. doi: 10.1210/en.2014-1830

Wongprayoon, P., and Govitrapong, P. (2017). Melatonin as a mitochondrial protector in neurodegenerative diseases. *Cell Mol. Life Sci.* 74, 3999–4014. doi: 10.1007/s00018-017-2614-x

Woodward, L. J., Anderson, P. J., Austin, N. C., Howard, K., and Inder, T. E. (2006). Neonatal MRI to predict neurodevelopmental outcomes in preterm infants. *New Engl. J. Med.* 355, 685–694. doi: 10.1056/NEJMoa053792

Wu, Y. W., Bauer, L. A., Ballard, R. A., Ferriero, D. M., Glidden, D. V., Mayock, D. E., et al. (2012). Erythropoietin for neuroprotection in neonatal encephalopathy: safety and pharmacokinetics. *Pediatrics* 130, 683–691. doi: 10.1542/peds.2012-0498

Xiao, Y., Luo, M., Luo, H., and Wang, J. (2014). Creatine for Parkinson's disease. *Cochr. Datab. Syst. Rev.* 6:Cd009646. doi: 10.1002/14651858.CD009646.pub2

Yata, K., Matchett, G. A., Tsubokawa, T., Tang, J., Kanamaru, K., and Zhang, J. H. (2007). Granulocyte-colony stimulating factor inhibits apoptotic neuron loss after neonatal hypoxia-ischemia in rats. *Brain Res.* 1145, 227–238. doi: 10.1016/j.brainres.2007.01.144

Yokobori, S., Hosein, K., Burks, S., Sharma, I., Gajavelli, S., and Bullock, R. (2013). Biomarkers for the clinical differential diagnosis in traumatic brain injury–a systematic review. *CNS Neurosci. Ther.* 19, 556–565. doi: 10.1111/cns.12127

Yong, V. W., Wells, J., Giuliani, F., Casha, S., Power, C., and Metz, L. M. (2004). The promise of minocycline in neurology. *Lancet Neurol.* 3, 744–751. doi: 10.1016/S1474-4422(04)00937-8

Zhang, C., Ling, C. L., Pang, L., Wang, Q., Liu, J. X., Wang, B. S., et al. (2017a). Direct macromolecular drug delivery to cerebral ischemia area using neutrophil-mediated nanoparticles. *Theranostics* 7, 3260–3275. doi: 10.7150/thno.19979

Zhang, J., Wang, Q., Xiang, H., Xin, Y., Chang, M., and Lu, H. (2014). Neuroprotection with erythropoietin in preterm and/or low birth weight infants. *J. Clin. Neurosci.* 21, 1283–1287. doi: 10.1016/j.jocn.2013.10.040

Zhang, Y., Chopp, M., Meng, Y., Katakowski, M., Xin, H., Mahmood, A., et al. (2015). Effect of exosomes derived from multipluripotent mesenchymal stromal cells on functional recovery and neurovascular plasticity in rats after traumatic brain injury. *J. Neurosurg.* 122, 856–867. doi: 10.3171/2014.11.JNS14770

Zhang, Y., Chopp, M., Zhang, Z. G., Katakowski, M., Xin, H., Qu, C., et al. (2017b). Systemic administration of cell-free exosomes generated by human bone marrow derived mesenchymal stem cells cultured under 2D and 3D conditions improves functional recovery in rats after traumatic brain injury. *Neurochem. Int.* 111, 69–81. doi: 10.1016/j.neuint.2016.08.003

Zhu, Y., Wendler, C. C., Shi, O., and Rivkees, S. A. (2014). Diazoxide promotes oligodendrocyte differentiation in neonatal brain in normoxia and chronic sublethal hypoxia. *Brain Res.* 1586, 64–72. doi: 10.1016/j.brainres.2014.08.046

14

Emerging Roles of miRNAs in Brain Development and Perinatal Brain Injury

Kenta Hyeon Tae Cho[1]*, Bing Xu*[1]*, Cherie Blenkiron*[2] *and Mhoyra Fraser*[1*]

[1] *Department of Physiology, Faculty of Medical Health and Sciences, University of Auckland, Auckland, New Zealand,*

[2] *Departments of Molecular Medicine and Pathology, Faculty of Medical Health and Sciences, University of Auckland, Auckland, New Zealand*

Correspondence:
Mhoyra Fraser
m.fraser@auckland.ac.nz

In human beings the immature brain is highly plastic and depending on the stage of gestation is particularly vulnerable to a range of insults that if sufficiently severe, can result in long-term motor, cognitive and behavioral impairment. With improved neonatal care, the incidence of major motor deficits such as cerebral palsy has declined with prematurity. Unfortunately, however, milder forms of injury characterized by diffuse non-cystic white matter lesions within the periventricular region and surrounding white matter, involving loss of oligodendrocyte progenitors and subsequent axonal hypomyelination as the brain matures have not. Existing therapeutic options for treatment of preterm infants have proved inadequate, partly owing to an incomplete understanding of underlying post-injury cellular and molecular changes that lead to poor neurodevelopmental outcomes. This has reinforced the need to improve our understanding of brain plasticity, explore novel solutions for the development of protective strategies, and identify biomarkers. Compelling evidence exists supporting the involvement of microRNAs (miRNAs), a class of small non-coding RNAs, as important post-transcriptional regulators of gene expression with functions including cell fate specification and plasticity of synaptic connections. Importantly, miRNAs are differentially expressed following brain injury, and can be packaged within exosomes/extracellular vesicles, which play a pivotal role in assuring their intercellular communication and passage across the blood–brain barrier. Indeed, an increasing number of investigations have examined the roles of specific miRNAs following injury and regeneration and it is apparent that this field of research could potentially identify protective therapeutic strategies to ameliorate perinatal brain injury. In this review, we discuss the most recent findings of some important miRNAs in relation to the development of the brain, their dysregulation, functions and regulatory roles following brain injury, and discuss how these can be targeted either as biomarkers of injury or neuroprotective agents.

Keywords: perinatal, development, brain injury, miRNAs, biomarkers, exosomes, therapies

INTRODUCTION

MicroRNAs (miRNAs) are a class of endogenous small single-stranded non-protein coding RNA molecules (20–24 nucleotides), often phylogenetically conserved, which play a critical role in the control of gene expression at the post-transcriptional level. Specifically, miRNAs mainly function post-transcriptionally by binding to the 3′ untranslated region (3′UTR) of target messenger RNAs (mRNA) and induce mRNA degradation or translational repression (Bartel, 2009). In addition to their repressive role there is considerable evidence to support post-transcriptional stimulation of gene expression by miRNAs either in specific situations by direct or indirect mechanisms (Vasudevan, 2012).

Given their abundance in the central nervous system (CNS) and their specific patterns of expression within all of the major cell types during development (Sempere et al., 2004; Cao et al., 2006; Cherubini et al., 2006; Narayan et al., 2015), it is unsurprising that a number of miRNAs have emerged as potential regulators of CNS development and homeostatic function and under pathological conditions of hypoxia-ischemia, as mediators of neuroinflammation and neurodegeneration (Bhalala et al., 2013; Moon et al., 2013). Investigation of the possible relationships between miRNAs and their importance to the developing brain, however, remain in its infancy, since the majority of studies have not biologically validated the effects of miRNAs beyond the predicted mRNA targets. Nevertheless, a growing body of studies have demonstrated a critical role of miRNAs in the maturation of oligodendrocytes and myelin formation including the pathophysiology of hypoxia-ischemia-induced brain injury in the developing brain (Barca-Mayo and Lu, 2012; Fitzpatrick et al., 2015; Galloway and Moore, 2016; Su et al., 2016). In relation to the latter, it is presently unknown whether the roles of specific miRNAs or their profiles differ in response to injury with increasing gestational age. However, it is plausible that differences do indeed exist given their importance developmentally and since the neuropathology of brain injury differs as a function of gestational age. Among term infants the spectrum of injuries is dominated by selective necrosis, accompanied by parasagittal cerebral injury involving the paracentral cerebral cortex and associated white matter and represents a watershed injury in a vascular distribution (Ferriero, 2016; Kinney and Volpe, 2018b). In contrast, preterm infants born between 23 and 32 weeks gestation are at greatest risk of injury to the cerebral white matter. Depending on the severity of the insult, the spectrum of white matter injury in the preterm population can differ markedly. In its most severe form, all cell types are affected including oligodendrocytes, glia and axons resulting in focal cystic necrotic lesions (periventricular leukomalacia) forming within regions of the periventricular white matter adjacent to the lateral ventricular wall, which can extend into the centrum semiovale and the subcortical white matter (Back et al., 2002; Kinney, Volpe, 2018a). Milder forms are typically of a diffuse non-cystic variety and are now the most common type of injury observed in the preterm population. Moreover, the predominant pathology underlying diffuse white matter injury in the preterm infant is loss and subsequent arrested differentiation of pre-myelinating oligodendrocyte progenitors, (Volpe et al., 2011; Buser et al., 2012; Back and Miller, 2014; van Tilborg et al., 2016) which results in reduced brain myelination and potentially could be an avenue for miRNA targeted therapy.

In addition to the aforementioned role of miRNAs in the pathophysiology of perinatal brain injury evidence now suggests CNS cells secrete stable miRNAs into the plasma, which are bound to protein, HDL, or packaged within exosomes/microvesicles following stroke (Rao et al., 2013; Chen et al., 2015; Mondello et al., 2018). As their release is intimately related to genomic changes in the brain, they have immense potential as biomarkers of perinatal brain injury and may lead to early diagnosis, thereby allowing early implementation of treatment. This section will review emerging concepts associated with miRNA control of brain development and discuss their connection to perinatal brain injury impacted by inflammation and hypoxia-ischemia and those, which may serve as potential diagnostic biomarkers of injury and therapeutic targets.

miRNAs IN CNS DEVELOPMENT

Development of the mammalian CNS involves a series of intricately coordinated events that requires precise spatial and temporal control of gene expression at both the transcriptional and translational levels (Taverna et al., 2014; Gotz et al., 2016). As previously mentioned, the brain has an abundance of miRNAs; many are specific to a given cell lineage or cell type with some being shown to vary dynamically within the brain both prior to and after birth, suggesting a need for different miRNAs throughout development (Lagos-Quintana et al., 2003; Miska et al., 2004; Bak et al., 2008; Smith et al., 2010; Podolska et al., 2011; Ziats and Rennert, 2014; Chen and Qin, 2015). The interplay between miRNAs and their target mRNAs have a critical regulatory role during neural development, from early neurogenesis to synaptogenesis as well as maintenance of neural function (**Figure 1**) (Davis et al., 2015). miRNAs interact mainly through downregulation of expression of both intrinsic and extrinsic factors and activities of cell-specific signaling mechanisms, and therefore regulate the establishment and maintenance of cell fate specification and differentiation of neural stem cells and neurogenic niches (Shi et al., 2010; Brett et al., 2011; Barca-Mayo and Lu, 2012).

miRNAs in Neuronal Cortical Development

The biological importance of miRNAs in neural development was first demonstrated by conditional knockout experiments of enzymes involved in miRNA biogenesis (Bernstein et al., 2003). The double-stranded RNA (dsRNA) nuclease Dicer is essential to this process (Petri et al., 2014). In mice, targeted ablation of the *Dicer1* gene affects brain development including impaired cortical neuron migration, microcephaly, and precursor differentiation in the spinal cord (Davis et al., 2008; De Pietri Tonelli et al., 2008). However, such studies do not readily assign roles for specific miRNAs since a deficiency in Dicer will affect the full complement of miRNAs in the targeted cells. Moreover, knockouts of specific miRNAs are often complicated, since bioinformatics analyses predict hundreds of targets for

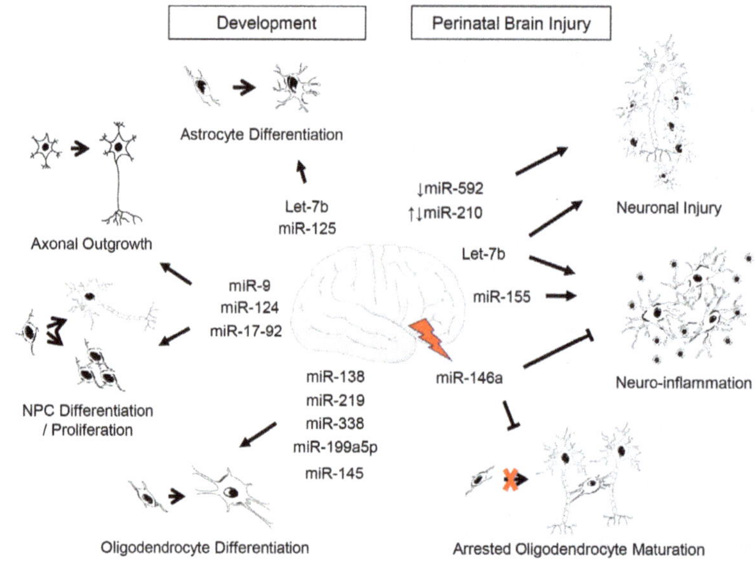

FIGURE 1 | Putative roles of miRNAs in CNS development and perinatal brain injury. Listed are miRNAs covered in this review. *Supporting citations are reviewed in text and summarised below.* **Development:** Let-7b and miR-125 are regulators of astrocyte differentiation (Shenoy et al., 2015). miR-17-92 cluster is involved in neural progenitor cell (NPC) proliferation (Bian et al., 2013) and axonal growth (Zhang et al., 2013). miR-124 regulates neurogenesis (Krichevsky et al., 2006; Makeyev et al., 2007) and axonal growth of retinal ganglion cells (He et al., 2018). miR-9 is implicated in the regulation of NPC differentiation and proliferation (Krichevsky et al., 2006; Radhakrishnan and Alwin Prem Anand, 2016) as well as axonal development and neuronal migration (Dajas-Bailador et al., 2012; Otaegi et al., 2011). miR-219 (Dugas et al., 2010; Shin et al., 2009), miR-338 (Zhao et al., 2010), miR-138 (Dugas et al., 2010), miR-199a-5p (Letzen et al., 2010), miR-145 (Letzen et al., 2010) regulate oligodendrocyte (OL) differentiation. **Perinatal brain injury:** The downregulation of miR-210 is associated with an increase in neuronal apoptosis following hypoxic-ischemic injury (Qiu et al., 2013b) and the upregulation of miR-210 exacerbates cortical injury (Ma et al., 2016; Wang et al., 2017). Post-injury, miR-146a negatively regulates inflammation (Gaudet et al., 2018; Omran et al., 2012) and promotes oligodendrogenesis (Liu et al., 2017). Silencing or inhibition of miR-155 ameliorates inflammation post-injury (Ashhab et al., 2013; Caballero-Garrido et al., 2015; Pena-Philippides et al., 2016; Roitbak, 2018). Let-7b released from neurons and immune cells following injury exacerbates neuronal cell death and induces neuroinflammation (Lehmann et al., 2012; Mueller et al., 2014). The downregulation of miR-592 following hypoxic-ischemic injury induces apoptosis in hippocampal neurons (Sun et al., 2018).

mammalian miRNAs, and it seems likely that many are indeed true targets (Lewis et al., 2003; Lim et al., 2005).

Despite these drawbacks, valuable information has been deemed regarding numerous miRNAs during brain development through loss-of-function and gain-of-function experiments (**Figure 1**). Evidence suggests that miRNAs play an important role in cortical development. For example, the miR-17-92 cluster, together with its paralogs miR-106a-363 and miR-106b-25, is required for appropriate development of embryonic fetal cells (Suh et al., 2004; Ventura et al., 2008). It consists of six miRNAs, processed from a common precursor transcript and grouped in four subfamilies, miR-17, miR-18, miR-19, and miR-92 (Ventura et al., 2008; Bian et al., 2013). A role for miR-17-92 in proliferation has been suggested since phosphatase and tensin homolog (*PTEN*; tumor suppressor gene) is one of its targets (Concepcion et al., 2012). Further, functional role studies have revealed that overexpression of the miR-17-92 cluster in axons of embryonic cortical cells modulates PTEN protein levels and increases axonal growth (Zhang et al., 2013). To confirm additional roles knockout studies of the miR-17-92 cluster and its paralogs have demonstrated an essential role of the miR-17-92 cluster in controlling expansion of neural stem cells and radial glial cells, and transition to intermediate progenitors, which are critical for normal cortical development and function (Bian et al., 2013). Moreover, knockout of miR-17-92 was associated with an upregulation of miR-17-92 target RNAs, *PTEN* and T-box transcription factor Eomes/*Tbr2* (*Tbr2*; a key regulator of neurogenesis in the SVZ), resulting in an increase in intermediate progenitors and suppression of cortical radial glial cells, respectively (Bian et al., 2013).

miR-124, the most abundant miRNA in the brain, is another well-studied regulator of neurogenesis, whose expression increases with commencement of neural differentiation and peaks in mature neurons (Krichevsky et al., 2006; Makeyev et al., 2007; Visvanathan et al., 2007; Cheng et al., 2009; Maiorano and Mallamaci, 2009; Ponomarev et al., 2011; Sanuki et al., 2011; Åkerblom et al., 2012; Sun et al., 2015). Targets of miR-124 include protein jagged-1 (Jag-1), Sry-type high mobility group box 9 (Sox9; involved in adult neurogenesis) and *DLX2* (transcription factor regulating neuronal subtype specification) (Cheng et al., 2009; Liu et al., 2011). Inhibition *in vivo* of miR-124 blocks neurogenesis resulting in a switch to gliogenesis, specifically inducing formation of ectopic astrocytes in the olfactory bulb derived from the subventricular zone (Åkerblom et al., 2012). Furthermore, overexpression experiments both *in vivo* and *in vitro* suggest that miR-124 plays a role in neural fate specification (Smirnova et al., 2005; Krichevsky et al., 2006; Silber et al., 2008; Åkerblom et al., 2012; Xia et al., 2012; Akerblom and Jakobsson, 2014) and most recently promotes axon growth of retinal ganglion cells differentiated from retinal stem cells (He et al., 2018).

Similarly, miR-9, a neuronal specific miRNA, with a prominent role in development, has also been implicated in the regulation of whether neural precursors will adopt a neuronal or glial fate (Krichevsky et al., 2006; Radhakrishnan and Alwin Prem Anand, 2016). miR-9 is highly expressed within the brain, primarily within neural precursors where it controls neural stem cell numbers (Delaloy et al., 2010; Akerblom et al., 2013; Coolen et al., 2013). Overexpression of miR-9 negatively regulates proliferation and accelerates neural differentiation through suppression of the orphan receptor TLX (human homolog of the tailless gene; also known as nuclear receptor subfamily 2, group E member 1 [Nr2e1]) suggesting that TLX and miR-9 participate in a feedback regulatory loop (Zhao et al., 2009). miR-9 is also involved in cortical axonal development via its target, microtubule-associated protein 1b (*Map1b*) (Dajas-Bailador et al., 2012). Furthermore, neuronal migration and outgrowth is also controlled by miR-9 through its interaction with forkhead transcription factors 1 and 2 (*Foxp1* and *Foxp2*) (Otaegi et al., 2011; Clovis et al., 2012).

miRNAs in Oligodendrocyte Development

Due to the critical roles of miRNAs in neurogenesis, it is unsurprising that miRNAs have also emerged as important regulators of oligodendrocyte development (**Figure 1**). Microarray analysis of miRNA profiles in normal CNS development and *Dicer1* knockout models have identified miR-219 as a crucial regulator of oligodendrocyte differentiation (Shin et al., 2009; Dugas et al., 2010; Zhao et al., 2010). miR-219 is highly expressed in the white matter areas of the brain and expression persists in mature oligodendrocytes (Dugas et al., 2010). Its mechanism of action is via direct repression of expression of its predicted targets, namely platelet-derived growth factor receptor alpha (PDGFRα), SRY-box containing gene 6 (Sox6), forkhead box J3 (FoxJ3), and zinc finger protein 238 (ZFP238), all of which promote oligodendrocyte proliferation and inhibit oligodendrocyte differentiation (Barres et al., 1994; Stolt et al., 2006; Dugas et al., 2010). Transfecting purified oligodendrocytes with miR-219 mimic increases expression levels of early (2′,3′-cyclic nucleotide 3′-phosphodiesterase, CNP; myelin basic protein, MBP) and late (myelin oligodendrocyte glycoprotein, MOG) oligodendrocyte specific differentiation markers (Dugas et al., 2010; Zhao et al., 2010). Furthermore, addition of miR-219 mimic to oligodendrocyte progenitor cells lacking functional *Dicer1* expression and which display deficits in myelin gene expression (CNP, MBP, and MOG), markedly enhanced maturation and restored their expression levels to control transfected cells (Dugas et al., 2010; Zhao et al., 2010). Cumulatively, these data indicate that miR-219 is critical for the coordinated transition of oligodendrocyte progenitor cells to oligodendrocytes and subsequent myelin formation and thus may have potential as a therapeutic strategy to promote myelination following injury.

Other important regulators of oligodendrocyte progenitor differentiation are miR-338 and miR-138 (Lau et al., 2008; Dugas et al., 2010). miR-338 is equally as significant as miR-219 in controlling oligodendrogenesis and shares common targets notably Sox6 and Hes Family BHLH Transcription Factor 5 (Hes5); both of which are negative regulators of myelin gene expression (Liu et al., 2006; Stolt et al., 2006; Dugas et al., 2010; Zhao et al., 2010). Furthermore, miR-338 is upregulated in mature oligodendrocytes (Lau et al., 2008) and its overexpression increases oligodendrocyte differentiation (Zhao et al., 2010). However, the role of miR-138 is somewhat incongruous. While miR-138 expression is also elevated in oligodendrocyte precursors its impact on oligodendrocyte development is less significant than miR-219 and miR-338 (Dugas et al., 2010). In contrast to miR-219, oligodendrocyte progenitors induced to differentiate by miR-138 mimic, only express early oligodendrocyte differentiation markers (CNP, MBP) but not late differentiation markers (Dugas et al., 2010). Moreover, miR-138 inhibits Sox4 transcription factor, a repressor of oligodendrocyte maturation (Potzner et al., 2007; Yeh et al., 2013). Together these findings suggest that miR-138 may play a role in extending the period oligodendrocytes are maintained in the early phase of oligodendrocyte differentiation thereby providing a suitable time frame for terminally differentiating oligodendrocytes to myelinate neighboring axons.

Elegant studies by Letzen et al. (2010), using human embryonic stem cells to investigate miRNA expression profiles have revealed unique patterns of expression during the various stages of oligodendrocyte differentiation and maturation. Specifically, four main clusters of miRNA expression were identified encompassing the breadth of the oligodendrocyte lineage scheme (early, mid, and late progenitors and mature oligodendrocytes). Predicted targets of the top differentially expressed genes included myelin-associated genes namely chromosome 11 open reading frame 9 (*C11Orf9*), myelin gene regulatory factor (*MRF*), claudin-11 (*CLDN11*), myelin transcription factor 1-like (*MYTL1*), myelin-associated oligodendrocyte basic protein (*MOBP*), myelin protein zero-like 2 (*MPZL2*), and discoidin domain receptor tyrosine kinase 1 (*DDR1*). Of interest, the authors showed that within the top 10 differentially expressed miRNAs, spanning early to mid-oligodendrocyte progenitor stages, both miR-199a-5p and miR-145 were strongly biased to *C11Orf9*, a gene considered to play a critical role in oligodendrocyte maturation and myelin production.

Evidence discussed above, thus highlights the need to define the role of miRNAs in normal neurodevelopment since they may lay the foundations for novel miRNA-based therapies for preterm infants at risk of brain injury.

miRNAs in Astroglial and Microglial Development

Within cells of the neural lineage, information on the function of miRNAs is predominately limited to neuronal and oligodendrocyte differentiation. Only a relatively few studies have been conducted to investigate the role of miRNAs in astrogliogenesis. This is somewhat surprising given astrocytes represent a major glial cell type in the CNS and are powerful homeostatic regulators of brain function (Giaume et al., 2010). Presumably, the difficulty encountered in isolating astrocyte progenitors *in vivo* has been a major constraint when investigating the functions of astrocyte miRNAs. However, in a recent study of glial progenitors induced to differentiate into astrocytes, deletion of all canonical miRNAs by conditional knockout of Dgcr8 (the RNA binding protein involved in processing of all canonical miRNAs) blocked astrocyte differentiation *in vitro* (Shenoy et al., 2015). Such results were also in keeping with Dicer-knockout studies of *in vivo* derived multipotent neural stem cells (Andersson et al., 2010). Furthermore, in the study conducted by Shenoy et al. (2015), let-7 and miR-125, operating through several targets, restored astrocyte differentiation. Additional studies of disruption of both astrogliogenesis and oligodendrogenesis with inhibition of miRNA formation in ventral spinal progenitors from $Olig1^{Cre}$ – mediated Dicer conditional knockout mice provide further support for miRNAs role in gliogenesis (Zheng et al., 2010, 2012). It is also important to note that a recent study has provided unprecedented evidence of miRNA expression profiles of astrocytes isolated by laser capture microdissection from various regions within the human second trimester fetal brain (17–20 weeks gestation) and adult brain (24–76 years) with no discernible pathology (Rao et al., 2016). Regional differences were noted in these studies, as well as lower expression of miRNAs in fetal vs. adult white matter astrocytes and high expression of miRNAs in the fetal germinal matrix, which presumably is of relevance in pathological conditions.

Microglia are another major glial population. Depending on their location within the CNS, microglia can vary in morphology and density and have important functions in immune surveillance, mediating innate immune responses. In recent years there has been an exponential increase in investigations focussing on the function and regulation of microglia by intrinsic and extrinsic factors within the developing and adult brain under both normal and abnormal physiological conditions (Baburamani et al., 2014; Katsumoto et al., 2014; Nayak et al., 2014; Hagberg et al., 2015; Michell-Robinson et al., 2015; Reemst et al., 2016; Li et al., 2017; Tay et al., 2017; Thion et al., 2018). However, to date, Ponomarev et al. (2011, 2013) have performed the only studies thus far on the role of miRNAs in microgliogenesis within the CNS and have demonstrated that miR-124 is highly expressed in normal CNS-resident microglia, but absent in peripheral monocytes and macrophages. As discussed previously (see section "miRNAs in Neuronal Cortical Development"), miR-124 is also highly expressed in other regions of the CNS and is an important regulator of neurogenesis and neuronal differentiation through its regulation of neuronal gene expression.

Ponomarev et al. (2011, 2013) also showed that miR-124 is a key promoter of the quiescent state of microglia. By forced overexpression of miR-124 in macrophages they were able to demonstrate that miR-124 negatively modulates CCAAT/enhancer-binding protein-α (C/EBP-α) transcription factor, and its downstream target PU.1, resulting in their transformation from an activated to a quiescent phenotype (Ponomarev et al., 2011, 2013). Furthermore, knockdown of miR-124 in microglia and macrophages returned both cells into an activated state (Ponomarev et al., 2011). Thus, this supports a role for miR-124 in the maintenance of a resting phenotype through targeting of the CEBPα/PU.1 pathway and possibly is a way to establish an "alternative" activation (M2) phenotype in resident microglia as part of the reparative response to hypoxia-ischemia- or infection-related neuroinflammation (see section "miRNAs and Neuroinflammation"). Finally, it is apparent that there is a need to identify other candidate miRNAs who may participate in developmental regulation of astrocytes and microglia.

ROLE OF miRNAs IN PERINATAL BRAIN INJURY

An extensive body of literature is now available to suggest dysregulation of miRNA biogenesis and their regulatory role is a common theme associated with the development of neurological injury and disorders from adult experimental models and patients (Dharap et al., 2009; Tan et al., 2009; Liu et al., 2010; Yuan et al., 2010; Bhalala et al., 2013; Eacker et al., 2013; Khanna et al., 2013; Moon et al., 2013; Wang and Yang, 2013; Ouyang et al., 2014). Accordingly, given this and evidence of miRNAs regulatory role during all stages of CNS development, there has been an emerging interest into the implications of miRNAs in perinatal brain injury (**Figure 1**).

HypoxamiRs

Insults such as impaired oxygen delivery or hypoxia has the potential to elicit expression of a distinct group of miRNAs known as hypoxamiRs, that according to the miRbase database (Griffiths-Jones, 2006; Kozomara and Griffiths-Jones, 2014) are in excess of a 100. Importantly, the specific hypoxamiR signature in response to hypoxia varies according to cell type affected and physiological response (Kulshreshtha et al., 2007; Nallamshetty et al., 2013).

Hypoxic regulation of miR-210, considered to be the master hypoxamiR, was first identified by miRNA microarray over a decade ago (Kulshreshtha et al., 2007) and has been shown to be consistently upregulated under various hypoxic conditions (Huang et al., 2010; Chan et al., 2012). Indeed, multiple studies involving adult models of ischemic stroke have consistently shown that miR-210 induction is a feature of the hypoxic response (Jeyaseelan et al., 2008; Dharap et al., 2009; Qiu et al., 2013b; Liu et al., 2018; Meng et al., 2018). Furthermore, in terms of neurogenesis, studies are contradictory in relation as to whether miR-210 inhibition increases neurogenesis following ischemia (Zeng et al., 2014; Ma et al., 2016; Voloboueva et al., 2017). Such differences presumably relate to timing of miR-210 inhibition, since evidence points to a reduction in proliferation with early post-ischemic inhibition, whereas later it increases neurogenesis (Voloboueva et al., 2017).

Similar controversy exists in relation to the immature brain, as evidence from various neonatal stroke models suggest miR-210 may play either a protective or a detrimental role

(Ma et al., 2016). For instance, Qiu et al. (2013a), using a PC12 cell model of oxygen glucose deprivation reported that miR-210 reduced PC12 cell death. The same group demonstrated that in PD (postnatal day; day of birth = postnatal day 0) 7 neonatal rats, miR-210 expression is downregulated in response to hypoxia-ischemia in association with increased brain edema (Qiu et al., 2013b) and that pretreatment with miR-210 mimic significantly reduced edema indicating a possible protective role in response to ischemia.

In contrast, Ma et al. (2016) reported that miR-210 is upregulated following a 2.5 h period of hypoxia-ischemia in PD10 neonatal rats. Furthermore, they demonstrated that miR-210 directly targets the 3′UTR region of the glucocorticoid receptor (GR) in the neonatal rat brain and down regulates GR protein following hypoxia-ischemia resulting in increased susceptibility to injury. In the same study, silencing of miR-210 by intracerebroventricular (ICV) administration of complementary locked nucleic oligonucleotides (miR-210-LNA, miR-210 inhibitor), 4 h after hypoxia-ischemia, significantly ameliorated neuronal injury and infarct size in association with a reduction in brain miR-210 levels. Interestingly, intranasal administration of miR-210-LNA under the same conditions resulted in similar effects. Additional studies by Ma et al. (2017), revealed ICV administration of miR-210 mimic in neonatal rats 48 h prior to hypoxic-ischemic injury compromised blood–brain barrier integrity by suppressing junction proteins, thus resulting in increased susceptibility to brain edema and immunoglobulin G (IgG) parenchyma leakage across the blood–brain barrier.

Finally, in a neonatal rat model of perinatal nicotine-sensitized hypoxic-ischemic brain injury, prior treatment with nicotine was associated with increased miR-210 expression, decreased brain-derived neurotrophic factor/tropomyosin receptor kinase B (BDNF/TRKB) protein expression, and increased susceptibility to hypoxic-ischemic injury (Wang et al., 2017). Moreover, ICV administration of miR-210-LNA 48 h before hypoxia-ischemia significantly decreased brain infarct size in both saline control and nicotine-treated cohorts to levels comparable. To conclude, since a number of verified and putative targets have been identified for miR-210 (Chan and Loscalzo, 2010), it is likely that there are contradictions found with respect to miR-210-specific effects as mentioned above. Such putative roles in relation to perinatal brain injury await corroboration that is more definitive.

miRNAs and Oligodendroglial Response to Hypoxia-Ischemia

Studies highlighting miRNAs as key regulators of oligodendrocyte development may have significant clinical implications with respect to further understanding the pathogenesis of preterm hypoxia-ischemia brain injury, since loss and subsequent arrested differentiation of oligodendrocyte progenitors is a hallmark of injury. Presently, there is a paucity of information with regard to how miRNA expression contributes to critical events of oligodendrogenesis occurring in response to hypoxia-ischemia within the developing brain.

Recently, however, the role of miRNAs in perinatal hypoxia-ischemia has been evaluated in NG2 specific *Dicer1* knockout mice (Birch et al., 2014). Loss of Dicer within oligodendrocyte progenitors following hypoxia-ischemia increased both the number of mature oligodendrocytes and MBP expression, which was associated with improved motor co-ordination performance. Furthermore, in the same study, miRNA profiling within lesion sites of wild-type mice, demonstrated delayed but significant increases in miR-138 and miR-338, 7 days following hypoxia-ischemia. These findings are difficult to resolve since *Dicer1* knockout would normally result in myelin loss and since miR-138 and miR-338 increases with oligodendrocyte differentiation, which was shown to be impaired with hypoxia-ischemia. The authors, however, proposed that mature miRNAs upregulated in response to hypoxia-ischemia may increase oligodendrocyte progenitor proliferation rate and thus decrease inversely differentiation. Further studies are required to address the roles of these miRNAs in this model of perinatal hypoxia-ischemia.

miRNAs and Neuroinflammation

Inflammatory responses play key roles in the regulation of neurodevelopment, neurodegeneration and injury. Due to their capacity to regulate simultaneously a cascade of different genes, miRNAs are well placed as key regulators of neuroinflammation and their dysfunction is equally recognized as contributing to adverse neuroinflammatory processes (Su et al., 2016). Depending upon the target mRNAs and stimulant involved, miRNAs can exhibit functions that are either pro-inflammatory, anti-inflammatory, and/or mixed immunomodulatory in nature.

The most notable of these miRNAs are miR-155 and miR-146a. While miR-155 has both pro- and anti-inflammatory functions (Duan et al., 2016), it is widely considered to be the most potent pro-inflammatory miRNA (Gaudet et al., 2018), and recognized as a key regulator of microglial-mediated immune responses (Cardoso et al., 2012; Butovsky et al., 2015). In the context of adult cerebral ischemia, there is substantial evidence that silencing or inhibition of miR-155 ameliorates the damaging effects of neuroinflammation (Liu et al., 2010; Caballero-Garrido et al., 2015; Pena-Philippides et al., 2016; Roitbak, 2018). Importantly, miR-146a, a negative regulator of inflammation, is characteristically upregulated in the pathogenesis of various neurological conditions (Gaudet et al., 2018) and considered to play a key role in the regulation of cell survival responses by negative regulation of Toll-like receptor 4 (TLR4) through targeting tumor necrosis factor (TNF) receptor-associated factor 6 (*TRAF6*) and interleukin-1 receptor-associated kinase 1 (*IRAK1*) genes in innate and adaptive immune cells (Taganov et al., 2006; Baltimore et al., 2008; Mann et al., 2017). In addition, miR-146a is a key of regulator of oligodendrogenesis both in the normal (Galloway and Moore, 2016) and ischemic brain (Liu et al., 2017) and a negative-feedback regulator of astrocyte-mediated inflammation (Taganov et al., 2006; Iyer et al., 2012).

While growing evidence has revealed that several miRNAs including miR-155 and miR-146a regulate the extent and timing of TLR responses and innate immune pathways (Taganov et al., 2006; O'Connell et al., 2007; Nahid et al., 2011; O'Neill et al., 2011; Quinn and O'Neill, 2011; Lehmann et al., 2012), little is known about their roles in modulation of neuroinflammation within the immature brain following injury. A study to examine the effect of inflammation on epileptogenesis revealed that miR-146a is upregulated in both a PD11 neonatal rat pilocarpine model of mesial temporal lobe epilepsy (MTLE) and children with MTLE and suggest miR-146a modulates the inflammatory response triggered by interleukin-1β (IL-1β) by inhibiting its expression level thus supporting a neuroprotective role for miR-146a (Omran et al., 2012). Further, studies from the same group and animal model revealed that miR-155 and TNF-alpha (TNF-α) is upregulated in seizure-related acute and chronic stages of MTLE (Ashhab et al., 2013). Similar dysregulation was also observed in children with MTLE, thus supporting a role for miR-155 and TNF-α in the development of seizure susceptibility in the immature brain.

Additional support for miR-146a pro-survival functions is also provided by a recent study conducted in PD1 neonatal rats exposed to hypoxia, in conjunction with BV-2 cells (Zhou et al., 2015). The authors showed that treatment with thymosin β4 (Tβ4), a major actin-sequestering protein, known to reduce inflammation and stimulate remyelination after neurological injury (Morris et al., 2010; Xiong et al., 2012), inhibited microglial activation and was associated with *in vitro* upregulation of miR-146a expression (Zhou et al., 2015). Interestingly, Tβ4 upregulation of miR-146a has been shown to promote oligodendrocyte differentiation and suppression of TLR pathways, thus adding to its therapeutic implications (Santra et al., 2014). Furthermore, lipopolysaccharide (LPS) *in vitro* stimulation of newborn cord blood results in upregulation of miR-146a expression in monocytes implicating its involvement in neonatal innate immune responses (Lederhuber et al., 2011). Similarly, studies of miRNA expression profiles from leukocytes isolated from newborn whole cord blood following LPS *in vitro* stimulation show a total of 85 miRNAs are differentially expressed of which several are proposed to modulate TLR inflammatory pathways (Chen J. et al., 2014). As previously discussed (see section "miRNAs in Astroglial and Microglial Development"), miR-124 is another example of a miRNA that regulates CNS inflammation and is highly expressed in microglia and can reduce CNS inflammation through promotion of microglia quiescence via the C/EBP-α-PU.1 pathway. Consequently, overexpression of miR-124 in microglia can induce a switch to M2 polarization, shown by expression of interleukin-10 (IL-10) and transforming growth factor β (TGF-β) (Ponomarev et al., 2011, 2013). Indeed, miR-124 could potentially become a powerful therapeutic strategy for alleviating brain injury in the perinatal period.

Let-7b, a highly abundant miRNA (Pena et al., 2009) and regulator of gene expression in the CNS, released from injured neurons and immune cells, has been demonstrated to exacerbate CNS injury through activation of TLR7 and induce neurodegeneration through neuronal TLR7 (Lehmann et al., 2012). Furthermore, ICV administration of an antagomir to let-7f, another let-7 family member, has been demonstrated to reduce cortical and striatal infarcts in an adult rat stroke model and be preferentially expressed in microglia within the ischemic boundary zone (Selvamani et al., 2012). Recently Mueller et al. (2014), demonstrated that a synthetic peptide analogous to the mammalian preimplantation factor (PIF) secreted by embryos and which is present in the maternal circulation during pregnancy inhibits let-7 miRNA biogenesis in both murine N2a neuroblastoma cells and RAW 264.7 macrophage cell lines. Using a PD3 neonatal rat hypoxic-ischemic brain injury model these authors then showed that subcutaneous administration of synthetic PIF 3 days after injury, significantly abolished the cortical volume reduction, neuronal loss and microgliosis associated with injury in this model 10 days after injury. Although the neuroprotective mechanism remains unclear these authors provided data to suggest that TLR4 may play an important role in synthetic PIF-induced let-7 repression and that KH-type splicing regulatory protein (KSRP) known to be involved with the biogenesis of the let-7 family of miRNAs and a mediator of mRNA decay (Repetto et al., 2012) may be an interacting cofactor involved with this process. Characterization of the specific signaling pathways activated is required to elucidate the significance of this potential pathway in mediating neuroprotection of the developing brain.

miRNAs AS POTENTIAL BIOMARKERS

There are numerous other brain-specific miRNAs known to play potentially crucial roles in the pathological processes of adult brain injury, whose roles in relation in perinatal brain injury have yet to be determined. Nevertheless, recent studies have focussed on identification of several miRNAs as potential biomarkers of perinatal brain injury to enable early diagnosis of the severity of injury (**Table 1**).

Studies, conducted by Looney et al. (2015), involving the analysis of umbilical cord blood miRNA profiles from a cohort of 70 newborn infants [18 controls, 33 with perinatal asphyxia in the absence of hypoxic ischemic encephalopathy (HIE), and 19 infants with HIE analysis], have revealed 70 miRNAs that are differentially expressed with injury. Notably, miR-374a was significantly downregulated in infants with electroencephalographic (EEG) confirmed HIE vs. controls, and further substantiated by quantitative real-time PCR analysis. While no functional mechanism of action and pathways were confirmed, target analysis revealed specific pathways and biological processes associated with neurological injury. Further research from the same group identified several potential downstream targets of this miRNA, namely activin-A receptor type IIb (*ACVR2B*) (Looney et al., 2017). Despite the lack of confirmation of a significant increase in activin-A levels, as previously demonstrated in biological fluids following perinatal asphyxia and HIE (Florio et al., 2004; Florio et al., 2007; Douglas-Escobar and Weiss, 2012), significantly increased levels of ACVR2B were detected in infants with severe HIE. Of interest, however, is the recent demonstration by Dillenburg et al. (2018) that overexpression of Acvr2b in oligodendroglial lineage cells impairs Acvr2a-regulated oligodendrocyte differentiation and myelin formation, thus supporting the possibility of restoration of Acvr2a-mediated signaling as a strategy to combat perinatal white matter injury.

Aside from the above clinical investigation, a recent study of global hypoxia-ischemia in newborn piglets has also provided

TABLE 1 | Potential miRNA biomarkers of perinatal hypoxia-ischemia.

miRNA biomarkers of perinatal HI	Studied cohorts/subjects	Sampling source	Techniques employed for miRNA detection	References
↓ miR-374a	70 newborn infants 18 controls, 33 with perinatal asphyxia in the absence of HIE, 19 infants with HIE	Umbilical cord blood	Microarray, qRT-PCR	Looney et al., 2015
↑ miR-374a ↑ miR-210	13 newborn piglets 5 controls, 8 with transient global HI	Plasma sample	qRT-PCR	Garberg et al., 2016
↑ miR-210	P10 rat pups 4 controls, 4 with right carotid ligation induced HI	Ipsilateral hemisphere	qRT-PCR	Ma et al., 2016
↑ miR-21	78 newborn infants 29 controls, 49 with asphyxia	Serum sample	qRT-PCR	Chen and Yang, 2015
↑ miR-210 ↑ miR-424 ↑ miR-21 ↑ miR-199a ↑ miR-20b	24 infants 12 controls, 12 severely growth restricted preterms	Maternal whole blood sample	qRT-PCR	Whitehead et al., 2013

HIE: hypoxic-ischemic encephalopathy, HI: hypoxia-ischemia, qRT-PCR: quantitative real-time polymerase chain reaction.

evidence to support circulating plasma miR-374a and the hypoxamiR miR-210 as potential biomarkers (Garberg et al., 2016). However, in contrast to Looney et al. (2015), these authors reported a significant upregulation of miR-374a 9.5 h after hypoxia-ischemia and noted that correlations were found between miR-374a and arterial pH, base excess and lactate levels over the study period. Since miR-374a is directly regulated by lactate dehydrogenase A with hypoxia (Wang et al., 2015), the authors concluded that miR-374a might play a role in metabolic adaptive responses to hypoxia-ischemia. Nevertheless, the increase in miR-210 is in congruence with previous studies under a hypoxic environment (Huang et al., 2010; Chan et al., 2012) and those observed by Ma et al. (2016) following hypoxia-ischemia in PD10 neonatal rats.

Other candidate miRNAs have been investigated, namely let7b, miR-29b, miR-124, miR-155, and miR-21 (Ponnusamy et al., 2016). Quantification of these miRNAs in dried blood spots, EDTA-blood, plasma and urine collected from a small cohort of newborns, failed to demonstrate significant differences with injury. However, miR-21, which is expressed in astrocytes, and been shown in adult plasma to be a potential early stage marker of acute cerebral infarction (Zhou and Zhang, 2014), was found to be elevated in serum of 49 neonates with HIE, thus providing support also for an early diagnosis biomarker of neonatal HIE (Chen and Yang, 2015).

Additional studies that warrant mention are preliminary studies conducted by Whitehead et al. (2013). An analysis was made of maternal whole blood expression levels of six miRNAs known to be associated with hypoxia in which fetuses had either experienced acute hypoxia during labor or chronic hypoxia associated with fetal growth retardation. Compared to gestational matched controls there was an upregulation of miR-210, miR-424, miR-21, miR-199a, and miR-20b. Furthermore, correlation with Doppler velocimetry assessments of hypoxia, confirmed the increase was associated with increased severity of hypoxia. The changes observed in miR-210 agree well with that of Ma et al. (2016) and those conducted in the piglet (Garberg et al., 2016) thus supporting the use as a maternally based biomarker of fetal hypoxia.

A caveat: while the field of miRNA research is constantly expanding one must appreciate that the endogenous source of miRNAs within available body fluids including, plasma, serum, urine and saliva can be from a diverse array of peripheral tissue cellular types including those of the brain, thus decreasing in essence the reliability of results. The other point to note is the problem of cell specification of miRNAs; the reality for many miRNAs as biomarkers in body fluids is that they may not be expressed exclusively within one particular cell type. In the last few years, however, since the identification of exosomes [cell-derived vesicles; typically ~40–100 nm in diameter (Raposo and Stoorvogel, 2013)], as a carrier of protein, lipids, mRNAs and miRNAs, with an important role in cell–cell-communication, there has been intense interest into whether brain-derived exosomes could serve better as biomarkers in the clinical diagnosis and management of brain injury (Valadi et al., 2007; Ludwig and Giebel, 2012; Patz et al., 2013; Taylor and Gercel-Taylor, 2014; Werner and Stevens, 2015). Additionally, unlike free circulating miRNAs, miRNAs are inherently enriched and stable within exosomes (Cheng et al., 2014). In the adult, increased levels of exosomes are released from cells following stroke and traumatic brain injury (Patz et al., 2013; Chiva-Blanch et al., 2016). Based on current information, it is apparent that brain-derived exosomes can traverse across the blood–brain barrier following injury. Their presence in the peripheral circulation places them in an ideal position to provide an informative platform for real-time assessment of newborns who have sustained brain injury or those who are at risk of adverse outcomes and to spearhead therapeutic discovery. However, such enthusiasm must be tempered by the harsh reality that proportionally brain-derived exosomes may represent only a small population of circulating exosomes whereas the contribution from peripheral sources may be relatively high in comparison. Although still in its infancy, platforms that employ microscale structures (e.g., microfluidics or acoustofluidics) (Contreras-Naranjo et al., 2017; Guo et al., 2018; Hisey et al., 2018; Li et al., 2018; Wu et al., 2018) and high-throughput phenotypic and functional analyses (e.g., advanced imaging flow cytometry) (Mastoridis et al., 2018) could circumvent this problem. If advanced to such a degree as to provide a rapid and effective means to selectively sort and detect brain-derived exosomes at a nanoscale level they would be of significant value for clinical evaluation.

In the adult, only a few clinical studies have been performed to assess the potential of exosomal-derived miRNAs as biomarkers of acute brain injury. Studies by Chen et al. (2017) demonstrated there was an association between increased circulating levels of exosomal miR-223 and acute ischemic stroke occurrence, stroke severity, and short-term outcomes. Furthermore, studies conducted by Ji et al. (2016) showed that serum exosomal miR-9 and miR-124 levels were positively associated with adverse scores of acute stroke injury, infarct volumes, and serum concentrations of the pro-inflammatory cytokine, interleukin-6 (IL-6). Currently, however, little is known of the usefulness of exosomal-derived miRNAs in the diagnosis of perinatal brain injury. Nevertheless, in a recent study conducted to investigate whether exosomal protein biomarkers would be valuable in the diagnosis of brain injury and assessment of the effectiveness of hypothermia, it was shown that neutral or decreasing serum neuronally derived exosomal synaptopodin protein levels occurred in neonates with abnormal neuroimaging scores (Goetzl et al., 2018).

There is also a growing interest as to the regenerative utility of exosomal-derived contents with and without loading with therapeutics (Doeppner et al., 2015; Luarte et al., 2016; Xiong et al., 2017; Kim et al., 2018). Several studies have also documented the neuron healing and protective abilities of stem cell derived exosomes (Lee et al., 2013; Zhang et al., 2015b; Long et al., 2017; Willis et al., 2017). Importantly, studies recently reported highlight the regenerative potential of mesenchymal stem cell (MSC)-derived extracellular vesicles in a preterm fetal sheep model of hypoxia-ischemia (Ophelders et al., 2016). In these studies, systemic administration to the fetus of MSC-extracellular vesicles resulted in improved brain activity namely a reduction in duration and number of seizures. Finally, as discussed later in Section "*In vivo* Evidence," it warrants mentioning that because exosomes can potentially act as a therapeutic delivery system they hold great promise in revolutionizing the way we can effectively treat perinatal brain injury.

miRNAs AS POTENTIAL THERAPEUTIC TARGETS

In alliance with the discovery of miRNAs as functional regulators of cell development, miRNAs have also been shown to orchestrate a variety of critical signaling pathways involved in injury progression and recovery (Shi et al., 2010; Gaudet et al., 2017). Given the recent demonstration that modulation of miRNA expression occurs following a hypoxic-ischemic insult in the developing brain, several therapeutic targets have emerged (**Figure 2**).

In vitro Evidence

In vitro studies have provided insights into the therapeutic potential of miRNAs that regulate reparative processes following a hypoxic-ischemic insult. For example, stroke-induced downregulation of miR-9 and miR-200b expression in the ischemic white matter region mediated serum response factor (SRF) induced differentiation of oligodendrocyte precursor cells (OPCs) into oligodendrocytes (Buller et al., 2012). Accordingly, *in vitro* overexpression of miR-9 and miR-200b suppressed SRF expression and inhibited OPC differentiation (Buller et al., 2012). Upon validation *in vivo*, the inhibition of miR-9 and miR-200b following injury may indicate a potential therapeutic strategy in the future given that myelination disturbances in the cerebral white matter represent a hallmark of perinatal brain injury (Pandit et al., 2013; Back and Miller, 2014).

Chondroitin sulfate proteoglycans (CSPGs) are well-characterized inhibitory extracellular matrix molecules expressed by reactive astrocytes, endothelial and oligodendrocyte progenitor cells that inhibit axonal regeneration after injury and are associated with adverse neurological outcome in preterm infants (McKeon et al., 1999; Jones et al., 2002, 2003; Chow et al., 2005). *In vitro* overexpression of miR29c and miR-17-92 cluster in embryonic cortical neurons has been shown to attenuate the inhibitory effect of CSPG by stimulating intrinsic axonal signals, suppressing Ras homolog gene family, member A (RhoA) and phosphate and tensin homolog (PTEN) protein levels, thereby promoting axonal outgrowth (Park et al., 2008; Zhang et al., 2013, 2015a). Thus, the potential loss or impaired axonal growth observed in focal necrotic white matter injury in the preterm brain could be feasibly targeted (Riddle et al., 2012).

miR-592 was originally suggested as a possible target for promoting cell apoptosis in various cancers (Liu M. et al., 2015; Liu Z. et al., 2015; Fu et al., 2016). Unsurprisingly, recent studies have also supported its regulatory role of cell death following cerebral ischemic injury (Irmady et al., 2014; Sun et al., 2018). In two studies carried out by Irmady et al. (2014) and Sun et al. (2018), both authors observed reduced expression of miR-592 following cerebral ischemic injury in the hippocampus of neonatal and juvenile mice, respectively. Concordantly, overexpression of miR-592 in cultured hippocampal neurons attenuated the activation of pro-apoptotic signaling and cell death (Irmady et al., 2014; Sun et al., 2018). The mechanism underlying this protective mechanism speculates the multi-functional role of miR-592. Sun et al. (2018) demonstrated that miR-592 affords neuroprotection by selectively targeting prostaglandin D2 receptor (PTGDR) and inhibiting prostaglandin D2 (PGD2)-DP signaling, an inflammatory pathway involving the release of glutamate (Weaver-Mikaere et al., 2013). Irmady et al. (2014), on the other hand revealed that vector mediated transfection of miR-592 in embryonic hippocampal neurons attenuated the level of neurotrophin receptor (NTR) p75 induced by ischemic injury and subsequent apoptotic cell death. The NTR p75 is a member

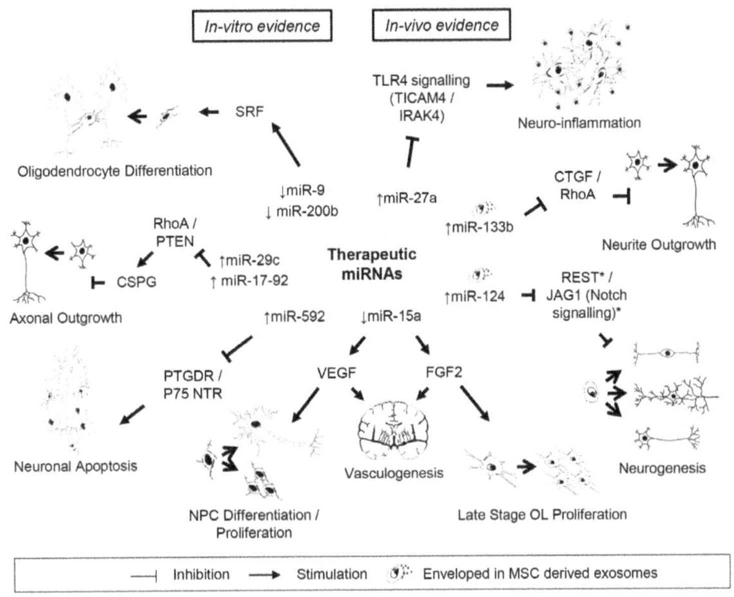

FIGURE 2 | Potential candidates of miRNA-based therapy against perinatal hypoxic-ischemic brain injury. Listed are miRNAs and their downstream targets supporting potentially beneficial outcomes after perinatal hypoxic-ischemic brain injury. *Supporting citations are reviewed in text and summarised below.* ***In-vitro* evidence:** Downregulation of miR-9 and miR-200b mediates serum response factor (SRF) induced oligodendrocyte progenitor cell (OPC) differentiation (Buller et al., 2012). miR-29c (Yi Zhang et al., 2015) and miR-17-92 cluster (Zhang et al., 2013) attenuates the inhibitory effect of chondroitin sulphate proteoglycans (CSPG) on axonal regrowth by stimulating ras homolog family member A (RhoA) and phosphate and tensin homolog (PTEN) protein levels. miR-592 attenuates the activation of pro-apoptotic signalling and neuronal death by targeting the prostaglandin D2 receptor (PTGDR) and neurotrophin receptor (NTR) p75 (Irmady et al., 2014; Sun et al., 2018). ***In-vivo* evidence:** miR-27a reduces TLR4-mediated inflammation (Li et al., 2015). Downregulation of miR-15a expression promote vasculogenesis by stimulating neurotrophic factors, fibroblast growth factor 2 (FGF2) and vascular endothelial growth factor (VEGF) (Yin et al., 2012), which can further support late stage oligodendrocyte (OL) proliferation/migration (Shindo et al., 2016) and neural progenitor cell (NPC) differentiation/proliferation (Teng et al., 2008), respectively. Mesenchymal stem cell (MSC) derived exosomal transfer of miR-133b enhanced neurite outgrowth by inhibiting connective tissue growth factor (CTGF) and RhoA expression (Xin et al., 2012, 2013). Exosome mediated neuronal delivery of miR-124 induces neurogenesis (Yang et al., 2017) speculatively via Usp14-dependent REST degradation (Doeppner et al., 2013) and inhibition of the JAG/Notch signalling pathway (Liu et al., 2011).

of the TNF receptor superfamily closely implicated with neuronal apoptosis following experimental perinatal brain injury (Volosin et al., 2006; Griesmaier et al., 2010). Given the prospective dual anti-apoptotic mechanism of miR-592, results of future *in vivo* studies are eagerly awaited.

In vivo Evidence

miR-27 is a potential regulator of cortical neuronal apoptosis whose expression in embryonic mouse cerebral cortices is attenuated in response to maternal hypoxia (Chen Q. et al., 2014). Furthermore, neuron-specific over-expression of miR-27b in the mouse cortex increased resistance to hypoxia induced apoptosis by inhibiting apoptotic protease-activating factor 1 (Apaf-1) (Chen Q. et al., 2014). Similar observations have been reported in rat primary embryonic hippocampal neuron cultures (Cai et al., 2016) and further potential targets and mechanisms of the miR-27 family have been alluded. For example, miR-27a, directly modulates components of the TLR4 signaling cascade, including TIR domain-containing adaptor molecule-2 (TICAM2) and interleukin-1 receptor-associated kinase 4 (IRAK4), cytoplasmic proteins that link TLR4 and recruit to adaptor protein MyD88 following TLR4 activation, respectively, and coordinates gene transcription and inflammation (Li et al., 2015; Lv et al., 2017). Prophylaxis treatment with miR-27a mimics in an ischemic reperfusion model results in reduced mRNA and protein expression of TICAM2 accompanied by attenuation of TLR4 activation and pro-inflammatory cytokine production, while pretreatment with miR-27a inhibitory oligonucleotides show opposite effects (Li et al., 2015). Comparable anti-inflammatory effects of miR-27a have also been observed in cultured neonatal microglial cells which were achieved by targeting IRAK4 and TLR4 (Lv et al., 2017). Speculatively, miR-27a can target multiple genes and regulate the TLR4 signaling pathway to prevent an excessive inflammatory response to injury. Indeed, various animal models of perinatal brain injury have shown that TLR4 activation and the ensuing inflammatory response can result in cell death and a pattern of injury similar to that seen in human infants, including hypomyelination, glia activation and disruption of thalamocortical function (Dean et al., 2011; Kannan et al., 2011; Dhillon et al., 2015). Therefore, the anti-apoptotic and anti-inflammatory effects of miR-27a/b may prove to be a potential therapeutic target in the future.

Cerebral angiogenesis is a critical reparative process of the microvasculature following hypoxic-ischemic injury, involving cellular cross-talk through neurotropic factors, improving regional blood supply, and facilitating the migration of neurons toward damaged regions (Ohab et al., 2006; Yin et al., 2015). Modulating this reparative process holds promise since the perinatal brain has the greatest potential for repair and recovery (Dzietko et al., 2013). miR-15a in vascular endothelial cells has emerged as a key regulator of angiogenesis, such that downregulation of miR-15a promotes vasculogenesis by increasing neurotrophic factors, including fibroblast growth factor 2 (FGF2) and vascular endothelial growth factor (VEGF) (Yin et al., 2012). Critically, VEGF released by angiogenic endothelial cells can promote proliferation and differentiation of neural progenitor cells via vascular endothelial growth factor receptor 2 (VEGFR2) (Teng et al., 2008). FGF2 is also an important growth factor involved in neurogenesis and gliogenesis during embryonic and postnatal development (Vaccarino et al., 1999). Crosstalk between cerebral endothelium and oligodendrocytes can promote proliferation and migration of late-stage OPCs through FGF2 (Shindo et al., 2016). Given that delayed treatment with VEGF and FGF2 have proven to be neuroprotective in perinatal models of brain injury (Monfils et al., 2006; Dzietko et al., 2013), miR-15a may be an attractive therapeutic target in the tertiary phase of injury (Fleiss and Gressens, 2012). In fact, it may pose advantages given its ability to target multiple genes in addition to delivering a synergistic effect.

MSCs have been extensively applied in both experimental and clinical settings of CNS diseases owing to their immunomodulatory, regenerative and reparative properties including stroke (Koh et al., 2008; Steinberg et al., 2016), multiple sclerosis (Zhang et al., 2005; Gerdoni et al., 2007; Uccelli et al., 2011) and perinatal brain injury (van Velthoven et al., 2010; Jellema et al., 2013; Drommelschmidt et al., 2017). Currently, it is proposed that MSCs exert their therapeutic potency at least in part through a paracrine mechanism involving the release of extracellular vesicles, which based on their size and intracellular origin include microvesicles (~100–1000 nm in diameter) and exosomes (~40–100 nm in diameter) (Hass and Otte, 2012; Mokarizadeh et al., 2012; Xin et al., 2012; Lee et al., 2013; Koniusz et al., 2016). Indeed, MSCs are prolific producers of extracellular vesicles; a feature that is maintained with immortalization of cells to generate permanent cell lines, making them an ideal option for biological tissue replacement regeneration (Yeo et al., 2013).

MSC-derived extracellular vesicles are enriched with a variety of proteins and different RNA species (mainly mRNA and miRNA) as well as trophic factors whose functions are linked to MSCs biological effects. Importantly, evidence now suggests that specific miRNAs are necessary to mediate MSC-derived extracellular vesicles neuroprotective effect (Xin et al., 2012). While miRNAs encapsulated within MSC derived microvesicles are predominantly in their precursor form (pre-miRNAs) (Chen et al., 2009), studies have demonstrated the presence and biological functional roles of exosomal mature miRNAs (Koh et al., 2010; Katakowski et al., 2013; Ono et al., 2014). The transfer of miR-133b from exosomal MSCs directly enhanced neurite outgrowth and functional recovery in adult stroke models (Xin et al., 2012, 2013). Given the putative occurrence of impaired neurite outgrowth in perinatal brain injury (Robinson et al., 2006; Dean et al., 2013), exosomal miR-133b may be important for brain connectivity and function. In an elegant series of studies conducted by Xin et al. (2012), miR-133b was substantially downregulated in the ischemic rat brain and increased following MSC intravenous administration. Connective tissue growth factor (CTGF) and RhoA are both inhibitors of neurite growth and are selective targets of miR-133b (Xin et al., 2014). Critically, administration of MSC-derived exosomes enriched with miR-133b reduced CTGF and RhoA expression and exhibited enhanced axonal plasticity, neurite remodeling and functional recovery compared to naturally occurring MSC-derived exosomes (Xin et al., 2013). These changes were confirmed in primary cultured neurons and astrocytes (Xin et al., 2013). Transfer of miR-133b enriched MSC derived exosomes in cultured neurons, inhibited RhoA expression and stimulated neurite outgrowth, while the transfer in astrocytes, downregulated CTGF expression, a known inhibitor of axonal growth and contributor to glial scar formation in human cerebral infarction (Schwab et al., 2000; Xin et al., 2013).

In a recent conducted study by Yang et al. (2017), rabies virus glycoprotein modified exosomes were employed to achieve neuron-specific delivery of miR-124 across the blood–brain barrier. Previously, invasive cerebral administration of miR-124, a regulator of neurogenesis (Makeyev et al., 2007; Cheng et al., 2009; Åkerblom et al., 2012), was reported to reduce infarct area and improve neuronal survival against ischemic injury in mice (Liu et al., 2011; Doeppner et al., 2013). In the study conducted by Yang et al. (2017), rabies virus glycoprotein exosomes effectively carried miR-124 to neurons of the ischemic region and supported neuronal identity of cortical neural progenitors and reduced ischemic cortical injury by robust neurogenesis. Thus the above evidence supports the therapeutic potential to ameliorate neuronal injury by exploiting the neurodevelopmental function of miRNAs.

Additionally, in concordance with Xin et al. (2012, 2013), MSC derived exosomes provide a therapeutically viable delivery of gene drugs to the brain and possibly specific cells across the blood–brain barrier. Since MSCs produce an abundant source of extracellular vesicles that contain a selection of miRNAs with the potential to elicit neuroprotective biological processes in response to injury, including the ability to modulate the action of neighboring cells, it seems worthwhile to investigate whether MSC-extracellular vesicles would be a promising therapy to promote neurological functional recovery in the developing brain following injury. Indeed, recent *in vivo* investigations using animal models of perinatal and neonatal brain injury support their application (Drommelschmidt et al., 2017); however, further investigations are required to characterize what specific miRNA profiles potentially contribute to protection.

Finally, it is pertinent to mention that exosomes/extracellular vesicles, viewed as potent vehicles by which to deliver potentially therapeutic miRNAs to the brain, can equally participate in the pathophysiological processes of blood-CSF-brain-communication. Recent studies undertaken in both an *in vivo*, *in vitro*, and *ex vivo* mouse model of endotoxemia have shown that miRNA-containing extracellular vesicles originating from the choroid plexus epithelium can enter brain parenchymal cells and via astrocytic and microglial processes induce miRNA target repression and inflammatory gene expression (Balusu et al., 2016). The transfer of potentially adverse proinflammatory driven extracellular vesicle-derived miRNAs to the brain via this route of communication would seem of considerable importance for the advancement of our understanding of the pathophysiological mechanisms of intrauterine infection-related preterm brain injury (Dammann and Leviton, 1997; Malaeb and Dammann, 2009), including the role of placental vesicle-derived miRNAs (Ilekis et al., 2016; Wei et al., 2017; Salomon et al., 2018) in this process and warrants further investigation.

CONCLUSION AND FUTURE DIRECTIONS

In the past decade, numerous articles have been published on the role of miRNAs within the brain. As post-transcriptional regulators of gene expression, miRNAs most definitely play a crucial role in the development of the brain. Nevertheless, research conducted to define their impact on the developing and injured brain is still in its infancy. Given specific miRNAs can exhibit diverse functional roles throughout development and can act synergistically, identification of their precise functional roles is fraught with difficulties. This is particularly relevant when considering adopting specific miRNAs as biomarkers of perinatal brain injury. Thus, careful interpretation of data is required not only in the context of biomarker potential, but also application as a therapeutic strategy since off-target effects can confound the latter. One attractive possibility to ensuring, at least targeted delivery, is the fast developing field of research involving exosome-based miRNA therapies for neurological injuries and disorders. Exosomes are considered a key carrier of circulating miRNAs. Since they mediate the exchange of miRNAs between cells, readily cross the blood–brain barrier and fuse with cell membranes, they hold promise not only as a miRNA biomarker carrier, but also as a means to deliver miRNA-based therapies to the developing injured brain. Clearly, continued developments in this field of research has the potential to enhance future prospects of effectively treating perinatal brain injury especially those vulnerable to premature injury.

AUTHOR CONTRIBUTIONS

KHTC and MF devised main conceptual ideas and outlines and took the lead in writing the manuscript. All authors contributed to the manuscript and provided feedback and discussed the manuscript.

FUNDING

This work was supported in part by the Neurological Foundation of NZ 1519-PG (MF), Health Research Council of New Zealand 18/183 (MF), Cure Kids 3581 (MF), Auckland Medical Research Foundation 1117009 (MF), and the Barbara Basham Doctoral Scholarship - Auckland Medical Research Foundation 1216004 (KHTC).

ACKNOWLEDGMENTS

We apologize to those authors whose excellent studies we have not dealt with within the scope and limitation of this review.

REFERENCES

Akerblom, M., and Jakobsson, J. (2014). MicroRNAs as neuronal fate determinants. *Neuroscientist* 20, 235–242. doi: 10.1177/1073858413497265

Åkerblom, M., Sachdeva, R., Barde, I., Verp, S., Gentner, B., Trono, D., et al. (2012). MicroRNA-124 is a subventricular zone neuronal fate determinant. *J. Neurosci.* 32, 8879–8889. doi: 10.1523/JNEUROSCI.0558-12.2012

Akerblom, M., Sachdeva, R., Quintino, L., Wettergren, E. E., Chapman, K. Z., Manfre, G., et al. (2013). Visualization and genetic modification of resident brain microglia using lentiviral vectors regulated by microRNA-9. *Nat. Commun.* 4:1770. doi: 10.1038/ncomms2801

Andersson, T., Rahman, S., Sansom, S. N., Alsio, J. M., Kaneda, M., Smith, J., et al. (2010). Reversible block of mouse neural stem cell differentiation in the absence of dicer and microRNAs. *PLoS One* 5:e13453. doi: 10.1371/journal.pone.0013453

Ashhab, M. U., Omran, A., Kong, H., Gan, N., He, F., Peng, J., et al. (2013). Expressions of tumor necrosis factor alpha and microRNA-155 in immature rat model of status epilepticus and children with mesial temporal lobe epilepsy. *J. Mol. Neurosci.* 51, 950–958. doi: 10.1007/s12031-013-0013-9

Baburamani, A. A., Supramaniam, V. G., Hagberg, H., and Mallard, C. (2014). Microglia toxicity in preterm brain injury. *Reprod. Toxicol.* 48, 106–112. doi: 10.1016/j.reprotox.2014.04.002

Back, S. A., Luo, N. L., Borenstein, N. S., Volpe, J. J., and Kinney, H. C. (2002). Arrested oligodendrocyte lineage progression during human cerebral white matter development: dissociation between the timing of progenitor differentiation and myelinogenesis. *J. Neuropathol. Exp. Neurol.* 61, 197–211. doi: 10.1093/jnen/61.2.197

Back, S. A., and Miller, S. P. (2014). Brain injury in premature neonates: a primary cerebral dysmaturation disorder? *Ann. Neurol.* 75, 469–486. doi: 10.1002/ana.24132

Bak, M., Silahtaroglu, A., Moller, M., Christensen, M., Rath, M. F., Skryabin, B., et al. (2008). MicroRNA expression in the adult mouse central nervous system. *RNA* 14, 432–444. doi: 10.1261/rna.783108

Baltimore, D., Boldin, M. P., O'Connell, R. M., Rao, D. S., and Taganov, K. D. (2008). MicroRNAs: new regulators of immune cell development and function. *Nat. Immunol.* 9, 839–845. doi: 10.1038/ni.f.209

Balusu, S., Van Wonterghem, E., De Rycke, R., Raemdonck, K., Stremersch, S., Gevaert, K., et al. (2016). Identification of a novel mechanism of blood-brain communication during peripheral inflammation via choroid plexus-derived extracellular vesicles. *EMBO Mol. Med.* 8, 1162–1183. doi: 10.15252/emmm.201606271

Barca-Mayo, O., and Lu, Q. R. (2012). Fine-tuning oligodendrocyte development by microRNAs. *Front. Neurosci.* 6:13. doi: 10.3389/fnins.2012.00013

Barres, B. A., Lazar, M. A., and Raff, M. C. (1994). A novel role for thyroid hormone, glucocorticoids and retinoic acid in timing oligodendrocyte development. *Development* 120, 1097–1108.

Bartel, D. P. (2009). MicroRNAs: target recognition and regulatory functions. *Cell* 136, 215–233. doi: 10.1016/j.cell.2009.01.002

Bernstein, E., Kim, S. Y., Carmell, M. A., Murchison, E. P., Alcorn, H., Li, M. Z., et al. (2003). Dicer is essential for mouse development. *Nat. Genet.* 35, 215–217. doi: 10.1038/ng1253

Bhalala, O. G., Srikanth, M., and Kessler, J. A. (2013). The emerging roles of microRNAs in CNS injuries. *Nat. Rev. Neurol.* 9, 328–339. doi: 10.1038/nrneurol.2013.67

Bian, S., Hong, J., Li, Q., Schebelle, L., Pollock, A., Knauss, J. L., et al. (2013). MicroRNA cluster miR-17-92 regulates neural stem cell expansion and transition to intermediate progenitors in the developing mouse neocortex. *Cell Rep.* 3, 1398–1406. doi: 10.1016/j.celrep.2013.03.037

Birch, D., Britt, B. C., Dukes, S. C., Kessler, J. A., and Dizon, M. L. (2014). MicroRNAs participate in the murine oligodendroglial response to perinatal hypoxia-ischemia. *Pediatr. Res.* 76, 334–340. doi: 10.1038/pr.2014.104

Brett, J. O., Renault, V. M., Rafalski, V. A., Webb, A. E., and Brunet, A. (2011). The microRNA cluster miR-106b~25 regulates adult neural stem/progenitor cell proliferation and neuronal differentiation. *Aging* 3, 108–124. doi: 10.18632/aging.100285

Buller, B., Chopp, M., Ueno, Y., Zhang, L., Zhang, R. L., Morris, D., et al. (2012). Regulation of serum response factor by miRNA-200 and miRNA-9 modulates oligodendrocyte progenitor cell differentiation. *Glia* 60, 1906–1914. doi: 10.1002/glia.22406

Buser, J. R., Maire, J., Riddle, A., Gong, X., Nguyen, T., Nelson, K., et al. (2012). Arrested preoligodendrocyte maturation contributes to myelination failure in premature infants. *Ann. Neurol.* 71, 93–109. doi: 10.1002/ana.22627

Butovsky, O., Jedrychowski, M. P., Cialic, R., Krasemann, S., Murugaiyan, G., Fanek, Z., et al. (2015). Targeting miR-155 restores abnormal microglia and attenuates disease in SOD1 mice. *Ann. Neurol.* 77, 75–99. doi: 10.1002/ana.24304

Caballero-Garrido, E., Pena-Philippides, J.C., Lordkipanidze, T., Bragin, D., Yang, Y., Erhardt, E.B., et al. (2015). In vivo inhibition of miR-155 promotes recovery after experimental mouse stroke. *J. Neurosci.* 35, 12446–12464. doi: 10.1523/JNEUROSCI.1641-15.2015

Cai, Q., Wang, T., Yang, W.-J., and Fen, X. (2016). Protective mechanisms of microRNA-27a against oxygen-glucose deprivation-induced injuries in hippocampal neurons. *Neural Regen. Res.* 11:1285. doi: 10.4103/1673-5374.189194

Cao, X., Yeo, G., Muotri, A. R., Kuwabara, T., and Gage, F. H. (2006). Noncoding RNAs in the mammalian central nervous system. *Annu. Rev. Neurosci.* 29, 77–103. doi: 10.1146/annurev.neuro.29.051605.112839

Cardoso, A. L., Guedes, J. R., Pereira de Almeida, L., and Pedroso de Lima, M. C. (2012). miR-155 modulates microglia-mediated immune response by down-regulating SOCS-1 and promoting cytokine and nitric oxide production. *Immunology* 135, 73–88. doi: 10.1111/j.1365-2567.2011.03514.x

Chan, S. Y., and Loscalzo, J. (2010). MicroRNA-210: a unique and pleiotropic hypoxamir. *Cell Cycle* 9, 1072–1083. doi: 10.4161/cc.9.6.11006

Chan, Y. C., Banerjee, J., Choi, S. Y., and Sen, C. K. (2012). miR-210: the master hypoxamir. *Microcirculation* 19, 215–223. doi: 10.1111/j.1549-8719.2011.00154.x

Chen, F., Du, Y., Esposito, E., Liu, Y., Guo, S., Wang, X., et al. (2015). Effects of focal cerebral ischemia on exosomal versus serum miR126. *Transl. Stroke Res.* 6, 478–484. doi: 10.1007/s12975-015-0429-3

Chen, H., and Yang, T. T. (2015). Expression and significance of serum miRNA-21 control HIF-1a in newborn with asphyxia. *Chin. J. Child Health Care* 23, 32–34.

Chen, J., Liu, Z., and Yang, Y. (2014). In vitro screening of LPS-induced miRNAs in leukocytes derived from cord blood and their possible roles in regulating TLR signals. *Pediatr. Res.* 75, 595–602. doi: 10.1038/pr.2014.18

Chen, Q., Xu, J., Li, L., Li, H., Mao, S., Zhang, F., et al. (2014). MicroRNA-23a/b and microRNA-27a/b suppress Apaf-1 protein and alleviate hypoxia-induced neuronal apoptosis. *Cell Death Dis.* 5:e1132. doi: 10.1038/cddis.2014.92

Chen, T. S., Lai, R. C., Lee, M. M., Choo, A. B. H., Lee, C. N., and Lim, S. K. (2009). Mesenchymal stem cell secretes microparticles enriched in pre-microRNAs. *Nucleic Acids Res.* 38, 215–224. doi: 10.1093/nar/gkp857

Chen, W., and Qin, C. (2015). General hallmarks of microRNAs in brain evolution and development. *RNA Biol.* 12, 701–708. doi: 10.1080/15476286.2015.1048954

Chen, Y., Song, Y., Huang, J., Qu, M., Zhang, Y., Geng, J., et al. (2017). Increased circulating exosomal miRNA-223 is associated with acute ischemic stroke. *Front. Neurol.* 8:57. doi: 10.3389/fneur.2017.00057

Cheng, L., Sharples, R. A., Scicluna, B. J., and Hill, A. F. (2014). Exosomes provide a protective and enriched source of miRNA for biomarker profiling compared to intracellular and cell-free blood. *J. Extracell. Vesicles* 3:10.3402/jev.v3.23743. doi: 10.3402/jev.v3.23743

Cheng, L.-C., Pastrana, E., Tavazoie, M., and Doetsch, F. (2009). miR-124 regulates adult neurogenesis in the subventricular zone stem cell niche. *Nat. Neurosci.* 12:399. doi: 10.1038/nn.2294

Cherubini, E., Gustincich, S., and Robinson, H. (2006). The mammalian transcriptome and the cellular complexity of the brain. *J. Physiol.* 575(Pt 2), 319–320. doi: 10.1113/jphysiol.2006.118364

Chiva-Blanch, G., Suades, R., Crespo, J., Pena, E., Padro, T., Jimenez-Xarrie, E., et al. (2016). Microparticle shedding from neural progenitor cells and vascular compartment cells is increased in ischemic stroke. *PLoS One* 11:e0148176. doi: 10.1371/journal.pone.0148176

Chow, L. C., Soliman, A., Zandian, M., Danielpour, M., and Krueger, R. C. Jr (2005). Accumulation of transforming growth factor-β2 and nitrated chondroitin sulfate proteoglycans in cerebrospinal fluid correlates with poor neurologic outcome in preterm hydrocephalus. *Neonatology* 88, 1–11. doi: 10.1159/000083945

Clovis, Y. M., Enard, W., Marinaro, F., Huttner, W. B., and De Pietri Tonelli, D. (2012). Convergent repression of Foxp2 3′UTR by miR-9 and miR-132 in embryonic mouse neocortex: implications for radial migration of neurons. *Development* 139, 3332–3342. doi: 10.1242/dev.078063

Concepcion, C. P., Bonetti, C., and Ventura, A. (2012). The microRNA-17-92 family of microRNA clusters in development and disease. *Cancer J.* 18, 262–267. doi: 10.1097/PPO.0b013e318258b60a

Contreras-Naranjo, J. C., Wu, H. J., and Ugaz, V. M. (2017). Microfluidics for exosome isolation and analysis: enabling liquid biopsy for personalized medicine. *Lab. Chip* 17, 3558–3577. doi: 10.1039/c7lc00592j

Coolen, M., Katz, S., and Bally-Cuif, L. (2013). miR-9: a versatile regulator of neurogenesis. *Front. Cell Neurosci.* 7:220. doi: 10.3389/fncel.2013.00220

Dajas-Bailador, F., Bonev, B., Garcez, P., Stanley, P., Guillemot, F., and Papalopulu, N. (2012). microRNA-9 regulates axon extension and branching by targeting Map1b in mouse cortical neurons. *Nat. Neurosci.* doi: 10.1038/nn.3082 [Epub ahead of print].

Dammann, O., and Leviton, A. (1997). Maternal intrauterine infection, cytokines, and brain damage in the preterm newborn. *Pediatr. Res.* 42, 1–8. doi: 10.1203/00006450-199707000-00001

Davis, G. M., Haas, M. A., and Pocock, R. (2015). MicroRNAs: not "fine-tuners" but key regulators of neuronal development and function. *Front. Neurol.* 6:245. doi: 10.3389/fneur.2015.00245

Davis, T. H., Cuellar, T. L., Koch, S. M., Barker, A. J., Harfe, B. D., McManus, M. T., et al. (2008). Conditional loss of Dicer disrupts cellular and tissue morphogenesis in the cortex and hippocampus. *J. Neurosci.* 28, 4322–4330. doi: 10.1523/JNEUROSCI.4815-07.2008

De Pietri Tonelli, D., Pulvers, J. N., Haffner, C., Murchison, E. P., Hannon, G. J., and Huttner, W. B. (2008). miRNAs are essential for survival and differentiation of newborn neurons but not for expansion of neural progenitors during early neurogenesis in the mouse embryonic neocortex. *Development* 135, 3911–3921. doi: 10.1242/dev.025080

Dean, J. M., McClendon, E., Hansen, K., Azimi-Zonooz, A., Chen, K., Riddle, A., et al. (2013). Prenatal cerebral ischemia disrupts MRI-defined cortical microstructure through disturbances in neuronal arborization. *Sci. Transl. Med.* 5:168ra167. doi: 10.1126/scitranslmed.3004669

Dean, J. M., Van De Looij, Y., Sizonenko, S. V., Lodygensky, G. A., Lazeyras, F., Bolouri, H., et al. (2011). Delayed cortical impairment following lipopolysaccharide exposure in preterm fetal sheep. *Ann. Neurol.* 70, 846–856. doi: 10.1002/ana.22480

Delaloy, C., Liu, L., Lee, J. A., Su, H., Shen, F., Yang, G. Y., et al. (2010). MicroRNA-9 coordinates proliferation and migration of human embryonic stem cell-derived neural progenitors. *Cell Stem Cell* 6, 323–335. doi: 10.1016/j.stem.2010.02.015

Dharap, A., Bowen, K., Place, R., Li, L. C., and Vemuganti, R. (2009). Transient focal ischemia induces extensive temporal changes in rat cerebral microRNAome. *J. Cereb. Blood Flow Metab.* 29, 675–687. doi: 10.1038/jcbfm.2008.157

Dhillon, S. K., Gunn, A. J., Jung, Y., Mathai, S., Bennet, L., and Fraser, M. (2015). Lipopolysaccharide-induced preconditioning attenuates apoptosis and differentially regulates TLR4 and TLR7 gene expression after ischemia in the preterm ovine fetal brain. *Dev. Neurosci.* 37, 497–514. doi: 10.1159/000433422

Dillenburg, A., Ireland, G., Holloway, R. K., Davies, C. L., Evans, F. L., Swire, M., et al. (2018). Activin receptors regulate the oligodendrocyte lineage in health and disease. *Acta Neuropathol.* 135, 887–906. doi: 10.1007/s00401-018-1813-3

Doeppner, T. R., Doehring, M., Bretschneider, E., Zechariah, A., Kaltwasser, B., Müller, B., et al. (2013). MicroRNA-124 protects against focal cerebral ischemia via mechanisms involving Usp14-dependent REST degradation. *Acta Neuropathol.* 126, 251–265. doi: 10.1007/s00401-013-1142-5

Doeppner, T. R., Herz, J., Gorgens, A., Schlechter, J., Ludwig, A. K., Radtke, S., et al. (2015). Extracellular vesicles improve post-stroke neuroregeneration and prevent postischemic immunosuppression. *Stem Cells Transl. Med.* 4, 1131–1143. doi: 10.5966/sctm.2015-0078

Douglas-Escobar, M., and Weiss, M. D. (2012). Biomarkers of brain injury in the premature infant. *Front. Neurol.* 3:185. doi: 10.3389/fneur.2012.00185

Drommelschmidt, K., Serdar, M., Bendix, I., Herz, J., Bertling, F., Prager, S., et al. (2017). Mesenchymal stem cell-derived extracellular vesicles ameliorate inflammation-induced preterm brain injury. *Brain Behav. Immun.* 60, 220–232. doi: 10.1016/j.bbi.2016.11.011

Duan, Q., Mao, X., Xiao, Y., Liu, Z., Wang, Y., Zhou, H., et al. (2016). Super enhancers at the miR-146a and miR-155 genes contribute to self-regulation of inflammation. *Biochim. Biophys. Acta* 1859, 564–571. doi: 10.1016/j.bbagrm.2016.02.004

Dugas, J. C., Cuellar, T. L., Scholze, A., Ason, B., Ibrahim, A., Emery, B., et al. (2010). Dicer1 and miR-219 Are required for normal oligodendrocyte differentiation and myelination. *Neuron* 65, 597–611. doi: 10.1016/j.neuron.2010.01.027

Dzietko, M., Derugin, N., Wendland, M., Vexler, Z., and Ferriero, D. (2013). Delayed VEGF treatment enhances angiogenesis and recovery after neonatal focal rodent stroke. *Transl. Stroke Res.* 4, 189–200. doi: 10.1007/s12975-012-0221-6

Eacker, S. M., Dawson, T. M., and Dawson, V. L. (2013). The interplay of microRNA and neuronal activity in health and disease. *Front. Cell Neurosci.* 7:136. doi: 10.3389/fncel.2013.00136

Ferriero, D. M. (2016). The vulnerable newborn brain: imaging patterns of acquired perinatal injury. *Neonatology* 109, 345–351. doi: 10.1159/000444896

Fitzpatrick, J. M., Anderson, R. C., and McDermott, K. W. (2015). MicroRNA: key regulators of oligodendrocyte development and pathobiology. *Int. J. Biochem. Cell Biol.* 65, 134–138. doi: 10.1016/j.biocel.2015.05.021

Fleiss, B., and Gressens, P. (2012). Tertiary mechanisms of brain damage: a new hope for treatment of cerebral palsy? *Lancet Neurol.* 11, 556–566. doi: 10.1016/S1474-4422(12)70058-3

Florio, P., Luisi, S., Bruschettini, M., Grutzfeld, D., Dobrzanska, A., Bruschettini, P., et al. (2004). Cerebrospinal fluid activin a measurement in asphyxiated full-term newborns predicts hypoxic ischemic encephalopathy. *Clin. Chem.* 50, 2386–2389. doi: 10.1373/clinchem.2004.035774

Florio, P., Luisi, S., Moataza, B., Torricelli, M., Iman, I., Hala, M., et al. (2007). High urinary concentrations of activin A in asphyxiated full-term newborns with moderate or severe hypoxic ischemic encephalopathy. *Clin. Chem.* 53, 520–522. doi: 10.1373/clinchem.2005.062604

Fu, Q., Du, Y., Yang, C., Zhang, D., Zhang, N., Liu, X., et al. (2016). An oncogenic role of miR-592 in tumorigenesis of human colorectal cancer by targeting Forkhead Box O3A (FoxO3A). *Expert Opin. Ther. Targets* 20, 771–782. doi: 10.1080/14728222.2016.1181753

Galloway, D. A., and Moore, C. S. (2016). miRNAs as emerging regulators of oligodendrocyte development and differentiation. *Front. Cell Dev. Biol.* 4:59. doi: 10.3389/fcell.2016.00059

Garberg, H. T., Huun, M. U., Baumbusch, L. O., Asegg-Atneosen, M., Solberg, R., and Saugstad, O. D. (2016). Temporal profile of circulating microRNAs after global hypoxia-ischemia in newborn piglets. *Neonatology* 111, 133–139. doi: 10.1159/000449032

Gaudet, A. D., Fonken, L. K., Watkins, L. R., Nelson, R. J., and Popovich, P. G. (2017). MicroRNAs: roles in regulating neuroinflammation. *Neuroscientist* 24, 221–245. doi: 10.1177/1073858417721150

Gaudet, A. D., Fonken, L. K., Watkins, L. R., Nelson, R. J., and Popovich, P. G. (2018). MicroRNAs: roles in regulating neuroinflammation. *Neuroscientist* 24, 221–245. doi: 10.1177/1073858417721150

Gerdoni, E., Gallo, B., Casazza, S., Musio, S., Bonanni, I., Pedemonte, E., et al. (2007). Mesenchymal stem cells effectively modulate pathogenic immune response in experimental autoimmune encephalomyelitis. *Ann. Neurol.* 61, 219–227. doi: 10.1002/ana.21076

Giaume, C., Koulakoff, A., Roux, L., Holcman, D., and Rouach, N. (2010). Astroglial networks: a step further in neuroglial and gliovascular interactions. *Nat. Rev. Neurosci.* 11, 87–99. doi: 10.1038/nrn2757

Goetzl, L., Merabova, N., Darbinian, N., Martirosyan, D., Poletto, E., Fugarolas, K., et al. (2018). Diagnostic potential of neural exosome cargo as biomarkers for acute brain injury. *Ann. Clin. Transl. Neurol.* 5, 4–10. doi: 10.1002/acn3.499

Gotz, M., Nakafuku, M., and Petrik, D. (2016). Neurogenesis in the developing and adult brain-similarities and key differences. *Cold Spring Harb. Perspect. Biol.* 8:a018853. doi: 10.1101/cshperspect.a018853

Griesmaier, E., Schlager, G., Wegleiter, K., Hermann, M., Urbanek, M., Simbruner, G., et al. (2010). Role of p75NTR in NMDAR-mediated excitotoxic brain injury in neonatal mice. *Brain Res.* 1355, 31–40. doi: 10.1016/j.brainres.2010.07.095

Griffiths-Jones, S. (2006). miRBase: the microRNA sequence database. *Methods Mol. Biol.* 342, 129–138. doi: 10.1385/1-59745-123-1:129

Guo, S. C., Tao, S. C., and Dawn, H. (2018). Microfluidics-based on-a-chip systems for isolating and analysing extracellular vesicles. *J. Extracell. Vesicles* 7:1508271. doi: 10.1080/20013078.2018.1508271

Hagberg, H., Mallard, C., Ferriero, D. M., Vannucci, S. J., Levison, S. W., Vexler, Z. S., et al. (2015). The role of inflammation in perinatal brain injury. *Nat. Rev. Neurol.* 11, 192–208. doi: 10.1038/nrneurol.2015.13

Hass, R., and Otte, A. (2012). Mesenchymal stem cells as all-round supporters in a normal and neoplastic microenvironment. *Cell Commun. Signal.* 10:26. doi: 10.1186/1478-811X-10-26

He, Y., Li, H. B., Li, X., Zhou, Y., Xia, X. B., and Song, W. T. (2018). MiR-124 promotes the growth of retinal ganglion cells derived from muller cells. *Cell Physiol. Biochem.* 45, 973–983. doi: 10.1159/000487292

Hisey, C. L., Dorayappan, K. D. P., Cohn, D. E., Selvendiran, K., and Hansford, D. J. (2018). Microfluidic affinity separation chip for selective capture and release of label-free ovarian cancer exosomes. *Lab. Chip* 18, 3144–3153. doi: 10.1039/c8lc00834e

Huang, X., Le, Q.T., and Giaccia, A.J. (2010). MiR-210–micromanager of the hypoxia pathway. *Trends Mol. Med.* 16, 230–237. doi: 10.1016/j.molmed.2010.03.004

Ilekis, J. V., Tsilou, E., Fisher, S., Abrahams, V. M., Soares, M. J., Cross, J. C., et al. (2016). Placental origins of adverse pregnancy outcomes: potential molecular targets: an Executive Workshop Summary of the Eunice Kennedy Shriver National Institute of Child Health and Human Development. *Am. J. Obstet. Gynecol.* 215(Suppl. 1), S1–S46. doi: 10.1016/j.ajog.2016.03.001

Irmady, K., Jackman, K. A., Padow, V. A., Shahani, N., Martin, L. A., Cerchietti, L., et al. (2014). Mir-592 regulates the induction and cell death-promoting activity of p75NTR in neuronal ischemic injury. *J. Neurosci.* 34, 3419–3428. doi: 10.1523/JNEUROSCI.1982-13.2014

Iyer, A., Zurolo, E., Prabowo, A., Fluiter, K., Spliet, W. G., van Rijen, P. C., et al. (2012). MicroRNA-146a: a key regulator of astrocyte-mediated inflammatory response. *PLoS One* 7:e44789. doi: 10.1371/journal.pone.0044789

Jellema, R. K., Wolfs, T. G., Passos, V. L., Zwanenburg, A., Ophelders, D. R., Kuypers, E., et al. (2013). Mesenchymal stem cells induce T-cell tolerance and protect the preterm brain after global hypoxia-ischemia. *PLoS One* 8:e73031. doi: 10.1371/journal.pone.0073031

Jeyaseelan, K., Lim, K. Y., and Armugam, A. (2008). MicroRNA expression in the blood and brain of rats subjected to transient focal ischemia by middle cerebral artery occlusion. *Stroke* 39, 959–966. doi: 10.1161/STROKEAHA.107.500736

Ji, Q., Ji, Y., Peng, J., Zhou, X., Chen, X., Zhao, H., et al. (2016). Increased Brain-Specific MiR-9 and MiR-124 in the serum exosomes of acute ischemic stroke patients. *PLoS One* 11:e0163645. doi: 10.1371/journal.pone.0163645

Jones, L. L., Sajed, D., and Tuszynski, M. H. (2003). Axonal regeneration through regions of chondroitin sulfate proteoglycan deposition after spinal cord injury: a balance of permissiveness and inhibition. *J. Neurosci.* 23, 9276–9288. doi: 10.1523/JNEUROSCI.23-28-09276.2003

Jones, L. L., Yamaguchi, Y., Stallcup, W. B., and Tuszynski, M. H. (2002). NG2 is a major chondroitin sulfate proteoglycan produced after spinal cord injury and is expressed by macrophages and oligodendrocyte progenitors. *J. Neurosci.* 22, 2792–2803. doi: 10.1523/JNEUROSCI.22-07-02792.2002

Kannan, S., Saadani-Makki, F., Balakrishnan, B., Dai, H., Chakraborty, P. K., Janisse, J., et al. (2011). Decreased cortical serotonin in neonatal rabbits exposed to endotoxin in utero. *J. Cereb. Blood Flow Metab.* 31, 738–749. doi: 10.1038/jcbfm.2010.156

Katakowski, M., Buller, B., Zheng, X., Lu, Y., Rogers, T., Osobamiro, O., et al. (2013). Exosomes from marrow stromal cells expressing miR-146b inhibit glioma growth. *Cancer Lett.* 335, 201–204. doi: 10.1016/j.canlet.2013.02.019

Katsumoto, A., Lu, H., Miranda, A. S., and Ransohoff, R. M. (2014). Ontogeny and functions of central nervous system macrophages. *J. Immunol.* 193, 2615–2621. doi: 10.4049/jimmunol.1400716

Khanna, S., Rink, C., Ghoorkhanian, R., Gnyawali, S., Heigel, M., Wijesinghe, D. S., et al. (2013). Loss of miR-29b following acute ischemic stroke contributes to neural cell death and infarct size. *J. Cereb. Blood Flow Metab.* 33, 1197–1206. doi: 10.1038/jcbfm.2013.68

Kim, H. Y., Kumar, H., Jo, M. J., Kim, J., Yoon, J. K., Lee, J. R., et al. (2018). Therapeutic efficacy-potentiated and diseased organ-targeting nanovesicles derived from mesenchymal stem cells for spinal cord injury treatment. *Nano Lett.* 18, 4965–4975. doi: 10.1021/acs.nanolett.8b01816

Kinney, H.C., Volpe, J.J. (2018a). "Encephalopathy of prematurity: neuropathology," in *Volpe's Neurology of the Newborn*, 6th Edn, eds J. Joseph,

M. D. Volpe, T. Basil, S. Darras Linda, J. Adré, J, Jeffrey et al (Amsterdam: Elsevier), 389–404.

Kinney, H.C., and Volpe, J.J. (2018b). "Hypoxic-ischemic injury in the term infant: neuropathology," in *Volpe's Neurology of the Newborn*, 6th Edn, eds J.J. Volpe, T.E. Inder, B.T. Darras, L.S. de Vries, A.J. du Plessis, J.J. Neil et al (Amsterdam: Elsevier), 484–499. doi: 10.1016/B978-0-323-42876-7.00018-1

Koh, S.-H., Kim, K. S., Choi, M. R., Jung, K. H., Park, K. S., Chai, Y. G., et al. (2008). Implantation of human umbilical cord-derived mesenchymal stem cells as a neuroprotective therapy for ischemic stroke in rats. *Brain Res.* 1229, 233–248. doi: 10.1016/j.brainres.2008.06.087

Koh, W., Sheng, C. T., Tan, B., Lee, Q. Y., Kuznetsov, V., Kiang, L. S., et al. (2010). Analysis of deep sequencing microRNA expression profile from human embryonic stem cells derived mesenchymal stem cells reveals possible role of let-7 microRNA family in downstream targeting of hepatic nuclear factor 4 alpha. *BMC Genomics* 11:S6. doi: 10.1186/1471-2164-11-S1-S6

Koniusz, S., Andrzejewska, A., Muraca, M., Srivastava, A. K., Janowski, M., and Lukomska, B. (2016). Extracellular vesicles in physiology, pathology, and therapy of the immune and central nervous system, with focus on extracellular vesicles derived from mesenchymal stem cells as therapeutic tools. *Front. Cell Neurosci.* 10:109. doi: 10.3389/fncel.2016.00109

Kozomara, A., and Griffiths-Jones, S. (2014). miRBase: annotating high confidence microRNAs using deep sequencing data. *Nucleic Acids Res.* 42(Database issue), D68–D73. doi: 10.1093/nar/gkt1181

Krichevsky, A. M., Sonntag, K. C., Isacson, O., and Kosik, K. S. (2006). Specific microRNAs modulate embryonic stem cell-derived neurogenesis. *Stem Cells* 24, 857–864. doi: 10.1634/stemcells.2005-0441

Kulshreshtha, R., Ferracin, M., Wojcik, S. E., Garzon, R., Alder, H., Agosto-Perez, F. J., et al. (2007). A microRNA signature of hypoxia. *Mol. Cell Biol.* 27, 1859–1867. doi: 10.1128/MCB.01395-06

Lagos-Quintana, M., Rauhut, R., Meyer, J., Borkhardt, A., and Tuschl, T. (2003). New microRNAs from mouse and human. *RNA* 9, 175–179. doi: 10.1261/rna.2146903

Lau, P., Verrier, J. D., Nielsen, J. A., Johnson, K. R., Notterpek, L., and Hudson, L. D. (2008). Identification of dynamically regulated microRNA and mRNA networks in developing oligodendrocytes. *J. Neurosci.* 28, 11720–11730. doi: 10.1523/JNEUROSCI.1932-08.2008

Lederhuber, H., Baer, K., Altiok, I., Sadeghi, K., Herkner, K. R., and Kasper, D. C. (2011). MicroRNA-146: tiny player in neonatal innate immunity? *Neonatology* 99, 51–56. doi: 10.1159/000301938

Lee, J.-K., Park, S.-R., Jung, B.-K., Jeon, Y.-K., Lee, Y.-S., Kim, M.-K., et al. (2013). Exosomes derived from mesenchymal stem cells suppress angiogenesis by down-regulating VEGF expression in breast cancer cells. *PLoS One* 8:e84256. doi: 10.1371/journal.pone.0084256

Lehmann, S. M., Kruger, C., Park, B., Derkow, K., Rosenberger, K., Baumgart, J., et al. (2012). An unconventional role for miRNA: let-7 activates Toll-like receptor 7 and causes neurodegeneration. *Nat. Neurosci.* 15, 827–835. doi: 10.1038/nn.3113

Letzen, B. S., Liu, C., Thakor, N. V., Gearhart, J. D., All, A. H., and Kerr, C. L. (2010). MicroRNA expression profiling of oligodendrocyte differentiation from human embryonic stem cells. *PLoS One* 5:e10480. doi: 10.1371/journal.pone.0010480

Lewis, B. P., Shih, I. H., Jones-Rhoades, M. W., Bartel, D. P., and Burge, C. B. (2003). Prediction of mammalian microRNA targets. *Cell* 115, 787–798. doi: 10.1016/S0092-8674(03)01018-3

Li, B., Concepcion, K., Meng, X., and Zhang, L. (2017). Brain-immune interactions in perinatal hypoxic-ischemic brain injury. *Prog. Neurobiol.* 159, 50–68. doi: 10.1016/j.pneurobio.2017.10.006

Li, K., Rodosthenous, R. S., Kashanchi, F., Gingeras, T., Gould, S. J., Kuo, L. S., et al. (2018). Advances, challenges, and opportunities in extracellular RNA biology: insights from the NIH exRNA Strategic Workshop. *JCI Insight* 3:98942. doi: 10.1172/jci.insight.98942

Li, X.-Q., Lv, H.-W., Wang, Z.-L., Tan, W.-F., Fang, B., and Ma, H. (2015). MiR-27a ameliorates inflammatory damage to the blood-spinal cord barrier after spinal cord ischemia: reperfusion injury in rats by downregulating TICAM-2 of the TLR 4 signaling pathway. *J. Neuroinflam.* 12:25. doi: 10.1186/s12974-015-0246-3

Lim, L. P., Lau, N. C., Garrett-Engele, P., Grimson, A., Schelter, J. M., Castle, J., et al. (2005). Microarray analysis shows that some microRNAs downregulate large numbers of target mRNAs. *Nature* 433, 769–773. doi: 10.1038/nature03315

Liu, A., Li, J., Marin-Husstege, M., Kageyama, R., Fan, Y., Gelinas, C., et al. (2006). A molecular insight of Hes5-dependent inhibition of myelin gene expression: old partners and new players. *EMBO J.* 25, 4833–4842. doi: 10.1038/sj.emboj.7601352

Liu, D. Z., Tian, Y., Ander, B. P., Xu, H., Stamova, B. S., Zhan, X., et al. (2010). Brain and blood microRNA expression profiling of ischemic stroke, intracerebral hemorrhage, and kainate seizures. *J. Cereb. Blood Flow Metab.* 30, 92–101. doi: 10.1038/jcbfm.2009.186

Liu, J., Zhang, K. S., Hu, B., Li, S. G., Li, Q., Luo, Y. P., et al. (2018). Systematic analysis of RNA regulatory network in rat brain after ischemic stroke. *Biomed. Res. Int.* 2018:8354350. doi: 10.1155/2018/8354350

Liu, M., Zhi, Q., Wang, W., Zhang, Q., Fang, T., and Ma, Q. (2015). Up-regulation of miR-592 correlates with tumor progression and poor prognosis in patients with colorectal cancer. *Biomed. Pharmacother.* 69, 214–220. doi: 10.1016/j.biopha.2014.12.001

Liu, X. S., Chopp, M., Pan, W. L., Wang, X. L., Fan, B. Y., Zhang, Y., et al. (2017). MicroRNA-146a promotes oligodendrogenesis in stroke. *Mol. Neurobiol.* 54, 227–237. doi: 10.1007/s12035-015-9655-7

Liu, X. S., Chopp, M., Zhang, R. L., Tao, T., Wang, X. L., Kassis, H., et al. (2011). MicroRNA profiling in subventricular zone after stroke: MiR-124a regulates proliferation of neural progenitor cells through Notch signaling pathway. *PLoS One* 6:e23461. doi: 10.1371/journal.pone.0023461

Liu, Z., Wu, R., Li, G., Sun, P., Xu, Q., and Liu, Z. (2015). MiR-592 inhibited cell proliferation of human colorectal cancer cells by suppressing of CCND3 expression. *Int. J. Clin. Exp. Med.* 8:3490.

Long, Q., Upadhya, D., Hattiangady, B., Kim, D. K., An, S. Y., Shuai, B., et al. (2017). Intranasal MSC-derived A1-exosomes ease inflammation, and prevent abnormal neurogenesis and memory dysfunction after status epilepticus. *Proc. Natl. Acad. Sci. U.S.A.* 114, E3536–E3545. doi: 10.1073/pnas.1703920114

Looney, A. M., Ahearne, C. E., Hallberg, B., Boylan, G. B., and Murray, D. M. (2017). Downstream mRNA target analysis in neonatal hypoxic-ischaemic encephalopathy identifies novel marker of severe injury: a proof of concept paper. *Mol. Neurobiol.* 54, 8420–8428. doi: 10.1007/s12035-016-0330-4

Looney, A. M., Walsh, B. H., Moloney, G., Grenham, S., Fagan, A., O'Keeffe, G. W., et al. (2015). Downregulation of umbilical cord blood levels of miR-374a in neonatal hypoxic ischemic encephalopathy. *J. Pediatr.* 167, 269–273.e2. doi: 10.1016/j.jpeds.2015.04.060

Luarte, A., Batiz, L. F., Wyneken, U., and Lafourcade, C. (2016). Potential therapies by stem cell-derived exosomes in cns diseases: focusing on the neurogenic niche. *Stem Cells Int.* 2016:5736059. doi: 10.1155/2016/5736059

Ludwig, A. K., and Giebel, B. (2012). Exosomes: small vesicles participating in intercellular communication. *Int. J. Biochem. Cell Biol.* 44, 11–15. doi: 10.1016/j.biocel.2011.10.005

Lv, Y.-N., Ou-yang, A.-J., and Fu, L.-S. (2017). MicroRNA-27a negatively modulates the inflammatory response in lipopolysaccharide-stimulated microglia by targeting TLR4 and IRAK4. *Cell. Mol. Neurobiol.* 37, 195–210. doi: 10.1007/s10571-016-0361-4

Ma, Q., Dasgupta, C., Li, Y., Bajwa, N. M., Xiong, F., Harding, B., et al. (2016). Inhibition of microRNA-210 provides neuroprotection in hypoxic-ischemic brain injury in neonatal rats. *Neurobiol. Dis.* 89, 202–212. doi: 10.1016/j.nbd.2016.02.011

Ma, Q., Dasgupta, C., Li, Y., Huang, L., and Zhang, L. (2017). MicroRNA-210 suppresses junction proteins and disrupts blood-brain barrier integrity in neonatal rat hypoxic-ischemic brain injury. *Int. J. Mol. Sci.* 18:E1356. doi: 10.3390/ijms18071356

Maiorano, N. A., and Mallamaci, A. (2009). Promotion of embryonic cortico-cerebral neuronogenesis by miR-124. *Neural Dev.* 4:40. doi: 10.1186/1749-8104-4-40

Makeyev, E. V., Zhang, J., Carrasco, M. A., and Maniatis, T. (2007). The MicroRNA miR-124 promotes neuronal differentiation by triggering brain-specific alternative pre-mRNA splicing. *Mol. Cell* 27, 435–448. doi: 10.1016/j.molcel.2007.07.015

Malaeb, S., and Dammann, O. (2009). Fetal inflammatory response and brain injury in the preterm newborn. *J. Child Neurol.* 24, 1119–1126. doi: 10.1177/0883073809338066

Mann, M., Mehta, A., Zhao, J. L., Lee, K., Marinov, G. K., Garcia-Flores, Y., et al. (2017). An NF-kappaB-microRNA regulatory network tunes macrophage inflammatory responses. *Nat. Commun.* 8:851. doi: 10.1038/s41467-017-00972-z

Mastoridis, S., Bertolino, G. M., Whitehouse, G., Dazzi, F., Sanchez-Fueyo, A., and Martinez-Llordella, M. (2018). Multiparametric analysis of circulating exosomes and other small extracellular vesicles by advanced imaging flow cytometry. *Front. Immunol.* 9:1583. doi: 10.3389/fimmu.2018.01583

McKeon, R. J., Jurynec, M. J., and Buck, C. R. (1999). The chondroitin sulfate proteoglycans neurocan and phosphacan are expressed by reactive astrocytes in the chronic CNS glial scar. *J. Neurosci.* 19, 10778–10788. doi: 10.1523/JNEUROSCI.19-24-10778.1999

Meng, Z. Y., Kang, H. L., Duan, W., Zheng, J., Li, Q. N., and Zhou, Z. J. (2018). MicroRNA-210 promotes accumulation of neural precursor cells around ischemic foci after cerebral ischemia by regulating the SOCS1-STAT3-VEGF-C Pathway. *J. Am. Heart Assoc.* 7:e005052. doi: 10.1161/JAHA.116.005052

Michell-Robinson, M. A., Touil, H., Healy, L. M., Owen, D. R., Durafourt, B. A., Bar-Or, A., et al. (2015). Roles of microglia in brain development, tissue maintenance and repair. *Brain* 138(Pt 5), 1138–1159. doi: 10.1093/brain/awv066

Miska, E. A., Alvarez-Saavedra, E., Townsend, M., Yoshii, A., Sestan, N., Rakic, P., et al. (2004). Microarray analysis of microRNA expression in the developing mammalian brain. *Genome Biol.* 5:R68. doi: 10.1186/gb-2004-5-9-r68

Mokarizadeh, A., Delirezh, N., Morshedi, A., Mosayebi, G., Farshid, A.-A., and Mardani, K. (2012). Microvesicles derived from mesenchymal stem cells: potent organelles for induction of tolerogenic signaling. *Immunol. Lett.* 147, 47–54. doi: 10.1016/j.imlet.2012.06.001

Mondello, S., Thelin, E. P., Shaw, G., Salzet, M., Visalli, C., Cizkova, D., et al. (2018). Extracellular vesicles: pathogenetic, diagnostic and therapeutic value in traumatic brain injury. *Expert Rev. Proteomics* 15, 451–461. doi: 10.1080/14789450.2018.1464914

Monfils, M. H., Driscoll, I., Kamitakahara, H., Wilson, B., Flynn, C., Teskey, G. C., et al. (2006). FGF-2-induced cell proliferation stimulates anatomical, neurophysiological and functional recovery from neonatal motor cortex injury. *Eur. J. Neurosci.* 24, 739–749. doi: 10.1111/j.1460-9568.2006.04939.x

Moon, J. M., Xu, L., and Giffard, R. G. (2013). Inhibition of microRNA-181 reduces forebrain ischemia-induced neuronal loss. *J. Cereb. Blood Flow Metab.* 33, 1976–1982. doi: 10.1038/jcbfm.2013.157

Morris, D. C., Chopp, M., Zhang, L., Lu, M., and Zhang, Z. G. (2010). Thymosin beta4 improves functional neurological outcome in a rat model of embolic stroke. *Neuroscience* 169, 674–682. doi: 10.1016/j.neuroscience.2010.05.017

Mueller, M., Zhou, J., Yang, L., Gao, Y., Wu, F., Schoeberlein, A., et al. (2014). PreImplantation factor promotes neuroprotection by targeting microRNA let-7. *Proc. Natl. Acad. Sci. U.S.A.* 111, 13882–13887. doi: 10.1073/pnas.1411674111

Nahid, M. A., Satoh, M., and Chan, E. K. (2011). MicroRNA in TLR signaling and endotoxin tolerance. *Cell Mol. Immunol.* 8, 388–403. doi: 10.1038/cmi.2011.26

Nallamshetty, S., Chan, S.Y., and Loscalzo, J. (2013). Hypoxia: a master regulator of microRNA biogenesis and activity. *Free Radic. Biol. Med.* 64, 20–30. doi: 10.1016/j.freeradbiomed.2013.05.022

Narayan, A., Bommakanti, A., and Patel, A. A. (2015). High-throughput RNA profiling via up-front sample parallelization. *Nat. Methods* 12, 343–346. doi: 10.1038/nmeth.3311

Nayak, D., Roth, T. L., and McGavern, D. B. (2014). Microglia development and function. *Annu. Rev. Immunol.* 32, 367–402. doi: 10.1146/annurev-immunol-032713-120240

O'Connell, R. M., Taganov, K. D., Boldin, M. P., Cheng, G., and Baltimore, D. (2007). MicroRNA-155 is induced during the macrophage inflammatory response. *Proc. Natl. Acad. Sci. U.S.A.* 104, 1604–1609. doi: 10.1073/pnas.0610731104

Ohab, J. J., Fleming, S., Blesch, A., and Carmichael, S. T. (2006). A neurovascular niche for neurogenesis after stroke. *J. Neurosci.* 26, 13007–13016. doi: 10.1523/JNEUROSCI.4323-06.2006

Omran, A., Peng, J., Zhang, C., Xiang, Q. L., Xue, J., Gan, N., et al. (2012). Interleukin-1beta and microRNA-146a in an immature rat model and children with mesial temporal lobe epilepsy. *Epilepsia* 53, 1215–1224. doi: 10.1111/j.1528-1167.2012.03540.x

O'Neill, L. A., Sheedy, F. J., and McCoy, C. E. (2011). MicroRNAs: the fine-tuners of Toll-like receptor signalling. *Nat. Rev. Immunol.* 11, 163–175. doi: 10.1038/nri2957

Ono, M., Kosaka, N., Tominaga, N., Yoshioka, Y., Takeshita, F., Takahashi, R.-U., et al. (2014). Exosomes from bone marrow mesenchymal stem cells contain a microRNA that promotes dormancy in metastatic breast cancer cells. *Sci. Signal.* 7:ra63 doi: 10.1126/scisignal.2005231

Ophelders, D. R., Wolfs, T. G., Jellema, R. K., Zwanenburg, A., Andriessen, P., Delhaas, T., et al. (2016). Mesenchymal stromal cell-derived extracellular vesicles protect the fetal brain after hypoxia-ischemia. *Stem Cells Transl. Med.* 5, 754–763. doi: 10.5966/sctm.2015-0197

Otaegi, G., Pollock, A., Hong, J., and Sun, T. (2011). MicroRNA miR-9 modifies motor neuron columns by a tuning regulation of FoxP1 levels in developing spinal cords. *J. Neurosci.* 31, 809–818. doi: 10.1523/JNEUROSCI.4330-10.2011

Ouyang, Y. B., Xu, L., Yue, S., Liu, S., and Giffard, R. G. (2014). Neuroprotection by astrocytes in brain ischemia: importance of microRNAs. *Neurosci. Lett.* 565, 53–58. doi: 10.1016/j.neulet.2013.11.015

Pandit, A. S., Ball, G., Edwards, A. D., and Counsell, S. J. (2013). Diffusion magnetic resonance imaging in preterm brain injury. *Neuroradiology* 55, 65–95. doi: 10.1007/s00234-013-1242-x

Park, K. K., Liu, K., Hu, Y., Smith, P. D., Wang, C., Cai, B., et al. (2008). Promoting axon regeneration in the adult CNS by modulation of the PTEN/mTOR pathway. *Science* 322, 963–966. doi: 10.1126/science.1161566

Patz, S., Trattnig, C., Grunbacher, G., Ebner, B., Gully, C., Novak, A., et al. (2013). More than cell dust: microparticles isolated from cerebrospinal fluid of brain injured patients are messengers carrying mRNAs, miRNAs, and proteins. *J. Neurotrauma* 30, 1232–1242. doi: 10.1089/neu.2012.2596

Pena, J. T., Sohn-Lee, C., Rouhanifard, S. H., Ludwig, J., Hafner, M., Mihailovic, A., et al. (2009). miRNA in situ hybridization in formaldehyde and EDC-fixed tissues. *Nat. Methods* 6, 139–141. doi: 10.1038/nmeth.1294

Pena-Philippides, J.C., Caballero-Garrido, E., Lordkipanidze, T., and Roitbak, T. (2016). In vivo inhibition of miR-155 significantly alters post-stroke inflammatory response. *J. Neuroinflam.* 13:287. doi: 10.1186/s12974-016-0753-x

Petri, R., Malmevik, J., Fasching, L., Akerblom, M., and Jakobsson, J. (2014). miRNAs in brain development. *Exp. Cell Res.* 321, 84–89. doi: 10.1016/j.yexcr.2013.09.022

Podolska, A., Kaczkowski, B., Kamp Busk, P., Sokilde, R., Litman, T., Fredholm, M., et al. (2011). MicroRNA expression profiling of the porcine developing brain. *PLoS One* 6:e14494. doi: 10.1371/journal.pone.0014494

Ponnusamy, V., Kapellou, O., Yip, E., Evanson, J., Wong, L. F., Michael-Titus, A., et al. (2016). A study of microRNAs from dried blood spots in newborns after perinatal asphyxia: a simple and feasible biosampling method. *Pediatr. Res.* 79, 799–805. doi: 10.1038/pr.2015.276

Ponomarev, E. D., Veremeyko, T., Barteneva, N., Krichevsky, A. M., and Weiner, H. L. (2011). MicroRNA-124 promotes microglia quiescence and suppresses EAE by deactivating macrophages via the C/EBP-alpha-PU.1 pathway. *Nat. Med.* 17, 64–70. doi: 10.1038/nm.2266

Ponomarev, E. D., Veremeyko, T., and Weiner, H. L. (2013). MicroRNAs are universal regulators of differentiation, activation, and polarization of microglia and macrophages in normal and diseased CNS. *Glia* 61, 91–103. doi: 10.1002/glia.22363

Potzner, M. R., Griffel, C., Lutjen-Drecoll, E., Bosl, M. R., Wegner, M., and Sock, E. (2007). Prolonged Sox4 expression in oligodendrocytes interferes with normal myelination in the central nervous system. *Mol. Cell Biol.* 27, 5316–5326. doi: 10.1128/MCB.00339-07

Qiu, J., Zhou, X. Y., Zhou, X. G., Cheng, R., Liu, H. Y., and Li, Y. (2013a). Neuroprotective effects of microRNA-210 against oxygen-glucose deprivation through inhibition of apoptosis in PC12 cells. *Mol. Med. Rep.* 7, 1955–1959. doi: 10.3892/mmr.2013.1431

Qiu, J., Zhou, X. Y., Zhou, X. G., Cheng, R., Liu, H. Y., and Li, Y. (2013b). Neuroprotective effects of microRNA-210 on hypoxic-ischemic encephalopathy. *Biomed. Res. Int.* 2013:350419. doi: 10.1155/2013/350419

Quinn, S. R., and O'Neill, L. A. (2011). A trio of microRNAs that control Toll-like receptor signalling. *Int. Immunol.* 23, 421–425. doi: 10.1093/intimm/dxr034

Radhakrishnan, B., and Alwin Prem Anand, A. (2016). Role of miRNA-9 in Brain Development. *J. Exp. Neurosci.* 10, 101–120. doi: 10.4137/JEN.S32843

Rao, P., Benito, E., and Fischer, A. (2013). MicroRNAs as biomarkers for CNS disease. *Front. Mol. Neurosci.* 6:39. doi: 10.3389/fnmol.2013.00039

Rao, V. T., Ludwin, S. K., Fuh, S. C., Sawaya, R., Moore, C. S., Ho, M. K., et al. (2016). MicroRNA expression patterns in human astrocytes in relation to anatomical location and age. *J. Neuropathol. Exp. Neurol.* 75, 156–166. doi: 10.1093/jnen/nlv016

Raposo, G., and Stoorvogel, W. (2013). Extracellular vesicles: exosomes, microvesicles, and friends. *J. Cell Biol.* 200, 373–383. doi: 10.1083/jcb.2012 11138

Reemst, K., Noctor, S. C., Lucassen, P. J., and Hol, E. M. (2016). The indispensable roles of microglia and astrocytes during brain development. *Front. Hum. Neurosci.* 10:566. doi: 10.3389/fnhum.2016.00566

Repetto, E., Briata, P., Kuziner, N., Harfe, B. D., McManus, M. T., Gherzi, R., et al. (2012). Let-7b/c enhance the stability of a tissue-specific mRNA during mammalian organogenesis as part of a feedback loop involving KSRP. *PLoS Genet.* 8:e1002823. doi: 10.1371/journal.pgen.1002823

Riddle, A., Maire, J., Gong, X., Chen, K. X., Kroenke, C. D., Hohimer, A. R., et al. (2012). Differential susceptibility to axonopathy in necrotic and non-necrotic perinatal white matter injury. *Stroke* 43, 178–184. doi: 10.1161/STROKEAHA. 111.632265

Robinson, S., Li, Q., DeChant, A., and Cohen, M. L. (2006). Neonatal loss of γ-aminobutyric acid pathway expression after human perinatal brain injury. *J. Neurosurg.* 104, 396–408. doi: 10.3171/ped.2006.104.6.396

Roitbak, T. (2018). Silencing a Multifunctional microrna is beneficial for stroke recovery. *Front. Mol. Neurosci.* 11:58. doi: 10.3389/fnmol.2018.00058

Salomon, C., Nuzhat, Z., Dixon, C. L., and Menon, R. (2018). Placental exosomes during gestation: liquid biopsies carrying signals for the regulation of human parturition. *Curr. Pharm. Des.* 24, 974–982. doi: 10.2174/ 1381612824666180125164429

Santra, M., Zhang, Z. G., Yang, J., Santra, S., Santra, S., Chopp, M., et al. (2014). Thymosin beta4 up-regulation of microRNA-146a promotes oligodendrocyte differentiation and suppression of the Toll-like proinflammatory pathway. *J. Biol. Chem.* 289, 19508–19518. doi: 10.1074/jbc.M113.529966

Sanuki, R., Onishi, A., Koike, C., Muramatsu, R., Watanabe, S., Muranishi, Y., et al. (2011). miR-124a is required for hippocampal axogenesis and retinal cone survival through Lhx2 suppression. *Nat. Neurosci.* 14, 1125–1134. doi: 10.1038/nn.2897

Schwab, J. M., Postler, E., Nguyen, T. D., Mittelbronn, M., Meyermann, R., and Schluesener, H. J. (2000). Connective tissue growth factor is expressed by a subset of reactive astrocytes in human cerebral infarction. *Neuropathol. Appl. Neurobiol.* 26, 434–440. doi: 10.1046/j.1365-2990.2000.00271.x

Selvamani, A., Sathyan, P., Miranda, R. C., and Sohrabji, F. (2012). An antagomir to microRNA Let7f promotes neuroprotection in an ischemic stroke model. *PLoS One* 7:e32662. doi: 10.1371/journal.pone.0032662

Sempere, L. F., Freemantle, S., Pitha-Rowe, I., Moss, E., Dmitrovsky, E., and Ambros, V. (2004). Expression profiling of mammalian microRNAs uncovers a subset of brain-expressed microRNAs with possible roles in murine and human neuronal differentiation. *Genome Biol.* 5:R13. doi: 10.1186/gb-2004-5-3-r13

Shenoy, A., Danial, M., and Blelloch, R. H. (2015). Let-7 and miR-125 cooperate to prime progenitors for astrogliogenesis. *EMBO J.* 34, 1180–1194. doi: 10.15252/ embj.201489504

Shi, Y., Zhao, X., Hsieh, J., Wichterle, H., Impey, S., Banerjee, S., et al. (2010). MicroRNA regulation of neural stem cells and neurogenesis. *J. Neurosci.* 30, 14931–14936. doi: 10.1523/JNEUROSCI.4280-10.2010

Shin, D., Shin, J. Y., McManus, M. T., Ptacek, L. J., and Fu, Y. H. (2009). Dicer ablation in oligodendrocytes provokes neuronal impairment in mice. *Ann. Neurol.* 66, 843–857. doi: 10.1002/ana.21927

Shindo, A., Maki, T., Itoh, K., Miyamoto, N., Egawa, N., Liang, A. C., et al. (2016). "Crosstalk between cerebral endothelium and oligodendrocyte after stroke," in *Non-Neuronal Mechanisms of Brain Damage and Repair After Stroke*, eds J. Chen, J. Zhang, and X. Hu (Cham: Springer), 151–170.

Silber, J., Lim, D. A., Petritsch, C., Persson, A. I., Maunakea, A. K., Yu, M., et al. (2008). miR-124 and miR-137 inhibit proliferation of glioblastoma multiforme cells and induce differentiation of brain tumor stem cells. *BMC Med.* 6:14. doi: 10.1186/1741-7015-6-14

Smirnova, L., Grafe, A., Seiler, A., Schumacher, S., Nitsch, R., and Wulczyn, F. G. (2005). Regulation of miRNA expression during neural cell specification. *Eur. J. Neurosci.* 21, 1469–1477. doi: 10.1111/j.1460-9568.2005.03978.x

Smith, B., Treadwell, J., Zhang, D., Ly, D., McKinnell, I., Walker, P. R., et al. (2010). Large-scale expression analysis reveals distinct microRNA profiles at different stages of human neurodevelopment. *PLoS One* 5:e11109. doi: 10.1371/journal. pone.0011109

Steinberg, G. K., Kondziolka, D., Wechsler, L. R., Lunsford, L. D., Coburn, M. L., Billigen, J. B., et al. (2016). Clinical outcomes of transplanted modified bone marrow-derived mesenchymal stem cells in stroke: a phase 1/2a study. *Stroke* 47, 1817–1824. doi: 10.1161/STROKEAHA.116.012995

Stolt, C. C., Schlierf, A., Lommes, P., Hillgartner, S., Werner, T., Kosian, T., et al. (2006). SoxD proteins influence multiple stages of oligodendrocyte development and modulate SoxE protein function. *Dev. Cell* 11, 697–709. doi: 10.1016/j.devcel.2006.08.011

Su, W., Aloi, M. S., and Garden, G. A. (2016). MicroRNAs mediating CNS inflammation: small regulators with powerful potential. *Brain Behav. Immun.* 52, 1–8. doi: 10.1016/j.bbi.2015.07.003

Suh, M. R., Lee, Y., Kim, J. Y., Kim, S. K., Moon, S. H., Lee, J. Y., et al. (2004). Human embryonic stem cells express a unique set of microRNAs. *Dev. Biol.* 270, 488–498. doi: 10.1016/j.ydbio.2004.02.019

Sun, L.-Q., Guo, G.-L., Zhang, S., and Yang, L.-L. (2018). Effects of MicroRNA-592-5p on hippocampal neuron injury following hypoxic-ischemic brain damage in neonatal mice-involvement of PGD2/DP and PTGDR. *Cell. Physiol. Biochem.* 45, 458–473. doi: 10.1159/000486923

Sun, Y., Luo, Z. M., Guo, X. M., Su, D. F., and Liu, X. (2015). An updated role of microRNA-124 in central nervous system disorders: a review. *Front. Cell Neurosci.* 9:193. doi: 10.3389/fncel.2015.00193

Taganov, K. D., Boldin, M. P., Chang, K. J., and Baltimore, D. (2006). NF-kappaB-dependent induction of microRNA miR-146, an inhibitor targeted to signaling proteins of innate immune responses. *Proc. Natl. Acad. Sci. U.S.A.* 103, 12481–12486. doi: 10.1073/pnas.0605298103

Tan, K. S., Armugam, A., Sepramaniam, S., Lim, K. Y., Setyowati, K. D., Wang, C. W., et al. (2009). Expression profile of MicroRNAs in young stroke patients. *PLoS One* 4:e7689. doi: 10.1371/journal.pone.0007689

Taverna, E., Gotz, M., and Huttner, W. B. (2014). The cell biology of neurogenesis: toward an understanding of the development and evolution of the neocortex. *Annu. Rev. Cell Dev. Biol.* 30, 465–502. doi: 10.1146/annurev-cellbio-101011-155801

Tay, T. L., Savage, J. C., Hui, C. W., Bisht, K., and Tremblay, M. E. (2017). Microglia across the lifespan: from origin to function in brain development, plasticity and cognition. *J. Physiol.* 595, 1929–1945. doi: 10.1113/JP272134

Taylor, D. D., and Gercel-Taylor, C. (2014). Exosome platform for diagnosis and monitoring of traumatic brain injury. *Philos. Trans. R. Soc. Lond. B Biol. Sci.* 369:20130503. doi: 10.1098/rstb.2013.0503

Teng, H., Zhang, Z. G., Wang, L., Zhang, R. L., Zhang, L., Morris, D., et al. (2008). Coupling of angiogenesis and neurogenesis in cultured endothelial cells and neural progenitor cells after stroke. *J. Cereb. Blood Flow Metab.* 28, 764–771. doi: 10.1038/sj.jcbfm.9600573

Thion, M. S., Low, D., Silvin, A., Chen, J., Grisel, P., Schulte-Schrepping, J., et al. (2018). Microbiome influences prenatal and adult microglia in a sex-specific manner. *Cell* 172, 500–516.e16. doi: 10.1016/j.cell.2017.11.042

Uccelli, A., Laroni, A., and Freedman, M. S. (2011). Mesenchymal stem cells for the treatment of multiple sclerosis and other neurological diseases. *Lancet Neurol.* 10, 649–656. doi: 10.1016/S1474-4422(11)70121-1

Vaccarino, F. M., Schwartz, M. L., Raballo, R., Rhee, J., and Lyn-Cook, R. (1999). Fibroblast growth factor signaling regulates growth and morphogenesis at multiple steps during brain development. *Curr. Top. Dev. Biol.* 46, 179–200. doi: 10.1016/S0070-2153(08)60329-4

Valadi, H., Ekstrom, K., Bossios, A., Sjostrand, M., Lee, J. J., and Lotvall, J. O. (2007). Exosome-mediated transfer of mRNAs and microRNAs is a novel mechanism of genetic exchange between cells. *Nat. Cell Biol.* 9, 654–659. doi: 10.1038/ncb1596

van Tilborg, E., Heijnen, C. J., Benders, M. J., van Bel, F., Fleiss, B., Gressens, P., et al. (2016). Impaired oligodendrocyte maturation in preterm infants: potential therapeutic targets. *Prog. Neurobiol.* 136, 28–49. doi: 10.1016/j.pneurobio.2015. 11.002

van Velthoven, C. T., Kavelaars, A., van Bel, F., and Heijnen, C. J. (2010). Mesenchymal stem cell treatment after neonatal hypoxic-ischemic brain injury improves behavioral outcome and induces neuronal and oligodendrocyte regeneration. *Brain Behav. Immun.* 24, 387–393. doi: 10.1016/j.bbi.2009. 10.017

Vasudevan, S. (2012). Posttranscriptional upregulation by microRNAs. *Wiley Interdiscip. Rev. RNA* 3, 311–330. doi: 10.1002/wrna.121

Ventura, A., Young, A. G., Winslow, M. M., Lintault, L., Meissner, A., Erkeland, S. J., et al. (2008). Targeted deletion reveals essential and overlapping functions of the miR-17 through 92 family of miRNA clusters. *Cell* 132, 875–886. doi: 10.1016/j.cell.2008.02.019

Visvanathan, J., Lee, S., Lee, B., Lee, J. W., and Lee, S. K. (2007). The microRNA miR-124 antagonizes the anti-neural REST/SCP1 pathway during embryonic CNS development. *Genes Dev.* 21, 744–749. doi: 10.1101/gad.1519107

Voloboueva, L. A., Sun, X., Xu, L., Ouyang, Y. B., and Giffard, R. G. (2017). Distinct Effects of miR-210 reduction on neurogenesis: increased neuronal survival of inflammation but reduced proliferation associated with mitochondrial enhancement. *J. Neurosci.* 37, 3072–3084. doi: 10.1523/JNEUROSCI.1777-16.2017

Volosin, M., Song, W., Almeida, R. D., Kaplan, D. R., Hempstead, B. L., and Friedman, W. J. (2006). Interaction of survival and death signaling in basal forebrain neurons: roles of neurotrophins and proneurotrophins. *J. Neurosci.* 26, 7756–7766. doi: 10.1523/JNEUROSCI.1560-06.2006

Volpe, J. J., Kinney, H. C., Jensen, F. E., and Rosenberg, P. A. (2011). The developing oligodendrocyte: key cellular target in brain injury in the premature infant. *Int. J. Dev. Neurosci.* 29, 423–440. doi: 10.1016/j.ijdevneu.2011.02.012

Wang, J., Wang, H., Liu, A., Fang, C., Hao, J., and Wang, Z. (2015). Lactate dehydrogenase A negatively regulated by miRNAs promotes aerobic glycolysis and is increased in colorectal cancer. *Oncotarget* 6, 19456–19468. doi: 10.18632/oncotarget.3318

Wang, L., Ke, J., Li, Y., Ma, Q., Dasgupta, C., Huang, X., et al. (2017). Inhibition of miRNA-210 reverses nicotine-induced brain hypoxic-ischemic injury in neonatal rats. *Int. J. Biol. Sci.* 13, 76–84. doi: 10.7150/ijbs.17278

Wang, Y., and Yang, G. Y. (2013). MicroRNAs in Cerebral Ischemia. *Stroke Treat.* 2013:276540. doi: 10.1155/2013/276540

Weaver-Mikaere, L., Gunn, A. J., Mitchell, M. D., Bennet, L., and Fraser, M. (2013). LPS and TNF alpha modulate AMPA/NMDA receptor subunit expression and induce PGE2 and glutamate release in preterm fetal ovine mixed glial cultures. *J. Neuroinflam.* 10:916. doi: 10.1186/1742-2094-10-153

Wei, J., Blenkiron, C., Tsai, P., James, J. L., Chen, Q., Stone, P. R., et al. (2017). Placental trophoblast debris mediated feto-maternal signalling via small RNA delivery: implications for preeclampsia. *Sci. Rep.* 7:14681. doi: 10.1038/s41598-017-14180-8

Werner, J. K., and Stevens, R. D. (2015). Traumatic brain injury: recent advances in plasticity and regeneration. *Curr. Opin. Neurol.* 28, 565–573. doi: 10.1097/WCO.0000000000000265

Whitehead, C. L., Teh, W. T., Walker, S. P., Leung, C., Larmour, L., and Tong, S. (2013). Circulating MicroRNAs in maternal blood as potential biomarkers for fetal hypoxia in-utero. *PLoS One* 8:e78487. doi: 10.1371/journal.pone.0078487

Willis, G. R., Kourembanas, S., and Mitsialis, S. A. (2017). Toward exosome-based therapeutics: isolation, heterogeneity, and fit-for-purpose potency. *Front. Cardiovasc. Med.* 4:63. doi: 10.3389/fcvm.2017.00063

Wu, M. L., Zhu, C. C., Qi, Y. Y., Shi, Y. X., Xu, H. N., and Yang, J. R. (2018). [Isolation, Identification and Degradation Characteristics of a 17beta-estradiol Degrading Strain Fusarium sp. KY123915]. *Huan Jing Ke Xue* 39, 4802–4808. doi: 10.13227/j.hjkx.201711077

Xia, H., Cheung, W. K., Ng, S. S., Jiang, X., Jiang, S., Sze, J., et al. (2012). Loss of brain-enriched miR-124 microRNA enhances stem-like traits and invasiveness of glioma cells. *J. Biol. Chem.* 287, 9962–9971. doi: 10.1074/jbc.M111.332627

Xin, H., Li, Y., Buller, B., Katakowski, M., Zhang, Y., Wang, X., et al. (2012). Exosome-mediated transfer of miR-133b from multipotent mesenchymal stromal cells to neural cells contributes to neurite outgrowth. *Stem Cells* 30, 1556–1564. doi: 10.1002/stem.1129

Xin, H., Li, Y., and Chopp, M. (2014). Exosomes/miRNAs as mediating cell-based therapy of stroke. *Front. Cell. Neurosci.* 8:377. doi: 10.3389/fncel.2014.00377

Xin, H., Li, Y., Liu, Z., Wang, X., Shang, X., Cui, Y., et al. (2013). MiR-133b promotes neural plasticity and functional recovery after treatment of stroke with multipotent mesenchymal stromal cells in rats via transfer of exosome-enriched extracellular particles. *Stem Cells* 31, 2737–2746. doi: 10.1002/stem.1409

Xiong, Y., Mahmood, A., and Chopp, M. (2017). Emerging potential of exosomes for treatment of traumatic brain injury. *Neural Regen. Res.* 12, 19–22. doi: 10.4103/1673-5374.198966

Xiong, Y., Mahmood, A., Meng, Y., Zhang, Y., Zhang, Z. G., Morris, D. C., et al. (2012). Neuroprotective and neurorestorative effects of thymosin beta4 treatment following experimental traumatic brain injury. *Ann. N. Y. Acad. Sci.* 1270, 51–58. doi: 10.1111/j.1749-6632.2012.06683.x

Yang, J., Zhang, X., Chen, X., Wang, L., and Yang, G. (2017). Exosome mediated delivery of miR-124 promotes neurogenesis after ischemia. *Mol. Ther. Nucleic Acids* 7, 278–287. doi: 10.1016/j.omtn.2017.04.010

Yeh, Y. M., Chuang, C. M., Chao, K. C., and Wang, L. H. (2013). MicroRNA-138 suppresses ovarian cancer cell invasion and metastasis by targeting SOX4 and HIF-1alpha. *Int. J. Cancer* 133, 867–878. doi: 10.1002/ijc.28086

Yeo, R. W., Lai, R. C., Zhang, B., Tan, S. S., Yin, Y., Teh, B. J., et al. (2013). Mesenchymal stem cell: an efficient mass producer of exosomes for drug delivery. *Adv. Drug Deliv. Rev.* 65, 336–341. doi: 10.1016/j.addr.2012.07.001

Yin, K.-J., Hamblin, M., and Eugene Chen, Y. (2015). Angiogenesis-regulating microRNAs and ischemic stroke. *Curr. Vasc. Pharmacol.* 13, 352–365. doi: 10.2174/15701611113119990016

Yin, K.-J., Olsen, K., Hamblin, M., Zhang, J., Schwendeman, S. P., and Chen, Y. E. (2012). Vascular endothelial cell-specific microRNA-15a inhibits angiogenesis in hindlimb ischemia. *J. Biol. Chem.* 287, 27055–27064. doi: 10.1074/jbc.M112.364414

Yuan, Y., Wang, J. Y., Xu, L. Y., Cai, R., Chen, Z., and Luo, B. Y. (2010). MicroRNA expression changes in the hippocampi of rats subjected to global ischemia. *J. Clin. Neurosci.* 17, 774–778. doi: 10.1016/j.jocn.2009.10.009

Zeng, L., He, X., Wang, Y., Tang, Y., Zheng, C., Cai, H., et al. (2014). MicroRNA-210 overexpression induces angiogenesis and neurogenesis in the normal adult mouse brain. *Gene Ther.* 21, 37–43. doi: 10.1038/gt.2013.55

Zhang, J., Li, Y., Chen, J., Cui, Y., Lu, M., Elias, S. B., et al. (2005). Human bone marrow stromal cell treatment improves neurological functional recovery in EAE mice. *Exp. Neurol.* 195, 16–26. doi: 10.1016/j.expneurol.2005.03.018

Zhang, Y., Chopp, M., Liu, X. S., Kassis, H., Wang, X., Li, C., et al. (2015a). MicroRNAs in the axon locally mediate the effects of chondroitin sulfate proteoglycans and cGMP on axonal growth. *Dev. Neurobiol.* 75, 1402–1419. doi: 10.1002/dneu.22292

Zhang, Y., Chopp, M., Meng, Y., Katakowski, M., Xin, H., Mahmood, A., et al. (2015b). Effect of exosomes derived from multipluripotent mesenchymal stromal cells on functional recovery and neurovascular plasticity in rats after traumatic brain injury. *J. Neurosurg.* 122, 856–867. doi: 10.3171/2014.11.Jns14770

Zhang, Y., Ueno, Y., Liu, X. S., Buller, B., Wang, X., Chôpp, M., et al. (2013). The MicroRNA-17-92 cluster enhances axonal outgrowth in embryonic cortical neurons. *J. Neurosci.* 33, 6885–6894. doi: 10.1523/JNEUROSCI.5180-12.2013

Zhao, C., Sun, G., Li, S., and Shi, Y. (2009). A feedback regulatory loop involving microRNA-9 and nuclear receptor TLX in neural stem cell fate determination. *Nat. Struct. Mol. Biol.* 16, 365–371. doi: 10.1038/nsmb.1576

Zhao, X., He, X., Han, X., Yu, Y., Ye, F., Chen, Y., et al. (2010). MicroRNA-mediated control of oligodendrocyte differentiation. *Neuron* 65, 612–626. doi: 10.1016/j.neuron.2010.02.018

Zheng, K., Li, H., Huang, H., and Qiu, M. (2012). MicroRNAs and glial cell development. *Neuroscientist* 18, 114–118. doi: 10.1177/1073858411398322

Zheng, K., Li, H., Zhu, Y., Zhu, Q., and Qiu, M. (2010). MicroRNAs are essential for the developmental switch from neurogenesis to gliogenesis in the developing spinal cord. *J. Neurosci.* 30, 8245–8250. doi: 10.1523/JNEUROSCI.1169-10.2010

Zhou, J., and Zhang, J. (2014). Identification of miRNA-21 and miRNA-24 in plasma as potential early stage markers of acute cerebral infarction. *Mol. Med. Rep.* 10, 971–976. doi: 10.3892/mmr.2014.2245

Zhou, T., Huang, Y. X., Song, J. W., and Ma, Q. M. (2015). Thymosin beta4 inhibits microglia activation through microRNA 146a in neonatal rats following hypoxia injury. *Neuroreport* 26, 1032–1038. doi: 10.1097/WNR.0000000000000463

Ziats, M. N., and Rennert, O. M. (2014). Identification of differentially expressed microRNAs across the developing human brain. *Mol. Psychiatry* 19, 848–852. doi: 10.1038/mp.2013.93

15

Human Umbilical Cord Therapy Improves Long-Term Behavioral Outcomes Following Neonatal Hypoxic Ischemic Brain Injury

*Tayla R. Penny[1,2], Amy E. Sutherland[1], Jamie G. Mihelakis[1], Madison C. B. Paton[1,2], Yen Pham[1], Joohyung Lee[3], Nicole M. Jones[4], Graham Jenkin[1,2], Michael C. Fahey[5], Suzanne L. Miller[1,2] and Courtney A. McDonald[1]**

[1] The Ritchie Centre, Hudson Institute of Medical Research, Clayton, VIC, Australia, [2] Department of Obstetrics and Gynaecology, Monash University, Clayton, VIC, Australia, [3] Centre for Endocrinology and Metabolism, Hudson Institute of Medical Research, Clayton, VIC, Australia, [4] Department of Pharmacology, School of Medical Sciences, University of New South Wales, Sydney, NSW, Australia, [5] Department of Paediatrics, Monash University, Clayton, VIC, Australia

***Correspondence:**
Courtney A. McDonald
courtney.mcdonald@hudson.org.au;
courtney.mcdonald@monash.edu

Background: Hypoxic ischemic (HI) insult in term babies at labor or birth can cause long-term neurodevelopmental disorders, including cerebral palsy (CP). The current standard treatment for term infants with hypoxic ischemic encephalopathy (HIE) is hypothermia. Because hypothermia is only partially effective, novel therapies are required to improve outcomes further. Human umbilical cord blood cells (UCB) are a rich source of stem and progenitor cells making them a potential treatment for neonatal HI brain injury. Recent clinical trials have shown that UCB therapy is a safe and efficacious treatment for confirmed cerebral palsy. In this study, we assessed whether early administration of UCB to the neonate could improve long-term behavioral outcomes and promote brain repair following neonatal HI brain injury.

Methods: HI brain injury was induced in postnatal day (PND) 7 rat pups via permanent ligation of the left carotid artery, followed by a 90 min hypoxic challenge. UCB was administered intraperitoneally on PND 8. Behavioral tests, including negative geotaxis, forelimb preference and open field test, were performed on PND 14, 30, and 50, following brains were collected for assessment of neuropathology.

Results: Neonatal HI resulted in decreased brain weight, cerebral tissue loss and apoptosis in the somatosensory cortex, as well as compromised behavioral outcomes. UCB administration following HI improved short and long-term behavioral outcomes but did not reduce long-term histological evidence of brain injury compared to HI alone. In addition, UCB following HI increased microglia activation in the somatosensory cortex compared to HI alone.

Conclusion: Administration of a single dose of UCB cells 24 h after HI injury improves behavior, however, a single dose of cells does not modulate pathological evidence of long-term brain injury.

Keywords: umbilical cord blood, behavior, hypoxia ischemia, hypoxic ischemic encephalopathy, cerebral palsy, stem cells

INTRODUCTION

Neonatal brain injury underlies long-term neurological deficits, including cerebral palsy (CP) and other cognitive and behavioral deficits that may become apparent months to years after birth (Vannucci, 2000; Ferrari et al., 2010). A significant cause of neonatal brain injury is severe and/or prolonged hypoxia-ischemia (HI) in utero, at labor or at birth, resulting in a lack of oxygen supply to the brain (Vannucci, 2000). Resulting brain injury is termed hypoxic-ischemic encephalopathy (HIE) which can be diagnosed through routine testing through use of Apgar and Sarnat scores, and MRI, however, the latter is usually performed outside of the early intervention critical treatment window. Because of this, some infants are not diagnosed within the early stages of HIE, thus early intervention therapies cannot be administered (Aridas et al., 2014; Ahearne et al., 2016). Of all neonates with HIE, 10–15% will die shortly after birth, 10–15% will develop cerebral palsy, and 40% will develop other disabilities, such as autism, epilepsy and impairment of cognition, motor abilities and behavioral problems (Cerio et al., 2013). Currently, the only treatment for HIE is therapeutic hypothermia which is effective but also restricted in scope (Cerio et al., 2013) in that treatment needs to commence within 6 h of birth (Chiang et al., 2017), is best applied in well-equipped tertiary hospitals, and is not a suitable treatment for babies born preterm (Bennet et al., 2012). These limitations indicate the need for the development of novel treatment/s, that could be used in conjunction with hypothermia or as a standalone treatment if required. The motor and behavioral impairments associated with HIE may not be diagnosed until many months after birth. For example, cerebral palsy may not be confirmed until 12–24 months of age, when a child is not reaching developmental milestones (Rosenbaum, 2003). It is therefore critical to assess long-term structural and functional outcomes in animal models of early intervention therapies for neonatal HI, with the aim of implementing a therapy that is beneficial for improving long-term neurodevelopmental outcomes.

Human umbilical cord blood cells (UCB) are an abundant source of naïve stem cells that can be easily harvested and feasibly be delivered to newborns within the first day of life, or be banked for later use (Cotten et al., 2014). UCB contains a large population of stem and progenitor cells, including endothelial progenitor cells and haematopoietic stem cells, as well as immunosuppressive cells, such as regulatory T cells and monocyte derived suppressor cells (Torelli et al., 2012; Jaing, 2014). UCB can be administered with little risk of rejection, even when used allogeneically (Maeda et al., 2005). This is partly due to a reduced presence of HLA antigens and, as such, there is a low risk of graft-versus-host disease, when compared to adult-derived cells, such as those derived from bone marrow (Knutsen and Wall, 2000). UCB is already an established treatment option for many conditions and is now under investigation for early intervention (within the first week after injury) in pre-clinical models of neurological injury (Aridas et al., 2016; Li et al., 2016; McDonald et al., 2018). In addition, there are a number of clinical trials underway that are investigating UCB therapy in children and adolescents with established cases of CP, treating months to years after the initial injury. Kang et al. (2015) demonstrated that a high dose of 20 million cells per kg administered to patients between 6 and 20 years old, results in improved motor functions and muscle strength within 6 months of treatment. Min et al. (2013) also showed that patients aged between 10 months and 10 years of age, treated with 30 million cells/kg also showed an improvement in gross motor function and cognitive scores. Data from clinical trials is promising, however, it is still unclear what long-term effects these cells have on behavioral and neuropathological outcomes, particularly following early intervention, when cells are delivered soon after injury.

This study aimed to assess the therapeutic use of human UCB for the treatment of HI brain injury in term-equivalent newborn rats, focused in particular on the analysis of long-term behavioral outcomes, as well as neuropathological outcomes. We hypothesized that a single dose of UCB at 24 h post neonatal HI insult would improve behavioral outcomes, as well as decrease neuronal damage and inflammation in the brain.

MATERIALS AND METHODS

Ethics Statement

All experiments in this project were performed with human ethics approval from Monash Health Human Ethics Committee (12387B) and Animal ethics approval from Monash Medical Centre Animal Ethics Committee A (MMCA/2015/42). Written informed consent was obtained from all participants prior to collection of UCB. All experiments were performed in accordance with the Australian National Health and Medical Research Council guidelines.

Isolation, Cryopreservation and Preparation of Cells

Human umbilical cord blood was collected via the umbilical vein of healthy term cesarean section births (>37 weeks), into a collection bag containing anticoagulant (Macopharma). The patients gave written informed consent for the collection and research use of cord blood. On average, ~125 ml of blood was collected from each patient. Blood was stored at room temperature on a shaker for <72 h before processing. To separate the mononuclear cell population, the blood was evenly separated into falcon tubes, diluted with equal amounts of phosphate buffered saline (PBS; Gibco Life Technologies) and centrifuged for 12 min at 3100 RPM at room temperature (RT), with no brake. The mononuclear cell layer was collected and washed with 20 ml PBS and centrifuged at 800 g at RT for 5 min. 20 ml of red blood cell lysis buffer [155 Mm ammonium chloride (NH4Cl: Sigma-Aldrich), 10 mM potassium bicarbonate (KHCO3: Sigma-Aldrich) and 0.1 mM EDTA (Sigma-Aldrich) dissolved in distilled water] was added to the cell pellet to lyse any remaining red blood cells in the sample. The lysis was stopped after 3 min with 30 ml media [10% fetal bovine serum (FBS), 1% antibiotic, 1% L-glutamine in DMEM/F12; all from Gibco Life Technologies] and centrifuged at 400 *g* at RT for 5 min. The cells were counted using trypan blue exclusion dye (Gibco) with a haemocytometer. Samples were then cryopreserved at an approximate density of 20–50 million cells/ml. UCB cells suspended in media were transferred to 2 ml cryopreservation vials and an equal volume of cryopreservation media [80% FBS (Gibco Life Technologies) containing 20% dimethyl sulfoxide (DMSO; Sigma-Aldrich)] was added dropwise, resulting in a final concentration of 10% DMSO. Vials were placed in a freezing container (Mr. Frosty, Thermo Fisher Scientific) and stored at −80°C overnight. Cells were then moved to liquid nitrogen for long-term storage.

Animals

Animal Ethics, Selection and Welfare

Time-mated pregnant Sprague-Dawley (SD) rat dams were sourced from Monash Animal Research Platform and transported to Monash Medical Centre Animal Facility 1 week prior to birth. They were housed in individual boxes in standard housing conditions in rooms with a 12-h light/dark cycle. The dams were allowed to birth naturally and were only disturbed to count the pups on PND 2–3.

A total of 36 rat pups (from 8 dams) were used in this study. Rat pups were randomly assigned to experimental groups, based on surgery times, to control for any neuroprotective effects associated with prolonged isoflurane exposure. 17 animals were exposed to HI (HI, $n = 11$: 3 males and 8 females; HI + UCB, $n = 6$: 3 males and 3 females) and 19 animals received sham surgery with no HI (Sham, $n = 19$: 8 males, 11 females). Sex of the animal was not taken into consideration when performing analysis.

Animal Surgery to Induce HI

A permanent unilateral carotid artery ligation was performed on post-natal day (PND) 7, followed by exposure to hypoxia, as previously described (McDonald et al., 2018). The pups were separated from their mother and placed on a 37°C heat pad before and after surgery. The pups were anesthetized by inhalation of 4% isoflurane which was maintained at 1–2% for the duration of the surgery. A small incision was made in the neck, and the left carotid artery was exteriorised before being occluded with an electrocautery device. The wound was sutured closed using 6-0 polypropylene suture and isoflurane was stopped. Bupivacaine was applied to the surgery site for pain management. The pups were returned to their dam for a 1 h recovery period. Following this, the pups that underwent artery ligation were placed in a humidified hypoxic chamber for 90 min at 8% oxygen, balanced with 92% nitrogen, and the chamber was maintained at 35–36°C. Control pups underwent a sham surgery, in which the artery was not ligated. Following surgery, they were returned to their dam for a 1 h recovery period and were then placed on a 37°C heating pad and exposed to normal room air for the same duration as the injury group that underwent hypoxia. Following the hypoxic treatment, the pups were returned to the dam for recovery. For the remainder of the experiment, the pups were health checked daily and weighed 3–4 times a week.

Preparation and Administration of UCB Cells

Rat pups received UCB cells 24 h post insult (PND8), via intraperitoneal injection. Cells were thawed rapidly in a 37°C water bath. UCB cells from three different donors were pooled and washed with media to remove DMSO within the freeze media. The cells were counted and viability determined using trypan blue exclusion. Before administration, cells were washed in PBS and resuspended in PBS at a final concentration of 5 million cells/ml. Cells were stored on ice until administration to rat pups.

Pups received 1 million UCB cells (equivalent to 61×10^6 cells/kg) via an intraperitoneal injection in a volume of 200 μl of PBS using a 30-gauge insulin syringe. HI control pups received an injection of 200 μl of PBS only, using a 30-guage insulin syringe.

Behavioral Testing

Negative Geotaxis Analysis

As previously described (McDonald et al., 2018), on PND14 the pups were placed head-down on a 45-degree inclined slope covered with a standard laboratory bench pad. The time taken for them to turn 180 degrees was recorded, and then the time taken to walk ~15 cm up the slope to cross a line was also recorded. This test was performed 3 times per pup. If the pup took longer than 90 s to complete the test, or if they climbed off the board, it was considered a fail and not included in the analysis. No pups were excluded from analysis in this study.

Open Field Test

The open field test was completed on PND 30 and 50 using the Topscan behavioral analysis program to track the movement of the rat. Distance, speed and time moved were recorded for both the inside area and the perimeter of the box. Before testing, the rats were acclimatized to the room for 1–2 h, and the open field boxes were disinfected to remove foreign smells that could influence behavior. For the open field test, the rats were placed in the large open box, approximately 50 cm × 50 cm, for 10 min and allowed to explore the box freely. This test assesses the anxiety behaviors of the rats, as a more anxious rat will spend the time walking the perimeter of the box (Gould et al., 2009).

Cylinder Test

On PND 30 and 50, the rats completed the cylinder test to analyze forelimb preference. The rats were placed in a clear glass beaker and video recorded from overhead for 2 min. The cylinder was disinfected between trials to remove foreign smells that could influence behavior. The videos were then analyzed to assess, upon rearing, how often the right and left foot touched the wall of the cylinder. This test assesses if the HI injury has impaired limb use and caused asymmetric motor control.

Behavioral Composite Z-Score

All behavioral outcomes were converted into a Z-score which was compared to the Z-score generated from the sham group. Z-score was calculated by subtracting the mean test score of the control group from the individual test score, divided by the standard deviation of the control group.

For the negative geotaxis z-score data was transformed from the time to turn and time to cross the line results (**Supplementary Figures S1A,B**) to generate z-scores. For the open field z-score data from average time spent in the center of the box (**Supplementary Figures S1C,D**) was used to generate z-scores. For the cylinder test z-score data from the percentage of left foot touches (**Supplementary Figures S1E,F**) was used to generate z-scores. These Z-scores were summed across the included tests (negative geotaxis analysis, open field test and cylinder test) to give a final cumulative score as an overall indication of behavioral deficits across both motor control and anxiety-like behavior.

Post-mortem and Brain Processing

On PND 50, following behavioral testing, the rats were culled by lethal inhalation of carbon dioxide, followed by decapitation. Brains were collected and fixed in 10% formalin (Grale Scientific) for 3–4 days, then processed and embedded in paraffin wax. For histological analysis, the embedded brains were coronally sectioned in 6 μm slices.

Histology

Gross Brain Morphology

Gross brain morphology and tissue area were assessed with Haematoxylin and Eosin (H&E, Amber Scientific, Australia). For each animal, triplicate slides over two regions approximately 0.2 and −3.3 mm Bregma were examined and data averaged across groups. Images were acquired by Aperio digital scanning (Leica Biosystems, Germany) and the volume of the left (ipsilateral to the injury) and right (contralateral to the injury) hemisphere were measured using Aperio ImageScope (Leica Biosystems, Germany). For percentage tissue loss, the difference in volume between the contralateral and ipsilateral hemispheres over the contralateral hemisphere volume was calculated, using the following formula [(volume of contralateral-volume of ipsilateral)/volume of contralateral], as previously described (Teo et al., 2017).

Immunohistochemistry

Microglia were identified using ionized calcium-binding adapter molecule 1 (Iba-1; 1:1000, Wako Pure Chemical Industries, Ltd., Osaka, Japan), apoptotic cell death was assessed using activated caspase 3 (Cas3; 1:800, R&D Systems, Minneapolis, MN, United States), myelin was assessed using Myelin Basic Protein (MBP; 1:250, Merck, Darmstadt, Germany), neuronal cell counts were assessed using NeuN (1:1000, Millipore, Burlington, MA, United States) and astrocytes were assessed using glial fibrillary acidic protein (GFAP; 1:400, Sigma-Aldrich, Castle Hill, NSW, Australia).

Briefly, brain sections were dewaxed in alcohol (xylene and ethanol), followed by antigen retrieval in heated citric acid buffer. Endogenous peroxidases were blocked by incubating sections with hydrogen peroxide in 50% methanol/dH_2O. The sections were blocked with serum [Iba1 and MBP: 10% normal goat serum (NGS); GFAP: 5% NGS; Cas3: 5% NGS + 2% Bovine serum albumin (BSA); NeuN: 5% NGS + 1% BSA]. Slides were incubated overnight at 4°C in the specific primary antibody. Sections were exposed to a secondary antibody for 1 h (Iba1 and Cas3: Goat anti-Rabbit IgG, 1:200; Vector Laboratories, Burlingame, CA, United States; MBP: Goat anti-Rat IgG, 1:200; Vector Laboratories, Burlingame, CA, United States; GFAP and NeuN: Goat anti- Mouse IgG, 1:200; Vector Laboratories, Burlingame, CA, United States). Staining was visualized using 3,3-diaminobenzidine (MP Biomedicals, Santa Ana, CA, United States).

Coronal brain sections were imaged using bright field microscopy on the Olympus BX-41 microscope (Olympus, Tokyo, Japan). For immunohistochemical analysis, images were acquired at 400×, with three random non-overlapping fields of view analyzed per region, on two non-adjacent duplicate slides per brain, averaged for each animal. The regions of interest examined included the somatosensory cortex (0.2 mm bregma) and the motor cortex (+3 mm bregma). Cell counts (Iba-1, NeuN, Caspase-3) and densitometry (MBP, GFAP) were preformed using Image J (NIH, Bethesda, MD, United States). Quantification of microglia cell types was achieved by classing the microglia as either resting (ramified, with branching projections protruding from the cell body) or active (amoeboid, no projections seen, cell body is round) (Kettenmann et al., 2011). Aggregates of microglia were observed as dense patches of microglia cell bodies and branching projections. All assessments were conducted on coded slides and images, with the examiner blinded to the experimental groups.

Statistical Analysis

Statistical analysis was performed using GraphPad Prism 7.0 (GraphPad Software, San Diego, CA, United States). Statistical significance was set at a P-value of <0.05, and all data was presented as the mean the standard error of the mean (SEM). Parametric data was analyzed using a one-way ANOVA with Tukey's *post hoc* analysis. Non-parametric data was analyzed using a Kruskal–Wallis test with Dunn's multiple comparisons *post hoc* analysis.

RESULTS

The Effect of HI Injury and UCB Administration on Behavioral Outcomes

Behavioral test scores from negative geotaxis analysis, open field test and cylinder test, were combined to form a Z-score such that overall effects of HI and UCB treatment could be compared relative to sham. Non-transformed behavioral data is included in **Supplementary Figure S1**. Regarding negative geotaxis analysis, which evaluates both motor strength and the vestibular reflex, the HI group was the only cohort to show a positive z-score compared to sham, where a positive score is indicative of worse outcomes, but overall there were no significant differences (**Figure 1A**). For the open field test, which assesses anxiety/exploratory behaviors, the same group relationships were observed, but also with no significant differences (**Figure 1B**). The cylinder test assesses forelimb asymmetry, and a significant increase in the Z-score in the HI group ($P < 0.05$, **Figure 1C**) was observed when compared to sham, where the UCB treated group showed no difference to sham (**Figure 1C**).

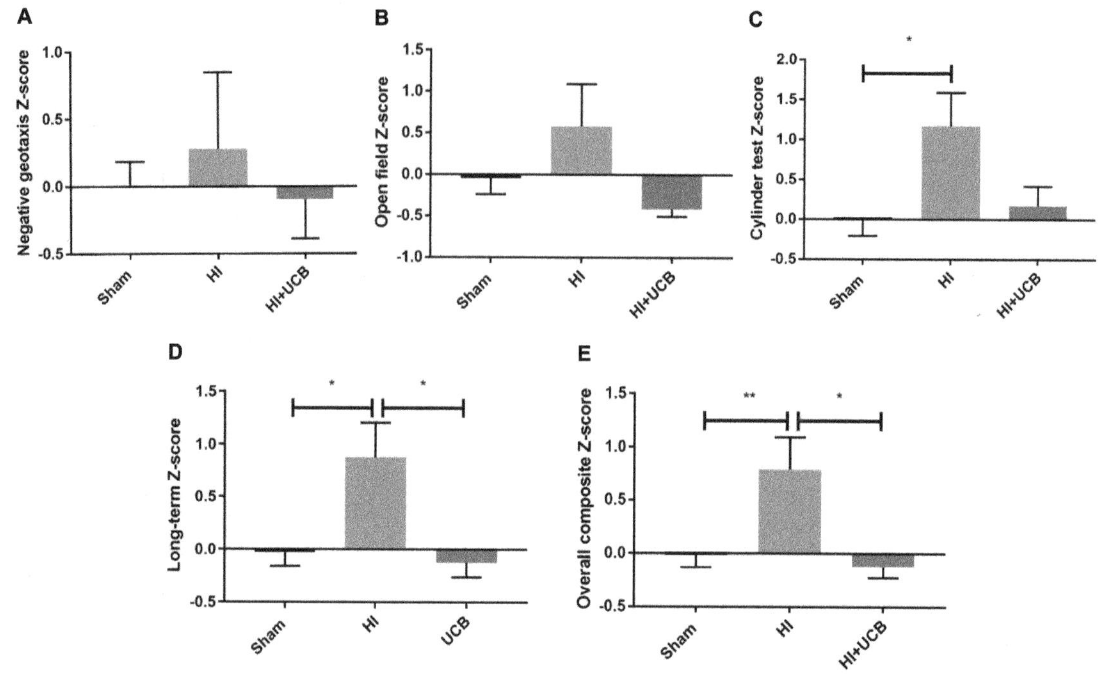

FIGURE 1 | Behavior is impaired by HI injury and is significantly restored following UCB administration. **(A)** *Z*-score of the negative geotaxis analysis at PND 14. **(B)** *Z*-score of overall open field test score from PND 30 and 50. **(C)** *Z*-score of overall cylinder test score from PND 30 and 50. **(D)** A combination of PND 30 and 50 data from the open field test and cylinder test. **(E)** Overall Composite *Z*-score combining data from the negative geotaxis analysis, cylinder test and open field test, from PND 14, 30, and 50 (Data expressed as mean ± SEM, n = 6–19 pups per group, *$P < 0.05$, **$P < 0.01$).

In order to ascertain the long term and overall behavioral burden, a long-term composite behavior score was calculated by combining data from D30 and D50 behavioral tests (**Figure 1D**) and an overall behavioral burden score was calculated by combining each of the individual test *Z*-scores for all behavioral tests (**Figure 1E**). This overall behavioral burden score incorporated motor strength, anxiety/exploratory behaviors and limb asymmetry. For both the long-term composite *z*-score and the overall behavioral burden, we observed a significant impairment following HI injury when compared to sham ($P < 0.05$ **Figure 1D**; $P < 0.01$ **Figure 1E**, respectively). Administration of UCB significantly reduced long-term outcomes ($P < 0.05$, **Figure 1D**) and the overall behavioral burden ($P < 0.05$, **Figure 1E**) compared to HI.

Effect of HI Injury and UCB Administration on Tissue Loss and Apoptotic Cell Death

The HI brain injury and UCB treatment had no effect on body weight over the course of the experiment, compared to sham (data not shown). At PND 50 (43 days post HI) a significant decrease in brain weight in both the HI and UCB groups ($P < 0.05$; **Figure 2A**), was observed when compared to the sham group. This brain injury was further confirmed by the substantial loss of brain tissue in the HI and UCB group, with significant tissue loss in the left hemisphere of the UCB group ($P < 0.05$; **Figures 2B,D,E**), compared to sham (**Figure 2C**). In addition to these morphological changes, we also saw a trend toward an increase in apoptosis in the somatosensory cortex in the HI ($P = 0.06$, **Figures 2F,I**) and a significant increase in the UCB group ($P < 0.05$; **Figures 2F,J**) compared to sham (**Figure 2H**). There was no significant change in apoptosis between groups in the motor cortex (**Figure 2G**). There was no significant change in the number of neurons, seen by NeuN immunohistochemistry, and the white matter density between groups in the somatosensory cortex and motor cortex, seen by MBP immunohistochemistry (data not shown).

Inflammatory Response Following HI Injury and UCB Cell Treatment

The inflammatory response following HI injury involves activation and proliferation of several immune cell types, including microglia (Liu and McCullough, 2013) and astrocytes and while this was thought to occur acutely, there is emerging evidence that the tertiary phase of inflammation plays a role in long-term outcomes (Fleiss and Gressens, 2012). Our results show that administration of UCB cells resulted in a significant increase in activated microglia (Iba1-positive staining) in the somatosensory cortex when compared to sham ($P < 0.05$; **Figure 3A**) and this increase was not seen in the HI group. There was no difference observed in resting microglia in the somatosensory cortex between any groups (**Figure 3B**). When looking at the motor cortex, there was no significant difference in the number of activated or resting microglia in this area (**Figures 3C,D**). In addition, there was no

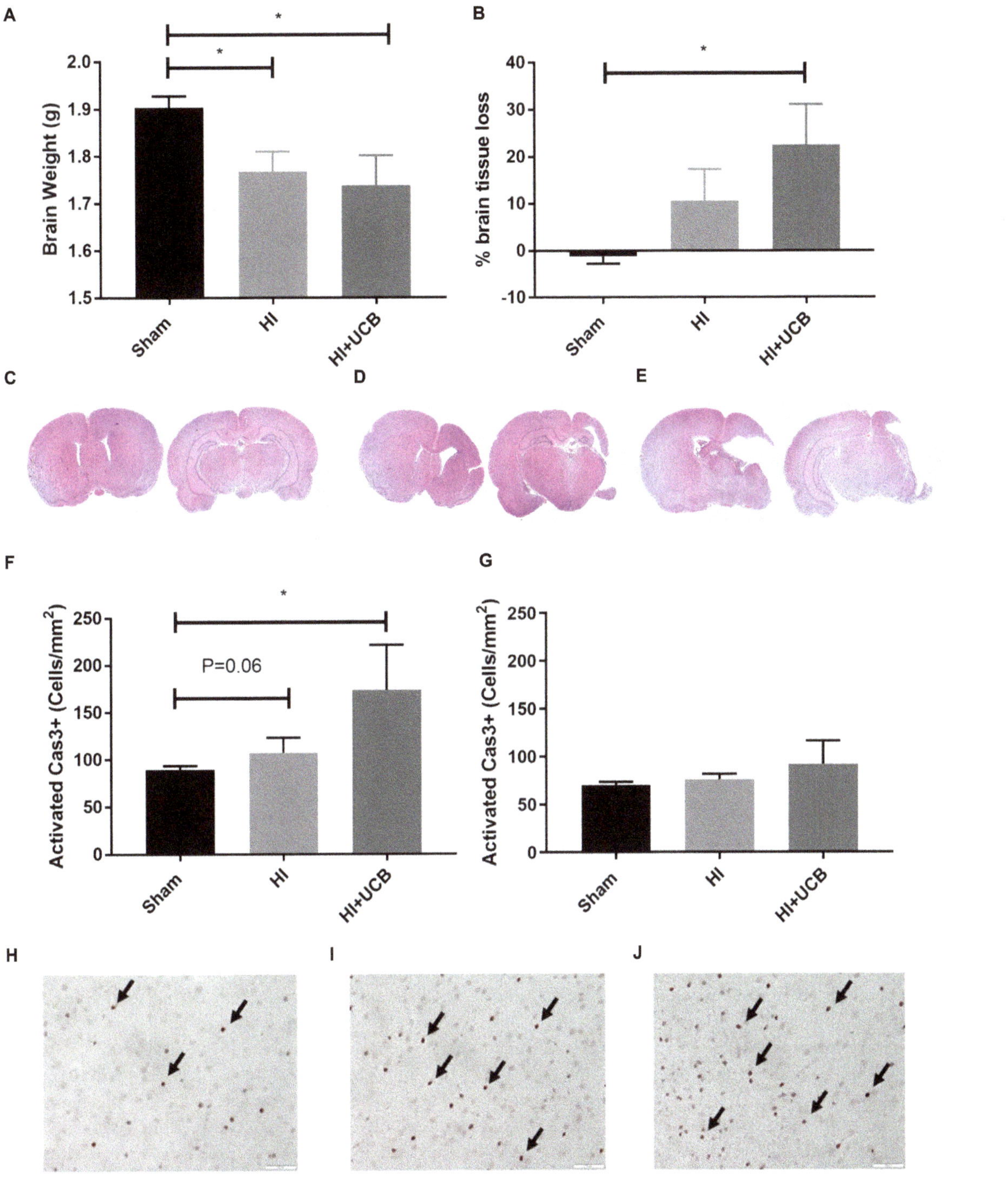

FIGURE 2 | HI injury causes tissue loss and cell death which is exacerbated by UCB administration. **(A)** Brain weights. **(B)** Percentage of left hemisphere volume of the total brain. Representative images of haematoxylin and eosin stained brain sections used for volumetric analysis for sham **(C)**, HI **(D)**, and UCB **(E)** groups. **(F)** Number of activated Caspase 3 positive cells in the somatosensory cortex of the brain. **(G)** Number of activated Caspase 3 positive cells in the motor cortex of the brain. Representative images of Cas3 positive cells (indicated by black arrows) in the somatosensory cortex of the brain in sham **(H)**, HI **(I)**, and UCB **(J)** animals (Data expressed as mean ± SEM, n = 6–19 pups per group, *$P < 0.05$, Scale bar = 50 μm).

significant difference in the number of microglia aggregates between groups in both the somatosensory and motor cortex (Data not shown).

Following HI injury and UCB treatment, we observed no significant changes in astrogliosis, as indicated by GFAP staining, for either astrocyte cell number or percentage coverage in both

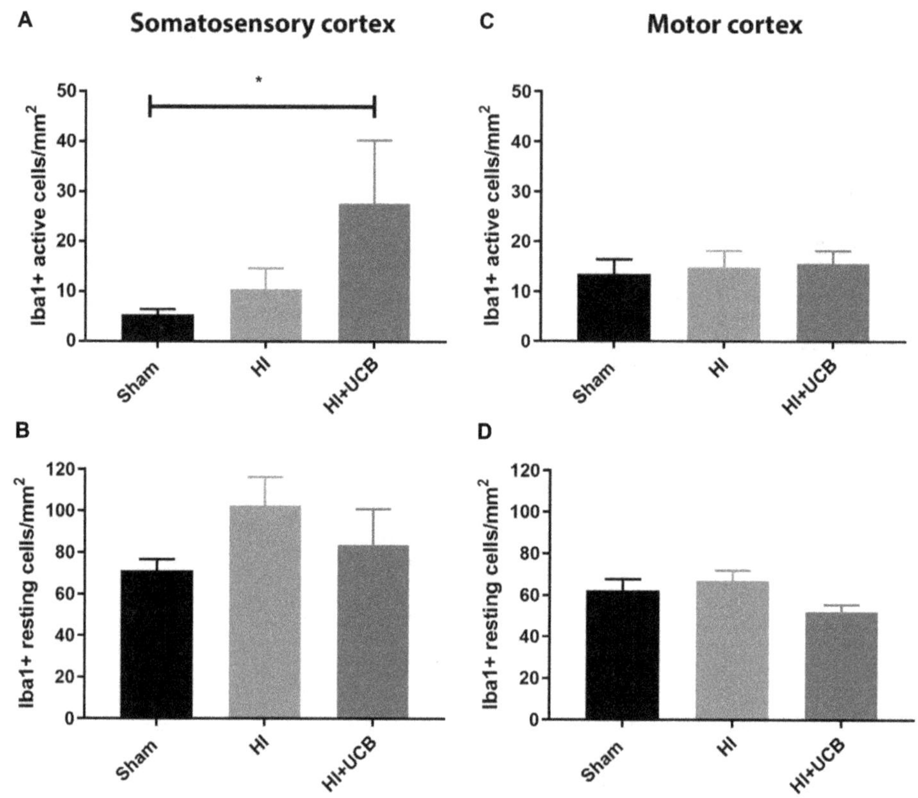

FIGURE 3 | Umbilical cord blood cells delivery increases microglia activation in the somatosensory cortex. **(A)** Number of activated Iba1 positive cells in the somatosensory cortex (SSC) in the brain. **(B)** Number of resting Iba1 positive cells in the SSC. **(C)** Number of activated Iba1 positive cells in the motor cortex (MC) of the brain. **(D)** Number of resting Iba1 positive cells in the MC (Data expressed as mean ± SEM, $n = 6–19$ pups per group, $^*P < 0.05$).

the somatosensory cortex (**Figures 4A,B**, respectively) and motor cortex (**Figures 4C,D**, respectively).

DISCUSSION

In this study, we investigated the long-term effects of UCB administration for term HI brain injury, particularly regarding behavior, and neuropathology. UCB therapy for HIE and CP has been explored in many preclinical studies and clinical trials and has been shown to improve short-term motor function, muscle strength and cognitive abilities (Kang et al., 2015; Romanov et al., 2015; Jensen and Hamelmann, 2016). In addition, we have previously shown that UCB reduces neuroinflammation and short-term behavioral outcomes in animal models (Aridas et al., 2016; McDonald et al., 2018); however, the long-term effects of UCB administration, particularly regarding behavioral outcomes, have not been widely investigated. It is important that these aspects are investigated to ensure that UCB is not only an effective treatment, but that it is also a sustainable treatment that will show benefits throughout the patient's life.

This study shows for the first time that UCB cell treatment significantly improves behavioral outcomes in the long-term. However, contrary to these positive behavioral effects, a single dose of UCB cells 24 h after a HI insult did not mitigate neuropathology. We provide evidence that UCB cell treatment may even exacerbate injury in particular regions, such as the somatosensory cortex where we observed increased tissue loss, apoptosis and microglial activation compared to the sham group. Nevertheless, this potential exacerbation of injury appeared to be region specific and importantly, was not significantly increased compared to the HI group.

CP is an umbrella term referring to a group of permanent movement disorders with associated deficits in cognition, perception and behavior (Novak et al., 2012). These commonly seen impairments highlight the need to investigate a therapy that will not only target injurious mechanisms, such as inflammation, and repair brain injury but will also improve behavioral outcomes. In this study, we standardized and transformed individual behavior scores into Z-scores, which were then combined to create an overall behavioral burden score. This composite scoring method is standard practice in neurological clinical trials to evaluate changes in motor ability over time in patients with multiple sclerosis (Fischer et al., 1999) and Parkinson's disease (Stocchi et al., 2018). Our previous study analyzed short-term behavioral deficits following HI and a single dose of UCB cells and found that 7 days after injury, UCB cells resolved impairments seen in the negative geotaxis test, indicating improved muscle strength and coordination (McDonald et al., 2018). In this study, we

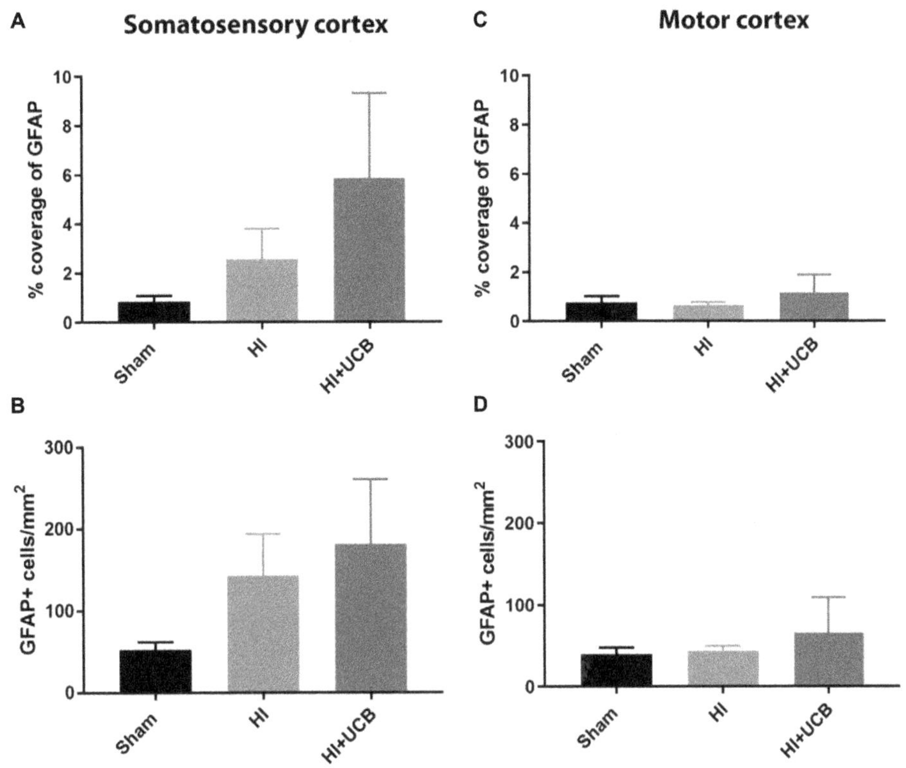

FIGURE 4 | Effects of HI injury and UCB administration on astrogliosis in the somatosensory and motor cortex. **(A)** Percentage coverage of GFAP in the somatosensory cortex (SSC) in the brain. **(B)** Number of GFAP positive cells in the SSC. **(C)** Percentage coverage of GFAP in the motor cortex (MC) of the brain. **(D)** Number of GFAP positive cells in the MC (Data expressed as mean ± SEM, n = 6–19 pups per group).

investigated the overall effects on behavior by examining the functional outcomes at 7, 23, and 43 days post injury and also the long-term subset at 23 and 43 days post injury. These time points were chosen as they correlate to the toddler stage (Colver et al., 2014), pre-pubescent and pubescent stages, respectively, in human development (Bolton et al., 2015). It is important that we look at these timepoints as motor and behavioral deficits associated with CP are often undetected until 12–24 months of age (Rosenbaum, 2003), but persist throughout an individual's life. This study showed that forelimb asymmetry was present after HI injury, which resulted in preference of the left forelimb. UCB administration reduced this asymmetry, where treated animals were mostly supporting on both forelimbs. In addition, the increased composite Z-score for the HI group reveals poor behavioral outcomes and highlights deficits in vestibular reflex, motor strength, coordination, anxiety behaviors, exploratory behaviors and symmetric limb use. UCB administration significantly reversed these behavioral deficits compared to the HI group, thus returning the Z-score to sham level. These results indicate that early administration of a single dose of UCB cells effectively treats motor and behavioral deficits following HI brain injury. These results are consistent with current clinical trial data to show that administration of UCB cells to children with established CP can improve motor function, strength and cognition (Kang et al., 2015; Jensen and Hamelmann, 2016). Given the lack of correlation between our behavioral outcomes and neuropathology, it may be worth considering other neurological tests that may be more relevant in future studies. These could include adhesive removal test and novel object recognition (Patel et al., 2015), however, it has been shown that spontaneous recovery in tests such as adhesive removal test is possible, while deficits in novel object recognition appear to be sustained long-term (Liguz-Lecznar et al., 2014).

Despite these beneficial effects of UCB in restoring motor and behavioral deficits, this improvement was not associated with a decrease in brain injury. We showed that HI significantly reduced brain weight and led to tissue loss and a trend toward increased apoptosis in the somatosensory cortex. Treatment with UCB did not restore brain weight or reduce tissue loss or apoptosis and may even exacerbate injury in specific regions, however, this was not significant compared to HI. Our previous study showed that, when UCB treatment was assessed 6 days after administration, UCB cells recovered tissue loss and reduced apoptosis (McDonald et al., 2018). Together our results indicate a single dose of UCB cells may be able to mediate injury early on, but this effect may not be sustained and as such increased doses and timing of administration needs to be examined. The development of HIE and cell degeneration after a severe asphyxic insult at birth is known to progress over time and is traditionally divided into different phases; the *primary*, *latent*, *secondary*, and *tertiary*. The primary phase of injury, which hypothermia targets, describes the period at which the injury is sustained (Gunn and Thoresen, 2006) and is shortly followed by the latent phase at 6–15 h after injury (Gunn and Thoresen, 2006). The secondary phase of injury is the point at which the majority of the damage is thought to occur, due to the acute upregulation of inflammatory pathways, oedema formation, cell death and breakdown of the blood–brain barrier (Gunn and Thoresen, 2006; Kaur et al., 2006; Thornton et al., 2012). This phase has been shown to last as little as 6 h and as long as 3 days in humans, and is a critical window of opportunity for treatment of HIE (Drury et al., 2010). This is the phase that we chose to target in this study by administering UCB cells at 24 h. The tertiary phase of injury can last weeks to years following the initial insult (Fleiss and Gressens, 2012), and is characterized by persisting brain lactic acidosis, epigenetic changes, persistent inflammation and aberrant gliosis, which may inhibit remyelination and regrowth of axons (Thornton et al., 2012; Hassell et al., 2015). One of the key contributing processes to injury during this phase is persistent inflammation. This inflammation has been shown to impede proliferation of cells in the brain, as well as synaptogenesis (Hassell et al., 2015). These prolonged injurious mechanisms could indicate that only targeting the secondary phase of injury with UCB cells is not sufficient for long term repair of the injured brain, and additional doses of UCB cells during the tertiary phase may be required for long-term neuropathological improvements.

Neuroinflammation plays a crucial role in mediating brain injury following a HI event, and is known to persist for many years after the initial injury (Fleiss and Gressens, 2012; Liu and McCullough, 2013). Despite the importance of microglia in the inflammatory response, there have been very few long-term studies looking at long-term microglial activation in any animal models or human cases of HIE (Fleiss and Gressens, 2012), thus we do not know how the microglia act at these long-term time points, or what their morphology might be. In this study, we showed that 43 days after injury, microglial activation remained increased compared to sham in the somatosensory cortex following UCB administration. This increase was not seen in the motor cortex, and there were no differences in resting microglia in either region. The presence of activated microglia for an extended period after injury indicates that there is either ongoing inflammation or repair; thus, microglia may be either in their classically activated M1 state, or in their alternatively activated M2 state. M1 microglia are pro-inflammatory and are activated in response to brain injury or inflammation (Lull and Block, 2010; Cherry et al., 2014). They are classified by their release of pro-inflammatory cytokines, reactive oxygen species and reactive nitrogen species (MacMicking et al., 1997; Cherry et al., 2014). M2 microglia are anti-inflammatory microglia, and express receptors that work to downregulate the inflammatory response and initiate tissue repair (Varin and Gordon, 2009). We hypothesize that the increase in activated microglia in the somatosensory cortex following UCB administration may be contributed by M2 activated microglia which could be working to activate reparative mechanisms. However, given we also observe increased apoptosis and tissue loss in the same region, this may be incorrect. Further investigation is needed to ascertain the long-term role of microglia following UCB cell treatment.

Our results demonstrate that there was an overall improvement in long-term behavioral outcomes following UCB administration, but this was not reflected in improvement in brain pathology, however, it also didn't exacerbate the injury compared to HI. In our study, the infarct was primarily localized to the somatosensory regions of the brain as is common in this model of injury. The damage to the motor cortex region of the brain was less severe, which may reflect improved coordination, motor control and learning abilities (Kawai et al., 2015), that were assessed with our behavioral tests, which could explain the disparity between pathological and behavioral outcomes. Another reason for this difference, may be that a single dose of UCB may have been sufficient to improve neuronal connectivity, which led to improvement in behavior. In a recent human study investigating the potential of UCB cells for Autism (Carpenter et al., 2019), they demonstrated that single infusion of UCB improved white matter connectivity as shown with MRI. In the context of our model, where there is a significant degree of injury, it may be that a single dose can improve behavioral outcomes, possibly through improvements in connectivity, but is not enough to improve neuropathology outcomes. Further optimisation of this UCB cell therapy is needed. In particular, it is important to explore different dosing regimens and test multiple doses of cells in order for this therapy to be appropriate for use in a human clinical cohort. In light of the new evidence for improved connectivity, MRI analysis of connectivity should also be incorporated into these preclinical investigations.

Limitations of this study include the variability that occurs with the HI rodent model. Despite there being clear injury in the HI group, shown by a decrease in brain weight, there was large variation in the size of the infarct between individual pups in both the HI and UCB groups. This variability was also obvious in the UCB group that had large variations for both microglial and astrocyte analysis. This may be overcome by including more animals to examine these indices in future long-term studies. It is understood that cell populations found within UCB are not always consistent between samples with different proportions of stem/progenitor cells. While we did try to reduce the impact of donor variation by pooling cells from multiple UCB donors before administration of UCB, this is an additional limitation that may have added to variation in the UCB treatment group observed in some of our results. In future studies, it is also important to assess adjuvant cell therapies alongside hypothermia, as hypothermia is the current standard of care in cases of term HIE. Studies by Park et al. (2015) have shown that a combination therapy of hypothermia and UCB-derived mesenchymal stem cells was more effective at attenuating injury, as well as improving behavioral function, than either therapy alone.

CONCLUSION

In summary, we show that early administration of a single dose of UCB cells reduces long-term behavioral deficits following HI.

We also show that, when a single dose of human UCB cells are administered 24 h after injury, UCB cells are unable to reduce indices of neuropathology in all regions of the brain, despite improvements in behavioral outcomes. This study supports the use of UCB as a treatment for neonatal HI brain injury and shows that further investigation into long-term outcomes is needed. Given that a single dose of UCB cells does not prevent tissue injury, it is clear that multiple doses of UCB cells should be considered at different time points, particularly the tertiary phase where ingoing inflammation may still be contributing to injury. By doing this, UCB cells will be able to target both the secondary and tertiary phase of injury, thus maximizing the therapeutic efficacy of UCB cells for neonatal HI brain injury.

AUTHOR CONTRIBUTIONS

TP designed, performed, and analyzed all experiments and was a major contributor in writing the manuscript. AS, JM, MP, and YP performed UCB isolations and animal experiments. JL, NJ, GJ, MF, and SM designed experiments and interpreted the data. CM developed idea, sought funding for project, designed and performed experiments, and interpreted data. All authors contributed to the writing, editing, and final approval of the manuscript.

FUNDING

This work was funded by Inner Wheel Australia and the Victorian Government's Operational Infrastructure Support Program. CM was supported by a National Health and Medical Research Council and Cerebral Palsy Alliance Australia Early Career Fellowship. SM was supported by a National Health and Medical Research Council Senior Research Fellowship.

ACKNOWLEDGMENTS

The authors would like to acknowledge the assistance of the Monash Health and Translation Precinct Histology Platform for their assistance with experiments performed in this study.

REFERENCES

Ahearne, C. E., Boylan, G. B., and Murray, D. M. (2016). Short and long term prognosis in perinatal asphyxia: an update. *World J. Clin. Pediatr.* 5, 67–74. doi: 10.5409/wjcp.v5.i1.67

Aridas, J. D., McDonald, C. A., Paton, M. C., Yawno, T., Sutherland, A. E., Nitsos, I., et al. (2016). Cord blood mononuclear cells prevent neuronal apoptosis in response to perinatal asphyxia in the newborn lamb. *J. Physiol.* 594, 1421–1435. doi: 10.1113/JP271104

Aridas, J. D., Yawno, T., Sutherland, A. E., Nitsos, I., Ditchfield, M., Wong, F. Y., et al. (2014). Detecting brain injury in neonatal hypoxic ischemic encephalopathy: closing the gap between experimental and clinical research. *Exp. Neurol.* 261, 281–290. doi: 10.1016/j.expneurol.2014.07.009

Bennet, L., Tan, S., Van, den Heuij L, Derrick, M., Groenendaal, F., van, Bel F, et al. (2012). Cell therapy for neonatal hypoxia-ischemia and cerebral palsy. *Ann. Neurol.* 71, 589–600. doi: 10.1002/ana.22670

Bolton, M. M., Heaney, C. F., Murtishaw, A. S., Sabbagh, J. J., Magcalas, C. M., and Kinney, J. W. (2015). Postnatal alterations in GABAB receptor tone produce sensorimotor gating deficits and protein level differences in adulthood. *Int. J. Dev. Neurosci.* 41, 17–27. doi: 10.1016/j.ijdevneu.2014.10.001

Carpenter, K. L. H., Samantha, M., Catherine, T., and Lyon, W. C. (2019). White matter tract changes associated with clinical improvement in an open-label trial assessing autologous umbilical cord blood for treatment of young children with autism. *Stem Cells Transl. Med.* 8, 138–147. doi: 10.1002/sctm.18-0251

Cerio, F. G. D., Lara-Celador, I., Antonia, A., and Enrique, H. (2013). Neuroprotective therapies after perinatal hypoxic-ischemic brain injury. *Brain Sci.* 3, 191–214. doi: 10.3390/brainsci3010191

Cherry, J. D., Olschowka, J. A., and O'Banion, M. K. (2014). Neuroinflammation and M2 microglia: the good, the bad, and the inflamed. *J. Neuroinflamm.* 11, 1–15. doi: 10.1186/1742-2094-11-98

Chiang, M.-C., Jong, Y.-J., and Lin, C.-H. (2017). Therapeutic hypothermia for neonates with hypoxic ischemic encephalopathy. *Pediatr. Neonatol.* 58, 475–483. doi: 10.1016/j.pedneo.2016.11.001

Colver, A., Fairhurst, C., and Pharoah, P. O. D. (2014). Cerebral palsy. *Lancet* 383, 1240–1249. doi: 10.1016/S0140-6736(13)61835-8

Cotten, C. M., Murtha, A. P., Goldberg, R. N., Grotegut, C. A., Smith, P. B., Goldstein, R. F., et al. (2014). Feasibility of autologous cord blood cells for infants with hypoxic-ischemic encephalopathy. *J. Pediatr.* 164:973-979.e1. doi: 10.1016/j.jpeds.2013.11.036

Drury, P. P., Bennet, L., and Gunn, A. J. (2010). Mechanisms of hypothermic neuroprotection. *Semin. Fetal Neonatal Med.* 15, 287–292. doi: 10.1016/j.siny.2010.05.005

Ferrari, D. C., Nesic, O., and Perez-polo, J. R. (2010). Perspectives on neonatal hypoxia/ischemia-induced edema formation. *Neurochem. Res.* 35, 1957–1965. doi: 10.1007/s11064-010-0308-y

Fischer, J. S., Richard, R., Gary, R. C., and Reingold, S. C. (1999). The Multiple Sclerosis Functional Composite measure (MSFC): an integrated approach to MS clinical outcome assessment. *Mult. Scler. J.* 5, 244–250. doi: 10.1177/135245859900500409

Fleiss, B., and Gressens, P. (2012). Tertiary mechanisms of brain damage: a new hope for treatment of cerebral palsy? *Lancet Neurol.* 11, 556–566. doi: 10.1016/S1474-4422(12)70058-3

Gould, T. D., Dao, D. T., and Kovacsics, C. E. (2009). "The Open Field Test," in *Mood and Anxiety Related Phenotypes in Mice*, ed. T. D. Gould (Berlin: Springer), 1–20. doi: 10.1007/978-1-60761-303-9

Gunn, A. J., and Thoresen, M. (2006). Hypothermic neuroprotection. *NeuroRx* 3, 154–169. doi: 10.1016/j.nurx.2006.01.007

Hassell, K. J., Ezzati, M., Alonso-Alconada, D., Hausenloy, D. J., and Robertson, N. J. (2015). New horizons for newborn brain protection: enhancing endogenous neuroprotection. *Arch. Dis. Child.* 100, F541–F552. doi: 10.1136/archdischild-2014-306284

Jaing, T.-H. (2014). Umbilical cord blood: a trustworthy source of multipotent stem cells for regenerative medicine. *Cell Transplant.* 23, 493–496. doi: 10.3727/096368914X678300

Jensen, A., and Hamelmann, E. (2016). First autologous cord blood therapy for pediatric ischemic stroke and cerebral palsy caused by cephalic molding during birth: individual treatment with mononuclear cells. *Case Rep. Transplant.* 2016:1717426. doi: 10.1155/2016/1717426

Kang, M., Min, K., Jang, J., Kim, S. C., Kang, M. S., Jang, S. J., et al. (2015). Involvement of immune responses in the efficacy of cord blood cell therapy for cerebral palsy. *Stem Cells Dev.* 24, 2259–2268. doi: 10.1089/scd.2015.0074

Kaur, C., Viswanathan, S., Lin, S. A., and Alamelu, S. (2006). Hypoxic damage to the periventricular white matter in neonatal brain: role of vascular endothelial growth factor, nitric oxide and excitotoxicity. *J. Neurochem.* 98, 1200–1216. doi: 10.1111/j.1471-4159.2006.03964.x

Kawai, R., Markman, T., Poddar, R., Ko, R., Fantana, A. L., Dhawale, A. K., et al. (2015). Motor cortex is required for learning but not for executing a motor skill. *Neuron* 86, 800–812. doi: 10.1016/j.neuron.2015.03.024

Kettenmann, H., Hanisch, U. K., Noda, M., and Verkhratsky, A. (2011). Physiology of microglia. *Physiol. Rev.* 91, 461–553. doi: 10.1152/physrev.00011.2010

Knutsen, A. P., and Wall, D. A. (2000). Umbilical cord blood transplantation in severe T-cell immunodeficiency disorders: two-year experience. *J. Clin. Immunol.* 20, 466–476. doi: 10.1023/A:1026463900925

Li, J., Yawno, T., Sutherland, A., Loose, J., Nitsos, I., Bischof, R., et al. (2016). Preterm white matter brain injury is prevented by early administration of umbilical cord blood cells. *Exp. Neurol.* 283, 179–187. doi: 10.1016/j.expneurol.2016.06.017

Liguz-Lecznar, M., Zakrzewska, R., Daniszewska, K., and Kossut, M. (2014). Functional assessment of sensory functions after photothrombotic stroke in the barrel field of mice. *Behav. Brain Res.* 261, 202–209. doi: 10.1016/j.bbr.2013.12.027

Liu, F., and McCullough, L. D. (2013). Inflammatory responses in hypoxic ischemic encephalopathy. *Acta Pharmacol. Sin.* 34, 1121–1130. doi: 10.1038/aps.2013.89

Lull, M. E., and Block, M. L. (2010). Microglial activation and chronic neurodegeneration. *Neurotherapeutics* 7, 354–365. doi: 10.1016/j.nurt.2010.05.014

MacMicking, J., Xie, Q. W., and Nathan, C. (1997). Nitric oxide and macrophage function. *Annu. Rev. Immunol.* 15, 323–350. doi: 10.1146/annurev.immunol.15.1.323

Maeda, A., Schwarz, A., Kernebeck, K., Gross, N., Aragane, Y., Peritt, D., et al. (2005). Intravenous infusion of syngeneic apoptotic cells by photopheresis induces antigen-specific regulatory T cells. *J. Immunol.* 174, 5968–5976. doi: 10.4049/jimmunol.174.10.5968

McDonald, C. A., Penny, T. R., Paton, M. C. B., Sutherland, A. E., Nekkanti, L., Yawno, T., et al. (2018). ffects of umbilical cord blood cells, and subtypes, to reduce neuroinflammation following perinatal hypoxic-ischemic brain injury. *J. Neuroinflamm.* 15:47. doi: 10.1186/s12974-018-1089-5

Min, K., Song, J., Kang, J. Y., Ko, J., Ryu, J. S., Kang, M. S., et al. (2013). Umbilical cord blood therapy potentiated with erythropoietin for children with cerebral palsy: a double-blind, randomized, placebo-controlled trial. *Stem Cells* 31, 581–591. doi: 10.1002/stem.1304

Novak, I., Hines, M., Goldsmith, S., and Barclay, R. (2012). Clinical prognostic messages from a systematic review on cerebral palsy. *Pediatrics* 130, e1285–e1312. doi: 10.1542/peds.2012-0924

Park, W. S., Sung, S. I., Ahn, S. Y., Yoo, H. S., Sung, D. K., Im, G. H., et al. (2015). Hypothermia augments neuroprotective activity of mesenchymal stem cells for neonatal hypoxic-ischemic encephalopathy. *PLoS One* 10:e0120893. doi: 10.1371/journal.pone.0120893

Patel, S. D., Leslie, P., Amber, C., Alexandra, H., Samuel, P., Eric, A., et al. (2015). Therapeutic hypothermia and hypoxia-ischemia in the term-equivalent neonatal rat: characterization of a translational preclinical model. *Pediatr. Res.* 78, 264–271. doi: 10.1038/pr.2015.100

Romanov, Y. A., Tarakanov, O. P., Radaev, S. M., Dugina, T. N., Ryaskina, S. S., Darevskaya, A. N., et al. (2015). Human allogeneic AB0/Rh-identical umbilical cord blood cells in the treatment of juvenile patients with cerebral palsy. *Cytotherapy* 17, 969–978. doi: 10.1016/j.jcyt.2015.02.010

Rosenbaum, P. (2003). Cerebral palsy: what parents and doctors want to know. *Br. Med. J.* 326, 970–974. doi: 10.1136/bmj.326.7396.970

Stocchi, F., Fabiana, G. R., Kallol, R. C., and Anders, J. (2018). The Parkinson's disease composite scale: results of the first validation study. *Eur. J. Neurol.* 25, 503–511. doi: 10.1111/ene.13529

Teo, J. D., Morris, M. J., and Jones, N. M. (2017). Maternal obesity increases inflammation and exacerbates damage following neonatal hypoxic-ischaemic brain injury in rats. *Brain Behav. Immun.* 63, 186–196. doi: 10.1016/j.bbi.2016.10.010

Thornton, C., Catherine, I. R., Anton, K., and Yasuka, M. (2012). Molecular mechanisms of neonatal brain injury. *Neurol. Res. Int.* 2012:16. doi: 10.1155/2012/506320

Torelli, G. F., Maggio, R., Peragine, N., Chiaretti, S., De Propris, M. S., Lucarelli, B., et al. (2012). unctional analysis and gene expression profile of umbilical cord blood regulatory T cells. *Ann. Hematol.* 91, 155–161. doi: 10.1007/s00277-011-1288-y

Vannucci, R. C. (2000). Hypoxic-ischemic encephalopathy. *Am. J. Perinatol.* 17, 113–120. doi: 10.1055/s-2000-9293

Varin, A., and Gordon, S. (2009). Alternative activation of macrophages: immune function and cellular biology. *Immunobiology* 214, 630–641. doi: 10.1016/j.imbio.2008.11.009

16

Evidence for Sexual Dimorphism in the Response to TLR3 Activation in the Developing Neonatal Mouse Brain

Raul Chavez-Valdez[1], Amin Mottahedin[2], Linnea Stridh[2], Tracylyn R. Yellowhair[1,3], Lauren L. Jantzie[1,3], Frances J. Northington[1] and Carina Mallard[2,4]*

[1] *Division of Neonatal-Perinatal Medicine, Department of Pediatrics, Johns Hopkins School of Medicine, Baltimore, MD, United States,* [2] *Institute of Neuroscience and Physiology, Sahlgrenska Academy, University of Gothenburg, Gothenburg, Sweden,* [3] *Department of Pediatrics and Department of Neurosciences, The University of New Mexico, Albuquerque, NM, United States,* [4] *Henan Key Laboratory of Child Brain Injury, The Third Affiliated Hospital of Zhengzhou University, Zhengzhou, China*

Correspondence:
Raul Chavez-Valdez
rchavez2@jhmi.edu

Toll-like receptor (TLR)3 activation during the neonatal period produces responses linked to the origins of neuropsychiatric disorders. Although there is sexual dimorphism in neuropsychiatric disorders, it is unknown if brain responses to TLR3 activation are sex-specific. We hypothesized that poly I:C in a post-natal day (P)8 model induces a sexually dimorphic inflammatory responses. C57BL6 mice received intraperitoneal injection of poly I:C (10 mg/kg) or vehicle [normal saline (NS)] at P8. Pups were killed at 6 or 14 h for caspase 3 and 8 activity assays, NFkB ELISA, IRF3, AP1, and GFAP western blotting and cytokines/chemokines gene expression real time qRT-PCR (4–6/group). A second group of pups were killed at 24 h (P9) or 7 days (P15) after poly I:C to assess astrocytic (GFAP) and microglia (Iba1) activation in the hippocampus, thalamus and cortex using immunohistochemistry, and gene and protein expression of cytokines/chemokines using real time RT-PCR and MSD, respectively (4–6/group). Non-parametric analysis was applied. Six hours after poly I:C, caspase-3 and -8 activities in cytosolic fractions were 1.6 and 2.8-fold higher in poly I:C-treated than in NS-treated female mice, respectively, while gene expressions of pro-inflammatory cytokines were upregulated in both sexes. After poly I:C, IRF3 nuclear translocation occurred earlier (6 h) in female mice and later (14 h) in male mice. At 14 h after poly I:C, only male mice also had increased nuclear NFκB levels (88%, $p < 0.001$) and GFAP expression coinciding with persistent IL-6 and FAS gene upregulation (110 and 77%, respectively; $p < 0.001$) and IL-10 gene downregulation (−42%, $p < 0.05$). At 24 h after poly I:C, IL-1β, CXCL-10, TNF-α, and MCP-1 were similarly increased in both sexes but at 7 days after exposure, CXCL-10 and INFγ were increased and IL-10 was decreased only in female mice. Accordingly, microglial activation persisted at 7 days after poly I:C in the hippocampus, thalamus and cortex of female mice. This preliminary study suggests that TLR3 activation may produce in the developing neonatal mouse brain a sexually dimorphic response with early activation of caspase-dependent pathways in female mice, activation of inflammatory cascades in both sexes, which then persists in female mice. Further well-powered studies are essential to confirm these sex-specific findings.

Keywords: poly I:C, inflammation, caspase, cytokines, astroglia, microglia, endoplasmic reticulum stress

INTRODUCTION

Toll-like receptors (TLRs) are a family of innate immune system receptors that react to both microbial stimulation and to molecules released upon tissue injury. TLR 3 modulates neuronal proliferation, differentiation, and axonal growth but also cell death in the developing brain (Cameron et al., 2007; Lathia et al., 2008; Sun et al., 2011). Neurons and glia cells express a broad variety of intracellular TLRs, including TLR3 in astrocytes and microglia (Bsibsi et al., 2002). In post-mortem specimens of preterm infants suffering periventricular white matter injury secondary to infectious or non-infectious inflammation, perinuclear TLR3 expression predominates in neurons and astrocytes (Vontell et al., 2013). Additionally, TLR3 activation increases the vulnerability to perinatal brain injury in neonatal mice (Stridh et al., 2013). In pathological conditions, TLR3 is activated by viral double stranded RNA or by endogenous ligands such as danger-associated molecular patterns (DAMPs) released from dying cells (Beg, 2002; Kariko et al., 2004). Following TLR3 activation, neuronal death may proceed via: (i) apoptosis with release of apoptotic bodies containing DNA fragments, or (ii) necrosis (or necrosis-like) with release of free suspended dead cell materials rich in DAMPs (Blasius and Beutler, 2010). In the injured developing brain, activated astrocytes and microglia engulf DAMPs forming intracellular vesicles, which fuse with TLR3-cointaing acidic endosomes (Rossi and Volterra, 2009; Ransohoff and Brown, 2012; Wakida et al., 2018). In astrocytes, TLR3 activation initiates a cytosolic TRIF-mediated cascade leading to translocation of NFκB, IRF3 and/or AP-1 to the nucleus upregulating transcription of pro-inflammatory mediators, which may perpetuate microglia activation and extend neuronal injury (Fitzgerald et al., 2003; Pobezinskaya et al., 2008).

Like most intracellular TLRs, TLR3 is a resident of the endoplasmic reticulum (ER) and traffics after uncoupling from chaperone proteins (e.g., GRP94) to the endosomal membrane (Blasius and Beutler, 2010). While chaperone proteins are essential for proper folding of TLR3 (Randow and Seed, 2001; Yang et al., 2007), other ER resident proteins are needed for translocation to the endosome (Tabeta et al., 2006). Consequently, persistent ER stress may modulate the response to many intracellular TLR ligands, including the TLR3 ligand polyinosine-polycytidylic acid (poly I:C) (Randow and Seed, 2001; Tabeta et al., 2006; Yang et al., 2007).

Activation of intracellular TLRs early in life is proposed as a mechanism leading to many neurodevelopmental and neuropsychiatric disorders (Brown, 2006; Arroyo et al., 2011; Kneeland and Fatemi, 2013), such as autism and schizophrenia (Fatemi et al., 1999). Although there is a significant male predominance in these disorders (McGrath, 2006; Loomes et al., 2017), sex differences in the mechanisms of TLR3-mediated brain injury early in life has not been reported. Since other models of neonatal brain injury suggest a greater proclivity to apoptosis in female mice and to necrosis-like cell death in male mice (Hagberg et al., 2004; Zhu et al., 2004, 2007; Northington et al., 2011; Chavez-Valdez et al., 2012; Chavez-Valdez et al., 2014), we hypothesized that poly I:C in the P8 mouse model will also induce greater caspase activation in female mice, and more prominent pro-inflammatory profile, astrogliosis, and injury in male mice. Additionally, we also studied the potential role of ER stress in sex-specific responses to TLR3 activation.

MATERIALS AND METHODS

Mice

Experiments were performed with approval by the Ethical Committee of the Sahlgrenska Academy, University of Gothenburg, Gothenburg, Sweden (No. 18-2015; 663/17) where the handling of animals was carried out. Handling was in accordance with the National Institute of Health Guide for the Care and Use of Laboratory Animals (NIH Publications No. 80-23) and the European Convention for the Protection of Vertebrate Animals Used for Experimental and Other Scientific Purposes, Council of Europe (ETS 123). All efforts were made to minimize the number of animals used. Both male and female mice were used for these experiments.

Wild type C57BL6J mice (The Jackson Laboratory, Scanbur, Denmark) were kept in a 12 h light/dark cycle at the animal facility at University of Gothenburg (Gothenburg, Sweden). Culling was performed in the last litter to equalize the sample size for each treatment group. In total 92 (48 male and 48 female) pups were used for these experiments. Litter size varied from 6 to 10 pups. At P8, pups were assigned to either sex group based on visual inspection of external characteristics. Animal received food and water *ad libitum*. Pups were weighed at P8, P9, and P15 to evaluate differences in growth by group. At P8 mice received intraperitoneal (IP) injection of the TLR3 agonist poly I:C (Poly I:C- Low Molecular Weight; InvivoGen, Toulouse, France) reconstituted in LPS-free normal saline (NS) to 1 mg/mL and injected at 10 mg/kg or vehicle (LPS-free NS). Pups were killed at 6 or 14 h for: (i) caspase 3 and 8 activity assays; (ii) NFkB ELISA; (iii) western blot for IRF3, AP1, and GFAP; and (iv) pro-inflammatory (IL-1β, TNFα, FAS, CXCL-1, CXCL-10, MCP-1, INF-β, INF-γ, and IL-6) and anti-inflammatory (IL-10) cytokines/chemokines gene expression by real time qRT-PCR. A second group of pups were killed at 24 h (P9) or 7 days (P15) after poly I:C exposure to evaluate: (i) microscopic injury using Nissl counterstaining; (ii) astroglia and microglia activation using GFAP and Iba1 IHC, respectively; and (iii) gene and protein expression of a similar battery of cytokines/chemokines as described above, by real-time RT-PCR and multiplex electrochemiluminescent immunoassay, respectively. All samples were coded and run by laboratory personnel blinded to treatments, sex, and times.

In all cases, mice were anesthetized and perfused intracardially with NS prior to brain dissection. Brains were snap frozen, and stored at −80°C until analysis except for the hemispheres used for histological evaluation, which were fixed in 4% paraformaldehyde (PFA) by immersion for 1 week followed by cryoprotection using 15 and 30% sucrose gradient prior to freezing at −80°C.

Caspase 3 and 8 Activity Assays

Cytoplasmic and nuclear fractions were prepared using a piece of brain from the same brains used for RNA isolation using a Subcellular Protein Fractionation Kit (Thermo Scientific, Rockford, IL, United States). Buffers were part of the kit and supplemented with protease and phosphatase inhibitors. Approximately 150 mg of tissue washed in ice-cold phosphate-buffered saline (PBS, pH 7.2) was homogenized in Cytoplasmic Extraction Buffer at 1:10 (w:v) using a standard tissue grinder and transferred to a tissue strainer. Following centrifugation at 500 × *g* for 5 min, supernatant (cytoplasmic fraction) was used for Caspase 3 and 8 activity assays. The pellet was sequentially resuspended in ice cold Membrane and Nuclear Extraction Buffers at 1:6.5 and 1:2.25 (w:v), respectively. The final supernatant, the nuclear fractions, were stored at −80°C for nuclear factor κB (NFκB) measurement. Twenty percent (w/v) glycerol was added to the fractions and protein concentrations were determined using the Bradford assay (Bradford, 1976). Cross-contamination between nuclear and cytosolic fractions was minimal following immunoblotting for Lamin B1 (nuclear protein) and HSP90 (cytosolic protein), details below. Cytosolic fractions were assayed for caspase 3 or caspase 8 activity using the respective Colorimetric Activity Assay Kits, (APT165 and APT129; Millipore, Billerica, MA, United States). Cytosolic fractions (400 μg) were plated in a 96-well culture plate and reconstituted in cell lysis buffer and diluted (1:1 v:v) in assay buffer provided by the manufacturer prior to incubation for 60 min at 37°C with the substrate Ac-DEVD-pNA (N-Acetyl-Asp-Glu-Val-Asp-*p*-nitroanilide) for caspase 3 or Ac-IETD- pNA (*N*-acetyl-Ile-Glu-Thr-Asp-ρ-nitroaniline) for caspase 8 activity assay. The chromophore ρ-NA was measured at 405 nm using a Model 680 Microplate Reader (Bio-Rad, Hercules, CA, United States). Semiquantitative measurement of ρNA concentrations in samples was determined indirectly using the linear model of absorbance.

Nuclear Factor-κB Transcription Factor Determination Using ELISA

Nuclear fractions were used to determine concentrations of NFκB bound to the consensus sequence 5′-GGGACTTTCC-3′ in the biotinylated capture probe and detected by exposure to the primary rabbit anti-NFκB p65 antibody (1:1000) followed by a horseradish peroxidase-conjugated goat anti-rabbit secondary detection antibody (1:500) using the EZ-TFA Transcription Factor Assay (Millipore, Temecula, CA, United States). Positive (TNFα-treated HeLa whole-cell extract), specific competitor (NFκB competitor oligonucleotide), and negative controls were used to establish specificity and sensitivity at λ450/ 650 nm using a microplate reader.

Western Blot for IRF3, AP1, GFAP, GRP94

Twenty μg-aliquots of cytosolic (for all protein targets) or nuclear fractions (for IRF3 and AP1) were diluted 3:1 (v:v) in 4X loading buffer under reducing conditions. Samples were loaded in 4–20% mini-protean TGX polyacrylamide precast protein gels (Biorad, Inc., Hercules, CA, United States) and transferred to nitrocellulose membrane using TransBlot Turbo Midi-size (Biorad, Inc.). Blots were stained with Ponceau S and blocked using 2.5% BSA with 0.1% Tween-20 in 50 mM Tris buffered saline (TBST, pH 7.4) before incubation overnight at 4°C in primary antibodies at 1:1000 (GFAP), and 1:500 (IRF3, AP1, and GRP94). After exposure blots were washed with TBST, exposed to secondary antibodies for 1 h and then developed using enhanced chemiluminescence (Clarity Western ECL Substrate, Biorad, Inc.). Loading control at 1:5000 was performed using β-actin for cytosolic fractions and histone H1.4 (both form Sigma). To quantify protein immunoreactivity, optical density (OD) was determined with ImageJ adjusted for background.

Antibodies

IRF3 (Proteintech Group, Inc. 11312-1-AP: RRID: AB_2127004): rabbit polyclonal IgG antibody raised against the IRF3 fusion protein Ag1858 detecting a single band at 49 to 55 kDa (2 μg/ml). AP1 (Proteintech Group, Inc. 22114-1-AP: RRID: AB_2750860): rabbit polyclonal IgG antibody raised against the p39 fusion protein Ag17419 detecting a single band at 40 to 46 kDa (2 μg/ml). GFAP (Proteintech Group, Inc. 16825-1-AP: RRID: AB_ 2109646): rabbit polyclonal IgG antibody raised against the GFAP fusion protein Ag10423 detecting a single band at 45 to 50 kDa (1 μg/ml). GRP94 (Proteintech Group, Inc. 60012-1-Ig: RRID: AB_2119056): mouse monoclonal IgM antibody raised against the GRP94 fusion protein Ag1439 detecting a single band at 95 kDa (2 μg/ml). For evaluation of nuclear-cytosol cross-contamination of the fractions, the following antibodies were used: (i) HSP90 (cytosolic protein, Cell Signaling Technology, Inc. 4875: RRID: AB_2233331): rabbit polyclonal antibody raised against the synthetic peptide surrounding Glu289 of the HSP protein of human origin detecting a single band at 90 kDa without cross-reactivity with other heat-shock proteins (1 μg/ml); and (ii) Lamin B1 (nuclear protein, Cell Signaling Technology, Inc. 13435: RRID: AB_2737428): rabbit monoclonal antibody produced by immunization with a synthetic peptide corresponding to residues surrounding Lys415 of lamin B1 protein of human origin detecting a band at 68 kDa (1 μg/ml).

Gene Expression Using Real Time qRT-PCR

Total RNA was extracted from two combined pieces from anterior and posterior brain from mice pups treated as described above. Tissues were obtained at 6, 14, 24 h (P9) and 7 days (P15) after normal saline or poly I:C exposure. PureLink™ RNA mini kit purification system (Invitrogen, Carlsbad, CA, United States) was used for RNA extraction and measured using a spectrophotometer at 260 nm absorbance. Total RNA (1 μg) was used for generation of complementary single strand DNA (cDNA) using iScript cDNA synthesis kit (BioRad). Reverse transcription protocol included 5 min at 25°C; 30 min at 42°C and 5 min at 85°C. cDNA was then used for gene amplification. The following SYBR Green Based primers from Qiagen (Germantown, MD, United States) were used: IL-6 (QT00098875), IL-1β (QT01048355), TNF-α (QT00104006), Fas (QT00095333), IFN-β (QT00249662), INF-γ (QT01038821), interferon-induced protein-10 (IP-10/CXCL-10) (QT00093436), CXCL-1 (QT00115647) monocyte chemoattractant protein-1 (MCP-1) (QT00167832), IL-10 (QT00106169), including the housekeeping genes GAPDH (QT01658692), and tyrosine 3-monooxygenase/tryptophan 5-monooxygenase activation protein, zeta polypeptide (YWHAZ; QT00105350). The amplification protocol included 40 cycles of 30 s at 95.0°C, 1 min at 60°C ending with 30 s at 72.0°C. Fold difference in gene expression was then corrected by the geometric mean of GAPDH and YWHAZ gene expression using the using the Pfaffl method (Pfaffl, 2001). Melting curves confirmed amplification of single PCR products.

Cytokine and Chemokine Measurement in Brain Crudes

To measure cytokine and chemokine concentrations in brain, a V-plex multi-plex electrochemiluminescent immunoassay platform (MesoScale Discovery, Gaithersburg, MD, United States) was used consistent with our prior studies (Maxwell et al., 2015; Robinson et al., 2016, 2018; Yellowhair et al., 2018). This system has been validated by traditional ELISA and produces measurements with high content validity and inter-assay variations less than 12%. Specifically, brain lysate (100 μg) or standard was loaded on to a 96-well plate in duplicate per manufacturer's specification. Plates were read on a Quickplex SQ 120 Imager (Mesoscale Discovery, Gaithersburg, MD, United States).

IHC for GFAP and Iba1

After intracardiac perfusion with NS and dissection, the brain hemispheres assigned for histological analysis were fixed by immersion in 4% PFA in 0.1 M PBS for 7 days. Tissues were cryoprotected with graded immersion in 15% and then 30% sucrose in PBS until the tissue sank, then frozen and stored in −80°C until cut at 50 μm on a freezing microtome. Sections obtained from animals killed 24 h or 7 days after normal saline or poly I:C exposure were used to assess astroglia (GFAP) and microglia (Iba1) activation and overall microscopic evidence of injury (Nissl counterstaining for GFAP IHC). Floating IHC was performed as previously described (Chavez-Valdez et al., 2018) with whole rabbit antisera anti-GFAP (DAKO/Agilent Technologies, Santa Clara, CA, United States; 1:1000), or anti-Iba1 (Wako Chemicals USA, Inc., Richmond, VA, United States; 1:500) followed by goat anti-rabbit antibody (1:200) used as the secondary antibody using DAB as the chromogen for GFAP and using Alexa Fluor 568 for immunofluorescence for Iba1. Cresyl-violet (CV) counterstaining was performed in those sections previously immunostained for GFAP to assess histological structure. GFAP IHC slides were imaged using a light microscope (Nikon Eclipse E400, Nikon, Minato, Japan), to produce high resolution photomicrographs (1344 × 1024 pixels). Percent area of GFAP immunostaining in the region of interest (hippocampal CA1 and DG, thalamic ventroposterior nuclei, and cingulate cortex) inserted within the 4 X × 20 X high-resolution photomicrographs was calculated using the color threshold function of ImageJ 1.8.0 software (NIH, Bethesda, MD, United States). Immunofluorescent images for Iba1 were captured at 512 × 512 pixels using a Laser Scanning Confocal Microscope LSM700 from Carl Zeiss AG (Oberkochen, Germany). Total Iba1 immunofluorescence signal was quantified using the histogram function in the Zen 2.3 blue edition (Carl Zeiss Microscopy GmbH, Jena, Germany).

Antibodies

GFAP (DAKO Z0334; RRID:AB_10013382): rabbit polyclonal antibody raised against GFAP isolated from cow spinal cord with no reported cross reactivity (1 μg/ml). *Iba1* (WAKO 019-19741; RRID:AB_839504): rabbit polyclonal antibody raised against a synthetic peptide corresponding to the C-terminus of Iba1 purified by antigen affinity chromatography, with no reported cross-reactivity with neuronal or astrocytic markers (1 μg/ml).

Statistical Analysis

For analysis of two related groups, such as the fold-change in gene expression relative to control (NS group) produced by the Pfaffl method, non-parametric Wilcoxon signed-rank test vs. control stratified by sex was applied. Data were presented as box and whisker plot, where the box was limited by the 25th and 75th percentiles and the solid line represented the median. The discontinued line sitting at 1 represented the relative expression of the comparison group (NS). For within sex and time group analysis of two independent treatments (NS and Poly I:C), Mann–Whitney U-test was applied. Significance was assigned by $p \leq 0.05$ in all cases. Analysis was performed using IBM SPSS Statistics 24V (IBM Corporation, Armonk, NY, United States).

RESULTS

Poly I:C Exposure and Growth

The median weight of the pups included in both treatment groups, NS and poly I:C, was similar prior to injection at P8 ($p = 0.76$ for males and $p = 0.84$ for females). By 24 h (P9) or 7 days (P15) after injection the rate of growth was 0.45 to 0.50 mg/day for pups in the NS and those in poly I:C treatment groups. No difference in growth rate by treatment group was documented in male pups ($p_{(24\ h)} = 0.70$, $p_{(7\ d)} = 0.31$) or female pups ($p_{(24\ h)} = 0.82$, $p_{(7\ d)} = 0.18$).

Sex Differences in Caspase 3 and Caspase 8 Activity in Mice After Poly I:C

Neither caspase 3 (**Figure 1A**), nor caspase 8 (**Figure 1B**) activity increased at 6 or 14 h after poly I:C exposure in male mice (n = 5/group). To the contrary, in female mice poly I:C increased caspase 3 activity by 57% from 0.28 (IQR 0.22–0.30) units to 0.44 (IQR 0.37–0.62) units at 6 h after exposure (p = 0.02 vs. NS exposed female mice, n = 4/group; **Figure 1A**). This increase in caspase-3 activity resolved at 14 h after poly I:C exposure. Accordingly, in female mice poly I:C also increased caspase-8 activity from 0.12 (IQR 0.05–0.22) units to 0.35 (0.32–0.42) units at 6 h after exposure (p = 0.02 vs. NS exposed female mice, n = 4/group; **Figure 1B**). Similar to caspase 3, caspase 8 increase resolved by 14 h after poly I:C exposure.

Sex Differences in NFκB and IRF3 Nuclear Translocation in Response to Poly I:C

While no difference in nuclear NFκB was observed 6 h after poly I:C (data not shown), 14 h after poly I:C exposure, NFκB nuclear levels increased by 28% in all mice (p = 0.04 vs. NS-exposed, n = 10/group, **Figure 1C**). When stratified by sex, no change in nuclear NFκB levels after poly I:C exposure was documented in female mice, while an increase of 76% (p = 0.04 vs. NS group, n = 5/group, **Figure 1C**) was documented in male mice at 14 h after poly I:C. Other pathways downstream of TLR3 activation were also studied. Nuclear translocation of IRF3 was temporally distinct between females and males. While IRF3 translocation to the nucleus occurred 6 h after poly I:C in female mice (p = 0.01 vs. NS, n = 6/group), this change was only observed at 14 h after poly I:C in the male mice (p = 0.01 vs. NS, n = 5–6/group; **Figure 1D**). No significant nuclear translocation of AP1 was observed at either 6 or 14 h after poly I:C in either sex (**Figure 1D**).

Increase Early Astrocytic Activation in Male Mice Exposed to Poly I:C

In activated astrocytes, TLR3 activation initiates a cytosolic cascade leading to nuclear translocation of NFκB, IRF3, and/or AP-1 and downstream transcription of pro-inflammatory mediators, which may perpetuate microglia activation and extend neuronal injury (Fitzgerald et al., 2003; Pobezinskaya et al., 2008). Expression of GFAP, an astrocytic marker, was unchanged 6 h after poly I:C exposure, while it was increased by 42.7% (p = 0.003 vs. NS-exposed mice, n = 8/group) at 14 h after exposure. Temporarily coinciding with their later nuclear translocation of NFκB and IRF3, only male mice responded with a 40% (p = 0.02, n = 4; **Figure 1E**) increase in GFAP expression at 14 h after poly I:C exposure, while female mice did not show any change.

Sexual Dimorphism in the Temporal Patterns of INF-β Gene Expression After Poly I:C

INF-β is the prime final product downstream of TLR3 activation. Six hours after poly I:C exposure, INF-β gene expression was upregulated by 8.8-fold in all mice (p = 0.005 vs. NS, n = 10; data not shown). INF-β gene upregulation derived from the early upregulation in female mice (11.3-fold, p = 0.03, n = 6; **Figure 1F**). Fourteen hours after poly I:C the gene expression of INF-β was upregulated by sevenfold (p = 0.005 vs. NS, n = 12; data not shown) in all mice, at this time point the increase derived from the upregulation in male mice (8.1-fold, p = 0.03, n = 6; **Figure 1F**). This pattern temporally mirrors the sexual dimorphism in IRF3 and NFκB nuclear translocations. By 24 h after poly I:C INF-β gene expression returns to levels similar to those seen in NS-treated mice. However, 7 days after poly I:C, INF-β becomes again upregulated in male mice (5.4-fold, p = 0.03 vs. NS, n = 6; **Figure 1F**).

Prolonged Pro-inflammatory Gene Profile After Poly I:C Exposure

Similar to INF-β, gene expression profile of many cytokines was sexually dimorphic following poly I:C exposure at P8. In male mice, poly I:C upregulated the mRNA level of the following pro-inflammatory genes at 6 h after exposure: IL-1β (5.1-fold, p = 0.04, n = 5; **Figure 2A**); CXCL-10 (345-fold p = 0.02, n = 6; **Figure 2B**); TNF-α (4.3-fold, p = 0.04, n = 6; **Figure 2C**); MCP-1 (14.3-fold, p = 0.04, n = 6; **Figure 2D**); FAS (twofold, p = 0.01, data not shown); and IL-6 (6.6-fold, p = 0.04, n = 5, **Figure 2E**); without changing the expression of the anti-inflammatory cytokine IL-10 (**Figure 2F**). Similarly, an early pro-inflammatory profile was documented 6 h after poly I:C exposure in female mice with upregulation of: IL-1β (sevenfold, p = 0.03, n = 6; **Figure 2A**); CXCL-10 (594-fold, p = 0.04, n = 5; **Figure 2B**); MCP-1 (46-fold, p = 0.03, n = 6; **Figure 2D**); FAS (2.8-fold, p = 0.04, data not shown); and IL-6 (sixfold, p = 0.03, n = 6; **Figure 2E**). In male mice, 14 h after poly I:C exposure all pro-inflammatory markers remained upregulated, including: IL-1β (3.5-fold, p = 0.02, n = 6; **Figure 2A**); CXCL-10 (51-fold, p = 0.02, n = 6; **Figure 2B**); TNF-α (5.3-fold, p = 0.02, n = 6, **Figure 2C**); MCP-1 (22-fold, p = 0.02, n = 6; **Figure 2D**), and FAS (1.8-fold, p = 0.01, n = 6; data not shown);but additionally IL-10 was downregulated by 42% (p = 0.04, n = 5; **Figure 2F**). Unlike male mice, the gene expression of several pro-inflammatory markers returned to normal in female mice at 14 h after poly I:C including, IL-6 and FAS and at 24 h after poly I:C, IL-1β. Additionally, the brains of female mice did not respond to poly I:C with down-regulation of IL-10 14 h after exposure, as documented in male mice (**Figure 2F**). As expected a trajectory to return to levels similar to those in NS-treated mice was observed between 24 h and 7 days after poly I:C. Thus, at 7 days after poly I:C IL-1β, TNF-α, and MCP-1 gene expressions were similar to those in NS-treated mice in both sexes. However, only in female mice, upregulation of the CXCL-10 (p = 0.03, n = 6) and

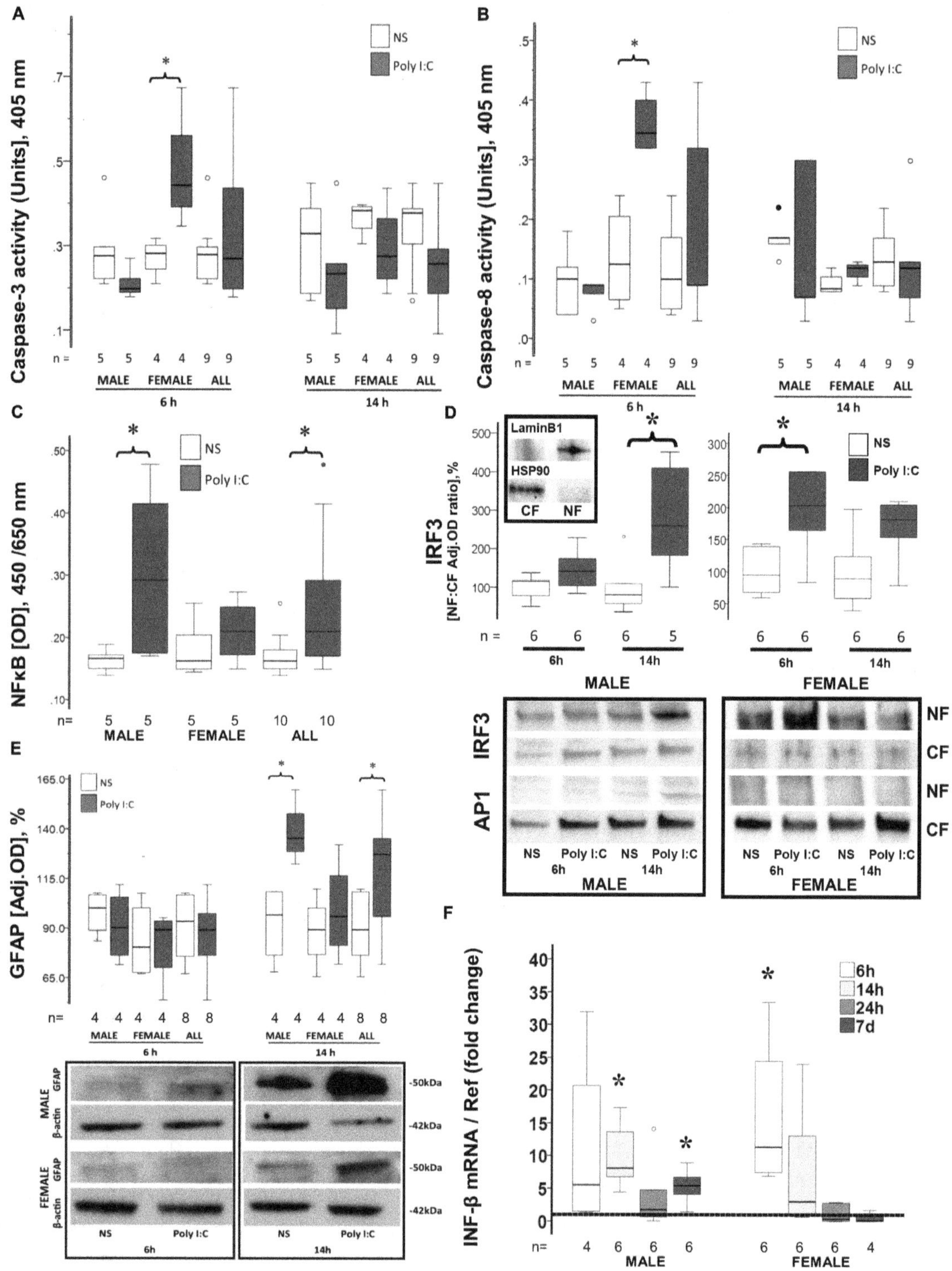

FIGURE 1 | Early sex-specific responses to poly I:C in the brain of P8 mice. Increased caspase-3 **(A)** and caspase-8 activity **(B)**, IRF3 nuclear translocation **(D)**, and INF-β gene upregulation **(F)** occur 6 h after poly I:C in the brain of female mice. Increased NFκB **(C)** and IRF3 **(D)** nuclear translocation, GFAP expression **(E)** and INF-β gene upregulation **(F)** occur 14 h after poly I:C in the brain of male mice. Data are presented using box and whiskers plots, where boxes are limited by the 75th and 25th percentiles interquartile range (IQR)] and whiskers are limited by the last data point within 1.5 times the IQR from the median (continuous line inside the box). **(A–E)** White boxes represent NS-treated pups, while gray boxes represent poly I:C-treated pups. **(D)** Representative immunoblots showing translocation of IRF3 and AP1 from the cytosolic fraction (CF) to the nuclear fraction (NF) in males and females at 6 and 14 h after poly I:C. Top immunoblots show purity of the NF and CF using Lamin B1 and HSP90, respectively. **(E)** Representative immunoblots showing GFAP expression in cytosolic fractions. **(F)** Shows the fold change in INF-β mRNA levels in the brain of male and female mice at 6, 14, 24 h and 7 days after poly I:C relative to NS-treated mice (discontinuous line sitting at 1). °, outlier (between 1.5 and 3 times the IQR); •, extreme (> 3 times the IQR); *$p < 0.05$.

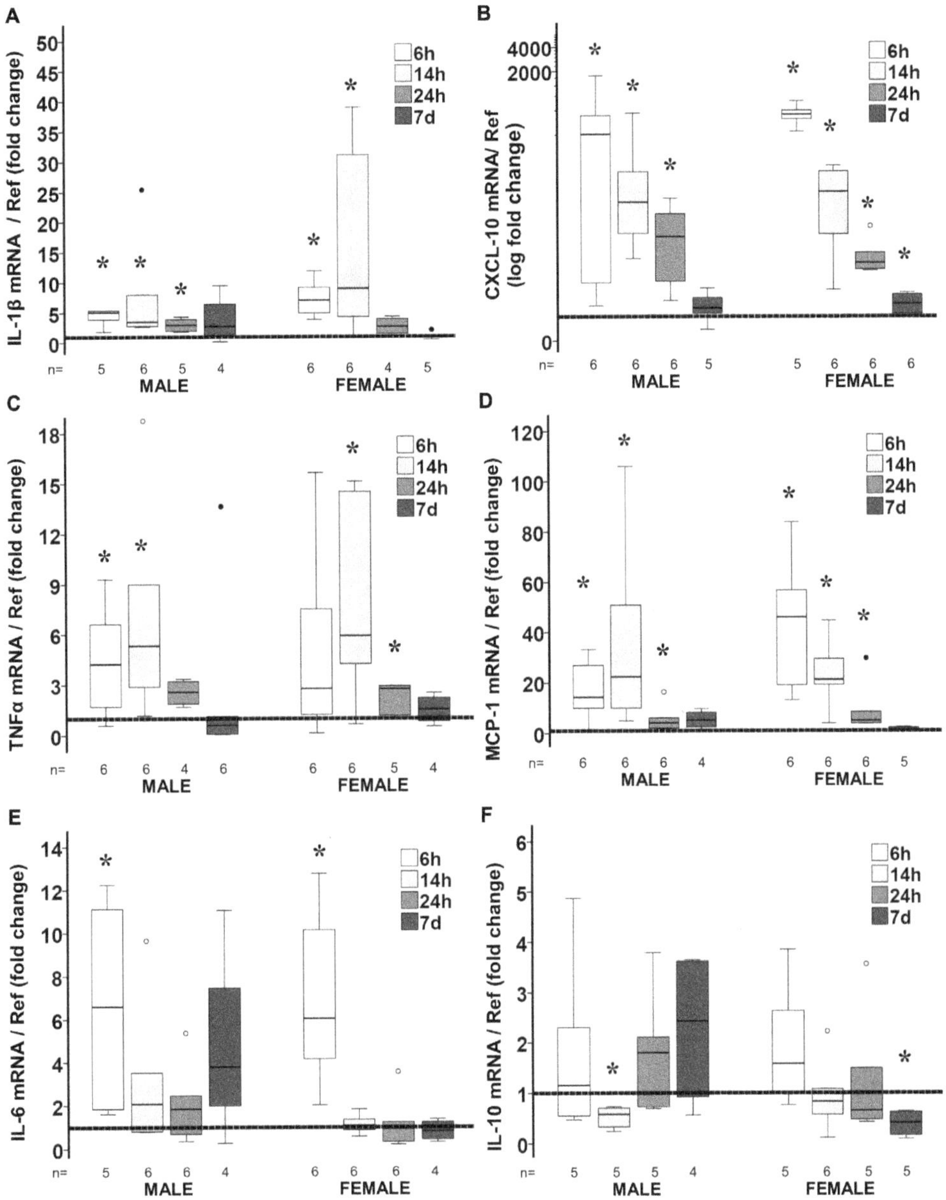

FIGURE 2 | Temporal changes in brain cytokine/ chemokine gene expression in response to poly I:C exposure at P8. Fold change in gene expression of IL-1β **(A)**, CXCL-10 **(B)**, TNFα **(C)**, MCP-1 **(D)**, IL-6 **(E)**, and IL-10 **(F)** in the brain of poly I:C treated mice relative to NS-treated mice. Data are shown using box and whiskers plots, where boxes are limited by the 75th and 25th percentiles (IQR) and whiskers are limited by the last data point within 1.5 times the IQR from the median (continuous line inside the box). Data from male and female mice at 6, 14, 24 h and 7 days after poly I:C relative to NS-treated mice (discontinuous line sitting at 1) is shown. °, outlier (between 1.5 and 3 times the IQR); •, extreme (>3 times the IQR); $^{*}p < 0.05$.

downregulation of IL-10 ($p = 0.04$, $n = 5$) genes were present at 7 days after poly I:C (**Figures 2B,F**).

An extensive battery of pro-inflammatory cytokines/chemokine protein levels were measured in poly I:C treated mice at 24 h and 7 days after HI (**Table 1**). Matching the gene expression data, IL-1β, CXCL-10, TNF-α, and MCP-1 were increased at 24 h after poly I:C exposure in both sexes. Also congruent with the gene expression results, 7 days after poly I:C the levels of CXCL-10 (63%, $p = 0.05$), CXCL-1 (19%, $p = 0.01$) and INF-γ (38%, $p = 0.006$) were elevated, while the level of IL-10 (−21%, $p = 0.05$) was decreased only in female mice (**Table 1**).

Astrocyte and Microglia Activation Following Poly I:C

Although by 14 h after poly I:C GFAP protein level was increased only in male mice, at 24 h after poly I:C GFAP expression was equally observed in the hippocampus (CA1 and dentate gyrus subfields) and cingulate cortex of both male and

TABLE 1 | Cytokine expression following poly I:C exposure stratified by sex.

		Males			Females		
		Saline	Poly I:C	*p*-value	Saline	Poly I:C	*p*-value
Pro-inflammatory (*n* = 6/group) (pg/100 μg protein)							
INF-γ Median [IQR]	**24 h**	0.103 [0.08–0.12]	0.119 [0.11–0.15]	0.10	0.091 [0.08–0.09]	0.096 [0.80–0.11]	0.52
	7 days	0.074 [0.06–0.09)	0.063 [0.04–0.07]	0.10	**0.045 [0.03–0.05]**	**0.062 [0.06–0.07]**	**0.006***
IL-1β Median [IQR]	**24 h**	**0.311 [0.27–0.37]**	**0.545 [0.44–0.64]**	**0.006***	**0.367 [0.29–0.45]**	**0.599 [0.47–0.74]**	**0.01***
	7 days	0.395 [0.34–0.43]	0.286 [0.24–0.43]	0.42	0.304 [0.27–0.35]	0.301 [0.26–0.33]	0.87
IL-2 Median [IQR]	**24 h**	0.101 [0.06–0.10]	0.095 [0.07–0.10]	0.56	0.108 [0.05–0.10]	0.106 [0.08–0.24]	0.43
	7 days	ND	ND	–	ND	ND	–
IL-5 Median [IQR]	**24 h**	**0.466 [0.40–0.58]**	**0.605 [0.53–0.64]**	**0.05***	0.483 [0.45–0.55]	0.634 [0.47–0.71]	0.10
	7 days	0.359 [0.29–0.39]	0.358 [0.26–0.38]	1.00	0.349 [0.33–0.37]	0.350 [0.28–0.39]	1.00
IL-12 Median [IQR]	**24 h**	18.16 [13.9–22.6]	23.92 [18.1–31.6]	0.26	20.48 [16.8–26.4]	24.49 [17.5–29.4]	0.42
	7 days	14.55 [9.71–18.9]	15.25 [7.62–19.9]	0.87	15.81 [6.39–18.4]	13.49 [9.62–16.4]	0.72
CXCL-1 Median [IQR]	**24 h**	2.79 [2.65–3.06]	3.19 [2.76–3.61]	0.10	2.66 [2.33–2.77]	3.04 [2.57–3.26]	0.10
	7 days	1.79 [1.39–1.99]	2.14 [1.73–2.34]	0.10	**1.76 [1.57–1.96]**	**2.09 [1.98–2.35]**	**0.01***
CXCL-10 Median [IQR]	**24 h**	**13.34 [10.8–13.3]**	**691.4 [521.1–1043]**	**0.004***	**13.92 [12.4–15.2]**	**480.9 [346.7–1782]**	**0.004***
	7 days	10.34 [9.6–13.7]	11.85 [10.6–12.6]	0.52	**9.45 [7.21–14.7]**	**15.42 [12.6–20.5]**	**0.05***
TNF-α Median [IQR]	**24 h**	**0.243 [0.21–0.31]**	**0.402 [0.37–0.46]**	**0.004***	**0.269 [0.25–0.32]**	**0.406 [0.38–0.43]**	**0.04***
	7 days	0.233 [0.21–0.26]	0.217 [0.18–0.26]	0.42	0.212 [0.18–0.24]	0.176 [0.16–0.23]	0.33
MCP-1 Median [IQR]	**24 h**	**2.14 [1.92–2.46]**	**40.88 [30.9–47.6]**	**0.004***	**1.819 [1.72–2.19]**	**38.58 [30.3–62.5]**	**0.004***
	7 days	1.546 [1.47–1.76]	1.662 [1.52–1.85]	0.42	1.509 [1.23–1.84]	1.706 [1.54–1.89]	0.10
Modulatory (*n* = 6/group) (pg/100 μg protein)							
IL-6 Median [IQR]	**24 h**	8.72 [8.05–10.5]	10.52 [9.21–10.8]	0.20	8.46 [7.91–10.4]	10.35 [8.53–11.4]	0.20
	7 days	7.62 [6.87–8.44]	7.54 [5.79–8.23]	0.75	7.02 [6.54–7.42]	7.26 [5.68–7.61]	1.00
Anti-inflammatory (*n* = 6/group) (pg/100 μg protein)							
IL-4 Median [IQR]	**24 h**	0.385 [0.23–0.66]	0.343 [0.28–0.39]	0.52	0.253 [0.18–0.42]	0.266 [0.20–0.36]	0.87
	7 days	0.149 [0.08–0.24]	0.139 [0.13–0.20]	0.87	0.148 [0.08–0.25]	0.132 [0.09–0.18]	0.75
IL-10 Median [IQR]	**24 h**	5.44 [4.52–6.26]	5.07 [4.42–5.91]	0.74	6.55 [5.64–7.09]	6.11 [5.75–6.74]	0.52
	7 days	4.64 [4.12–5.34]	4.63 [4.13–5.61]	0.87	**5.24 [5.05–5.42]**	**4.13 [3.32–5.17]**	**0.05***

Bold font signifies statistical significance.

female mice (**Figure 3** and **Table 2**). Seven days after poly I:C, evidence of astrocytic activation greatly diminished in both sexes in all regions (**Figures 3A,B,D**) with the exception of the ventroposterior nuclei of the thalamus, demonstrating greater number of reactive astrocytes at 7 days than at 24 h after poly I:C (**Figure 3C** and **Table 2**). Similar to GFAP staining, Iba-1 staining peaked at 24 h after poly I:C in the hippocampus and the cingulate cortex (**Figure 4**) but unlike GFAP-staining, residual Iba-1 immunofluorescence at 7 days after exposure show a sex specific pattern. While evidence of microglia activation was almost resolved in the hippocampus (**Figures 4A** [CA1] and **4B** [DG]), thalamus (**Figure 4C**) and cingulate cortex (**Figure 4D**) at 7 days after poly I:C in male mice; significant residual activation was present in all those brain regions in female mice (**Figure 4**). Semi-quantitative analysis of Iba1 immunofluorescence in those regions are shown in **Figure 4** and **Table 3**.

CHOP Expression Following Poly I:C

Both CHOP gene and protein expression were increased 24 h after poly I:C exposure in males and female mice (**Figure 5**). However, only in the male mice, 7 days after poly I:C sexual dimorphism in CHOP gene expression resulted in a threefold increase compared to NS treated mice suggesting persistent ER stress in male mice. Expression of GRP94, an important ER chaperone for TLR3 and a known protective factor against ER stress, was not different between treatment groups in either sex.

The full dataset analyzed and reported in the result section is available to the reader as **Supplementary Material**.

DISCUSSION

Our pilot results suggest that TLR3 activation affects the developing brain differently in male and female mice. Early caspase activation is more prominent in the brain of female mice 6 h after exposure to poly I:C at P8. Here, we also document sexually specific temporal patterns of pro-inflammatory cytokine/chemokine expression. Early IRF-3 nuclear translocation downstream of TLR3 activation leads to INF-β upregulation 6 h after poly I:C in female mice, while delayed NFκB-IRF-3 nuclear translocation leads to INF-β upregulation 14 h after exposure in male mice. Although, several pro-inflammatory cytokines such as IL-1β, CXCL-10, TNF-α, MCP-1, FAS, and IL-6 are increased by 6 h after poly I:C in both sexes, some of them, IL-6 and FAS, remain upregulated at 14 h after poly I:C in conjunction with IL-10 downregulation only in the male mice. Earlier activation of astrocytes after poly I:C may explain the increased pro-inflammatory profile seen in male mice at 14 h after exposure. While most of the pro-inflammatory markers return to levels similar to those seen in NS-treated mice sometime between 24 h and 7 days after poly I:C in male mice; late increase in INF-γ, CXCL-1, and CXCL-10, combined with decrease IL-10, and persistent microglia activation suggest a greater late pro-inflammatory state in female mice 7 days after poly I:C. We speculate that a second "wave" of INF-β upregulation documented in male mice 7 days after poly I:C, may prevent release of INF-γ, microglia activation, and downstream release of CXCL-10 in the male mice (Ottum et al., 2015; Kovarik et al., 2016). Mechanistically, delayed CHOP upregulation in male mice 7 days after poly I:C may prevent cytokine translation in male mice (Moon, 2014). Altogether, TLR3 activation produces early activation of apoptotic pathways predominantly in female mice, early pro-inflammatory cytokine profile in both sexes, which extends at least for 7 days after poly I:C exposure in female mice presumptively secondary to persistent microglia activation. The role of ER-stress in the sexual dimorphism in response to poly I:C is still unclear.

Sex differences in the mechanisms of cell death have been described after brain injury secondary to stroke (Liu et al., 2011) and hypoxia-ischemia (Hagberg et al., 2004; Zhu et al., 2007; Northington et al., 2011; Chavez-Valdez et al., 2012) and here, we provide preliminary evidence that these differences may also occur in response to TLR3 activation in the neonatal brain. In the developing brain, a greater acute proclivity to apoptotic cell death in females and to a pro-inflammatory necrotic-like cell death in males has been documented (Hurn et al., 2005; Vannucci and Hurn, 2009; Northington et al., 2011). Cultured female neurons are more sensitive to etoposide-induced apoptosis, while cultured male neurons are more sensitive to excitotoxic stress (Du et al., 2004). Accordingly, following perinatal hypoxia-ischemia or ischemic brain injury, inhibition of caspases provides protection to female rodents (Renolleau et al., 2007), while inhibition of PARP-1-mediated necrotic pathways provides protection to male rodents (Hagberg et al., 2004). Activation of TLR3 by poly I:C leads to both types of cell death. TLR3-mediated apoptotic cell death occurs via upregulation of death-receptors 4/5 and a transactivating p63 isoform α-mediated and IRF3-mediated initiation of the extrinsic pathway (Sun et al., 2011; Gambara et al., 2015) or via a death receptor devoted RIP1-mediated TLR3/caspase-8 complex formation (Estornes et al., 2012). On the other hand, TLR3-mediated necrotic-like cell death, such as programmed necrosis, occurs in the setting of caspase-8 inhibition via a RIP3 kinase-dependent mechanism that involves TRIF and MLKL, but independent of RIP1 (He et al., 2011; Kaiser et al., 2013; Lotzerich et al., 2018). Indirectly, TNF death receptor activation following exposure to TLR3 ligands may proceed via classic RIP1-RIP3 necroptosis pathway, which is also prominent in male mice in the P7 model of hypoxia-ischemia (Northington et al., 2011; Kaiser et al., 2013; Chavez-Valdez et al., 2014). Our results suggest that similar to stroke and hypoxia-ischemia, the mechanisms of cell death in the developing brain after TLR3 activation diverge by sex. The greater caspase 3 and caspase 8 activity documented in the brain of female mice 6 h after poly I:C suggest a preferential activation of the apoptotic extrinsic pathway compared to male mice. Furthermore, IRF3 mediated initiation of apoptotic extrinsic pathway is suggested by the increased IRF3 nuclear translocation demonstrated 6 h after poly I:C in female mice, and event that coincided with caspase activation.

There is also evidence for intrinsic sex-specific differences in inflammatory responses induced by activation of immune cells in the immature brain (Mallard et al., 2018). Additionally, peripheral inflammatory responses may also have an influence in severity of brain injury in a sex-specific manner. For example, peripheral depletion of circulating myeloid cells reduces brain inflammation and injury in male but not female mice (Smith et al., 2018). Further, in models of non-viral

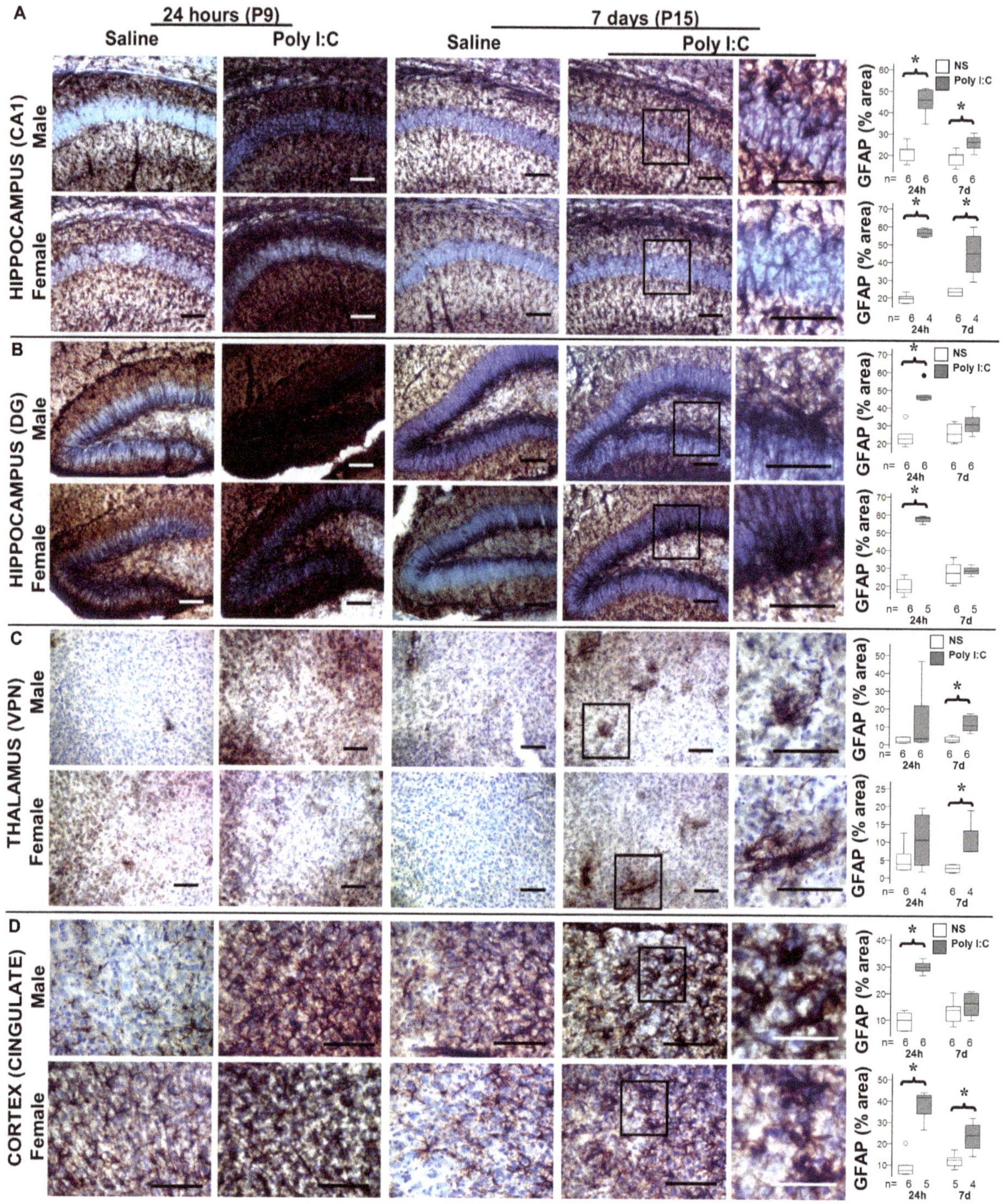

FIGURE 3 | Temporal changes in astrocytic activation after poly I:C exposure at P8. Representative photomicrographs of GFAP immunoreactivity in the CA1 **(A)** and dentate gyrus (DG, **B**) subfields of the hippocampus, ventroposterior nuclei (VPN) of the thalamus **(C)**, and cingulate cortex **(D)** of male and female mice at 24 h and 7 days after treated with normal saline or poly I:C. High magnification details are provided for 7 days after poly I:C. In all panels, bar represents 100 μm, with the exception of the detail higher magnification panel for the cingulate cortex at 7 days after poly I:C, where bar represent 50 μm. Semi-quantitative analyses of percent area of GFAP immunostaining per sex and region of interest are shown using box and whiskers plots, where boxes are limited by the 75th and 25th percentiles (IQR) and whiskers are limited by the last data point within 1.5 times the IQR from the median (continuous line inside the box). Data from male (top) and female (bottom) mice at 24 h and 7 days after treatment with NS (white boxes) or poly I:C (gray boxes) are shown. °, outlier (between 1.5 and 3 times the IQR); •, extreme (>3 times the IQR); *$p < 0.05$ ($n = 6$/ group). Twenty-four hours after poly I:C, significant astrocytic activation was observed in the hippocampus (CA1 and DG subfields) and cingulate cortex. At 7 days after poly I:C, astrocytic activation greatly diminished with the exception of the VPN of the thalamus, demonstrating greater evidence of astrocytosis at 7 days than at 24 h after poly I:C. No sex-specific differences were observed. Detailed information about percent area of GFAP immunoreactivity in each area of interest is provided in **Table 2**.

TABLE 2 | Percent area of GFAP immunostaining per region.

Region	Sex	24 h (P9)			7 days (P15)		
		Saline	Poly I:C	*p*-Value	Saline	Poly I:C	*p*-Value
Hippocampus CA1 Median % [IQR]	**Male**	22.6 [18.9–22.9]	45.9 [42.9–49.5]	**0.002**	20.3 [16.8–20.7]	26.4 [24–28.4]	**0.009**
	Female	19.7 [17.6–20.7]	56.5 [54.9–58.4]	**0.01**	23.6 [21.8–25.2]	45.2 [37.8–52.4]	**0.01**
Hippocampus DG Median % [IQR]	**Male**	22.6 [20.5–24.7]	46.2 [44.9–47.4]	**0.002**	24.4 [21.6–30.2]	30.8 [27.9–33.9]	NS
	Female	18.2 [16.6–22.8]	58.3 [57.1–58.8]	**0.004**	27.3 [22.9–31.1]	28.7 [27.1–30.5]	NS
Thalamus VPN Median % [IQR]	**Male**	1.8 [1–3.9]	3.3 [1.9–17.5]	NS	2.8 [1.9–4.2]	10.8 [8.7–15.2]	**0.002**
	Female	3.9 [2.4–6.3]	10.6 [4.5–16.7]	NS	2.7 [1.9–3.5]	7.6 [7.5–10.5]	**0.01**
Cingulate Cortex Median % [IQR]	**Male**	9.9 [6.8–12.2]	29.9 [28.9–31.1]	**0.002**	13.8 [10.6–15.1]	13.8 [10.6–15.1]	NS
	Female	7.5 [6.3–9.3]	41.7 [34.1–42.9]	**<0.001**	12.4 [9.9–13.6]	23.9 [19.9–27.4]	**0.003**

Data show as percent (%) area of GFAP immunoreactivity in the region of interest within high magnification photomicrograph. n = 4–6/group. Mann–Whitney U-test used for analysis. DG, dentate gyrus; NS, non-significant; VPN, ventroposterior nuclei. Bold font signifies statistical significance.

septic peritonitis and ischemic bowel injury, TLR3 genetic deletion attenuates the perpetuation of cytokines and chemokines release by macrophages, recruitment of neutrophils, systemic inflammation, and multiorgan injury (Cavassani et al., 2008). Similar role of TLR3 activation as an amplifier of the early inflammatory responses have been reported in the kidney and the liver (Patole et al., 2005; Lang et al., 2006). Activation of TLR3 with poly I:C induces a prolonged inflammatory response from cultured astrocytes (Chistyakov et al., 2018), microglia (Dupuis et al., 2016; Yousif et al., 2018), and brain endothelial cells (Johnson et al., 2018). The prolonged inflammatory response induced by TLR3 activation in microglia and astrocytes biologically serves to control or to enhance insidious viral infections such as Chikungunya (Priya et al., 2014) and HIV-1 (Bhargavan and Kanmogne, 2018) and non-viral infections such as Borrelia burgdorferi (Greenmyer et al., 2018). Sex differences in inflammatory responses depend on the specific intracellular TLR ligand used. Male peripheral mononuclear cells (PMNCs) treated with TLR7 ligands produce less INF than females cells, while male PMNCs treated with TLR8 and TLR9 agonists produce more IL-10 than female cells (Torcia et al., 2012). Thus, the activation of TLR7, 8, and 9 may provide a net anti-inflammatory effect in the males. However, the role of sex on the TLR3-mediated prolonged inflammatory response is unknown in the developing brain until now. Our experiments suggest persistent increase in pro-inflammatory cytokines IL-6, FAS and INF-β, and decrease in IL-10 in the brain of male mice up to 14 h after poly I:C, which contrast with the response in the brain of female mice. We speculate that this is the result of more acute/subacute pro-inflammatory necrotic type of cell death with earlier astrocytic activation in male mice. The pro-inflammatory response appears to resolve in the male mice sometime between 24 h and 7 days after poly I:C. In contrast, a pro-inflammatory profile persist at least until 7 days after poly I:C in female mice. The expression of INF-β after poly I:C may explain the lack of INF-γ expression in both males and female pups up to 24 h (Ottum et al., 2015). In contrast, the lack of INF-β upregulation documented in female mice 7 days after poly I:C, may explain the late upregulation of INF-γ, microglia activation and downstream CXCL-10 expression (Kovarik et al., 2016). However, the role of systemic inflammation in the persistent pro-inflammatory profile documented in the brain of female mice after poly I:C is still unclear.

We acknowledge limitations in this study. We have not dissect the few discrepancies between transcription and translation of certain markers, such as IL-1β or CHOP at 24 h, which shows sex dimorphism in gene expression. Further, we have not studied the influence of systemic inflammation in the brain. Knowing that the blood–brain barrier (BBB) integrity is altered by systemic inflammation, disrupting immune cell trafficking to the brain and leading to activation of astrocytes within the BBB (Banks, 2005; Abbott et al., 2006); our exposure paradigm using IP poly I:C will presumably induce both a primary inflammatory response, as well as a systemic-derived response in the brain secondary to glial activation by circulating cytokines released during TLR3 activation of cells in other organs (e.g., macrophages, adipocytes, keratinocytes). Although the complex interactions between systemic and brain inflammatory responses cannot be further elaborated with the reported set of experiments, TLR3 activation by poly I:C appears to produce only a modest systemic inflammatory short lasting response compared to responses to LPS (Packard et al., 2012), thus we speculate that the earlier GFAP peak at 14 h after poly I:C, may be the result of a greater influence of systemic inflammation in the brain of male mice as previously reported (Smith et al., 2018), which may also explain the increase IL-6, FAS and decrease IL-10 seen simultaneously in males. Similarly, we cannot conclude about the cellular source of the sexual dimorphism in cytokine expression documented in female

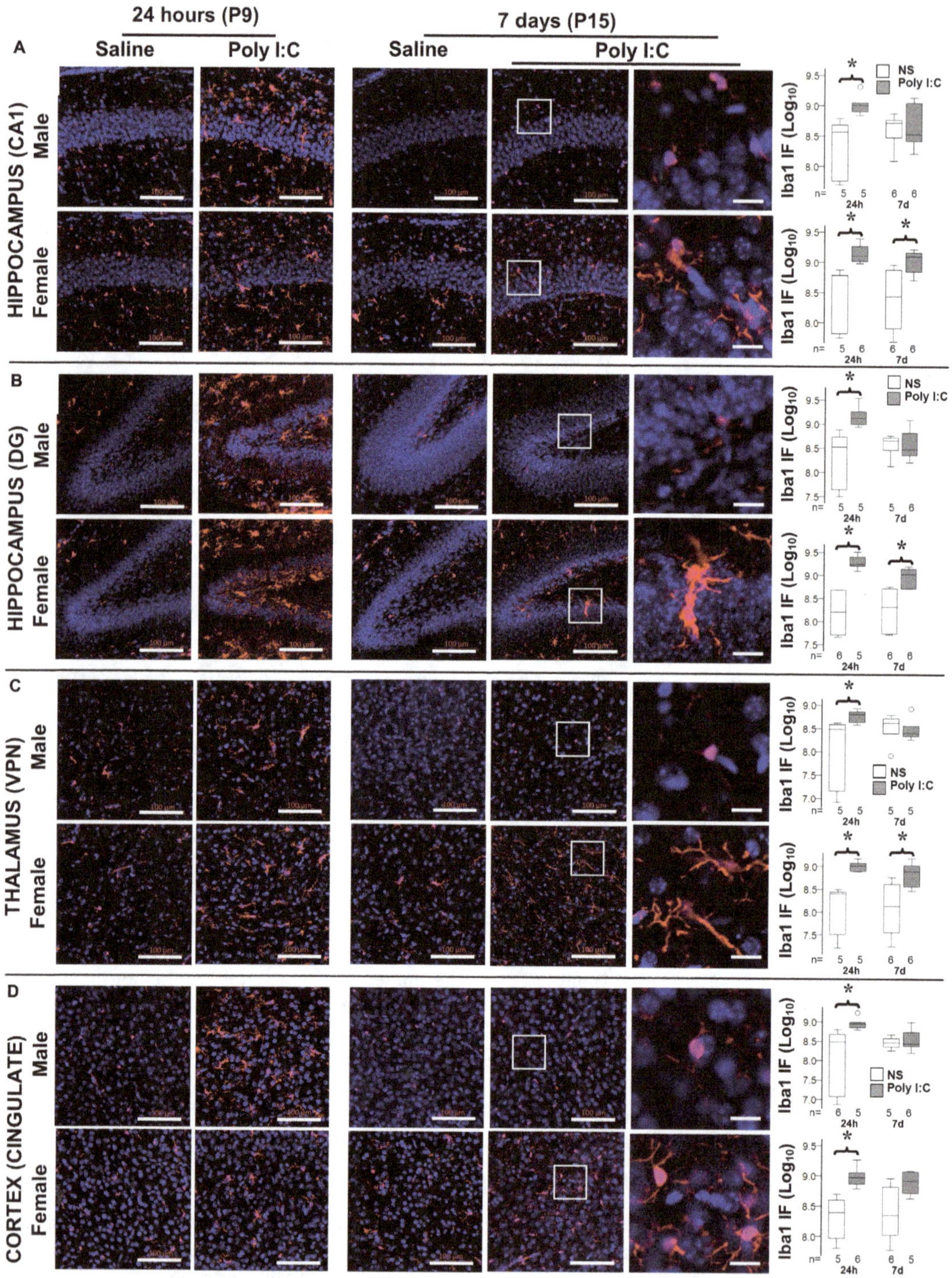

FIGURE 4 | Temporal changes in microglia activation after poly I:C exposure at P8. Representative photomicrographs of Iba1 immunofluorescence in the CA1 **(A)** and dentate gyrus (DG, **B**) subfields of the hippocampus, VPN of the thalamus **(C)**, and cingulate cortex **(D)** of male (top row) and female mice (bottom row) at 24 h and 7 days after treatment with normal saline (NS) or poly I:C. High magnification datails show at 7 d after poly I:C. In all panels, bar represents 100 μm, with the exception of the detail high magnification panels for 7 days after poly I:C, where bar represent 20 μm. Semi-quantitative analyses of Iba1 immunofluorescence per sex and region of interest are shown using box and whiskers plots, where boxes are limited by the 75th and 25th percentiles (IQR) and whiskers are limited by the last data point within 1.5 times the IQR from the median (continuous line inside the box). Data from male (top) and female (bottom) mice at 24 h and 7 days after treatment with NS (white boxes) or poly I:C (gray boxes) are shown. Data are presented as the decimal logarithmic transformation of the total immunofluorescence signal in arbitrary units. °, outlier (between 1.5 and 3 times the IQR); •, extreme (>3 times the IQR); *$p < 0.05$ (n = 4–6/group). Twenty-four hours after poly I:C, significant microglia activation was observed in all regions in both sexes. At 7 days after poly I:C, microglia activation significantly diminished in male mice (top), while persisted in all brain regions in female mice (bottom). Detailed information about immunofluorescence provided in **Table 3**.

TABLE 3 | Semi-quantitative analysis of Iba1 immunofluorescence per region.

Region	Sex	24 h (P9) Saline	24 h (P9) Poly I:C	24 h (P9) *p*-Value	7 days (P15) Saline	7 days (P15) Poly I:C	7 days (P15) *p*-Value
Hippocampus CA1 Median [IQR]	**Male**	370 [57–484]	1021 [801–1125]	**0.008**	527 [344–585]	341 [273–929]	NS
	Female	610 [66–617]	1283 [1070–1750]	**0.004**	404 [87–735]	1253 834–1412]	**0.04**
Hippocampus DG Median [IQR]	**Male**	333 [44–538]	1342 [993–1826]	**0.008**	455 [289–518]	296 [243–565]	NS
	Female	260 [52–479]	1748 [1601–2505]	**0.004**	285 [63–511]	1087 [597–1370]	**0.01**
Thalamus VPN Median [IQR]	**Male**	305 [14–388]	635 [434–734]	**0.03**	417 [250–519]	255 [219–365]	NS
	Female	254 [32–279]	1039 [773–1188]	**0.008**	187 [41–390]	824 [426–1059]	**0.04**
Cingulate Cortex Median [IQR]	**Male**	314 [70–458]	903 [728–988]	**0.009**	298 [239–390]	279 [250–482]	NS
	Female	249 [93–397]	899 [741–980]	**0.004**	284 [107–609]	830 [525–1186]	NS

Data show immunofluorescence arbitrary units (millions). n = 5–6/group. Mann-Whitney U-test used for analysis. DG, dentate gyrus; NS, non-significant; VPN, ventroposterior nuclei. Bold font signifies statistical significance.

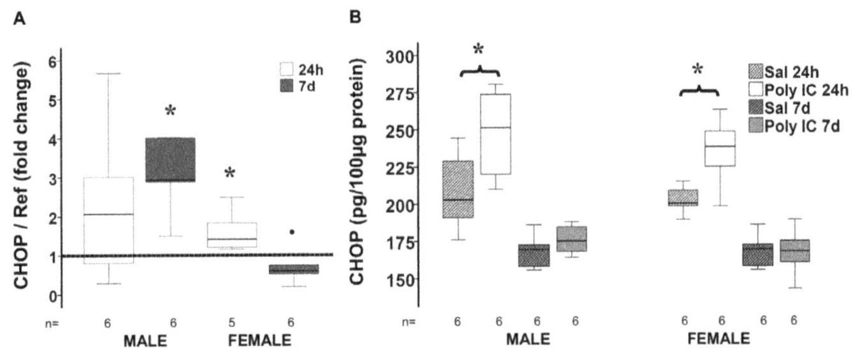

FIGURE 5 | Delayed sex-specific CHOP expression after poly I:C in P8 mice. Fold change in CHOP gene **(A)** and protein **(B)** expression at 24 h and 7 days after poly I:C exposure at P8. Data are shown using box and whiskers plots, where boxes are limited by the 75th and 25th percentiles (IQR) and whiskers are limited by the last data point within 1.5 times the IQR from the median (continuous line inside the box). Fold change was calculated relative to NS-treated mice shown as discontinuous line sitting at 1). °, outlier (between 1.5 and 3 times the IQR); •, extreme (>3 times the IQR); $^{*}p < 0.05$.

mice 7 days after poly I:C exposure. However, the simultaneous lack of INF-β gene upregulation, increase INF-γ levels, increase Iba-1 expression across brain regions, and increase CXCL-10 levels, allow us to speculate that persistently activated microglia may be the source of these changes. Other mechanisms by which poly I:C may also produce effects in the brain (e.g., activation of inflammasome) as suggested by others (Rajan et al., 2010; Franchi et al., 2014) need further studies. In rodents, IP injection of poly I:C at less than half of the dose used in our experiments (3–4 instead of 10 mg/kg) produces fever within 5 to 14 h after injection (Hopwood et al., 2009) and also impairs endothelial function (Zimmer et al., 2011). Since a decrease in core temperature may suppress microglial induction and attenuate inflammation, the evaluation of temperature changes in response to poly I:C also needs further investigation. Finally, our experiments are not powered to study differences within sexes and the analysis has been limited to differences between treatments within each sex group. Thus, larger studies, with 20–30 mice per group depending on the primary outcomes used for power calculation, are needed to confirm our preliminary observations between sexes.

Perinatal TLR3 activation is speculated as a mechanism leading to several neurodevelopmental, neurodegenerative, and neuropsychiatric disorders (Brown, 2006; De Miranda et al., 2010; Arroyo et al., 2011; Forrest et al., 2012; Kneeland and Fatemi, 2013). The male predominance in these disorders (McGrath, 2006; Loomes et al., 2017), matches the early sex differences documented within the first 24 h after TLR3 activation in our experiments. We propose that following exposure of the developing brain to TLR3 ligand, female cells acutely die via apoptosis, while male cells die via necrotic-like cell death (i.e., programmed necrosis), as suggested in other models of neonatal brain injury (Hagberg et al., 2004; Zhu et al., 2007; Northington et al., 2011; Chavez-Valdez et al., 2012). The early release of DAMPs from necrotic cells and the effects of systemic inflammation may intensify astrocytosis in male mice, with downstream nuclear translocation of transcription factors and production of pro-inflammatory mediators within the first 24 h. The role of the late pro-inflammatory response documented in female mice after TLR3 activation in the development of neurological disorders is unclear. However, emergent literature is suggesting a protective role of inflammatory mediators against neurodegenerative diseases (Lemere, 2007; Ottum et al., 2015; Le et al., 2016). Further experiments better powered to confirm our speculations are needed to then study the role of these potential sex differences in the sex dimorphism seen in many of neurological disorders linked to TLR3 activation early in life.

AUTHOR CONTRIBUTIONS

RC-V, FN, and CM: experimental design. AM and LS: animal works. RC-V, AM, LS, TY, and LJ: tissue processing. RC-V, TY, and LJ: immunohistochemistry, PCR, and biochemical assays. RC-V: statistical analysis and initial draft preparation. All authors: critical reviews of the manuscript and approval of final version.

FUNDING

Experiments and investigators were funded in part by grants from the National Institutes of Health (KO8NS096115 - RC-V; R01HL139492 - LJ; RO1HD070996, RO1HD086058 - FN; R01NS103483 - CM), the Johns Hopkins University-School of Medicine Clinician Scientist Award (RC-V), the Sutland-Pakula Endowment for Neonatal Research (RC-V) and Swedish Research Council (VR-2017-01409 - CM), Swedish state under the agreement between the Swedish government and the county councils, the ALF-agreement (ALFGBG-722491 - CM), Neurobid, HEALTH-F2-2009-241778 (CM), the Leducq foundation (DSRR_P34404 - CM), and the Swedish Brain Foundation (FO2017-0063).

ACKNOWLEDGMENTS

The authors thank Mrs. Deborah Flock, Ms. Elizabeth Krisanda, and Mr. Charles Lechner for their technical support and Mrs. Rosie Silva for her administrative assistance.

REFERENCES

Abbott, N. J., Ronnback, L., and Hansson, E. (2006). Astrocyte-endothelial interactions at the blood-brain barrier. *Nat. Rev. Neurosci.* 7, 41–53. doi: 10.1038/nrn1824

Arroyo, D. S., Soria, J. A., Gaviglio, E. A., Rodriguez-Galan, M. C., and Iribarren, P. (2011). Toll-like receptors are key players in neurodegeneration. *Int. Immunopharmacol.* 11, 1415–1421. doi: 10.1016/j.intimp.2011.05.006

Banks, W. A. (2005). Blood-brain barrier transport of cytokines: a mechanism for neuropathology. *Curr. Pharm. Des.* 11, 973–984.

Beg, A. A. (2002). Endogenous ligands of Toll-like receptors: implications for regulating inflammatory and immune responses. *Trends Immunol.* 23, 509–512.

Bhargavan, B., and Kanmogne, G. D. (2018). Toll-like receptor-3 mediates HIV-1-induced interleukin-6 expression in the human brain endothelium via TAK1 and JNK pathways: implications for viral neuropathogenesis. *Mol. Neurobiol.* 55, 5976–5992. doi: 10.1007/s12035-017-0816-8

Blasius, A. L., and Beutler, B. (2010). Intracellular toll-like receptors. *Immunity* 32, 305–315. doi: 10.1016/j.immuni.2010.03.012

Bradford, M. M. (1976). A rapid and sensitive method for the quantitation of microgram quantities of protein utilizing the principle of protein-dye binding. *Anal. Biochem.* 72, 248–254.

Brown, A. S. (2006). Prenatal infection as a risk factor for schizophrenia. *Schizophr. Bull.* 32, 200–202. doi: 10.1093/schbul/sbj052

Bsibsi, M., Ravid, R., Gveric, D., and van Noort, J. M. (2002). Broad expression of Toll-like receptors in the human central nervous system. *J. Neuropathol. Exp. Neurol.* 61, 1013–1021.

Cameron, J. S., Alexopoulou, L., Sloane, J. A., DiBernardo, A. B., Ma, Y., Kosaras, B., et al. (2007). Toll-like receptor 3 is a potent negative regulator of axonal growth in mammals. *J. Neurosci.* 27, 13033–13041. doi: 10.1523/JNEUROSCI.4290-06.2007

Cavassani, K. A., Ishii, M., Wen, H., Schaller, M. A., Lincoln, P. M., Lukacs, N. W., et al. (2008). TLR3 is an endogenous sensor of tissue necrosis during acute inflammatory events. *J. Exp. Med.* 205, 2609–2621. doi: 10.1084/jem.2008 1370

Chavez-Valdez, R., Emerson, P., Goffigan-Holmes, J., Kirkwood, A., Martin, L. J., and Northington, F. J. (2018). Delayed injury of hippocampal interneurons after neonatal hypoxia-ischemia and therapeutic hypothermia in a murine model. *Hippocampus* 28, 617–630. doi: 10.1002/hipo.22965

Chavez-Valdez, R., Martin, L. J., and Northington, F. J. (2012). Programmed necrosis: a prominent mechanism of cell death following neonatal brain injury. *Neurol. Res. Int.* 2012:257563. doi: 10.1155/2012/257563

Chavez-Valdez, R., Martin, L. J., Razdan, S., Gauda, E. B., and Northington, F. J. (2014). Sexual dimorphism in BDNF signaling after neonatal hypoxia-ischemia and treatment with necrostatin-1. *Neuroscience* 260, 106–119. doi: 10.1016/j.neuroscience.2013.12.023

Chistyakov, D. V., Azbukina, N. V., Lopachev, A. V., Kulichenkova, K. N., Astakhova, A. A., and Sergeeva, M. G. (2018). Rosiglitazone as a Modulator of TLR4 and TLR3 signaling pathways in rat primary neurons and astrocytes. *Int. J. Mol. Sci.* 19:E113. doi: 10.3390/ijms19010113

De Miranda, J., Yaddanapudi, K., Hornig, M., Villar, G., Serge, R., and Lipkin, W. I. (2010). Induction of Toll-like receptor 3-mediated immunity during gestation inhibits cortical neurogenesis and causes behavioral disturbances. *Mbio* 1, e00176–e00210. doi: 10.1128/mBio.00176-10

Du, L., Bayir, H., Lai, Y., Zhang, X., Kochanek, P. M., Watkins, S. C., et al. (2004). Innate gender-based proclivity in response to cytotoxicity and programmed cell death pathway. *J. Biol. Chem.* 279, 38563–38570. doi: 10.1074/jbc.M405461200

Dupuis, N., Mazarati, A., Desnous, B., Chhor, V., Fleiss, B., Le Charpentier, T., et al. (2016). Pro-epileptogenic effects of viral-like inflammation in both mature and immature brains. *J. Neuroinflamm.* 13:307. doi: 10.1186/s12974-016-0773-6

Estornes, Y., Toscano, F., Virard, F., Jacquemin, G., Pierrot, A., Vanbervliet, B., et al. (2012). dsRNA induces apoptosis through an atypical death complex associating TLR3 to caspase-8. *Cell Death Differ.* 19, 1482–1494. doi: 10.1038/cdd.2012.22

Fatemi, S. H., Emamian, E. S., Kist, D., Sidwell, R. W., Nakajima, K., Akhter, P., et al. (1999). Defective corticogenesis and reduction in reelin immunoreactivity in cortex and hippocampus of prenatally infected neonatal mice. *Mol. Psychiatry* 4, 145–154.

Fitzgerald, K. A., McWhirter, S. M., Faia, K. L., Rowe, D. C., Latz, E., Golenbock, D. T., et al. (2003). IKKepsilon and TBK1 are essential components of the IRF3 signaling pathway. *Nat. Immunol.* 4, 491–496. doi: 10.1038/ni921

Forrest, C. M., Khalil, O. S., Pisar, M., Smith, R. A., Darlington, L. G., and Stone, T. W. (2012). Prenatal activation of Toll-like receptors-3 by administration of the viral mimetic poly(I:C) changes synaptic proteins, N-methyl-D-aspartate receptors and neurogenesis markers in offspring. *Mol. Brain* 5:22. doi: 10.1186/1756-6606-5-22

Franchi, L., Eigenbrod, T., Munoz-Planillo, R., Ozkurede, U., Kim, Y. G., Arindam, C., et al. (2014). Cytosolic double-stranded RNA activates the NLRP3 inflammasome via MAVS-induced membrane permeabilization and K+ efflux. *J. Immunol.* 193, 4214–4222. doi: 10.4049/jimmunol.1400582

Gambara, G., Desideri, M., Stoppacciaro, A., Padula, F., De Cesaris, P., Starace, D., et al. (2015). TLR3 engagement induces IRF-3-dependent apoptosis in androgen-sensitive prostate cancer cells and inhibits tumour growth in vivo. *J. Cell Mol. Med.* 19, 327–339. doi: 10.1111/jcmm.12379

Greenmyer, J. R., Gaultney, R. A., Brissette, C. A., and Watt, J. A. (2018). Primary human microglia are phagocytically active and respond to *Borrelia burgdorferi* with upregulation of chemokines and cytokines. *Front. Microbiol.* 9:811. doi: 10.3389/fmicb.2018.00811

Hagberg, H., Wilson, M. A., Matsushita, H., Zhu, C., Lange, M., Gustavsson, M., et al. (2004). PARP-1 gene disruption in mice preferentially protects males from perinatal brain injury. *J. Neurochem.* 90, 1068–1075. doi: 10.1111/j.1471-4159.2004.02547.x

He, S., Liang, Y., Shao, F., and Wang, X. (2011). Toll-like receptors activate programmed necrosis in macrophages through a receptor-interacting kinase-3-mediated pathway. *Proc. Natl. Acad. Sci. U.S.A.* 108, 20054–20059. doi: 10.1073/pnas.1116302108

Hopwood, N., Maswanganyi, T., and Harden, L. M. (2009). Comparison of anorexia, lethargy, and fever induced by bacterial and viral mimetics in rats. *Can. J. Physiol. Pharmacol.* 87, 211–220. doi: 10.1139/y09-003

Hurn, P. D., Vannucci, S. J., and Hagberg, H. (2005). Adult or perinatal brain injury: does sex matter? *Stroke* 36, 193–195. doi: 10.1161/01.STR.0000153064.41332.f6

Johnson, R. H., Kho, D. T., O'Carroll, S. J., Angel, C. E., and Graham, E. S. (2018). The functional and inflammatory response of brain endothelial cells to toll-like receptor agonists. *Sci. Rep.* 8:10102. doi: 10.1038/s41598-018-28518-3

Kaiser, W. J., Sridharan, H., Huang, C., Mandal, P., Upton, J. W., Gough, P. J., et al. (2013). Toll-like receptor 3-mediated necrosis via TRIF, RIP3, and MLKL. *J. Biol. Chem.* 288, 31268–31279. doi: 10.1074/jbc.M113.462341

Kariko, K., Ni, H., Capodici, J., Lamphier, M., and Weissman, D. (2004). mRNA is an endogenous ligand for Toll-like receptor 3. *J. Biol. Chem.* 279, 12542–12550. doi: 10.1074/jbc.M310175200

Kneeland, R. E., and Fatemi, S. H. (2013). Viral infection, inflammation and schizophrenia. *Prog. Neuropsychopharmacol. Biol. Psychiatry* 42, 35–48. doi: 10.1016/j.pnpbp.2012.02.001

Kovarik, P., Castiglia, V., Ivin, M., and Ebner, F. (2016). Type I interferons in bacterial infections: a balancing act. *Front. Immunol.* 7:652. doi: 10.3389/fimmu.2016.00652

Lang, K. S., Georgiev, P., Recher, M., Navarini, A. A., Bergthaler, A., Heikenwalder, M., et al. (2006). Immunoprivileged status of the liver is controlled by toll-like receptor 3 signaling. *J. Clin. Invest.* 116, 2456–2463. doi: 10.1172/JCI28349

Lathia, J. D., Okun, E., Tang, S. C., Griffioen, K., Cheng, A., Mughal, M. R., et al. (2008). Toll-like receptor 3 is a negative regulator of embryonic neural progenitor cell proliferation. *J. Neurosci.* 28, 13978–13984. doi: 10.1523/JNEUROSCI.2140-08.2008

Le, W., Wu, J., and Tang, Y. (2016). Protective microglia and their regulation in parkinson's disease. *Front. Mol. Neurosci.* 9:89. doi: 10.3389/fnmol.2016.00089

Lemere, C. A. (2007). A beneficial role for IL-1 beta in Alzheimer disease? *J. Clin. Invest.* 117, 1483–1485. doi: 10.1172/JCI32356

Liu, F., Lang, J., Li, J., Benashski, S. E., Siegel, M., Xu, Y., et al. (2011). Sex differences in the response to poly(ADP-ribose) polymerase-1 deletion and caspase inhibition after stroke. *Stroke* 42, 1090–1096. doi: 10.1161/STROKEAHA.110.594861

Loomes, R., Hull, L., and Mandy, W. P. L. (2017). What is the male-to-female ratio in autism spectrum disorder? a systematic review and meta-analysis. *J. Am. Acad. Child Adolesc. Psychiatry* 56, 466–474. doi: 10.1016/j.jaac.2017.03.013

Lotzerich, M., Roulin, P. S., Boucke, K., Witte, R., Georgiev, O., and Greber, U. F. (2018). Rhinovirus 3C protease suppresses apoptosis and triggers caspase-independent cell death. *Cell Death Dis.* 9:272. doi: 10.1038/s41419-018-0306-6

Mallard, C., Tremblay, M. E., and Vexler, Z. S. (2018). Microglia and neonatal brain injury. *Neuroscience* doi: 10.1016/j.neuroscience.2018.01.023 [Epub ahead of print].

Maxwell, J. R., Denson, J. L., Joste, N. E., Robinson, S., and Jantzie, L. L. (2015). Combined in utero hypoxia-ischemia and lipopolysaccharide administration in rats induces chorioamnionitis and a fetal inflammatory response syndrome. *Placenta* 36, 1378–1384. doi: 10.1016/j.placenta.2015.10.009

McGrath, J. J. (2006). Variations in the incidence of schizophrenia: data versus dogma. *Schizophr. Bull.* 32, 195–197. doi: 10.1093/schbul/sbi052

Moon, Y. (2014). Ribosomal alteration-derived signals for cytokine induction in mucosal and systemic inflammation: noncanonical pathways by ribosomal inactivation. *Med. Inflamm.* 2014:708193. doi: 10.1155/2014/708193

Northington, F. J., Chavez-Valdez, R., Graham, E. M., Razdan, S., Gauda, E. B., and Martin, L. J. (2011). Necrostatin decreases oxidative damage, inflammation, and injury after neonatal HI. *J. Cereb. Blood Flow Metab.* 31, 178–189. doi: 10.1038/jcbfm.2010.72

Ottum, P. A., Arellano, G., Reyes, L. I., Iruretagoyena, M., and Naves, R. (2015). Opposing roles of interferon-gamma on cells of the central nervous system in autoimmune neuroinflammation. *Front. Immunol.* 6:539. doi: 10.3389/fimmu.2015.00539

Packard, A. E., Hedges, J. C., Bahjat, F. R., Stevens, S. L., Conlin, M. J., Salazar, A. M., et al. (2012). Poly-IC preconditioning protects against cerebral and renal ischemia-reperfusion injury. *J. Cereb. Blood Flow Metab.* 32, 242–247. doi: 10.1038/jcbfm.2011.160

Patole, P. S., Grone, H. J., Segerer, S., Ciubar, R., Belemezova, E., Henger, A., et al. (2005). Viral double-stranded RNA aggravates lupus nephritis through Toll-like receptor 3 on glomerular mesangial cells and antigen-presenting cells. *J. Am. Soc. Nephrol.* 16, 1326–1338. doi: 10.1681/ASN.2004100820

Pfaffl, M. W. (2001). A new mathematical model for relative quantification in real-time RT-PCR. *Nucleic Acids Res.* 29:e45.

Pobezinskaya, Y. L., Kim, Y. S., Choksi, S., Morgan, M. J., Li, T., Liu, C., et al. (2008). The function of TRADD in signaling through tumor necrosis factor receptor 1 and TRIF-dependent toll-like receptors. *Nat. Immunol.* 9, 1047–1054. doi: 10.1038/ni.1639

Priya, R., Patro, I. K., and Parida, M. M. (2014). TLR3 mediated innate immune response in mice brain following infection with chikungunya virus. *Virus Res.* 189, 194–205. doi: 10.1016/j.virusres.2014.05.010

Rajan, J. V., Warren, S. E., Miao, E. A., and Aderem, A. (2010). Activation of the NLRP3 inflammasome by intracellular poly I:C. *FEBS Lett.* 584, 4627–4632. doi: 10.1016/j.febslet.2010.10.036

Randow, F., and Seed, B. (2001). Endoplasmic reticulum chaperone gp96 is required for innate immunity but not cell viability. *Nat. Cell Biol.* 3, 891–896. doi: 10.1038/ncb1001-891

Ransohoff, R. M., and Brown, M. A. (2012). Innate immunity in the central nervous system. *J. Clin. Invest.* 122, 1164–1171. doi: 10.1172/JCI58644

Renolleau, S., Fau, S., Goyenvalle, C., Joly, L. M., Chauvier, D., Jacotot, E., et al. (2007). Specific caspase inhibitor Q-VD-OPh prevents neonatal stroke in P7 rat: a role for gender. *J. Neurochem.* 100, 1062–1071. doi: 10.1111/j.1471-4159.2006.04269.x

Robinson, S., Corbett, C. J., Winer, J. L., Chan, L. A. S., Maxwell, J. R., Anstine, C. V., et al. (2018). Neonatal erythropoietin mitigates impaired gait, social interaction and diffusion tensor imaging abnormalities in a rat model of prenatal brain injury. *Exp. Neurol.* 302, 1–13. doi: 10.1016/j.expneurol.2017.12.010

Robinson, S., Winer, J. L., Berkner, J., Chan, L. A., Denson, J. L., Maxwell, J. R., et al. (2016). Imaging and serum biomarkers reflecting the functional efficacy of extended erythropoietin treatment in rats following infantile traumatic brain injury. *J. Neurosurg. Pediatr.* 17, 739–755. doi: 10.3171/2015.10.PEDS15554

Rossi, D., and Volterra, A. (2009). Astrocytic dysfunction: insights on the role in neurodegeneration. *Brain Res. Bull.* 80, 224–232. doi: 10.1016/j.brainresbull.2009.07.012

Smith, P. L. P., Mottahedin, A., Svedin, P., Mohn, C. J., Hagberg, H., Ek, J., et al. (2018). Peripheral myeloid cells contribute to brain injury in male neonatal mice. *J. Neuroinflamm.* 15:301. doi: 10.1186/s12974-018-1344-9

Stridh, L., Mottahedin, A., Johansson, M. E., Valdez, R. C., Northington, F., Wang, X., et al. (2013). Toll-like receptor-3 activation increases the vulnerability of the neonatal brain to hypoxia-ischemia. *J. Neurosci.* 33, 12041–12051. doi: 10.1523/JNEUROSCI.0673-13.2013

Sun, R., Zhang, Y., Lv, Q., Liu, B., Jin, M., Zhang, W., et al. (2011). Toll-like receptor 3 (TLR3) induces apoptosis via death receptors and mitochondria by up-regulating the transactivating p63 isoform alpha (TAP63alpha). *J. Biol. Chem.* 286, 15918–15928. doi: 10.1074/jbc.M110.178798

Tabeta, K., Hoebe, K., Janssen, E. M., Du, X., Georgel, P., Crozat, K., et al. (2006). The Unc93b1 mutation 3d disrupts exogenous antigen presentation and signaling via toll-like receptors 3, 7 and 9. *Nat. Immunol.* 7, 156–164. doi: 10.1038/ni1297

Torcia, M. G., Nencioni, L., Clemente, A. M., Civitelli, L., Celestino, I., Limongi, D., et al. (2012). Sex differences in the response to viral infections: TLR8 and TLR9 ligand stimulation induce higher IL10 production in males. *PLoS One* 7:e39853. doi: 10.1371/journal.pone.0039853

Vannucci, S. J., and Hurn, P. D. (2009). Gender differences in pediatric stroke: is elevated testosterone a risk factor for boys? *Ann. Neurol.* 66, 713–714. doi: 10.1002/ana.21925

Vontell, R., Supramaniam, V., Thornton, C., Wyatt-Ashmead, J., Mallard, C., Gressens, P., et al. (2013). Toll-like receptor 3 expression in glia and neurons alters in response to white matter injury in preterm infants. *Dev. Neurosci.* 35, 130–139. doi: 10.1159/000346158

Wakida, N. M., Cruz, G. M. S., Ro, C. C., Moncada, E. G., Khatibzadeh, N., Flanagan, L. A., et al. (2018). Phagocytic response of astrocytes to damaged neighboring cells. *PLoS One* 13:e0196153. doi: 10.1371/journal.pone.0196153

Yang, Y., Liu, B., Dai, J., Srivastava, P. K., Zammit, D. J., Lefrancois, L., et al. (2007). Heat shock protein gp96 is a master chaperone for toll-like receptors and is important in the innate function of macrophages. *Immunity* 26, 215–226. doi: 10.1016/j.immuni.2006.12.005

Yellowhair, T. R., Noor, S., Maxwell, J. R., Anstine, C. V., Oppong, A. Y., Robinson, S., et al. (2018). Preclinical chorioamnionitis dysregulates CXCL1/CXCR2 signaling throughout the placental-fetal-brain axis. *Exp. Neurol.* 301(Pt B), 110–119. doi: 10.1016/j.expneurol.2017.11.002

Yousif, N. M., de Oliveira, A. C. P., Brioschi, S., Huell, M., Biber, K., and Fiebich, B. L. (2018). Activation of EP2 receptor suppresses poly(I: C) and LPS-mediated inflammation in primary microglia and organotypic hippocampal slice cultures: contributing role for MAPKs. *Glia* 66, 708–724. doi: 10.1002/glia.23276

Zhu, C., Wang, X., Huang, Z., Qiu, L., Xu, F., Vahsen, N., et al. (2007). Apoptosis-inducing factor is a major contributor to neuronal loss induced by neonatal cerebral hypoxia-ischemia. *Cell Death Differ.* 14, 775–784. doi: 10.1038/sj.cdd.4402053

Zhu, C., Wang, X., Qiu, L., Peeters-Scholte, C., Hagberg, H., and Blomgren, K. (2004). Nitrosylation precedes caspase-3 activation and translocation of apoptosis-inducing factor in neonatal rat cerebral hypoxia-ischaemia. *J. Neurochem.* 90, 462–471. doi: 10.1111/j.1471-4159.2004.02500.x

Zimmer, S., Steinmetz, M., Asdonk, T., Motz, I., Coch, C., Hartmann, E., et al. (2011). Activation of endothelial toll-like receptor 3 impairs endothelial function. *Circ. Res.* 108, 1358–1366. doi: 10.1161/CIRCRESAHA.111.243246

17

Transplanted Human Oligodendrocyte Progenitor Cells Restore Neurobehavioral Deficits in a Rat Model of Preterm White Matter Injury

Xiaohua Wang[1,2,3], Jing Zang[2], Yinxiang Yang[2], Siliang Lu[2], Qian Guan[2], Dou Ye[2], Zhaoyan Wang[2], Haipeng Zhou[2], Ke Li[2], Qian Wang[2], Youjia Wu[3] and Zuo Luan[1,2]**

[1] The Second School of Clinical Medicine, Southern Medical University, Guangzhou, China, [2] Department of Pediatrics, The Sixth Medical Center of PLA General Hospital, Beijing, China, [3] Department of Pediatrics, Affiliated Hospital of Nantong University, Nantong, China

***Correspondence:**
Youjia Wu
francis_nt@163.com
Zuo Luan
luanzuo@aliyun.com

Background: Preterm white matter injury (PWMI) is a common brain injury and a leading cause of life-long neurological deficits in premature infants; however, no effective treatment is available yet. This study aimed to investigate the fate and effectiveness of transplanted human oligodendrocyte progenitor cells (hOPCs) in a rat model of PWMI.

Methods: Hypoxia-ischemia was induced in rats at postnatal day 3, and hOPCs (6×10^5 cells/5 μL) were intracerebroventricularly transplanted at postnatal day 7. Neurobehavior was assessed 12 weeks post-transplant using the CatWalk test and Morris water maze test. Histological analyses, as well as immunohistochemical and transmission electron microscopy, were performed after transcardial perfusion.

Results: Transplanted hOPCs survived for 13 weeks in PWMI brains. They were widely distributed in the injured white matter, and migrated along the corpus callosum to the contralateral hemisphere. Notably, 82.77 ± 3.27% of transplanted cells differentiated into mature oligodendrocytes, which produced myelin around the axons. Transplantation of hOPCs increased the fluorescence intensity of myelin basic protein and the thickness of myelin sheaths as observed in immunostaining and transmission electron microscopy, while it reduced white matter atrophy at the level of gross morphology. With regard to neurobehavior, the CatWalk test revealed improved locomotor function and inter-paw coordination after transplantation, and the cognitive functions of hOPC-transplanted rats were restored as revealed by the Morris water maze test.

Conclusions: Myelin restoration through the transplantation of hOPCs led to neurobehavioral improvements in PWMI rats, suggesting that transplanting hOPCs may provide an effective and promising therapeutic strategy in children with PWMI.

Keywords: preterm white matter injury, oligodendrocyte progenitor cell, myelination, neurobehavioral deficit, cell therapy

INTRODUCTION

Although advances in intensive care have led to improved survival of preterm infants, they have coincided with an increased incidence of premature brain injury. Preterm white matter injury (PWMI) is the most prevalent form of brain injury in premature infants and is the leading cause of cerebral palsy and other permanent neurological deficits (1). Currently, diffuse WMI characterized by global white matter hypomyelination, has become the most common type of PWMI observed in preterm infants (2). Diffuse WMI, as measured by diffusion tensor imaging, is associated with white matter atrophy, ventriculomegaly, and structural alterations of critical white matter tracts (3, 4).

The key pathological mechanism underlying PWMI is delayed or disturbed maturation of oligodendrocytes (OLs) and subsequent myelination (5). OL lineage cells develop through oligodendrocyte progenitor cells (OPCs), immature pre-myelinating OLs (pre-OLs), and finally mature into myelinated OLs (4, 6). OPCs and pre-OLs are predominant in the white matter from the gestational age of 23–32 weeks. As these immature OL lineage cells are highly sensitive to preterm-related insults, infants born at this gestational age with exposure to inflammation and/or hypoxia are at a high risk of impaired OL differentiation and myelination (5, 7). Furthermore, a lack of proper myelination during brain development will ultimately result in axonal degeneration and impaired brain connectivity (8).

Currently, no effective treatment is available for WMI in the developing brain. Stem/progenitor cell-based therapies are promising for treating neurological disorders, with potential neuroprotective and/or regenerative effects on injured brain cells. Neural stem cells (NSCs) and mesenchymal stem cells (MSCs) have been reported to improve neurobehavioral outcomes in some animal models of WMI (9, 10), however, they mainly play a neuroprotective role rather than regenerative replacement, because the differentiation rate of NSCs into OL is very low, and MSCs cannot differentiate into OL. Among stem cells, OPCs are considered to be the optimal cells for WMI treatment, as it has the potential to self-renew and differentiate into myelin-producing OLs (11, 12).

To date, there has been little published work on OPC-based therapies for PWMI. A limited number of studies have demonstrated that transplanted mouse-derived OPCs have neuroprotective effects in a rat model of periventricular leukomalacia (PVL, another type of PWMI), by stimulating endogenous NSC proliferation, inhibiting neuronal apoptosis, and improving cognitive impairment (13, 14). Evidently, there are species differences in myelin development and myelin regeneration between human-derived OPCs and mouse-derived OPCs (15), and human OPCs are superior when it comes to translatability for clinical trials. In 2018, a study by Tae-Kyun et al. showed that human-derived F3.olig2 OPCs (established from an immortalized human NSC line) restored neurobehavioral functions by preventing axonal demyelination in a rat model of PVL (16). However, this study of human OPC treatment for PWMI described a possible neuroprotective effect of OPCs within 5 weeks, but not a regenerative effect. Thus, our study was designed to observe the migration and differentiation capacity of hOPCs during a 13-week observation period and to determine whether transplanted hOPCs could regenerate myelin and improve neurobehavioral outcomes in a rat model of PWMI.

MATERIALS AND METHODS

Animal Model of PWMI

This study was approved by the Animal Ethical and Welfare Committee of the Chinese PLA General Hospital (Beijing, China) (Ethics No. SCXK-2012-0001). The number and suffering of the animals were minimized as much as possible. The day of birth was defined as postnatal day (P) 0. Hypoxia-ischemia (HI) was induced in rats at P3 as previously described (17, 18). Briefly, 38 Sprague-Dawley pups of either sex from three litters were anesthetized by placing them on ice for 10 min, and the right common carotid artery was isolated and permanently occluded by electrocoagulation. Pups were allowed to recover for 30–60 min and then were placed in a container perfused with a humidified gas mixture (6% oxygen in nitrogen) at 37°C for 90 min. Thirty surviving pups were randomized into one of two groups: PWMI or PWMI+hOPCs ($n = 15$ per group). Animals in the control group ($n = 10$) underwent surgery without arterial occlusion or subsequent hypoxia.

Preparation of hOPCs

The hOPCs were prepared and provided by the Pediatric Laboratory at the Sixth Medical Center of the Chinese PLA General Hospital, according to the guidelines approved by the Hospital's Ethics Committee (Ethics No. 2015013). Briefly, hNSCs were isolated from the cortex of human embryos aged 10–13 weeks and amplified in the NSC medium. To generate hOPCs, hNSCs were cultured for 10 days to form neurospheres, which were dissociated into single cells and induced to differentiate in the differentiation medium (19). The purity of the hOPCs was 80–90%, as confirmed in our previous study (20). Before transplantation surgery, hOPCs were stained with specific markers such as PDGFR-α, A2B5, NG2, and O4 (see **Supplementary Figure 1**) and then resuspended in 5 μL of PBS to make a single-cell suspension containing 6×10^5 cells.

Transplantation of hOPCs

Four days after HI insult, pups in the PWMI+hOPCs group were intracerebroventricularly transplanted with hOPCs. Briefly, pups were placed in a stereotaxic device under isoflurane anesthesia (induction at 2.5% and then 1% for maintenance). An incision was made to the skin, and a needle was inserted through the skull at the following coordinates (from Bregma): anteroposterior, −0.5 mm; mediolateral, −1.5 mm; and dorsoventral, −2.0 ∼ −2.5 mm. Pups were injected with 6×10^5 cells (5 μL) over the course of 10 min. The syringe was left *in situ* for 5 min and then gradually withdrawn. The pups were placed on a heated blanket to recover before being returned to the dam. Animals in the PWMI group received an injection of 5 μL PBS at the same coordinates. All groups received cyclosporine A (10 mg/kg/day;

Sandimmun, Novartis) intraperitoneally for 4 weeks starting 3 days before transplantation, followed by 100 μg/mL in the drinking water until the perfusion.

Neurobehavioral Tests

Twelve weeks after transplantation, the rats were subjected to behavioral tests: the CatWalk test and Morris water maze test. These tests were performed between 8 am and 11 am by a well-trained investigator and an assistant who were blinded to the experimental groups.

CatWalk Test

The CatWalk test was used to objectively assess walking ability, and was carried out with an automated computer-assisted system (Noldus Information Technology, The Netherlands) (21, 22). An enclosed glass walkway was illuminated with fluorescent light coming from the side. The light reflected by the rats' paws as they contacted the walkway was captured by a high-speed video camera and then transformed into a digital image. Before the test, rats were trained to cross the glass walkway toward their home cage. The test was conducted in a dark, silent room. The runs with accepted step cycles were analyzed for each rat. If a rat failed to complete a run within 5 s, walked backward, or reared on the glass floor, it was given an additional run, and an alternative motivator such as food reward was used. Two rats in PWMI group and three rats in PWMI+hOPCs group were excluded because they failed to complete the run. The videos were analyzed using CatWalk XT 10.6, and footprints were automatically or manually labeled as right fore (RF), right hind (RH), left fore (LF), and left hind (LH) paws. After identification of individual footprints, data including individual paw statistics, comparative paw statistics, interlimb coordination, and temporal parameters were all automatedly analyzed and exported.

Morris Water Maze Test

The Morris water maze test was performed to evaluate spatial learning and memory, as previously described (13, 23). Briefly, this task was performed in a circular device with a diameter of 150 cm and a height of 50 cm and was filled with water (30 cm in depth, 22 ± 2°C). A black hidden platform (12 cm in diameter) was placed in Quadrant 2, ~1.5 cm beneath the water surface. Rats in their home cage were placed in the testing room for at least 1 h before the test to minimize the effects of stress on behavioral outcomes. For the navigation test, rats underwent four trials daily with different drop locations, over five consecutive days. Each trial ended when the rat rested on the platform for 3 s. If a rat could not find the platform within 60 s, it was led to the platform and allowed to rest for 10 s. The space probe trial, with the platform removed, took place on the sixth day over 60 s. Data were analyzed using the Morris water maze system (Labmaze V3.0; Zhongshidichuang Science and Technology Development Co., Ltd, Beijing, China). The latency to find the platform, number of platform crossings, number of platform quadrant crossings, and time spent in the platform quadrant were recorded.

Tissue Preparation and Histological Assessment

Thirteen weeks after transplantation, the rats were deeply anesthetized with 10% chloral hydrate and transcardially perfused with 0.9% saline followed by 4% paraformaldehyde (PFA). Brains were removed and post-fixed in 4% PFA at 4°C for 24 h, followed by cryoprotection in a graded series of sucrose (15% and 30%). Coronal sections were cut at 8 μm using a freezing microtome (Cm1850; Leica, Germany) and stored at −80°C. Brain sections (2.04, 1.32, 0.12, −0.84, −1.92, −3.00, and −5.40 mm from Bregma) were stained with hematoxylin and eosin (HE) and Luxol fast blue (LFB), as previously described (24, 25). All stained sections were scanned on a computer using an Axio scan (Z1 system; Zeiss, Germany).

To evaluate cerebral atrophy, on each section with HE staining, the areas of both hemispheres were measured by ImageJ software (NIH, USA), and the volume was calculated by multiplying the appropriate area by the section interval thickness. To minimize errors associated with tissue processing, the relative volume of cerebral atrophy was determined using the following formula: (contralateral cerebral volume—ipsilateral cerebral volume)/contralateral cerebral volume (26).

To evaluate white matter atrophy, in each section with LFB staining, the white matter areas (including the corpus callosum, external capsule, internal capsule, and striatum fiber bundles) within the ipsilateral and contralateral hemispheres were measured. The volume was calculated according to the same principle as above, and the relative volume of white matter atrophy was determined as follows: (contralateral white matter volume—ipsilateral white matter volume)/contralateral white matter volume.

Immunohistochemistry and Imaging

Frozen sections were blocked with 2% BSA/0.3% Triton X-100 in PBS for 1 h and incubated with the following primary antibodies overnight at 4°C: anti-hN (1:300, mouse monoclonal, Millipore) and anti-stem121 (1:500, mouse monoclonal, TaKaRa) for the detection of transplanted human cells; anti-GFAP (1:1,000, rabbit polyclonal, Abcam) for the detection of astrocytes; anti-Olig2 (1:200, rabbit polyclonal, Millipore) for the detection of oligodendrocytes; anti-NF (1:500, rabbit polyclonal, BioLegend) for axon staining; and anti-myelin basic protein (MBP) (1:100, rabbit polyclonal, Abcam) for myelin staining. Subsequently, the sections were washed in PBS and incubated in the appropriate secondary antibodies conjugated with Alexa Fluor-488 or−594 for 1 h at 37°C. Images were acquired immediately after staining using a fluorescence microscope (Olympus IX51, Japan). To quantify the differentiation capacity of hOPCs into Olig2$^+$ oligodendrocytes, the proportion of hN$^+$ cells that were also Olig2$^+$ was determined in five animals. Images were taken from three 20 × objective fields per section and from three sections (2.04, 0.12, and −5.40 mm from Bregma) per animal, namely, nine sampling regions per animal. To quantify the differentiation capacity of hOPCs into MBP$^+$ oligodendrocytes or GFAP$^+$ astrocytes, the area fraction of stem121$^+$/MBP$^+$ or stem121$^+$/GFAP$^+$ to stem121$^+$ was measured using ImageJ in five animals. Images were taken from nine 40 × objective fields of each animal according to the same principle as described above. To ascertain whether processes of human-derived cells were wrapped around host axons, a three-dimensional reconstruction by Z-stack scanning through regions of interest was acquired with a confocal microscope (Olympus FV300, Japan).

Immunostaining of MBP (1:100, rat monoclonal, Abcam) was performed to determine the integrity of the host myelin. Alexa Fluor-488 conjugated donkey anti-rat IgG (1:200, Abcam, UK) was used as the secondary antibody. To detect the MBP intensity of the ipsilateral cingulate gyrus and external capsule, region-specific images were taken from three adjacent sections (~0.12 mm from Bregma) in each animal, and the green intensity was analyzed using ImageJ.

Transmission Electron Microscopy (TEM)

The corpus callosum (~1 × 1 × 1 mm), adjacent to the transplant site, was isolated from the forebrain and fixed at 4°C in a solution containing 2.5% glutaraldehyde and 2% PFA. The samples were subsequently embedded in epoxy resin, sliced using an ultrathin microtome, and stained with uranium acetate and lead citrate. Ultrathin sections were observed under a transmission electron microscope and photographed for further analysis. These procedures were mostly performed at the Electron Microscopy Center of Tsinghua University. TEM images were analyzed for g-ratio using Image-Pro Plus 6.0 (Media Cybernetics, USA). G-ratio was defined as the ratio of the diameter of an axon to the diameter of the axon plus its myelin sheath (24). Quantification was performed in 50 randomly chosen myelinated axons at 6,000× magnification for each animal ($n = 4$ per group).

Statistical Analysis

Data are presented as mean ± SEM, unless stated otherwise. Continuous variables of the Morris water maze test were analyzed by repeated measures two-way analysis of variance (ANOVA), followed by Fisher's least significant difference (LSD) *post hoc* test when appropriate. Gait analysis data were compared using the Kruskal–Wallis non-parametric test, followed by a Mann-Whitney *U*-test when the results were significant. Other data were analyzed using one-way ANOVA. The statistical significance level was set at $P \leq 0.05$. Data analysis and statistical inference were performed using the SPSS 25.0 (IBM, Armonk, NY).

RESULTS

Migration and Differentiation of Transplanted hOPCs in PWMI Rats

At 13 weeks post-transplantation, stem121$^+$/hN$^+$ cells were widely distributed in injured white matter areas and migrated through the corpus callosum to the contralateral cingulate gyrus and external capsule. Scattered cells were also found in the lower layers of the cortex and fimbria of the hippocampus (**Figure 1**). The hN$^+$ cells were the most highly concentrated near the transplant site (522.67 ± 145.55), followed by the section at −5.40 mm from Bregma (387.11 ± 140.41) and the

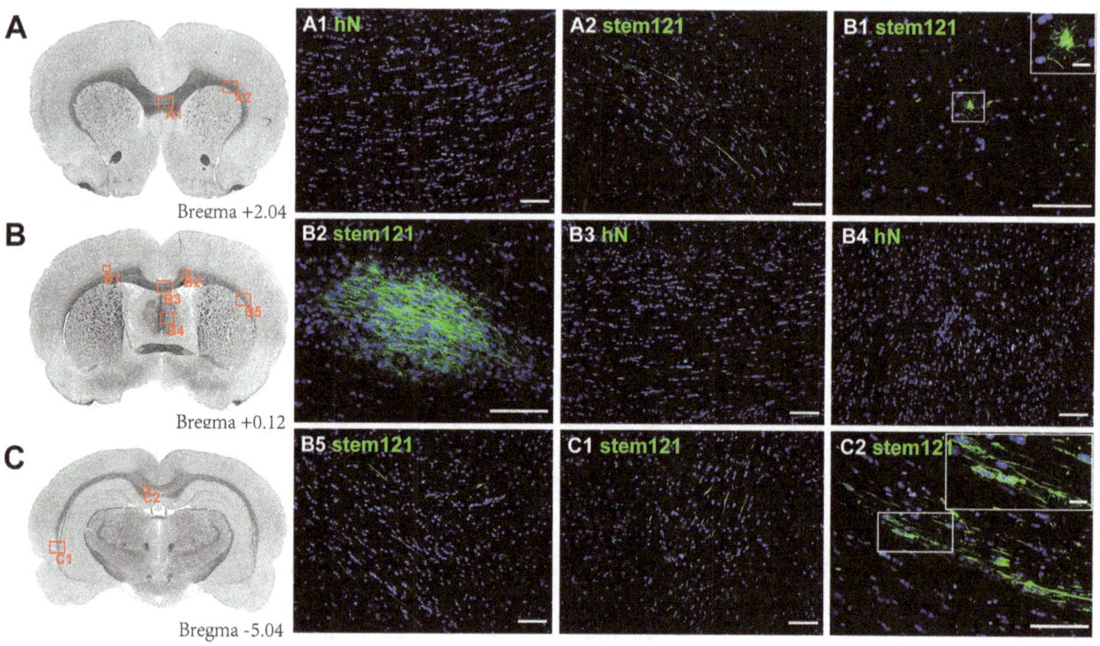

FIGURE 1 | Migration of transplanted hOPCs. **(A–C)** Stem121$^+$/hN$^+$ cells were widely distributed in the injured white matter and migrated to the contralateral brain in PWMI rats at 13 weeks after transplantation. Stem121$^+$ cells in the lower layers of the cortex were round with extensive and radial processes (B1), while cells in the corpus callosum were spindle-shaped with long parallel processes (C2). All coronal sections were counterstained with DAPI. Scale bar represents 100 μm in (A1-C2) and 15 μm in zoomed images of B1 and C2.

section at 2.04 mm from Bregma (270.00 ± 38.00); however, there was no statistical difference in hN^+ cell counts between these three sections [$F_{(2,6)} = 4.830$, $P = 0.056$; one-way ANOVA]. Interestingly, $stem121^+$ cells in the lower layers of the cortex were round with radial processes (**Figure 1B1**), consistent with type I morphology, while cells in the corpus callosum and external capsule were spindle-shaped with long parallel processes (**Figure 1C2**), consistent with type II/III morphology (27).

To identify and quantify the differentiation of transplanted cells, double immunostaining was performed. The majority (87.29 ± 1.75%) of hN^+ cells co-expressed Olig2, and the area fraction of $stem121^+MBP^+/stem121^+$ was up to 82.77 ± 3.27%, while the area fraction of $stem121^+GFAP^+/stem121^+$ was 0.97 ± 0.21% (**Figures 2A,B**), suggesting that most transplanted cells matured to be MBP-producing OLs in injured white matter, and only a few cells differentiated into astrocytes. Importantly, reconstructed confocal images showed a close, ensheathment-like position of NF^+ $stem121^-$ host axons with $stem121^+$ cells differentiated from hOPCs (**Figure 2C**).

hOPCs Restored Myelin Integrity of PWMI Rats

Compared with the control rats, HI-injured rats displayed decreased MBP intensity in both hemispheres 13 weeks post-transplantation, and the intensity in the ipsilateral hemisphere was lower than that in the contralateral hemisphere, especially in the external capsule (**Figure 3A**). Quantitative analysis revealed that MBP intensity in the ipsilateral cingulate gyrus and external capsule was significantly lower in HI-injured rats than in control rats [cingulate gyrus: $F_{(2,18)} = 3.550$, $P = 0.050$, PWMI vs. control, $P = 0.025$; external capsule: $F_{(2,18)} = 8.145$, $P = 0.003$, PWMI vs. control, $P = 0.001$; one-way ANOVA with LSD for multiple comparisons]. MBP in the cingulate gyrus of the PWMI+hOPCs group was comparable to that in both the control group and the PWMI group, while MBP expression in the external capsule of the PWMI+hOPCs group was more intense than that of the PWMI group ($P = 0.047$; LSD), but still lower than that of the control group ($P = 0.046$; LSD) (**Figure 3B**).

We next used TEM to visualize the ultrastructure of the demyelinated areas. In control animals, a large amount of thick and compact myelin sheaths was observed in the corpus callosum. In comparison, the myelin sheath was sparse in the PWMI rats, with a thin and disrupted structure. The hOPC-transplanted rats exhibited evidence of structural restoration, as observed in the density and thickness of the myelin sheath, but the restored myelin was thinner than the normal myelin sheath (**Figure 3C**). These findings were confirmed by the quantification of the g-ratio (0.625 ± 0.006 in the control group, 0.780 ± 0.002 in the PWMI group, and 0.647 ± 0.009 in the PWMI+hOPCs group) [$F_{(2,9)} = 4.622$, $P < 0.001$, PWMI vs. control, $P < 0.001$, PWMI+hOPCs vs. PWMI, $P < 0.001$, PWMI+hOPCs vs. control, $P = 0.027$; one-way ANOVA with LSD for multiple comparisons; **Figures 3D,E**]. Taken together, these results demonstrate that transplanted hOPCs restored the integrity of the myelin sheath in PWMI rats.

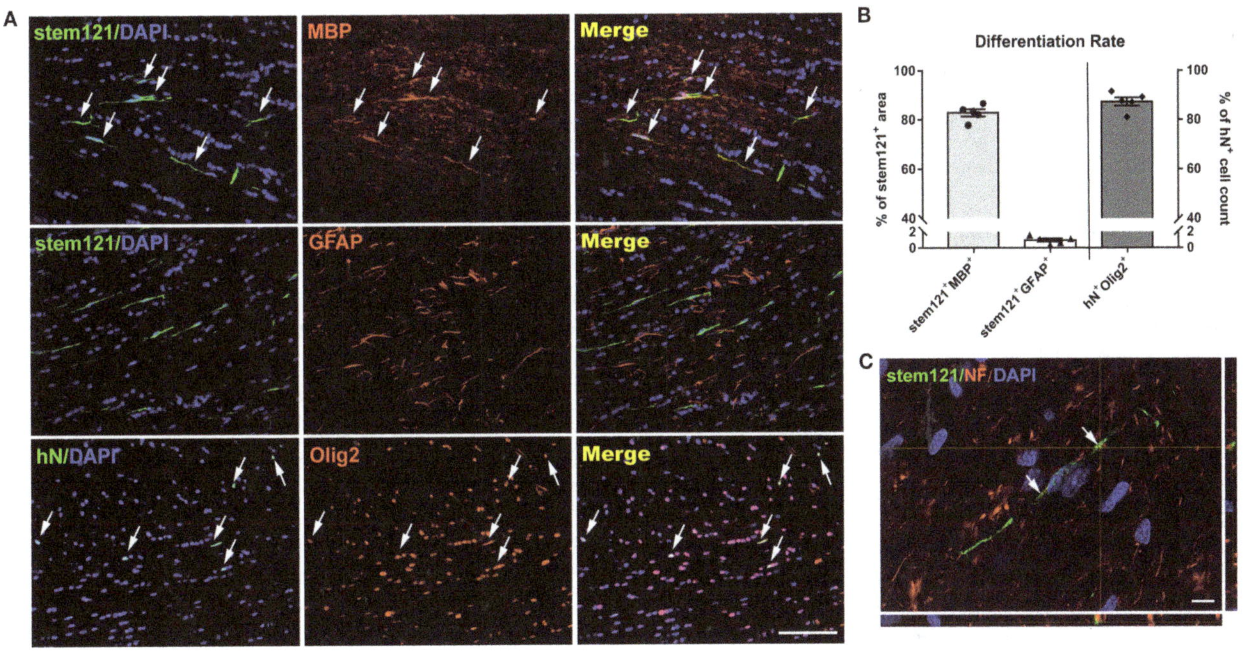

FIGURE 2 | Differentiation of transplanted hOPCs. **(A)** Representative images of hOPCs differentiation at 13 weeks post-transplantation. **(B)** More than 80% of transplanted cells co-expressed Olig2 and MBP, and little GFAP co-staining was observed in $stem121^+$ cells ($n = 5$ per group; three sections per rat, with three sites randomly sampled per section). **(C)** Confocal images showed the ensheathment of axons by $stem121^+$ OLs. Scale bar represents 50 μm in **(A)** and 10 μm in **(C)**. Data are presented as mean ± SEM.

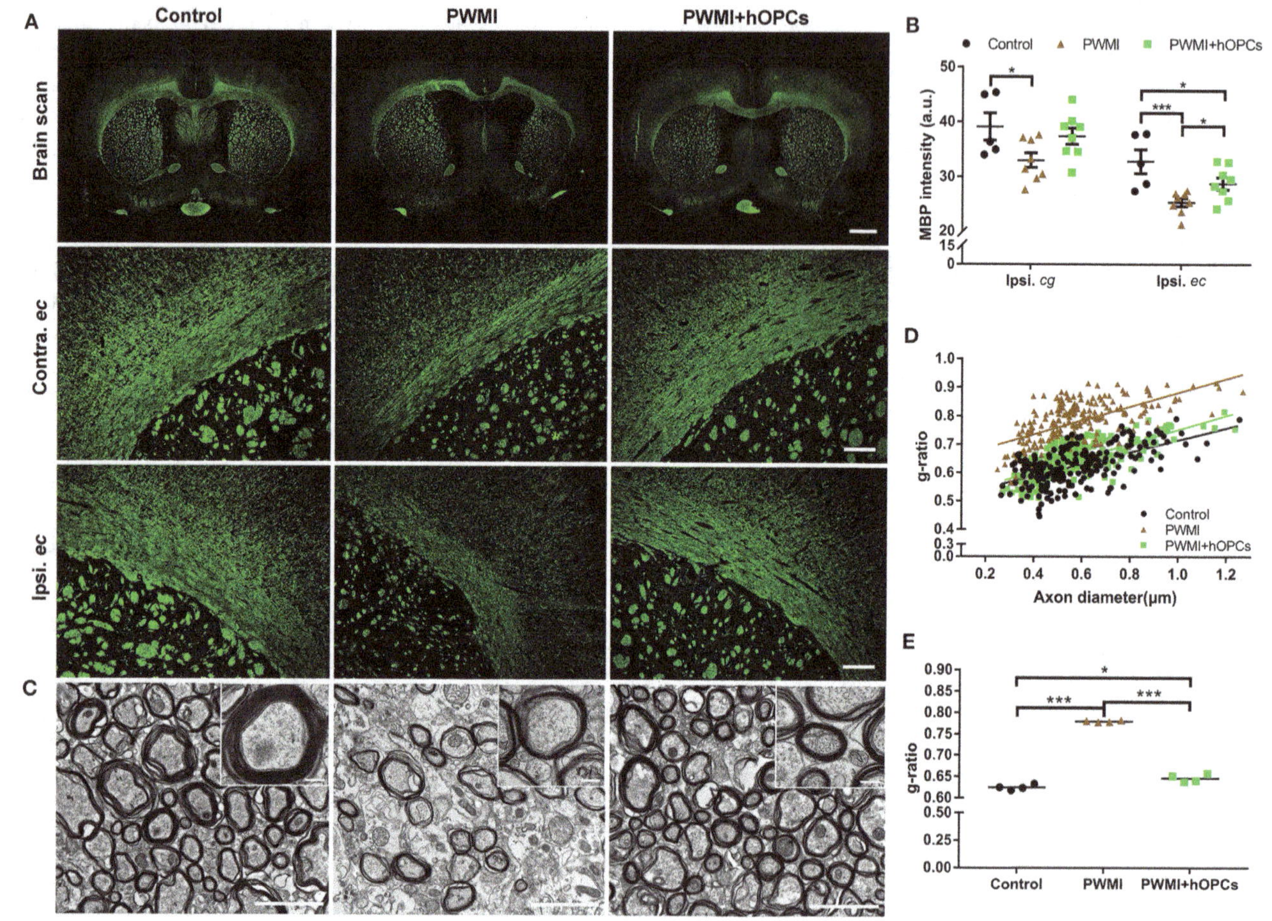

FIGURE 3 | Immunohistochemical and TEM analysis of myelin. **(A)** Representative images of MBP intensity in both hemispheres and external capsules at 13 weeks post-transplantation. Scale bar represents 2,000 μm in the top row and 200 μm in the two lower rows. **(B)** Quantification of MBP intensity in the ipsilateral cingulate gyrus (*cg*) and external capsule (*ec*) ($n = 5$ for control, $n = 8$ for PWMI and PWMI+hOPCs; three sections per rat; one-way ANOVA with LSD for multiple comparisons). **(C)** Representative TEM images of myelin sheath in the corpus callosum. Scale bar represents 2 μm in **(C)** and 200 nm for the insert pictures. **(D,E)** G-ratios of myelinated axons in the corpus callosum of the control, PWMI, and PWMI+hOPCs groups ($n = 4$ per group, one-way ANOVA with LSD for multiple comparisons). Data are presented as mean ± SEM. $^{*}P < 0.05$, $^{***}P < 0.001$.

hOPCs Improved Neuropathological Outcomes of PWMI Rats

At the level of gross morphology, PWMI rats showed prominent cerebral atrophy and white matter atrophy compared with control animals [cerebral atrophy, $F_{(2,20)} = 4.578$, $P = 0.031$, PWMI vs. control, $P = 0.033$; white matter atrophy, $F_{(2,20)} = 15.629$, $P = 0.001$, PWMI vs. control, $P = 0.002$; Brown-Forsythe test with Dunnett's T3 for multiple comparisons; **Figures 4A,B,D**]. Furthermore, cerebral atrophy along with white matter atrophy in PWMI rats was found to be relatively uniform across the rostro-caudal axis (**Figures 4C,E**), without specifically injured coronal levels. White matter atrophy volume was reduced in hOPC-transplanted rats ($P = 0.03$; Dunnett's T3), but the cerebral atrophy showed no significant change compared to PWMI animals. In addition, cerebral atrophy volume and white matter atrophy volume in hOPC-transplanted rats were still obvious compared to the control group (cerebral atrophy, $P = 0.043$; white matter atrophy, $P = 0.005$; Dunnett's T3; **Figures 4B,D**). In hOPCs-transplanted rats, the white matter of ipsilateral corpus callosum, external capsule and internal capsule was slightly sparse and structurally abnormal compared to the contralateral (see **Supplementary Figure 2**). These results indicated that transplantation of hOPCs can partially reserve the injured white matter tissue.

hOPCs Alleviated Neurobehavioral Deficits in PWMI Rats

Gait parameters in the CatWalk test selected for analysis between groups are listed and defined in **Supplementary Table 1**. Compared to control animals, a severe reduction was observed in parameters that reflect locomotor function of PWMI rats: print length [RF, $H_{(2)} = 11.110$, $P = 0.004$, PWMI vs. control, $P = 0.001$; RH, $H_{(2)} = 14.505$, $P = 0.001$, PWMI vs. control, $P < 0.001$; LF, $H_{(2)} = 13.009$, $P = 0.001$, PWMI vs. control, $P < 0.001$; LH, $H_{(2)} = 10.166$, $P = 0.006$, PWMI vs. control, $P < 0.001$],

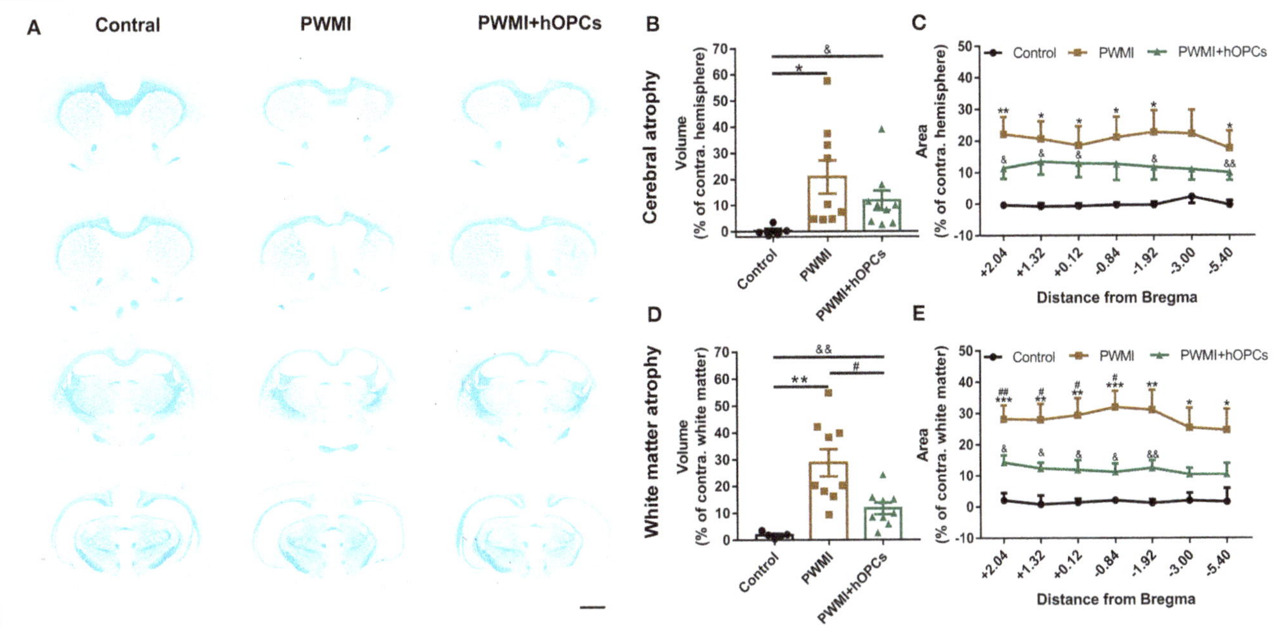

FIGURE 4 | Measurement of cerebral atrophy and white matter atrophy. **(A)** Representative coronal sections stained with LFB demonstrate prominent white matter atrophy in the PWMI group and restoration following transplant. Scale bar = 2 mm. **(B,C)** Cerebral atrophy area in specific coronal sections and cerebral atrophy volume were analyzed between groups ($n = 5$ for controls, $n = 9$ for PWMI and PWMI+hOPCs; seven sections per rat; Brown-Forsythe test with Dunnett's T3 for multiple comparisons). **(D,E)** White matter atrophy area in specific coronal sections and white matter atrophy volume were compared between groups ($n = 5$ for controls, $n = 9$ for PWMI and PWMI+hOPCs; seven sections per rat; Brown-Forsythe test with Dunnett's T3 for multiple comparisons). Data are presented as mean ± SEM; PWMI vs. control: $^{*}P < 0.05$, $^{**}P < 0.01$, $^{***}P < 0.001$; PWMI + hOPCs vs. PWMI: $^{\#}P < 0.05$, $^{\#\#}P < 0.01$; PWMI + hOPCs vs. control: $^{\&}P < 0.05$, $^{\&\&}P < 0.01$.

stride length [RF, $H_{(2)} = 15.759$, $P < 0.001$, PWMI vs. control, $P < 0.001$; RH, $H_{(2)} = 15.185$, $P = 0.001$, PWMI vs. control, $P < 0.001$; LF, $H_{(2)} = 16.520$, $P < 0.001$, PWMI vs. control, $P < 0.001$; LH, $H_{(2)} = 15.605$, $P < 0.001$, PWMI vs. control, $P < 0.001$], swing speed [RF, $H_{(2)} = 15.114$, $P = 0.001$, PWMI vs. control, $P < 0.001$; RH, $H_{(2)} = 17.746$, $P < 0.001$, PWMI vs. control, $P < 0.001$; LF, $H_{(2)} = 14.527$, $P = 0.001$, PWMI vs. control, $P < 0.001$; LH, $H_{(2)} = 16.258$, $P < 0.001$, PWMI vs. control, $P < 0.001$] and max contact area [RF, $H_{(2)} = 11.342$, $P = 0.003$, PWMI vs. control, $P < 0.001$; RH, $H_{(2)} = 8.694$, $P = 0.013$, PWMI vs. control, $P = 0.003$; LF, $H_{(2)} = 8.847$, $P = 0.012$, PWMI vs. control, $P = 0.001$; LH, $H_{(2)} = 11.413$, $P = 0.003$, PWMI vs. control, $P < 0.001$] of each paw. Furthermore, the coupling parameters LH->RH [$H_{(2)} = 3.847$, $P = 0.032$, PWMI vs. control, $P = 0.015$] and LF->LH [$H_{(2)} = 4.200$, $P = 0.024$, PWMI vs. control, $P = 0.01$], used as a measure of inter-paw coordination, changed significantly. hOPC-transplanted animals displayed marked improvement in gait parameters including print length of right paws (RF, $P = 0.039$; RH, $P = 0.004$; LF, $P = 0.121$; LH, $P = 0.121$), stride length (RF, $P = 0.012$; RH, $P = 0.014$; LF, $P = 0.024$; LH, $P = 0.026$), swing speed (RF, $P = 0.014$; RH, $P = 0.009$; LF, $P = 0.012$; LH, $P = 0.034$), and step cycle [RF, $H_{(2)} = 8.414$, $P = 0.015$, PWMI+hOPCs vs. PWMI, $P = 0.008$; RH, $H_{(2)} = 8.422$, $P = 0.015$, PWMI+hOPCs vs. PWMI, $P = 0.01$; LF, $H_{(2)} = 10.767$, $P = 0.005$, PWMI+hOPCs vs. PWMI, $P = 0.003$; LH, $H_{(2)} = 9.618$, $P = 0.008$, PWMI+hOPCs vs. PWMI, $P = 0.005$] of each paw, as well as LH->RH ($P = 0.045$) and LF->LH ($P = 0.044$) couplings (Kruskal-Wallis non-parametric test with Mann-Whitney U-test for multiple comparisons; **Figure 5**).

In the Morris water maze test, the PWMI group showed a much longer latency to find the platform compared to control animals from navigation test day 2 [Day 2, $F_{(2,37)} = 4.221$, $P = 0.022$, PWMI vs. control, $P = 0.018$; Day 3, $F_{(2,37)} = 5.196$, $P = 0.010$, PWMI vs. control, $P = 0.008$; Day 4, $F_{(2,37)} = 6.414$, $P = 0.004$, PWMI vs. control, $P = 0.003$; Day 5, $F_{(2,37)} = 12.655$, $P = 0.001$, PWMI vs. control, $P = 0.005$], suggesting impairment of spatial learning ability in these rats. By contrast, OPC-transplanted animals reduced the latency time to a near-normal level (Day 2, $P = 0.019$; Day 3, $P = 0.012$; Day 4, $P = 0.006$; Day 5, $P = 0.001$) (Repeated measures ANOVA with LSD *post-hoc* test; **Figure 6A**). In the probe trial, PWMI rats had much fewer platform crossings and platform quadrant crossings compared to control animals [platform crossings, $F_{(2,37)} = 3.645$, $P = 0.036$, PWMI vs. control, $P = 0.034$; platform quadrant crossings, $F_{(2,37)} = 4.798$, $P = 0.014$, PWMI vs. control, $P = 0.016$; one-way ANOVA with LSD], suggesting a spatial memory deficit. In hOPC-transplanted rats, the platform crossings and platform quadrant crossings, but not duration in the platform quadrant, were increased (platform crossings, $P = 0.023$; platform quadrant crossings, $P = 0.01$; LSD) (**Figures 6B–D**). Taken together, the above results indicate that locomotor and cognitive deficits of PWMI rats can be improved by engraftment of hOPCs.

DISCUSSION

The present study aimed to determine the fate and effectiveness of transplanted hOPCs in a rat model of PWMI. We found that hOPCs transplanted via the ventricle migrated widely

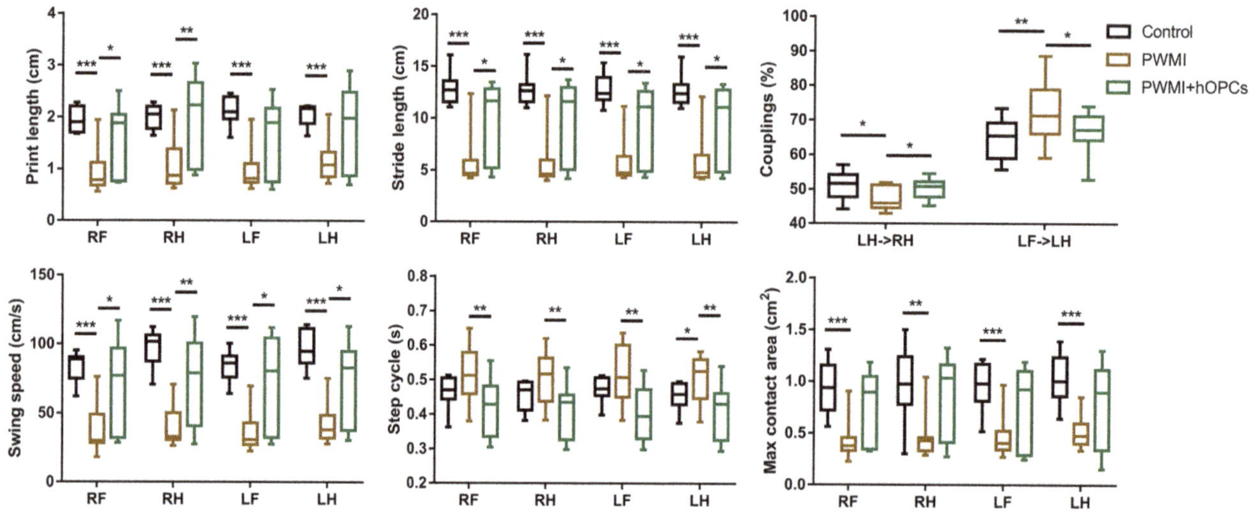

FIGURE 5 | Gait analysis between groups. HI injury-induced severe alternation in print length, stride length swing speed and max contact area of each paw, as well as coupling parameters LH->RH and LF->LH. Such alternation of gait parameters was improved following hOPCs-transplantation ($n = 10$ for controls, $n = 13$ for PWMI and $n = 12$ for PWMI+hOPCs; Kruskal–Wallis non-parametric test with Mann-Whitney *U*-test for multiple comparisons). Data are presented as median (IQR); *$P < 0.05$, **$P < 0.01$, ***$P < 0.001$.

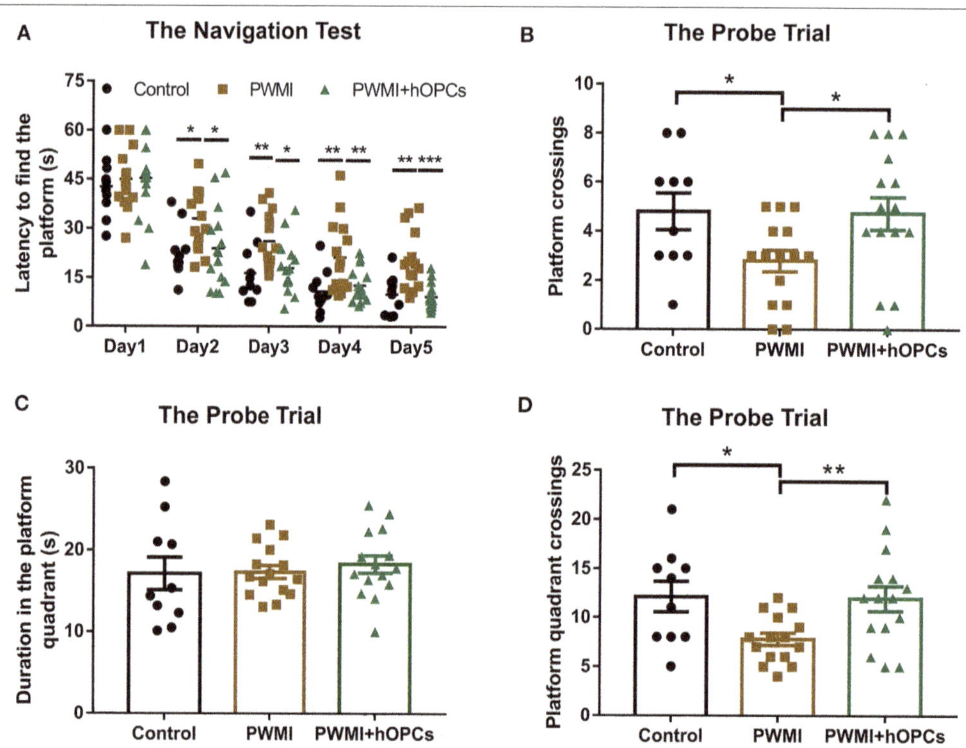

FIGURE 6 | Assessment of cognitive function. **(A)** In the navigation test, increased latency to find the platform of PWMI rats were reduced to a near-normal level after hOPCs-transplantation ($n = 10$ for the control, $n = 15$ for PWMI and PWMI+hOPCs; repeated measures ANOVA, followed by LSD *post-hoc* test). **(B–D)** In the probe trial, platform crossings and platform quadrant crossings, but not duration in the platform quadrant, decreased in PWMI group and improved after hOPCs-transplantation ($n = 10$ for the control, $n = 15$ for PWMI and PWMI+hOPCs; one-way ANOVA with LSD for multiple comparisons). Data are presented as mean ± SEM; *$P < 0.05$, **$P < 0.01$, ***$P < 0.001$.

and differentiated into myelin-forming OLs at 13 weeks after grafting. Transplantation of hOPCs restored myelin and rescued neurobehavioral deficits. Importantly, we first demonstrated the regenerative effect of hOPC in PWMI rats.

PWMI is a major neuropathological brain injury often seen in survivors of premature birth. In humans, the susceptibility to PWMI peaks between the gestational age of 23 and 32 weeks, which corresponds to P2 to P5 in rats with regard to white matter development (2, 17). Accordingly, OPCs and pre-OLs in neonatal rats are also vulnerable to ischemia, hypoxia, and inflammatory insults. Previous studies in neonatal rats have confirmed that ischemia (unilateral carotid artery ligation) combined with hypoxia (5–8% O_2 for 0.5–3.5 h) induces disturbed myelination and neurological deficits (17, 28). Consistent with previous work, HI-injured rats in our study displayed obvious myelin loss and structural alterations observed by TEM and immunohistochemistry, along with extensive white matter atrophy and an enlarged lateral ventricle on the gross morphology. PWMI can cause a wide range of neurological sequelae later in life, including severe motor disabilities such as cerebral palsy and subtle consequences such as impaired perceptual abilities and cognitive function, attention problems, and psychiatric conditions (29, 30). In our study, the HI-injured neonatal rats showed decreased locomotor function, abnormal inter-paw coordination, and cognitive dysfunctions, as revealed by neurobehavioral tests. The above-mentioned neuropathological and behavioral abnormalities in HI-injured rats were similar to the key characteristics of human PWMI (2, 4).

Sensitive behavioral tests that can detect long-term deficits in PWMI rats are critical for cell replacement studies, because exogenous cells may take months to proliferate, differentiate, and integrate into the host brain (27). The CatWalk is one of the most suitable methods for the quantitative assessment of impaired gait and locomotor function in rodents, as this automated system can quickly and objectively analyze a large number of gait parameters, particularly dynamic parameters such as swing duration, and interlimb coordination, which are difficult to quantify by any other method (21). The CatWalk test has been widely used in peripheral nerve injury, spinal cord injury, and ischemic brain injury models (31–33). PWMI model is also a kind of ischemic brain injury, so we introduced it into this experiment. Based on the strength and reliability of each parameter demonstrated in previous studies (21, 22, 33), 17 parameters were selected for functional evaluation in our study, and the results showed that print length, stride length, swing speed, max contact area, and couplings were changed in PWMI rats at 12 weeks post-transplant, suggesting a long-term impairment in locomotor function and coordination. The Morris water maze, a classic test for evaluating cognitive function, revealed impaired spatial learning and memory in PWMI rats, which was consistent with the results of previous studies (13, 16). We speculate that the deficits are associated not only with white matter atrophy, which interrupts brain connection, but also with a certain extent of gray matter damage, such as damage to cortical motor areas. Although this is an animal model of WMI, gray matter cannot be completely spared.

A number of preclinical studies have confirmed the effectiveness of OPC transplantation in other demyelinating diseases (24, 34–36), but there has been little published work on hOPC therapies for PWMI. Here we showed that hNSC-derived OPCs intracerebroventricularly transplanted 4 days after injury survived for 13 weeks, disseminated mostly to injured white matter areas, and migrated along white matter tracts. The distribution preference for white matter may be due to the fact that neonatal HI injury predominantly affects the white matter, and damaged white matter has a chemotactic effect on transplanted cells. This chemotaxis is believed to be mediated by trophic factors such as stromal cell-derived factor 1α, chemokine (C-X-C motif) receptor 4, and vascular endothelial growth factor (VEGF) (37, 38). Notably, up to 82.77% of our transplanted cells differentiated into mature OLs, as detected by double immunostaining for stem121 and MBP markers. By contrast, a study by Kuai et al. revealed that embryonic stem cell (ESC)-derived OPCs displayed poor survival and limited migration ability in twitcher mice, which led to remyelination failure (39). Webber et al. showed a low differentiation rate into mature OLs of rat-derived OPCs in PWMI animals (14). Compared with the above studies, the relatively extensive migration and high-efficiency differentiation of hOPCs observed here mainly attributed to the origin and stage of transplanted cells. The hOPCs grafted in our study were induced from human fetal NSCs, different from the ESC-derived or rat-derived OPCs, and 80–90% of our hOPCs expressed PDGF-αR, A2B5, and O4, consistent with a late OPC phenotype (20), while early OPCs, expressing NG2, Olig2, and A2B5, were used by Webber et al. Secondly, contrary to the above studies, we used cyclosporine for anti-rejection to ensure the survival of exogenous cells. According to previous studies, cyclosporine treatment can reduce xenogeneic cell rejection and prolong the survival of transplanted cells (40, 41).

Importantly, our study demonstrated that transplantation of hOPCs markedly restored myelination in PWMI rats, as an increase in myelin integrity was observed via immunostaining of host MBP and ultrastructural analysis by TEM, as well as a reduction in white matter atrophy at the level of gross morphology. The mechanisms underlying myelin repair include myelin regeneration and the neuroprotective effects of the transplanted grafts. Traditionally, cell-based therapies have been introduced to replace lost or damaged cells through targeted differentiation (42). In this study, a large fraction of transplanted hOPCs differentiated into OLs and produced myelin wrapping around axons, as confirmed by co-staining and confocal scanning. This implies that the implanted hOPCs generated new myelin sheaths by cell replacement. Moreover, a growing number of studies have indicated that grafted cells can release various neurotrophic factors such as brain-derived neurotrophic factor, ciliary neurotrophic factor, VEGF, and insulin-like growth factor-1, which exert favorable effects on angiogenesis, neurogenesis, neuronal survival, and myelination (43–45). We suspected that our transplanted hOPCs can secret neuroprotective factors into the local environment, thus preventing myelin loss and promoting endogenous myelination. However, a limitation here is that we cannot separately quantify exogenous myelination and endogenous myelination induced by hOPC transplantation.

Moreover, the transplantation of hOPCs significantly improved the behavioral performance of PWMI rats. Ameliorated cognitive deficits were achieved at 12 weeks after transplantation, as observed in the Morris water maze test. Automated gait analysis revealed that transplanted hOPCs restored locomotor function and inter-paw coordination in PWMI rats. It is believed that these improved neurological functions are associated with the repair of myelin and white matter structures, which restores saltatory conduction and brain connectivity (46).

In conclusion, the present study showed that transplanted hOPCs restored the myelin of injured white matter and eventually led to neurobehavioral improvements in PWMI rats. Importantly, we first demonstrated the regenerative effect of hOPCs in PWMI animals. These results suggest that the transplantation of hOPCs may be an effective and promising therapeutic strategy for children with PWMI. Our results are encouraging for further translational studies. In addition, others in our research group have found highly expressed neurotrophic factors in hOPCs by single-cell sequencing, our follow-up research is to identify neurotrophic factors secreted by hOPCs *in vivo,* which benefit endogenous remyelination or prevent myelin loss.

ETHICS STATEMENT

The studies involving human participants were reviewed and approved by Ethics Committee of the Chinese PLA General Hospital (Beijing, China). The patients/participants provided their written informed consent to participate in this study. The animal study was reviewed and approved by the Animal Ethical and Welfare Committee of the Chinese PLA General Hospital (Beijing, China).

AUTHOR CONTRIBUTIONS

YY, YW, and ZL designed the experiments. XW and JZ carried out HI operations and cell transplantation. ZW, DY, and QW were responsible for preparation of hOPCs. QG and KL conducted behavioral tests. SL, XW, and HZ performed histological staining and statistical analysis. XW and YY drafted the manuscript. All authors contributed to manuscript revision, read, and approved the submitted version.

FUNDING

This study was supported by the National Key R&D Programme of China [grant number 2017YFA0104200], funded by Ministry of Science and Technology of the People's Republic of China.

ACKNOWLEDGMENTS

The authors thank Jingjing Wang at the Center of Biomedical Analysis, Tsinghua University for the help with confocal microscopy. We also thank Editage (www.editage.cn) for English language editing.

REFERENCES

Back SA, Miller SP. Brain injury in premature neonates: a primary cerebral dysmaturation disorder? *Ann Neurol.* (2014) 75:469–86. doi: 10.1002/ana.24132

Back SA. White matter injury in the preterm infant: pathology and mechanisms. *Acta Neuropathol.* (2017) 134:331–49. doi: 10.1007/s00401-017- 1718-6

Alexandrou G, Mårtensson G, Skiöld B, Blennow M, Adén U, Vollmer B. White matter microstructure is influenced by extremely preterm birth and neonatal respiratory factors. *Acta Paediatrica.* (2014) 103:48–56. doi: 10.1111/apa. 12445

van Tilborg E, de Theije CGM, van Hal M, Wagenaar N, de Vries LS, Benders MJ, et al. Origin and dynamics of oligodendrocytes in the developing brain: Implications for perinatal white matter injury. *Glia.* (2018) 66:221–38. doi: 10.1002/glia. 23256

van Tilborg E, Heijnen CJ, Benders MJ, van Bel F, Fleiss B, Gressens P, et al. Impaired oligodendrocyte maturation in preterm infants: potential therapeutic targets. *Prog Neurobiol.* (2016) 136:28–49. doi: 10.1016/j.pneurobio.2015. 11.002

Emery B. Regulation of oligodendrocyte differentiation and myelination. *Science.* (2010) 330:779–82. doi: 10.1126/science.11 90927

Bennet L, Dhillon S, Lear CA, van den Heuij L, King V, Dean JM, et al. Chronic inflammation and impaired development of the preterm brain. *J Reprod Immunol.* (2018) 125:45–55. doi: 10.1016/j.jri.2017. 11.003

Vaes JEG, Vink MA, de Theije CGM, Hoebeek FE, Benders M, Nijboer CHA. The potential of stem cell therapy to repair white matter injury in preterm infants: lessons learned from experimental models. *Front Physiol.* (2019) 10:540. doi: 10.3389/fphys.2019. 00540

Oppliger B, Joerger-Messerli M, Mueller M, Reinhart U, Schneider P, Surbek DV, et al. Intranasal delivery of umbilical cord-derived mesenchymal stem cells preserves myelination in perinatal brain damage. *Stem Cells Dev.* (2016) 25:1234–42. doi: 10.1089/scd. 2016.0027

Uchida N, Chen K, Dohse M, Hansen KD, Dean J, Buser JR, et al. Human neural stem cells induce functional myelination in mice with severe dysmyelination. *Sci Transl Med.* (2012) 4:155ra36. doi: 10.1126/scitranslmed.3 004371

Nishiyama A, Boshans L, Goncalves CM, Wegrzyn J, Patel KD. Lineage, fate, and fate potential of NG2-glia. *Brain Res.* (2016) 1638:116–28. doi: 10.1016/j. brainres.2015.08.013

Sharp J, Frame J, Siegenthaler M, Nistor G, Keirstead HS. Human embryonic stem cell-derived oligodendrocyte progenitor cell transplants improve recovery after cervical spinal cord injury. *Stem Cells.* (2010) 28:152– 63. doi: 10.1002/stem.245

Chen LX, Ma SM, Zhang P, Fan ZC, Xiong M, Cheng GQ, et al. Neuroprotective effects of oligodendrocyte progenitor cell transplantation in premature rat brain following hypoxic-ischemic injury. *PLoS ONE.* (2015) 10:e0115997. doi: 10.1371/journal.pone.0 115997

Webber DJ, van Blitterswijk M, Chandran S. Neuroprotective effect of oligodendrocyte precursor cell transplantation in a long-term model of periventricular leukomalacia. *Am J Pathol.* (2009) 175:2332–42. doi: 10.2353/ajpath.2009.0 90051

Dietz KC, Polanco JJ, Pol SU, Sim FJ. Targeting human oligodendrocyte progenitors for myelin repair. *Exp Neurol.* (2016) 283:489–500. doi: 10.1016/j.expneurol.2016. 03.017

Kim TK, Park D, Ban YH, Cha Y, An ES, Choi J, et al. Improvement by human oligodendrocyte progenitor cells of neurobehavioral disorders in an experimental model of neonatal periventricular leukomalacia. *Cell Transplant.* (2018) 27:1168–77. doi: 10.1177/0963689718 781330

Back SA, Han BH, Luo NL, Chricton CA, Xanthoudakis S, Tam J, et al. Selective vulnerability of late oligodendrocyte progenitors to hypoxia-ischemia. *J Neurosci.* (2002) 22:455– 63. doi: 10.1523/ JNEUROSCI.22-02-00455.2002

Zhu LH, Bai X, Zhang N, Wang SY, Li W, Jiang L. Improvement of human umbilical cord mesenchymal stem cell transplantation on glial cell and behavioral function in a neonatal model of periventricular white matter damage. *Brain Res.* (2014) 1563:13–21. doi: 10.1016/j.brainres.2014. 03.030

Zhou H, He Y, Wang Z, Wang Q, Hu C, Wang X, et al. Identifying the functions of two biomarkers in human oligodendrocyte progenitor cell development. *J Transl Med.* (2021) 19:188. doi: 10.1186/s12967-021-0 2857-8

Wang C, Luan Z, Yang Y, Wang Z, Wang Q, Lu Y, et al. High purity of human oligodendrocyte progenitor cells obtained from neural stem cells: suitable for clinical application. *J Neurosci Methods.* (2015) 240:61– 6. doi: 10.1016/j.jneumeth.2014.10.017

Kappos EA, Sieber PK, Engels PE, Mariolo AV, D'Arpa S, Schaefer DJ, et al. Validity and reliability of the CatWalk system as a static and dynamic gait analysis tool for the assessment of functional nerve recovery in small animal models. *Brain Behav.* (2017) 7:e00723. doi: 10.1002/brb3.723

Parkkinen S, Ortega FJ, Kuptsova K, Huttunen J, Tarkka I, Jolkkonen J. Gait impairment in a rat model of focal cerebral ischemia. *Stroke Res Treat.* (2013) 2013:410972. doi: 10.1155/2013/410972

Park D, Lee SH, Bae DK, Yang YH, Yang G, Kyung J, et al. Transplantation of human adipose tissue-derived mesenchymal stem cells restores the neurobehavioral disorders of rats with neonatal hypoxic-ischemic encephalopathy. *Cell Med.* (2013) 5:17–28. doi: 10.3727/215517913X6 58936

Piao J, Major T, Auyeung G, Policarpio E, Menon J, Droms L, et al. Human embryonic stem cell-derived oligodendrocyte progenitors remyelinate the brain and rescue behavioral deficits following radiation. *Cell Stem Cell.* (2015) 16:198–210. doi: 10.1016/j.stem.2015.01.004

Tsuji M, Ohshima M, Taguchi A, Kasahara Y, Ikeda T, Matsuyama A novel reproducible model of neonatal stroke in mice: comparison with a hypoxia-ischemia model. *Exp Neurol.* (2013) 247:218–25. doi: 10.1016/j.expneurol.2013.04.015

Penny TR, Sutherland AE, Mihelakis JG, Paton MCB, Pham Y, Lee J, et al. Human umbilical cord therapy improves long-term behavioral outcomes following neonatal hypoxic ischemic brain injury. *Front Physiol.* (2019)
10:283. doi: 10.3389/fphys.2019.00283

Xu L, Ryu J, Hiel H, Menon A, Aggarwal A, Rha E, et al. Transplantation of human oligodendrocyte progenitor cells in an animal model of diffuse traumatic axonal injury: survival and differentiation. *Stem Cell Res Ther.* (2015) 6:93. doi: 10.1186/s13287-015-0087-0

Lee JA, Kim BI, Jo CH, Choi CW, Kim EK, Kim HS, et al. Mesenchymal stem- cell transplantation for hypoxic-ischemic brain injury in neonatal rat model. *Pediatr Res.* (2010) 67:42–6. doi: 10.1203/PDR.0b013e3181bf594b

Yang P, Chen YH, Yen CF, Chen HL. Psychiatric diagnoses, emotional- behavioral symptoms and functional outcomes in adolescents born preterm with very low birth weights. *Child Psychiatry Hum Dev.* (2015) 46:358– 66. doi: 10.1007/s10578-014-0475-1

Skranes J, Vangberg TR, Kulseng S, Indredavik MS, Evensen KA, Martinussen M, et al. Clinical findings and white matter abnormalities seen on diffusion tensor imaging in adolescents with very low birth weight. *Brain.* (2007) 130:654–66. doi: 10.1093/brain/awm001

Bozkurt A, Deumens R, Scheffel J, O'Dey DM, Weis J, Joosten EA, et al. CatWalk gait analysis in assessment of functional recovery after sciatic nerve injury. *J Neurosci Methods.* (2008) 173:91–8. doi: 10.1016/j.jneumeth.2008.05.020

Petrosyan HA, Hunanyan AS, Alessi V, Schnell L, Levine J, Arvanian VL. Neutralization of inhibitory molecule NG2 improves synaptic transmission, retrograde transport, and locomotor function after spinal cord injury in adult rats. *J Neurosci.* (2013) 33:4032–43. doi: 10.1523/JNEUROSCI.4702- 12.2013

Hetze S, Römer C, Teufelhart C, Meisel A, Engel O. Gait analysis as a method for assessing neurological outcome in a mouse model of stroke. *J Neurosci Methods.* (2012) 206:7–14. doi: 10.1016/j.jneumeth.2012.02.001

Givogri MI, Galbiati F, Fasano S, Amadio S, Perani L, Superchi D, et al. Oligodendroglial progenitor cell therapy limits central neurological deficits in mice with metachromatic leukodystrophy. *J Neurosci.* (2006) 26:3109– 19. doi: 10.1523/JNEUROSCI.4366-05.2006

Thiruvalluvan A, Czepiel M, Kap YA, Mantingh-Otter I, Vainchtein I, Kuipers J, et al. Survival and functionality of human induced pluripotent stem cell-derived oligodendrocytes in a nonhuman primate model for multiple sclerosis. *Stem Cells Transl Med.* (2016) 5:1550–61. doi: 10.5966/sctm.2016-0024

Wang S, Bates J, Li X, Schanz S, Chandler-Militello D, Levine C, et al. Human iPSC-derived oligodendrocyte progenitor cells can myelinate and rescue a mouse model of congenital hypomyelination. *Cell Stem Cell.* (2013) 12:252–64. doi: 10.1016/j.stem.2012.12.002

Robin AM, Zhang ZG, Wang L, Zhang RL, Katakowski M, Zhang L, et al. Stromal cell-derived factor 1alpha mediates neural progenitor cell motility after focal cerebral ischemia. *J Cereb Blood Flow Metab.* (2006) 26:125–34. doi: 10.1038/sj.jcbfm.9600172

Vaquero J, Zurita M, de Oya S, Coca S, Morales C, Salas C. Expression of vascular permeability factor in craniopharyngioma. *J Neurosurg.* (1999) 91:831–4. doi: 10.3171/jns.1999.91.5.0831

Kuai XL, Ni RZ, Zhou GX, Mao ZB, Zhang JF, Yi N, et al. Transplantation of mouse embryonic stem cell-derived oligodendrocytes in the murine model of globoid cell leukodystrophy. *Stem Cell Res Ther.* (2015) 6:30. doi: 10.1186/s13287-015-0024-2

Wennersten A, Holmin S, Al Nimer F, Meijer X, Wahlberg LU, Mathiesen Sustained survival of xenografted human neural stem/progenitor cells in experimental brain trauma despite discontinuation of immunosuppression. *Exp Neurol.* (2006) 199:339–47. doi: 10.1016/j.expneurol.2005.12.035

Hovakimyan M, Müller J, Wree A, Ortinau S, Rolfs A, Schmitt O. Survival of transplanted human neural stem cell line (ReNcell VM) into the rat brain with and without immunosuppression. *Ann Anat.* (2012) 194:429– 35. doi: 10.1016/j.aanat.2012.05.003

Pimentel-Coelho PM, Mendez-Otero R. Cell therapy for neonatal hypoxic-ischemic encephalopathy. *Stem Cells Dev.* (2010) 19:299– 310. doi: 10.1089/scd.2009.0403

Zhang YW, Denham J, Thies RS. Oligodendrocyte progenitor cells derived from human embryonic stem cells express neurotrophic factors. *Stem Cells Dev.* (2006) 15:943–52. doi: 10.1089/scd.2006.15.943

Kishida N, Maki T, Takagi Y, Yasuda K, Kinoshita H, Ayaki T, et al. Role of perivascular oligodendrocyte precursor cells in angiogenesis after brain ischemia. *J Am Heart Assoc.* (2019) 8:e011824. doi: 10.1161/JAHA.118.011824

Lu P, Jones LL, Snyder EY, Tuszynski MH. Neural stem cells constitutively secrete neurotrophic factors and promote extensive host axonal growth after spinal cord injury. *Exp Neurol.* (2003) 181:115–29. doi: 10.1016/S0014-4886(03)00037-2

Fünfschilling U, Supplie LM, Mahad D, Boretius S, Saab AS, Edgar J, et al. Glycolytic oligodendrocytes maintain myelin and long-term axonal integrity. *Nature.* (2012) 485:517–21. doi: 10.1038/nature11007

18

The Value of Diffusion Kurtosis Imaging in Detecting Delayed Brain Development of Premature Infants

Xin Zhao[1†], Chunxiang Zhang[1†], Bohao Zhang[1], Jiayue Yan[2], Kaiyu Wang[3], Zitao Zhu[4] and Xiaoan Zhang[1]*

[1] Department of Imaging, Third Affiliated Hospital of Zhengzhou University, Zhengzhou, China, [2] McGill University, Montreal, QC, Canada, [3] MRI Research, GE Healthcare, Beijing, China, [4] Wuhan University, Wuhan, China

***Correspondence:**
Xiaoan Zhang
zxa@zzu.edu.cn

[†] These authors have contributed equally to this work and share first authorship

Objective: Preterm infants are at high risk of the adverse neurodevelopmental outcomes. Our aim is to explore the value of diffusion kurtosis imaging (DKI) in diagnosing brain developmental disorders in premature infants.

Materials and Methods: A total of 52 subjects were included in this study, including 26 premature infants as the preterm group, and 26 full-term infants as the control group. Routine MRI and DKI examinations were performed. Mean kurtosis (MK), radial kurtosis (RK), fractional anisotropy (FA), and mean diffusivity (MD) values were measured in the brain regions including posterior limbs of the internal capsule (PLIC), anterior limb of internal capsule (ALIC), parietal white matter (PWM), frontal white matter (FWM), thalamus (TH), caudate nucleus (CN), and genu of the corpus callosum (GCC). The chi-squared test, *t*-test, Spearman's correlation analysis, and receiver operating characteristic curve were used for data analyses.

Results: In the premature infant group, the MK and RK values of PLIA, ALIC, and PWM were lower than those in the control group ($p < 0.05$). The FA values of PWM, FWM, and TH were also lower than those of the control group ($p < 0.05$). The area under curves of MK in PLIC and ALIC, MD in PWM, and FA in FWM were 0.813, 0.802, 0.842, and 0.867 ($p < 0.05$). In the thalamus and CN, the correlations between MK, RK values, and postmenstrual age (PMA) were higher than those between FA, MD values, and PMA.

Conclusion: Diffusion kurtosis imaging can be used as an effective tool in detecting brain developmental disorders in premature infants.

Keywords: brain, neurodevelopment, preterm infants, MRI, diffusion kurtosis imaging

INTRODUCTION

In the recent years, the birth rate of premature babies has increased significantly in many countries (1). At the same time, with the development of monitoring and treatment technology in the neonatal intensive care unit (NICU), the survival rate of premature babies has also been greatly improved. Compared with full-term babies, the brain developments of premature babies are impaired due to the young gestational age (GA) (2). To provide objective indicators for clinical evaluation of brain development status, it would be necessary to quantitatively analyze the brain development of preterm and full-term infants.

Traditional diffusion tensor imaging (DTI) technique has been used to study the brain development of premature infants. Although pathological specimens can directly show the degree of brain development, these cannot reflect the level of brain development in a living state. DTI technology can non-invasively provide quantitative parameters to reflect the development of white matter in the living body, with the integrity of tissue evaluated from the microscopic field and the white matter (WM) fibers and fiber bundles of the brain tissue being observed (3). Many studies have shown that the more mature the development of neonatal WM, the higher the fractional anisotropy (FA) value and the lower the diffusion coefficient apparent diffusion coefficient (ADC) value (4, 5). When applying diffusion-weighted imaging (DWI) and DTI to assess WM development, the theoretical premise of these two models is that the diffusion of water molecules is normally distributed (6). However, the diffusion distribution of human brain water molecules is dominated by non-normal distribution (7, 8). The current DWI and DTI evaluation methods still have certain limitations.

Diffusion kurtosis imaging (DKI) is an extension of DTI technology, which describes the degree of water diffusion deviating from the normal distribution in tissues. The kurtosis information reflects the non-Gaussian characteristics caused by the complex structure. It better reflects the changes in the microstructure of brain gray matter and WM (9), thus, be more suitable for grasping the microstructure changes. In the recent years, DKI has been used to evaluate brain development. The DKI has detected significant microstructural changes consistent with known patterns of brain maturation (10). In addition, study has shown that DKI shows potential advantages in detecting normal brain development in children (11), but few studies have focused on brain development in premature babies, which may help understand the early neurodevelopmental characteristics of premature babies. In this study, we aimed to discuss the value and advantages of DKI in evaluating the brain development of preterm infants with multiple parameters.

MATERIALS AND METHODS

Subjects

A total of 52 newborns underwent MRI examination from January 2020 to May 2021, including 26 premature infants and 26 full-term infants. Before the examination, the doctor informed the guardian of the purpose and potential risks and obtained informed parental consent. This study was approved by the Ethics Committee.

All the recruited infants met the following inclusion criteria: no chromosomes or major congenital diseases; no intracranial infection, sepsis and other infectious diseases; no hypoglycemic encephalopathy, bilirubin encephalopathy, and other encephalopathy. Imaging criteria: routine MRI showed normal results; no obvious motion artifacts. Groups were divided according to the following criteria. GA $\geq$ 37 weeks (mean GA: 38.67 $\pm$ 1.18 weeks) was considered as the term infant group (n = 26), and scanned at 40.57 $\pm$ 3.07 weeks; GA <37 weeks (mean GA: 34.22 $\pm$ 2.08 weeks) was the premature infant group (n = 26), and scanned at term equivalent age [mean postmenstrual age (PMA): 41.53 $\pm$ 2.22 weeks].

Magnetic Resonance Acquisition and Image Analysis

Each newborn was given an intravenous injection of 5 mg/kg of phenobarbital 30 min before the MRI scan. After the newborn fell asleep, he was escorted to the MRI room by the attending physician and his family. The nurse put the swaddled baby on the MRI scan bed, then used sponges to properly fix both the sides of the head. Finally, antinoise earplugs were placed in the external auditory canal to reduce the impact of MRI equipment noise.

All the MRI scan were carried out on 3.0 T MR scanner (Pioneer, GE Healthcare, Milwaukee, Wisconsin, USA) with T1WI flair, T2WI flair, DWI, and DKI (TR = 2,000 ms, TE = 2.32 ms, directions = 30, b-value = 0, 1,000, 2,000 mm^2/s).

The DKI parametric maps were calculated by using the iQuant software (GE Healthcare, Beijing, China). The iQuant is based on the commercial version of software Horos (https://horosproject.org/). Since the newest AW4.7 version cannot support the old platform for DKI processing, the GE development team moved the algorithms including the DKI images processing from AW4.6 FuncTool platform (GE Healthcare, Beijing) to the Horos and named as iQuant. The DKI algorithm was used as plugin in iQuant. Then, the two radiologists of physicists outline 7 regions of interest (ROI) including posterior limbs of the internal capsule (PLIC), anterior limb of internal capsule (ALIC), genu of the corpus callosum (GCC), parietal white matter (PWM), frontal white matter (FWM), thalamus (TH), and lenticular nucleus (LN) which were outlined manually. The ROIs were measured three times bilaterally and an average value was calculated to minimize the error value.

Statistical Analysis

The statistical analysis was performed on IBM SPSS Statistics 21.0 (IBM Corporation, Armonk, NY, USA). The Student's t-test or chi-squared test was used to compare the differences in clinical characteristics between groups. The receiver operating characteristic curve (ROC) was used to analyze the differences among different ROIs. Spearman's correlation analysis was used to analyze the correlation between DKI parameters and PMA. $p < 0.05$ indicated statistical significance.

RESULTS

General Demographics of Infants

There was no difference between the preterm group (11 males, 15 females) and term born (14 males, 12 females) in gender, delivery method, mean PMA at MRI, mean birth weight, and mean body weight at MRI ($p > 0.05$), as shown in **Table 1**. The DKI parameters showed good interobserver agreement, as shown in **Table 2**.

Comparison of DKI Parameters Between Preterm Infants and Term Infants

Figure 1 displayed T1WI flair, T_2WI flair, DWI, MK, and MD images of two newborns.

As shown in **Figure 2**, significant differences were found between preterm infants and term infants. In the preterm infant group, the MK value (0.605 $\pm$ 0.134 vs. 0.734 $\pm$ 0.133, $p = 0.001$)

and RK value (0.716 ± 0.148 vs. 0.821 ± 0.150, $p = 0.037$) of PLIC were significantly different from the term infant group. The MK and RK values of ALIC in the term infant group were significantly higher than those of the preterm infant group (0.601 ± 0.154 vs. 0.711 ± 0.121, $p = 0.006$; 0.708 ± 0.144 vs. 0.793 ± 0.142, $p = 0.039$). MK, RK, FA, and MD value were all significantly different from that of the term infant group in PWM (0.268 ± 0.100 vs. 0.355 ± 0.108, $p = 0.004$; 0.366 ± 0.134 vs. 0.489 ± 0.142, $p = 0.029$; 0.282 ± 0.114 vs. 0.386 ± 0.115, $p = 0.002$; $1.357 \pm 0.083 \times 10^{-3}$ mm^2/s vs. $1.221 \pm 0.106 \times 10^{-3}$ mm^2/s, $p = 0.002$, respectively). The FA values of FWM and TH were significantly lower than those of the term infant group (0.320 ± 0.129 vs. 0.392 ± 0.108, $p = 0.035$; 0.205 ± 0.043 vs. 0.275 ± 0.090, $p = 0.001$, respectively).

TABLE 1 | General demographics of infants.

	Preterm infants ($n = 26$)	Term infants ($n = 26$)
Male%	11 (42.3)	14 (53.8)
Cesarean delivery%	7 (27)	10 (38.5)
Mean GA (SD; week)	34.22 ± 2.08*	38.67 ± 1.18
Mean PMA at MRI (SD; week)	40.57 ± 3.07	41.53 ± 2.22
Mean birth weight (SD; kg)	2.66 ± 0.74	3.01 ± 0.31
Mean body weight at MRI (SD; kg)	3.55 ± 0.56	3.68 ± 0.63

There were no differences between preterm infants group ($n = 26$) and term born ($n = 26$) in gender, delivery method, mean PMA at MRI, mean birth weight and mean body weight at MRI($P > 0.05$). Mean GA in the preterm groups was lower than that in the term control group ($P < 0.05$). GA, gestational age; PMA, postmenstrual age.
**indicates $P < 0.05$.*

TABLE 2 | Inter-observer consistency of measurements.

Parameters	Intraclass correlation coefficient, 95% CI
MK	0.894 (0.635–0.993)
RK	0.880 (0.620–0.983)
FA	0.955 (0.716–0.994)
MD	0.903 (0.636–0.993)

95% CI = 95% confidence interval. MK, mean kurtosis; RK, radial kurtosis; FA, fractional anisotropy; MD, mean diffusivity.

Diagnostic Performance of DKI Parameters

By comparing the DKI parameters between the two groups in different regions, the region and parameter with significant differences were obtained. We performed ROC analyses on these regions and parameters. The area under curves (AUC) of MK in PLIC and ALIC were 0.813 and 0.802 with the sensitivity of 75.4, 77.7% and the specificity of 86.9, 80.8% (critical point: 0.703 and 0.649, respectively, $p < 0.05$). The AUC of MD in PWM was 0.842 with a sensitivity of 72.3% and a specificity of 87.8% (critical point: 1.419, $p < 0.05$). Similarly, the AUC of FA in FWM was 0.867 with a sensitivity of 78.5% and a specificity of 92.3% (critical point: 0.469, $p < 0.05$). Details are shown in **Table 3**.

Correlation Between DKI Parameters and PMA in the Gray Matter Areas

As shown in **Figure 3**, in the thalamus the correlation between MK, RK values, and PMA ($r = 0.643$ and 0.594, respectively, $p < 0.05$) was higher than the correlation between FA, MD values and PMA ($r = 0.347$ and -0.176, respectively, $p > 0.05$). Similarly, the correlation between MK, RK values, and PMA ($r = 0.519$ and

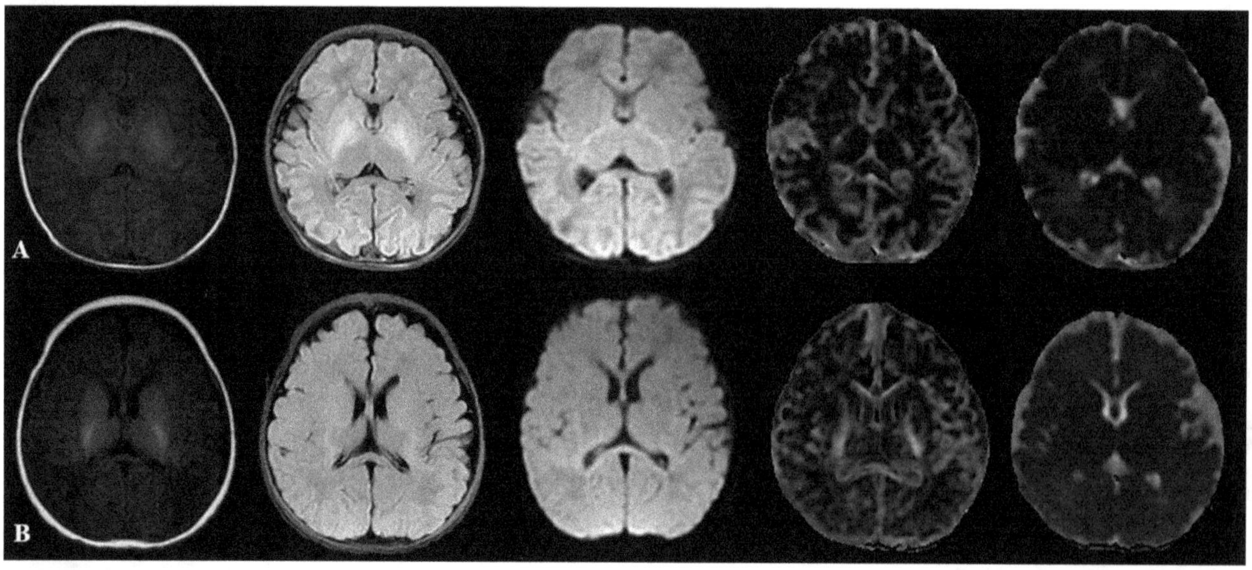

FIGURE 1 | Comparison of multiparameter images in different PMAs. **(A)** represented: male, GA 30 weeks, PMA 42 weeks. **(B)** represented: male, GA 37 weeks, PMA 43 weeks. From left to right: T1WI flair, T2WI flair, DWI, MK, and MD maps. DWI, diffusion-weighted imaging; PMA, postmenstrual age; GA, gestational age; MK, mean kurtosis; MD, mean diffusivity.

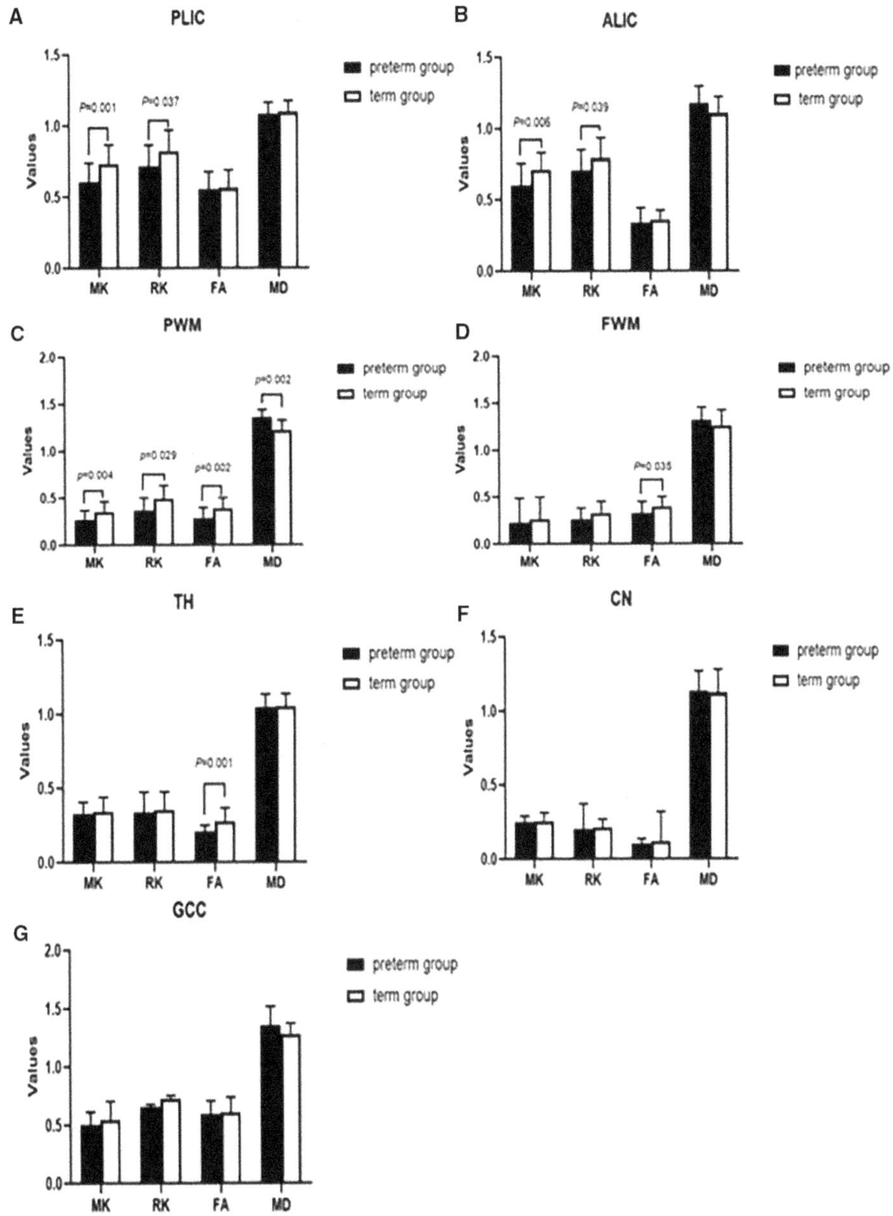

FIGURE 2 | Comparing the difference of parameter values between preterm infants (n = 26) and term infants (n = 26) in the different brain regions **(A–G)**. Black represented premature infants, white represented full-term infants. PLIC, posterior limbs of the internal capsule; ALIC, anterior limb of internal capsule; PWM, parietal white matter; FWM, frontal white matter; TH, thalamus; CN, caudate nucleus; GCC, genu of the corpus callosum; MK, mean kurtosis; RK, radial kurtosis; FA, fractional anisotropy; MD, mean diffusivity.

0.605, $p < 0.05$) was greater than the correlation between FA and MD values and PMA ($r = 0.450, p < 0.05; r = -0.300, p > 0.05$) in caudate nucleus (CN).

DISCUSSION

During the brain development of premature infants, DKI can reveal the microstructure changes and maturation processes in different brain regions. Through comparison with term infants, this study shows that DKI is helpful in diagnosing brain retardation in premature infants. Compared with the parameter FA, the parameters MK and RK of DKI can better capture microstructure changes. When describing gray matter structure, such as TH and CN, MK is better than FA. These results indicate that MK is superior to FA in diagnosing premature infants with delayed brain development. It is more advantageous in discovering changes in the microstructure of the brain.

Because premature birth may lead to relatively slow brain development in premature infants, there are some brain regions that are less developed than the full-term infants. In this study,

TABLE 3 | Diagnostic performance of DKI parameters in different ROIs.

ROI	Parameters	Specificity	Sensitivity	Critical point	AUC	*P*-value
PLIC	MK	86.90%	75.40%	0.703	0.813	<0.05*
	RK	80.80%	46.20%	0.882	0.638	>0.05
ALIC	MK	80.80%	77.70%	0.649	0.802	<0.05*
	RK	69.20%	60.40%	0.793	0.614	>0.05
PWM	MK	63.10%	55.40%	0.344	0.542	>0.05
	RK	73.10%	53.80%	0.42	0.571	>0.05
	FA	52.20%	35.70%	0.727	0.522	>0.05
	MD	87.80%	72.30%	1.419	0.842	<0.05*
FWM	FA	92.30%	78.50%	0.469	0.867	<0.05*
TH	FA	82.30%	11.50%	0.479	0.665	>0.05

Diagnostic manifestations of DKI parameters in different ROIs. The AUC of MK in PLIC and ALIC were 0.813 and 0.802 ($P < 0.05$). The AUC of MD in PWM was 0.842 ($P < 0.05$). The AUC of FA in FWM was 0.867 ($P < 0.05$). PLIC, posterior limbs of the internal capsule; ALIC, anterior limb of internal capsule; PWM, parietal white matter; FWM, frontal white matter; TH, thalamus; MK, mean kurtosis; RK, radial kurtosis; FA, fractional anisotropy; MD, mean diffusivity; AUC, area under curves.
**indicates $P < 0.05$.*

we found that the MK and RK values of PLIC and ALIC were lower than those of the full-term infants. The fibers that made up the internal capsule (IC) came from the descending fibers of the cerebral cortex. The following factors affected the development of the complex structure of IC (12, 13), i.e., the increase of nerve cell axon diameter, change of nerve cell membrane composition, *myelination of axons continued to improve*, increase in the number of microglia, and decreased extracellular space. The parameters of DKI, such as MK, RK can sensitively reflect these microstructure complexity. This is also in line with Paydar's view that MK and RK allow more comprehensive characterization of the microstructural changes during brain development of the children, especially in PLIC and ALIC (10). Frontal-parietal white matter (FWM, PWM) reflected the degree of brain development in the front and middle brain. In this study, the FA values of PWM and FWM were lower than those in the term infant group. FWM was the language and motor center (14), so it is speculated that the language and motor development of preterm infants is delayed than that of full-term infants. Similarly, when the PWM of premature babies was underdeveloped, the ability to the sense of touch and pain and language was also delayed. The thalamus was the gray matter nucleus, one of the areas where neonatal metabolism was vigorous. Its myelin development was also very active. At the same time, the thalamus was also the highest sensory center and the most important sensory conduction relay station (15–17). The results showed that the FA value of TH was lower than that in the term infants. It was assumed that premature babies were delayed in perception, cognition, and motor development. DKI can be used as an effective tool to assess brain developmental delay in the premature infants.

By comparing DKI parameters in the different brain regions between the two groups, we selected four ROIs with significant differences, including ALIC, PLIC, PWM, and FWM. Our results showed that the AUC of MK in ALIC and PLIC were statistically significant. Studies have shown that the neonatal brain development follows a backward-to-forward pattern. Due to the early myelination of ALIC and PLIC, the metabolism is vigorous and the oxygen demand is high. When exposed to risk factors for preterm birth, the metabolically active areas are the first to be damaged (18). At the same time, MK can reflect the backward development of PLIC and ALIC by capturing the changes in microstructure (19). When brain development is impaired, the decreased density of cells and axon membranes may also lead to decreased MK values, which are significantly different from those in the control group (16). In our study, FA did not show good diagnostic value in ALIC and PLIC. Because the IC acts as a WM plate connecting the upper and lower fibers of the cerebral cortex to the brainstem, the structure is more complicated (20). For this complex structure, the diffusion of water molecules actually deviates from the normal distribution, and MK can quantify this deviation.

Radial kurtosis represents the degree to which the molecular diffusion deviates radially from the Gaussian pattern. Compared with the FA value, RK changes more significantly in the premature brain of the infants (21), which is confirmed in this study. The diagnostic value of RK in PWM was statistically significant. We speculated that the RK value may more sensitively reflect the limited radial diffusion of PWM.

With the same view as Vasung, the FA value of FWM has a certain diagnostic value in premature infants with brain development disorders (22). There was a significant difference in the FA value of FWM. It may be because FA is mainly affected by cell changes and fiber bundle density, while MK is majorly affected by the complexity of the microstructure (23, 24). Therefore, as a major functional area of the brain, we believe that FA value is sensitive in FWM.

This study confirmed that the correlations between MK, RK, and PMA were higher than the correlations between FA, MD, and PMA in the TH or CN. For homogeneous structures, such as gray matter, MK and RK are more sensitive as compared with FA and MD. MK and RK played an important role in detecting the development of isotropic tissues (such as gray matter) (25). In the gray matter region, the changes of MK and RK parameters may be related to the increased concentration of mature neuronal macromolecules and the decrease of tissue water content (26, 27) or to other special structures occurring in the development of gray matter. As an advanced and sensitive imaging technique,

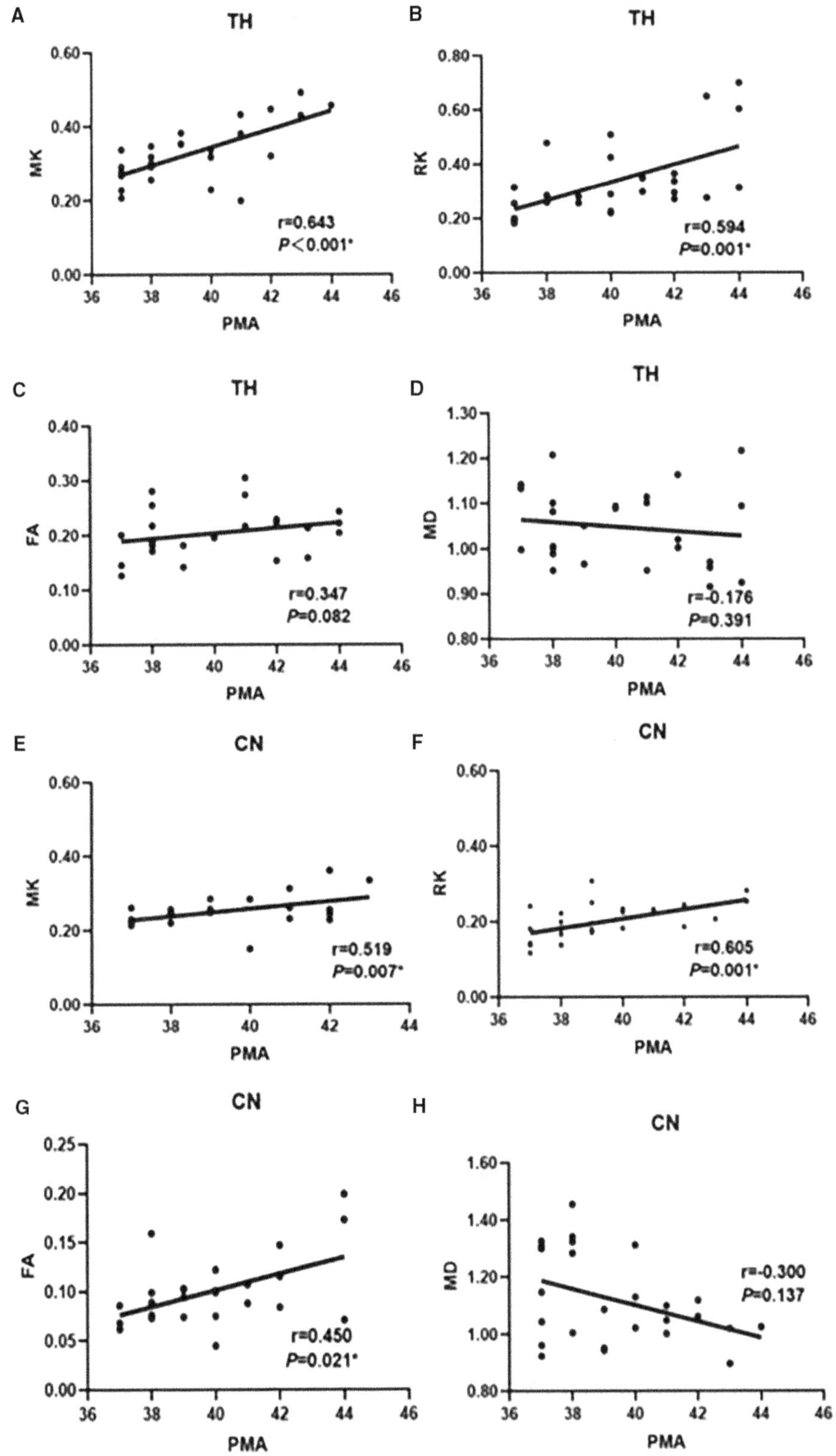

FIGURE 3 | Correlation between MK, RK, FA, MD, and PMA in TH **(A–D)**; Correlation between MK, RK, FA, MD, and PMA in CN **(E–H)** in the preterm infants ($n = 26$). MK and FA regression lines with correlational coefficient (r). correlation significance (P). The selected ROI are the thalamus and the caudate nucleus. PMA, postmenstrual age; TH, thalamus; CN, caudate nucleus; MK, mean kurtosis; RK, radial kurtosis; FA, fractional anisotropy; MD, mean diffusivity.

MK and RK can be used to detect the subtle structural changes of thalamic neurons in the premature infants. MK and RK can show hidden manifestations that FA and MD cannot detect *in vivo*. Therefore, we speculate that the MK and RK parameters have an advantage in reflecting the development of the deep nucleus in the premature infants. MK and RK parameters can better reflect the brain maturity of premature infants.

There were several limitations in this study. This study was only a cross-sectional study. Further verification of longitudinal data is still needed. In addition, the sample size was not large enough. Next, we will continue to enlarge the sample size. Finally, the PMA range of the study subjects was relatively large. If the same newborn brain template is used, the accuracy of image registration may be improved. The next step will be to establish brain templates for different segments of PMA.

CONCLUSION

In conclusion, this study found that MK of ALIC and PLIC, RK of PWM and FA of FWM have some diagnostic value in detecting the brain developmental disorders in the premature infants. The MK and RK values of TH and CN can better reflect the brain maturity of the deep gray matter in the premature infants. These parameters could be used as reliable imaging markers for the diagnosis of the brain developmental disorders in the premature infants.

AUTHOR CONTRIBUTIONS

XZ and CZ designed and wrote the research. BZ and JY performed the research and analyzed the data. KW modified language. ZZ collected data. XZ designed and funded the research. All authors contributed to the article and approved the submitted version.

FUNDING

This research was funded by the National Natural Science Foundation of China, Grant No. 81870983; sponsor: XZ.

REFERENCES

Ushida T, Kidokoro H, Nakamura N, Katsuki S, Imai K, Nakano- Kobayashi T, et al. Impact of maternal hypertensive disorders of pregnancy on brain volumes at term-equivalent age in preterm infants: a voxel-based morphometry study. *Pregnancy Hypertens.* (2021) 25:143–9. doi: 10.1016/j.preghy.2021.06.003

Baldoli C, Scola E, Della Rosa P, Pontesilli S, Longaretti R, Poloniato A, et al. Maturation of preterm newborn brains: a fMRI-DTI study of auditory processing of linguistic stimuli and white matter development. *Brain Struct Funct.* (2015) 220:3733–51. doi: 10.1007/s00429-014-0887-5

Hui E, Cheung M, Chan K, Wu E. B-value dependence of DTI quantitation and sensitivity in detecting neural tissue changes. *Neuroimage.* (2010) 49:2366–74. doi: 10.1016/j.neuroimage.2009.10.022

Li X, Gao J, Wang M, Zheng J, Li Y, Hui E, et al. Characterization of extensive microstructural variations associated with punctate white matter lesions in preterm neonates. *AJNR American journal of neuroradiology.* (2017) 38:1228–34. doi: 10.3174/ajnr.A5226

Fischi-Gómez E, Vasung L, Meskaldji D, Lazeyras F, Borradori-Tolsa C, Hagmann P, et al. Structural brain connectivity in school-age preterm infants provides evidence for impaired networks relevant for higher order cognitive skills and social cognition. *Cerebral cortex.* (2015) 25:2793– 805. doi: 10.1093/cercor/bhu073

Palacios E, Owen J, Yuh E, Wang M, Vassar M, Ferguson A, et al. The evolution of white matter microstructural changes after mild traumatic brain injury: a longitudinal DTI and NODDI study. *Sci Adv.* (2020) 6:eaaz6892. doi: 10.1126/sciadv.aaz6892

Lu H, Jensen J, Ramani A, Helpern J. Three-dimensional characterization of non-gaussian water diffusion in humans using diffusion kurtosis imaging. *NMR in biomedicine.* (2006) 19:236–47. doi: 10.1002/nbm.1020

Guan J, Ma X, Geng Y, Qi D, Shen Y, Shen Z, et al. Diffusion Kurtosis Imaging for detection of early brain changes in Parkinson's disease. *Front Neurol.* (2019) 10:1285. doi: 10.3389/fneur.2019.01285

Cheung M, Hui E, Chan K, Helpern J, Qi L, Wu E. Does diffusion kurtosis imaging lead to better neural tissue characterization? A rodent brain maturation study. *NeuroImage.* (2009) 45:386– 92. doi: 10.1016/j.neuroimage.2008.12.018

Paydar A, Fieremans E, Nwankwo J, Lazar M, Sheth H, Adisetiyo V, et al. Diffusional kurtosis imaging of the developing brain. *AJNR Am J Neuroradiol.* (2014) 35:808–14. doi: 10.3174/ajnr.A3764

Shi J, Yang S, Wang J, Huang S, Yao Y, Zhang S, et al. Detecting normal pediatric brain development with diffusional kurtosis imaging. *Eur J Radiol.* (2019) 120:108690. doi: 10.1016/j.ejrad.2019.108690

Dibble M, Ang J, Mariga L, Molloy E, Bokde A. Diffusion tensor imaging in very preterm, moderate-late preterm and term-born neonates: a systematic review. *J Pediatr.* (2021). doi: 10.1016/j.jpeds.2021.01.008

Choi Y, Lee J, Lee J, Lee J, Lee Y, Ahn J, Lee H. Delayed maturation of the middle cerebellar peduncles at near-term age predicts abnormal neurodevelopment in preterm infants. *Neonatology* 2021:1-10. doi: 10.1159/000512921

Rosch K, Mostofsky S. Development of the frontal lobe. *Handb Clin Neurol.* (2019) 163:351–67. doi: 10.1016/B978-0-12-804281-6.00019-7

Grossman E, Ge Y, Jensen J, Babb J, Miles L, Reaume J, et al. Thalamus and cognitive impairment in mild traumatic brain injury: a diffusional kurtosis imaging study. *J Neurotrauma.* (2012) 29:2318– 27. doi: 10.1089/neu.2011.1763

Mukherjee P, Miller J, Shimony J, Philip J, Nehra D, Snyder A, et al. Diffusion-tensor MR imaging of gray and white matter development during normal human brain maturation. *AJNR American journal of neuroradiology.* (2002) 23:1445–56.

Mukherjee P, Miller J, Shimony J, Conturo T, Lee B, Almli C, et al. Normal brain maturation during childhood: developmental trends characterized with diffusion-tensor MR imaging. *Radiology.* (2001) 221:349– 58. doi: 10.1148/radiol.2212001702

Ling X, Tang W, Liu G, Huang L, Li B, Li X, et al. Assessment of brain maturation in the preterm infants using diffusion tensor imaging (DTI) and enhanced T2 star weighted angiography (ESWAN). *Eur J Radiol.* (2013) 82:e476–483. doi: 10.1016/j.ejrad.2013.04.003

Dubois J, Dehaene-Lambertz G, Perrin M, Mangin J, Cointepas Y, Duchesnay E, et al. Asynchrony of the early maturation of white matter bundles in healthy infants: quantitative landmarks revealed noninvasively by diffusion tensor imaging. *Hum Brain Mapp.* (2008) 29:14–27. doi: 10.1002/hbm. 20363

Olivieri B, Rampakakis E, Gilbert G, Fezoua A, Wintermark P. Myelination may be impaired in neonates following birth asphyxia. *NeuroImage Clinical.* (2021) 31:102678. doi: 10.1016/j.nicl.2021.102678

Yoshida S, Oishi K, Faria A, Mori S. Diffusion tensor imaging of normal brain development. *Pediatric radiology.* (2013) 43:15–27. doi: 10.1007/s00247-012-2496-x

Vasung L, Fischi-Gomez E, Hüppi P. Multimodality evaluation of the pediatric brain: DTI and its competitors. *Pediatr Radiol.* (2013) 43:60– 8. doi: 10.1007/s00247-012-2515-y

Ouyang M, Jeon T, Sotiras A, Peng Q, Mishra V, Halovanic C, et al. Differential cortical microstructural maturation in the preterm human brain with diffusion kurtosis and tensor imaging. *Proc Natl Acad Sci USA.* (2019) 116:4681–8. doi: 10.1073/pnas. 1812156116

Nossin-Manor R, Card D, Raybaud C, Taylor M, Sled J. Cerebral maturation in the early preterm period-A magnetization transfer and diffusion tensor imaging study using voxel-based analysis. *Neuroimage.* (2015) 112:30– 42. doi: 10.1016/j.neuroimage.2015.02.051

McKenna F, Miles L, Donaldson J, Castellanos F, Lazar M. Diffusion kurtosis imaging of gray matter in young adults with autism spectrum disorder. *Sci Rep.* (2020) 10:21465. doi: 10.1038/s41598-020-78486-w

Das S, Wang J, Bing L, Bhetuwal A, Yang H. Regional values of diffusional kurtosis estimates in the healthy brain during normal aging. *Clin Neuroradiol.* (2017) 27:283–98. doi: 10.1007/s00062-015-0490-z

Gullion L, Stansell J, Moss H, Jenkins D, Aljuhani T, Coker-Bolt P. The impact of early neuroimaging and developmental assessment in a preterm infant diagnosed with cerebral palsy. *Case Rep Pediatr.* (2019) 2019:9612507. doi: 10.1155/2019/9612507

Permissions

 Every chapter published in this book has been scrutinized by our experts. Their significance has been extensively debated. The topics covered herein carry significant findings which will fuel the growth of the discipline. They may even be implemented as practical applications or may be referred to as a beginning point for another development.

The contributors of this book come from diverse backgrounds, making this book a truly international effort. This book will bring forth new frontiers with its revolutionizing research information and detailed analysis of the nascent developments around the world.

We would like to thank all the contributing authors for lending their expertise to make the book truly unique. They have played a crucial role in the development of this book. Without their invaluable contributions this book wouldn't have been possible. They have made vital efforts to compile up to date information on the varied aspects of this subject to make this book a valuable addition to the collection of many professionals and students.

This book was conceptualized with the vision of imparting up-to-date information and advanced data in this field. To ensure the same, a matchless editorial board was set up. Every individual on the board went through rigorous rounds of assessment to prove their worth. After which they invested a large part of their time researching and compiling the most relevant data for our readers.

The editorial board has been involved in producing this book since its inception. They have spent rigorous hours researching and exploring the diverse topics which have resulted in the successful publishing of this book. They have passed on their knowledge of decades through this book. To expedite this challenging task, the publisher supported the team at every step. A small team of assistant editors was also appointed to further simplify the editing procedure and attain best results for the readers.

Apart from the editorial board, the designing team has also invested a significant amount of their time in understanding the subject and creating the most relevant covers. They scrutinized every image to scout for the most suitable representation of the subject and create an appropriate cover for the book.

The publishing team has been an ardent support to the editorial, designing and production team. Their endless efforts to recruit the best for this project, has resulted in the accomplishment of this book. They are a veteran in the field of academics and their pool of knowledge is as vast as their experience in printing. Their expertise and guidance has proved useful at every step. Their uncompromising quality standards have made this book an exceptional effort. Their encouragement from time to time has been an inspiration for everyone.

The publisher and the editorial board hope that this book will prove to be a valuable piece of knowledge for researchers, students, practitioners and scholars across the globe.

List of Contributors

James P. Boardman
MRC Centre for Reproductive Health, The Queen's Medical Research Institute, The University of Edinburgh, Edinburgh, United Kingdom
Centre for Clinical Brain Sciences, Chancellor's Building, The University of Edinburgh, Edinburgh, United Kingdom

Graeme Ireland, Gemma Sullivan, Rozalia Pataky and Veronique Miron
MRC Centre for Reproductive Health, The Queen's Medical Research Institute, The University of Edinburgh, Edinburgh, United Kingdom

Bobbi Fleiss and Pierre Gressens
Centre for the Developing Brain, Division of Imaging Sciences and Biomedical Engineering, King's College London, London, United Kingdom
PROTECT, INSERM, Université Paris Diderot, Sorbonne Paris Cité, Paris, France
PremUP, Paris, France

Dietmar Spengler, Elisa Loewe and Martin F. Krause
Department of Pediatrics, University Hospital Schleswig-Holstein, Kiel, Germany

Eileen I. Chang, Miguel A. Zarate, Thomas J. Arndt and Charles E. Wood
Department of Physiology and Functional Genomics, University of Florida College of Medicine, Gainesville, FL, United States

Elaine M. Richards and Maureen Keller-Wood
Department of Pharmacodynamics, University of Florida College of Pharmacy, Gainesville, FL, United States

Maria B. Rabaglino
CEPROCOR, National Scientific and Technical Research Council (CONICET), Córdoba, Argentina

Dries Hendrikx, Mario Lavanga, Ofelie De Wel and Sabine Van Huffel
Department of Electrical Engineering, KU Leuven, Leuven, Belgium
IMEC, Leuven, Belgium

Anne Smits, Liesbeth Thewissen and Gunnar Naulaers
Department of Development and Regeneration, KU Leuven, Leuven, Belgium
Neonatal Intensive Care Unit, University Hospitals Leuven, Leuven, Belgium

Katrien Jansen
Department of Development and Regeneration, KU Leuven, Leuven, Belgium
Neonatal Intensive Care Unit, University Hospitals Leuven, Leuven, Belgium
Child Neurology, University Hospitals Leuven, Leuven, Belgium

Alexander Caicedo
Facultad de Ciencias Naturales y Matemáticas, Universidad del Rosario, Bogotá, Colombia

Eduardo Villamor-Martinez, Owais Mohammed Rahim, Pieter Degraeuwe and Eduardo Villamor
Department of Pediatrics, School for Oncology and Developmental Biology (GROW), Maastricht University Medical Center, Maastricht, Netherlands

Monica Fumagalli, Sofia Passera, Giacomo Cavallaro and Fabio Mosca
Neonatal Intensive Care Unit, Department of Clinical Sciences and Community Health, Fondazione IRCCS Cà Granda Ospedale Maggiore Policlinico, Università degli Studi di Milano, Milan, Italy

Frank van Bel and Floris Groenendaal
Department of Neonatology, Wilhelmina Children's Hospital and Brain Center Rudolf Magnus, University Medical Center Utrecht, Utrecht University, Utrecht, Netherlands

Josine Vaes
Laboratory of Neuroimmunology and Developmental Origins of Disease, University Medical Center Utrecht, Utrecht University, Utrecht, Netherlands

Kelly Q. Zhou, Laura Bennet, Alistair J. Gunn and Joanne O. Davidson
Department of Physiology, The University of Auckland, Auckland, New Zealand

Colin R. Green
Department of Ophthalmology, The University of Auckland, Auckland, New Zealand

Veronika Golubinskaya, Helena Gustafsson Carina Mallard and Holger Nilsson
Department of Physiology, Institute of Neuroscience and Physiology, The Sahlgrenska Academy, University of Gothenburg, Gothenburg, Sweden

Regina Vontell and Veena Supramaniam
Division of Imaging Sciences & Biomedical Engineering, Centre for the Developing Brain, King's College London, King's Health Partners, St Thomas' Hospital, London, United Kingdom

Josephine Wyatt-Ashmead
Wigglesworth Perinatal-Padiatric Pathology Service, Imperial College Healthcare NHS Trust, London, United Kingdom

Mary J. Berry and Melissa Schlegel
Department of Paediatrics and Child Health, University of Otago, Wellington, New Zealand
Capital and Coast District Health Board, Wellington, New Zealand

Greg M. Kowalski, Clinton R. Bruce and Rod J. Snow
School of Exercise Sciences, Institute for Physical Activity and Nutrition, Deakin University, Geelong, VIC, Australia

Damien L. Callahan
Centre for Cellular and Molecular Biology, School of Life and Environmental Science, Deakin University, Melbourne, VIC, Australia

Miranda L. Davies-Tuck, Hayley Dickinson and Stacey J. Ellery
The Ritchie Centre, Hudson Institute of Medical Research, and Department of Obstetrics and Gynaecology, Monash University, Clayton, VIC, Australia

Angus Goodson and Angie Slocombe
Capital and Coast District Health Board, Wellington, New Zealand

David W. Walker
School of Health and Biomedical Sciences, RMIT University, Melbourne, VIC, Australia

Rebecca A. Dorner and Marilee C. Allen
Neonatology, Johns Hopkins Hospital, Baltimore, MD, United States
Neurosciences Intensive Care Nursery, Johns Hopkins Hospital, Baltimore, MD, United States

Bruno P. Soares
Neurosciences Intensive Care Nursery, Johns Hopkins Hospital, Baltimore, MD, United States
Pediatric Radiology and Pediatric Neuroradiology, Johns Hopkins Hospital, Baltimore, MD, United States

Shenandoah Robinson
Neurosciences Intensive Care Nursery, Johns Hopkins Hospital, Baltimore, MD, United States
Pediatric Neurosurgery, Johns Hopkins Hospital, Baltimore, MD, United States

Jamie Perin
Biostatistics, Epidemiology, and Data Management Core, Johns Hopkins Hospital, Baltimore, MD, United States

Vera Joanna Burton
Neurology and Developmental Medicine, Kennedy Krieger Institute, Baltimore, MD, United States
Department of Neurology, The Johns Hopkins School of Medicine, Baltimore, MD, United States

Sofia Ryytty Stålnacke, Birgitta Böhm and Eric Herlenius
Department of Women's and Children's Health, Karolinska Institutet, Karolinska University Hospital, Stockholm, Sweden

Mesfin Tessma
Department of Learning, Informatics, Management and Ethics - LIME, Karolinska Institutet, Stockholm, Sweden

Claudia Sisa, Jordan Naylor and Mariya Hristova
Perinatal Brain Protection and Repair Group, EGA Institute for Women's Health, University College London, London, United Kingdom

Sharad Kholia, Stefania Bruno and Giovanni Camussi
Department of Medical Sciences, University of Turin, Turin, Italy

Maria Beatriz Herrera Sanchez and Maria Chiara Deregibus
2i3T, Incubator and Technology Transfer, Molecular Biotechnology Center, University of Turin, Turin, Italy

Jameel M. Inal
Extracellular Vesicle Research Unit and Bioscience Research Group, School of Life and Medical Sciences, University of Hertfordshire, Hatfield, United Kingdom

Sigrun Lange
Tissue Architecture and Regeneration Research Group, School of Life Sciences, University of Westminster, London, United Kingdom

Megan Finch-Edmondson, Catherine Morgan and Iona Novak
The Discipline of Child and Adolescent Health, The Children's Hospital at Westmead Clinical School, The University of Sydney Medical School, Sydney, NSW, Australia
Cerebral Palsy Alliance Research Institute, The University of Sydney, Sydney, NSW, Australia

Kenta Hyeon Tae Cho, Bing Xu and Mhoyra Fraser
Department of Physiology, Faculty of Medical Health and Sciences, University of Auckland, Auckland, New Zealand

Rod W. Hunt
Department of Neonatal Medicine, The Royal Children's Hospital, Melbourne, VIC, Australia
Department of Paediatrics, University of Melbourne, Melbourne, VIC, Australia
Neonatal Research, Murdoch Children's Research Institute, Melbourne, VIC, Australia
Department of Obstetrics and Gynaecology, Monash University, Melbourne, VIC, Australia

Cherie Blenkiron
Departments of Molecular Medicine and Pathology, Faculty of Medical Health and Sciences, University of Auckland, Auckland, New Zealand

Tayla R. Penny, Madison C. B. Paton, Graham Jenkin and Suzanne L. Miller
The Ritchie Centre, Hudson Institute of Medical Research, Clayton, VIC, Australia
Department of Obstetrics and Gynaecology, Monash University, Clayton, VIC, Australia

Amy E. Sutherland, Jamie G. Mihelakis, Yen Pham and Courtney A. McDonald
The Ritchie Centre, Hudson Institute of Medical Research, Clayton, VIC, Australia

Joohyung Lee
Centre for Endocrinology and Metabolism, Hudson Institute of Medical Research, Clayton, VIC, Australia

Nicole M. Jones
Department of Pharmacology, School of Medical Sciences, University of New South Wales, Sydney, NSW, Australia

Michael C. Fahey
Department of Paediatrics, Monash University, Clayton, VIC, Australia

Raul Chavez-Valdez and Frances J. Northington
Division of Neonatal-Perinatal Medicine, Department of Pediatrics, Johns Hopkins School of Medicine, Baltimore, MD, United States

Amin Mottahedin and Linnea Stridh
Institute of Neuroscience and Physiology, Sahlgrenska Academy, University of Gothenburg, Gothenburg, Sweden

Tracylyn R. Yellowhair and Lauren L. Jantzie
Division of Neonatal-Perinatal Medicine, Department of Pediatrics, Johns Hopkins School of Medicine, Baltimore, MD, United States
Department of Pediatrics and Department of Neurosciences, The University of New Mexico, Albuquerque, NM, United States

Carina Mallard
Institute of Neuroscience and Physiology, Sahlgrenska Academy, University of Gothenburg, Gothenburg, Sweden
Henan Key Laboratory of Child Brain Injury, The Third Affiliated Hospital of Zhengzhou University, Zhengzhou, China

Xiaohua Wang
The Second School of Clinical Medicine, Southern Medical University, Guangzhou, China
Department of Pediatrics, The Sixth Medical Center of PLA General Hospital, Beijing, China
Department of Pediatrics, Affiliated Hospital of Nantong University, Nantong, China

Jing Zang, Yinxiang Yang, Siliang Lu, Qian Guan, Dou Ye, Zhaoyan Wang, Haipeng Zhou, Ke Li and Qian Wang
Department of Pediatrics, The Sixth Medical Center of PLA General Hospital, Beijing, China

Youjia Wu
Department of Pediatrics, Affiliated Hospital of Nantong University, Nantong, China

Zuo Luan
The Second School of Clinical Medicine, Southern Medical University, Guangzhou, China
Department of Pediatrics, The Sixth Medical Center of PLA General Hospital, Beijing, China

Xin Zhao, Chunxiang Zhang, Bohao Zhang and Xiaoan Zhang
Department of Imaging, Third Affiliated Hospital of Zhengzhou University, Zhengzhou, China

Jiayue Yan
McGill University, Montreal, QC, Canada

Kaiyu Wang
MRI Research, GE Healthcare, Beijing, China

Zitao Zhu
Wuhan University, Wuhan, China

Index

www.ingramcontent.com/pod-product-compliance
Lightning Source LLC
LaVergne TN
LVHW081034210926
848485LV00004B/1018
* 9 7 8 1 6 3 9 2 7 9 4 3 2 *